Four Lost Links

Upper left: James M. Pryse, 1859–1942 (reprinted from William Q. Judge, "Faces of Friends," *Path*, vol. 9, June 1894)

Upper right: Cajzoran Ali / Amber Steen, 1895–1966 (reprinted from Cajzoran Ali, *Divine Posture*, 1928)

Lower left: Ivah Bergh Whitten, 1873–1947 (reprinted from Ivah Bergh Whitten, *What Color Means to You*, 1932)

Lower right: S. G. J. (Stephen Geoffrey John) Ouseley, 1903–57 (reprinted from Stephen Ouseley, *From Camaldoli to Christ*, 1931)

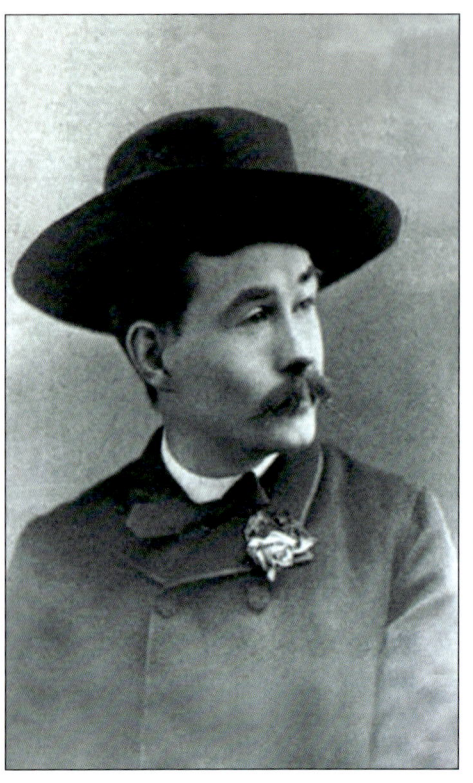
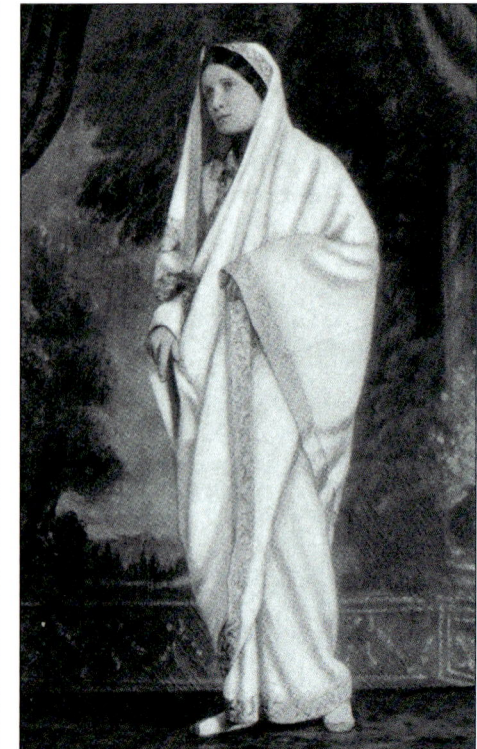
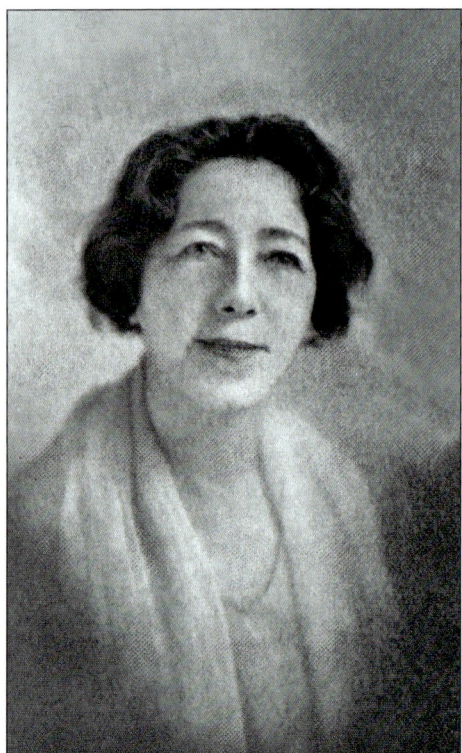
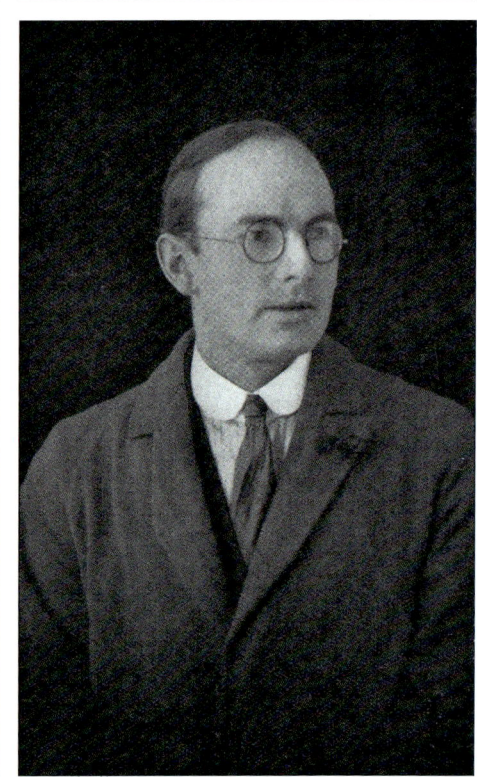

Scholars of Indian religions have long known that the chakra system seen in modern art and postural yoga are very modern and syncretic. What Kurt Leland shows us in this marvelous new book is just how modern and how syncretic they really are: we even get precise origin dates, authors, and texts. With an astonishing resume of historical research, Leland tells the story of the Western chakra system from its ancient Indian Tantric roots, through its definitive beginnings around 1880 in Bengal, to its most modern incarnations in color symbolism and energy healing. In a spirit of intellectual generosity, he does not demean or dismiss any of these cross-cultural creations. He sees them all as local relative attempts to harmonize with and activate a multidimensional "rainbow body" of consciousness that we all share and are.

—Jeffrey J. Kripal, author of *Esalen: America and the Religion of No Religion,* J. Newton Rayzor Professor of Religion, Rice University

RAINBOW BODY

*A History of the
Western Chakra System
from Blavatsky to Brennan*

KURT LELAND

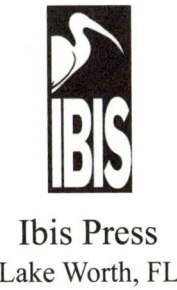

Ibis Press
Lake Worth, FL

Published in 2016 by Ibis Press
A division of Nicolas-Hays, Inc.
P. O. Box 540206
Lake Worth, FL 33454-0206
www.ibispress.net

Distributed to the trade by
Red Wheel/Weiser, LLC
65 Parker St. • Ste. 7
Newburyport, MA 01950
www.redwheelweiser.com

Copyright © 2016 by Kurt Leland
Edgar Cayce Readings © 1971, 1993–2007
by the Edgar Cayce Foundation

All rights reserved. No part of this publication may be reproduced or transmitted in any form or by any means, electronic or mechanical, including photocopying, recording, or by any information storage and retrieval system, without permission in writing from Nicolas-Hays, Inc. Reviewers may quote brief passages.

ISBN 978-0-89254-219-2
Ebook: ISBN 978-0-89254-634-3

Library of Congress Cataloging-in-Publication Data

Names: Leland, Kurt, author.
Title: Rainbow body : a history of the western chakra system from Blavatsky to Brennan / Kurt Leland.
Description: Lake Worth, FL: Ibis Press, 2016. | Includes bibliographical references and index.
Identifiers: LCCN 2016029377 (print) | LCCN 2016032718 (ebook) | ISBN 9780892542192 (alk. paper) | ISBN 9780892546343 ()
Subjects: LCSH: Chakras (Theosophy)--History. | Chakras--History.
Classification: LCC BP573.C5 L45 2016 (print) | LCC BP573.C5 (ebook) | DDC 299/.934--dc23
LC record available at https://lccn.loc.gov/2016029377

Book design and production by Studio 31
www.studio31.com

[BP]

Printed in the United States of America

Table of Contents

List of Illustrations and Plates	9
Acknowledgments	13
Introduction	17
Note on Sanskrit Transliteration	24
Evolution of the Eastern Chakra System: A Chronology	25
Part 1. East Is East and West Is West	**31**
Chapter 1. The Mysterious Maps of Bipin Behari Shom	33
"Errors" of Hinduism	36
East and West	41
Chapter 2. The Universe according to Tantra	44
The Eastern Chakra System	47
Chapter 3. Reversing Creation: Yoga and the Chakras	56
Hatha Yoga	59
Mantra Yoga	62
Nada Yoga	63
Laya Yoga	64
Chapter 4. The Western Chakra System	72
Typology of Expounders and Systems	76
Source Amnesia	79
Occult Correspondences	82
Researcher or Investigator?—My Position	86
Part 2. Esoteric Matrix: The Chakra Teachings of H. P. Blavatsky (1879–91)	**91**
Chapter 5. Journey to the West	93
Glimpses of Tantric Occultism	95
Tantric Anatomy	99
Chapter 6. Madame Blavatsky's Esoteric Instructions	102
Hatha versus Raja Yoga	103
The Pineal Gland	106

Chakras in the Head	109
Path of the Saints	110
The Seven Rays	112
The Aura	114
Chapter 7. Inner Group Teachings	117
The Kundalini Practice	122

Part 3. Whirling Wheels: Theosophical Clairvoyance (1890s–1920s) — 129

Chapter 8. Annie Besant and the Higher Planes	131
Astral Projection	136
Chapter 9. The Lotus Petals of Rudolf Steiner	141
Initiation and Its Results	141
Chapter 10. The Law of Breath and the Tree of Life	151
Subtle Forces (Rāma Prasād)	151
Kingly Yoga (Swami Vivekananda)	154
The Human Aura (Auguste Jean-Baptiste Marques)	157
Rhythmic Breathing (Ella Adelia Fletcher)	159
Flying Rolls (Golden Dawn)	161
Spheres, Pillars, and Paths (Kabbalah)	162
Chapter 11. Chakras of the Apocalypse (James Morgan Pryse)	170
The Kundalini Practice Revisited	173
Multiple Chakra Systems	174
The Snake and the Cross	176
Chapter 12. Charles W. Leadbeater and the Serpent Fire	183
The Inner Life	188
The Hidden Side of Things	191
Chapter 13. The Duel of Leadbeater and Woodroffe	197
The Serpent Power	197
The Chakras	201
Leadbeater's Legacy	207

Table of Contents 7

Part 4. Chromotherapy: Science of Rays, Colors, and Glands (1920s–1950s) — 211

Chapter 14. Alice Bailey and the Seven Rays — 213
Initiation: Human and Solar — 215
Letters on Occult Meditation — 217
The Light of the Soul — 220
The Soul and Its Mechanism — 221
Esoteric Healing — 222

Chapter 15. Mysterious Glands — 226
Chemistry of the Soul (Herman Harold Rubin) — 227
The Many Lives of Cajzoran Ali (Amber Steen) — 230
Steen's Legacy — 233

Chapter 16. The Sikh and the Psychic — 237
Edgar Cayce and the Glad Helpers — 237
Eastern Wisdom for Western Minds (Bhagat Singh Thind) — 241
The Lord's Prayer — 244
Cayce's Legacy — 249
A Question of Precedence — 250

Chapter 17. Lost Teachings of Cosmic Color — 254
Masters and Rays — 255
Ivah Bergh Whitten — 258
Color Awareness — 261
Fundamentals of Cosmic Color — 262
Color Correspondences — 265
Whitten's Legacy — 272

Chapter 18. Temples of Radiance — 277
Color Temple College (Roland Hunt) — 278
Cosmic Color Fellowship (S. G. J. Ouseley) — 283
Temple of Radiant Reflection (Mary L. Wiyninger) — 292

Part 5. Scholars and Swamis and Shrinks, Oh My! (1930s–70s) — 295

    Chapter 19. The Serpent's Brood — 297
        Jung and *The Serpent Power* — 298
        The Chakras at Mid-Century — 302
        Joseph Campbell and Sri Ramakrishna — 305

    Chapter 20. Kundalini Hot Springs—Esalen Institute — 312
        Michael Murphy and Sri Aurobindo — 313
        Esalen and Energy — 316

    Chapter 21. Handbooks to Higher Consciousness — 322
        Transcendent Needs (Abraham Maslow) — 322
        The Only Dance There Is (Ram Dass) — 324
        Here Comes Everybody (William Schutz) — 326
        The Handbook to Higher Consciousness (Ken Keyes Jr.) — 330
        Total Orgasm (Jack Lee Rosenberg) — 332

    Chapter 22. The Birth of the Western Chakra System — 334
        Yoga Psychology (Haridas Chaudhuri) — 334
        The Yogi and the Shrinks (Swami Rama) — 335
        Child of Bodymind (Ken Dychtwald) — 337

Part 6. Light-Wheels Roll On (1980s and Beyond) — 349

    Chapter 23. Way of the Dodo—Extinct Systems — 351
        Under the Hood (Peter Rendel) — 351
        Energy and Ecstasy (Bernard Gunther) — 352
        The Holy Grail (Jack Schwarz) — 355
        Mansions of Color (Christopher Hills) — 361

    Chapter 24. The Great Chakra Controversy — 367
        Wheels, Colors, and Crystals (Anodea Judith and Joy Gardner) — 370
        Chakra Science (Hiroshi Motoyama and Others) — 371
        German Developments (Klausbernd Vollmar and Others) — 372

Bailey Revisited (David Tansley and Zachary Lansdowne)	375
Pranic Healing (Choa Kok Sui)	376
Going Within (Shirley MacLaine)	380
Chapter 25. The Multidimensional Rainbow Body	384
Hands versus Wheels (Brennan and Bruyere)	386
Auras, Bodies, and Planes	392
Multiple Bodies and Systems	395
Multidimensional Chakras	399
The New Astral Projection	402
Chakras of the Future	404
Notes	407
Bibliography	474
Index	499
About the Author	517

Illustrations

Figures

1.	Mysterious Map A	34
2.	Mysterious Map B	35
3.	Chakras and Nadis	48
4.	*Anāhata-cakra*	53
5.	Correspondences from Blavatsky's Esoteric Instruction No. 1	119
6.	Kundalini Rising	155
7.	Chakra Locations according to Crowley	165
8.	Chakras and the Tree of Life	167
9.	Pryse's Chakras, Planets, and Signs	172
10.	Chakra Locations according to Pryse	178
11.	Chakra Functions according to Pryse	179
12.	Leadbeater's Chakra Functions	195
13.	Nadis and Caduceus	200
14.	Endocrine Glands	228

15.	Ali's Chakras and Glands	229
16.	The Lord's Prayer according to Cayce	246
17.	The Lord's Prayer according to Heindel	247
18.	Head Chakras according to Hodson	253
19.	Masters and Rays according to Whitten	263
20.	Chakras and Planes according to Whitten	281
21.	Mapping the Rays in Blavatsky's Esoteric Instruction No. 2	287
22.	Tibetan Chakras as Chorten	359
23.	Western Chakras as Holy Grail	359
24.	Front and Back Chakras	379

Tables

1.	The Sanskrit Alphabet	68
2.	Basu's Tantric Anatomy (1888)	100
3.	Basu's Chakras (1888)	100
4.	Blavatsky's Kundalini Practice Correspondences (1891)	121
5.	Planes, Bodies, and Principles according to Besant (1897–1912)	134
6.	Chakras according to Steiner (1908)	143
7.	Crowley's Chakra Correlations (1909)	164
8.	Chakras according to Pryse (1910)	181
9.	Leadbeater's Colors and Powers (1910)	192
10.	Leadbeater's Colors and Powers (1927)	204
11.	Bailey's Contributions to the Chakra System (1930–53)	223
12.	Cajzoran Ali on the Chakras (1928)	234
13.	Chakra/Gland Correspondences (1927–36)	251
14.	Whitten's Major Ray Correspondences (1932)	266
15.	Whitten's Types and Needs (1932)	268
16.	Whitten's Minor Ray Correspondences (1932)	269
17.	Tattvas, Symbols, and Colors	271
18.	Rays, Chakras, and Colors (1920s–30s)	273
19.	Ouseley's Correspondences (ca. 1950)	290

20. Evolution of Chakra Qualities (1970s) — 346
21. The *Voluntary Controls* Chakra System (1978) — 356
22. Chakras according to Christopher Hills (1977) — 364
23. The Western Chakra System (ca. 1990) — 382
24. Chakras according to Rosalyn Bruyere (1988) — 388
25. Brennan's and Besant's Planes — 396

Plates

Frontispiece. Four Missing Links

Color Insert follows page 256

1. Chakras East and West
2. Chakras according to Sabhapaty
3. Aura Layers and Principles
4. Pryse's Continuum of Human Potential
5. "The Chakras according to Gichtel"
6. Leadbeater's Chakras—Front View
7. Leadbeater's Chakras—Side View
8. Ali's Chakras and Glands

Acknowledgments

Just as it takes a village to raise a child, so it takes an intellectual community of people who may not know each other to bring to birth a book. I would like to thank the following individuals for the helpful roles they played at various stages of production of this *Rainbow Body*:

Dr. Karl Baier of the University of Vienna, for permission to cite a paper posted on the Internet in advance of print publication and for access to a German translation of Sabhapaty Swami's *The Philosophy and Science of Vedanta and Raja Yoga*
Mary Bergman of the Brookline Public Library, Brookline, MA, for interlibrary loan support
Keith Cantú, for the opportunity to pool resources and sort out various textual issues in the writings of Sabhapaty Swami, the subject of his PhD dissertation
Ashley Clements, Alan Goodwin, Harry Hobbs, and Jay Hovenesian, for furthering favors and friendship
Andrew Davies and Nancy Lehwalder, for reading and commenting on the manuscript
Jeannie S. Dean, for a reminder of Shirley MacLaine's demonstration of the chakras on the *Tonight* show
Sharron Dorr, Nancy Grace, and Richard Smoley of Quest Books / Theosophical Publishing House, for support in preparing the new "authoritative" version of Charles W. Leadbeater's *The Chakras*, an important stepping stone to the present book
Richard Dvorak, for his photographing and restoring the fragile, damaged, and problematically preserved image of Sabhapaty Swami, a detail of which appears as plate 2
Ken Dychtwald, for his reminiscences about Esalen and the writing of his first book, *Bodymind*
Brian Galford, for past and present author photos
Tinsley Galyean and Nicole Goott, Judson Scott and Susan Thornberg, Kevin and Sonora Thomas, for getaway opportunities

that allowed me to advance the research, writing, and revision stages of this project

Claire Gardner, archivist, and Laura Holt, librarian, of the Association for Research and Enlightenment, Virginia Beach, VA, for research support

Michael Gomes, librarian of the Emily Sellon Memorial Library, New York, NY, for research support

May Harshbarger, for the loan of a volume of *The Secret Doctrine* from the Ozark Theosophical Camp Library, Sulphur Springs, AR, that allowed me to produce a readable version of figure 5, after many failed attempts with earlier editions

Karl Friedrich Hörner, for sublime patience in the process of translating the book into German even as the final text was still evolving—and for his superior editing and fact-checking skills, which have saved me from a thousand minor embarrassments

Robert Hütwohl, for help in tracking down German versions of quotations by Blavatsky

Janet Kerschner, archivist of the Theosophical Society in America, Wheaton, IL, for material on Ivah Bergh Whitten and for sending out the call that allowed the image of Sabhapaty Swami to be found

Judith Kiely, librarian of the Rudolf Steiner Library in Hudson, NY, for aid in tracking down the original articles in German in which Steiner first presented his ideas on the chakras

Nancy Lehwalder, librarian of the Theosophical Library in Seattle, for research and editorial support

Marina Maestas, head librarian of the Olcott Memorial Library in Wheaton, IL, for research support and access to special collections

Dr. Peter Michel of Aquamarin Verlag, for being the first to see the possibilities of this book and offering to publish it in German

Lakshmi Narayan of the Krotona Library, Ojai, CA, for research support

Leslie Price, archivist of the College of Psychic Studies in London, UK, for his mentoring and collegial exchange of support, especially in connection with the work of Theosophical clairvoyant Phoebe Payne

Dr. James Santucci of the University of Southern California, Fullerton, CA, for the opportunity to publish an editorial report on my work on Leadbeater's *The Chakras* in his journal, *Theosophical History*, and for email exchanges that helped me clarify some of my ideas

Karen and Steve Schweizer, for rediscovering the long-lost book from 1880 in which the image of Sabhapaty Swami appeared while they were visiting the Theosophical Headquarters in Adyar, Chennai, India

Pablo Sender, reference librarian at Henry S. Olcott Memorial Library at the Theosophical Society in America, Wheaton, IL, for research support

Professor Shinde of the Adyar Library and Research Center at the Theosophical Society headquarters in Adyar, Chennai, India, for providing the circumstances under which the image of Sabhapaty Swami could be located and photographed

Dr. Mark Singleton, author of *Yoga Body* and moderator for the website modernyogaresearch.org, for support in connection with the material on Cajzoran Ali

Donald Weiser, Yvonne Paglia, and James Wasserman of Ibis Press, for their creative collaboration in making this book a reality—and especially to James for meeting its multitudinous design challenges with dignity and grace

Martha Woolverton, once again, for her brilliant editing skills on this and three earlier books

Introduction

On a summer day in 2014, while browsing among the bulk bins of the local food co-op, I came across a small advertising brochure that someone had abandoned. The cover showed a twenty-something white female dressed in a sheer white tunic and seated in a yogic meditation pose. Superimposed on her torso were seven colored medallions, each containing a letter of the Sanskrit alphabet. They ranged from red at her seat to purple at the crown of her head, following the order of the spectrum. Closer inspection revealed that each medallion had a different number of petal-like rays.

These medallions were representations of the seven chakras (Sanskrit for "wheels"), a schema that originated centuries ago in India in connection with a type of yoga that has become a staple of contemporary yoga classes and New Age metaphysics. The chakras are said to appear to clairvoyant vision as whirling discs or vortices of light, hence their name. Ancient texts taught that their activation through strenuous meditative and ritualistic practice would result in a seven-step process of consciousness expansion leading to enhanced spiritual powers, enlightenment, and liberation from the karmic law of rebirth.

The product in the advertising brochure was called "Organic Chakra Balancing Aromatherapy Roll-Ons." It was made by Aura Cacia, a company that markets scented essential oils manufactured from herbs and flowers for healing purposes—hence aromatherapy. The brochure opened into a vertical table of color-coded correspondences identifying the locations, qualities, and effects on emotion, mind, and spirit of chakras that have been "balanced" through the use of these aromatherapy roll-ons—one for each chakra, each compounded of a different formula of essential oils.

Several half-amused questions came to mind: Could a scent really "open the floodgates of compassion and understanding" associated with the heart chakra? Why was the "empowering" third chakra associated with a "delicate citrus blend"? How would a fully enlightened being smell when wearing all seven scents at once?

The predominant question was, How did we get *here* from *there*? The list of chakra qualities was familiar from dozens of New Age books on the subject: *grounding* in the first chakra, *sensuality* or *sexuality* in the second, *empowerment* in the third, *compassion* in the fourth, *communication* in the fifth, *intuitive insight* in the sixth, and *enlightenment* in the seventh. Yet anyone who looks into the origins of the chakra system in India may be astonished to find that the chakras have colors, but there is no rainbow; they have qualities and spiritual powers but not those on this list. No scents are involved. The idea of chakra balancing is never mentioned in the scriptures. The chakras are to be pierced, dissolved, and transcended to achieve a state of "liberation within life" rather than an emotionally and spiritually balanced lifestyle (whatever that might mean).

I first heard of the chakras in the late 1970s from a friend who was a disciple of an Indian yogi. I learned their locations and how to breathe to purify them. Through the metaphysical grapevine, I learned of a list of chakra qualities similar to the one in the Aura Cacia brochure. A few books on the subject were available in metaphysical bookstores, but I did not buy or read them.

Fast forward to 2002—I was asked to write a book on the spiritual effects of music. I considered using the chakra system as a framework for describing mystical or peak experiences associated with composing, performing, and listening to music. Dozens of books on the chakras were now available, with many variations in listing the colors and qualities. I wanted to work with the most authentic list of qualities I could find. But research into ancient Indian systems confused me—some had as few as four chakras, and others as many as forty-nine. Several questions drove me—though they were still unresolved when the book was published in 2005:

- When did the term *chakra* first come into the English language?
- When did the rainbow color scheme originate, and who was responsible for it?

- Where did the ubiquitous New Age list of chakra qualities come from, and how long has it been around?

In the summer of 2012, I was approached about annotating a new edition of a book on the chakras published in 1927 by Charles W. Leadbeater, a clairvoyant who worked within the Theosophical Society. His book *The Chakras* had been in print continuously for nearly ninety years. Though considered a classic in the field of New Age chakra studies, this book was not an easy read. Leadbeater used obscure terminology, assuming his Theosophical readership would understand it without explanation. There were several ways in which his clairvoyant perceptions of the chakras differed not only from ancient Indian texts, but also from recent New Age books. I tried to create an "authoritative," stand-alone text, with notes explaining all the terms and an afterword that placed the book in context within the evolution of the New Age version of the chakra system.

This project allowed me to solve the problem of where the rainbow color scheme came from. Being under a tight deadline, I was unable to pursue the other questions. However, in the summer of 2014, I received a request to give a talk on the chakra system. That opportunity allowed me to further my research. I was able to trace the first references to the chakra system in English. I was also able to track the century-long evolution of what I call the Western chakra system. This evolution began in the 1880s, in the writings of Madame Helena Petrovna Blavatsky, founder of the Theosophical Society, and was more or less complete by 1990, when actress Shirley MacLaine appeared on the *Tonight Show* and amused a national TV audience by affixing colored circles representing the chakra system onto Johnny Carson's clothing and head.

I have concluded that the evolution of the Western chakra system was an unintentional collaboration between the following:

- Esotericists and clairvoyants (many with a Theosophical background)

- Scholars of Indology (the study of Indian culture, including religious beliefs)
- Mythologist Joseph Campbell
- Psychologists (Carl Jung and the originators of the human potential movement at Esalen Institute in Big Sur, California)
- Indian yogis (some of whose "ancient" teachings made use of Leadbeater's color system)
- Energy healers (Barbara Brennan and others)

The two primary strands of this evolutionary sequence—the rainbow color scheme and the list of qualities—did not come together in print until 1977. Thus the much-vaunted "ancient" chakra system of the West was barely forty years old, its history obscured by the habit of New Age writers, both in print and on the Internet, not to include notes and sources for their information—a habit called source amnesia.

I have written this book for people who want to know about the *real* history of the Western chakra system—a wild and wacky story that somehow produced a body of spiritual and alternative healing practices that has profoundly influenced the lives of millions. Part 1, "East Is East and West Is West," deals with the early evolution of the chakra system. I examine the Indian background of this system and develop useful definitions of key Sanskrit terms, such as *Tantra*, *yoga*, *chakra*, *nadi*, and *kundalini*. I also indicate what I mean by Eastern and Western chakra systems and provide guidelines for classifying such systems.

In part 2, "Esoteric Matrix: The Chakra Teachings of H. P. Blavatsky (1879–91)," I demonstrate the key role played by Madame Blavatsky and the Theosophical Society (TS) in transmitting Eastern teachings on the chakras to the West—and radically altering them in the process.

Part 3, "Whirling Wheels: Theosophical Clairvoyance (1890s–1920s)," details the contributions of Theosophists such as Annie Besant and Charles W. Leadbeater to the Western chakra system, as well as those of Rudolf Steiner and lesser known figures, such as Rāma Prasād and Ella Adelia Fletcher, who produced early manuals of yoga practice. For context, I include discussions of the chakra teachings of several non-Theosophists, such as Swami Vivekananda and Sir John Woodroffe, whose translation and commentary on a key tantric description of the chakras, *The Serpent Power*, became a classic text in Western chakra studies.

Part 4, "Chromotherapy: Science of Rays, Colors, and Glands (1920s–1950s)," provides original research on how the rainbow colors and the endocrine glands became associated with the Western chakra system. Aside from Alice Bailey and Edgar Cayce, the figures covered here are mostly unknown: Ivah Bergh Whitten, S. G. J. Ouseley, and the mysterious American yogini Cajzoran Ali, whose true name and story are revealed here for the first time. Rare portraits of these missing links in the development of the Western chakra system appear in the frontispiece.

In part 5, "Scholars and Swamis and Shrinks, Oh My! (1930s–70s)," I present contributions to the evolution of the Western chakra system by European and American scholars, such as Carl Jung and Joseph Campbell, as well as those by several Indian spiritual teachers, from Ramakrishna and Sri Aurobindo to Swami Rama. In particular, I focus on the Esalen Institute's human potential movement, a loose-knit band of psychologists, philosophers, and bodyworkers—including Esalen's founder, Michael Murphy—who were instrumental in formulating the standard list of chakra qualities. In this section, I announce the birth of the Western chakra system as we know it, in June 1977, a result of Esalen's unique concatenation of Eastern mysticism, Western occultism, and European/American psychology.

Part 6, "Light-Wheels Roll On (1980s and Beyond)," deals with the fallout of this birth, which includes a number of competing systems, now forgotten, as well as controversies caused by differing numbers, names, locations, colors, and functions in these systems. In the 1980s, writers on the chakras, such as Anodea Judith (*Wheels of Life*), began consolidating information from various systems to resolve such controversies and reinforce the hegemony of the system we now consider traditional.

This was also the decade when innovative practitioners in the developing field of energy medicine began applying the chakra system to various forms of bodywork, including acupuncture, Polarity Therapy, and Reiki. Toward the end of the decade, bestselling author and actress Shirley MacLaine was offering public workshops on the chakras—and her October 4, 1990, appearance on the *Tonight Show* could be called the Western chakra system's coming-out party. It was no longer an esoteric yoga teaching but an aspect of popular culture.

In the 1990s, books, workshops, websites, and music based on the chakras proliferated, touching on many forms of spiritual and healing practice—though often repeating what had gone before. It would be self-defeating to track down every variation or innovation on the now standard association of rainbow colors and chakra qualities. Instead, I close the book with speculations on what could be considered the last stage in the development of the Western chakra system—the codifying of esoteric teachings on chakras, subtle bodies, and planes and their use in astral projection. Such speculations accompanied the development of the Western chakra system like a shadowy secondary rainbow during much of the twentieth century and emerged into their clearest presentation in the work of Barbara Brennan.

Because the chakra system represents a nexus of so many topics—from kundalini yoga to clairvoyant perception of the aura, psychotherapy to bodywork—I limit my explorations to material with direct relevance to the development of the Western chakra system. Thus I do not deal with techniques of kundalini yoga or practices for developing the chakras. For lack of space, I have left out many yogis, clairvoyants, scientific researchers, and kundalini experiencers who have worked within this tradition. Those I cite, especially in connection with the transmission of the chakra system into various types of bodywork, may represent only the earliest emergence into print of the developmental stages they represent. They may not have been the originators of the material they passed on—the latter may remain anonymous or may have published later.

A chronology of the development of the chakra system in India appears after this introduction to provide historical context. Extensive endnotes and a bibliography document my sources. Twenty-four figures and eight color plates show how the evolving Western chakra system was portrayed during the late nineteenth and early twentieth centuries. Some have never been reproduced beyond their initial publication. Furthermore, twenty-five tables summarize chakra teachings decade by decade, exposing the rich, though largely hidden, vein of metaphysical speculation that led to the development of the Western chakra system and highlighting when and how the key components of this system fell into place.

Contemporary historians of South Asian religions who specialize in fields in which the chakras play a part sometimes rail against Western New Age appropriation of these teachings.[1] Nevertheless, the unintentional collaboration of esotericists, clairvoyants, scholars, psychologists, yogis, and energy healers that produced the Western chakra system probably mirrors the spread of tantric teachings throughout East Asia over many centuries. In both cases, a constant selection and recombination of details determined what was left out and what was passed on from one generation to the next. If that spreading fulfilled ancient cultural and spiritual needs, the same thing could be said of the modern West—even if the result has been commodified in ways unimaginable in the India of a thousand years ago (as in the case of aromatherapy roll-ons).

I see the development of the Western chakra system as the embodiment of a deeply meaningful archetype of enlightenment, common to East *and* West—that of the spiritually perfected being, graphically represented by the image seen so often on covers of books on the chakras: a resplendent, meditating human form, shining with the rainbow-colored light of having fully realized our spiritual potential, each chakra representing an evolutionary stage on this sacred developmental journey.

Note on Sanskrit Transliteration

Because this is a book about the *Western* chakra system and the spelling of *chakra* with *ch* is normative for books on this subject, I use the proper transliteration *cakra* only in rare cases, as when appended to the transliterated Sanskrit name of a particular chakra—hence *anāhata-cakra*.

Other Sanskrit words are treated with the International Alphabet of Sanskrit Transliteration (IAST) on first appearance in the chronology, the body, the notes, and in certain illustrations—hence, *kuṇḍalinī* (first appearance) and *kundalini* (subsequent appearances). After the first appearance, I not only drop diacritical marks, but also form plurals with the addition of *s*, as is usual with English words—hence *nadis* rather than *nāḍī-s*.

In the case of Sanskrit terms commonly discussed in Western books on the chakras, I use the simplest Anglicized form, which often substitutes *sh* for *ś* or *ṣ*—hence *kosha* instead of *kośa*. Because I cite books from a century of scholarly and nonscholarly writing on the chakras, each using its own transliteration system (or none), I have chosen to treat quotations in the same simplified way, rather than reproducing them as they stand or updating them with IAST—hence *akasha* rather than *âkâsa* or *ākāsha* or *ākāśa*. This decision primarily affects quotations from works of H. P. Blavatsky and other early Theosophical writers who used now-outmoded transliteration systems—which subsequent editors often attempted to update in various ways. The one exception is the name of the second chakra, *svadhishthana* (IAST: *svādhiṣṭhāna*), which New Age books on the chakras often render as *svadisthana*.

Sanskrit names of religious cults and philosophies, gods and goddesses, locations, texts (such as Upanishads and Tantras), and authors are transliterated throughout with IAST—hence Sāṃkhya, Śiva, Nālandā, *Yoga Sūtra* of Patañjali.

Evolution of the Eastern Chakra System:

A Chronology

[Most dates are generalized, speculative, and subject to scholarly debate.[1]]

1500–1000 BCE. Compilation of the Vedas, the most sacred foundational texts of Hinduism.

1200s BCE. *Atharva Veda* compiled, from which the Āyurveda system of health and healing develops, including the principle of *marmāṇi* (vital points), some of which are located in areas of the physical body later associated with the chakras.

800s–200s BCE. Sāṃkhya (enumerating) philosophy under formation, one of six darshanas (*darśana*; "views") of later Hindu philosophy; includes concept of *tattva* ("thatness"; categories or essences), of which the five *mahā-bhūta* (gross elements) of earth, water, fire, air, and akasha (*ākāśa*; "radiance" or "space"; often translated as "ether") are key aspects, later linked to the chakras.

500s BCE. Earliest Upanishads. Vedānta (Vedas' end) under development—another of the six darshanas, derived from the Upanishads, considered the last revealed scriptures of Hinduism. First mentions of *nāḍī* (channels), nerve-like conductors of *prāṇa* (vital energy) in the subtle body, in *Bṛhadāraṇyaka Upaniṣad* (4.2.3; called *hita*, "healthful," instead of nadis) and *Chāndogya Upaniṣad* (8.6.1–5; includes relation of prana to sunlight and mentions five types and colors; also mentions a nadi going from heart to head through which the soul exits at death—a reference to the "central channel" of later texts). Life of Gautama Buddha (traditional date; current scholarship is trending toward the 400s).[2]

200s–00s BCE. Earliest definition of *yoga* (union) in *Kaṭha Upaniṣad* (6.10–11); yoga would become another of the six darshanas.

200 BCE–400 CE. Written form of *Mahābhārata*, India's great national epic, evolving following centuries of development in oral traditions.

100 BCE. Gautama Buddha's teachings first committed to writing in Sri Lanka as Theravāda canon in Pāli language. Mahāyāna Buddhism under development.

100s CE. *Caraka Saṃhitā*, an essential work of Āyurveda, lists several "major vital points" (*mahā-marmāṇi*) that may later form a basis for the chakra system (perhaps via the *Bhāgavata Purāṇa*; see below).[3]

200s. Śaivism, a branch of Hinduism focused on worship of Śiva—the benevolent "destroyer" aspect of godhead, whose function is to break down "the ego personality so it becomes pervious to the Divine light"[4]—developing in western India.

200–400. *Maitrī Upaniṣad*, sixth book (thought to be a later addition), mentions a lotus in the heart (6.1–2) and *suṣumṇā-nāḍī* ("gracious nadi"; 6.21; also called "central channel"). Yoga philosophy crystalizing in book 6 of *Mahābhārata*, which contains the *Bhagavad Gita*. Both Yoga and Sāṃkhya crystalizing in book 12 of *Mahābhārata*: *Mokṣadharma Parvan*, "Section on the Way of Liberation"—which may anticipate later teachings on chakras (i.e., concentration on navel, heart, throat, and head, locations of the third through sixth chakras).[5]

300s. *Viṣṇu Purāṇa* articulates a cosmology of seven heavenly realms (*loka*) and seven infernal realms (*tala*).

350–450. *Yoga Sūtra* of Patañjali (disputed date, sometimes cited as 2nd century BCE), and its commentary, *Yoga-Bāṣya* of Vedavyāsa, refer to nadis and chakras, highlighting four locations associated with the later chakra system (navel, heart, throat, and "the light in the head").[6]

400s–500s. Mahāyāna Buddhism and Brahmanism flourish side by side in India. Mahāyāna texts exported to China and thence to Japan; first translations of these texts from Sanskrit into Chinese (many surviving only in this form).

Evolution of the Eastern Chakra System 27

600s. Tantric Buddhism developing in eastern India. Śaivism replacing Buddhism in western and southern India.

600s–700s. *Śūraṅgama Sūtra*, known only in Chinese translations from 700s but possibly originating at Nālandā (major Indian Mahāyāna Buddhist monastic university), teaches the dissolution of six "knots" to achieve enlightenment—these knots are linked to elements and categories of perception, as in later tantric teachings on the chakras, but without being located as focal points for concentration in the body.[7]

700s. *Bhāgavata Purāṇa* references the central channel (sushumna); six "sites" (*sthāneṣu*) within the body (navel, heart, chest, root of palate [uvula?], brow, head), by which yogis liberate themselves from the body, and the gross and subtle senses and elements and realms of the universe perceived by these senses (2.2.19–31);[8] also mentions a four-chakra system (navel, heart, throat, and brow) (4.4.25). Vedānta fully crystalized in writings of Śaṅkara (788–820).[9] Tantric Buddhism spreading into China, where it is called Mìzōng (Esoteric School), and Tibet, where it is called Vajrayāna (Diamond Path). Four-chakra system (navel, heart, throat, and head) appears in tantric Buddhist texts, such as *Caryāgīti* and *Hevajra Tantra*.[10] Five-chakra system taught in Buddhist *Guhyasamāja Tantra*.

800s. Hindu Tantra emerges. Tantric Buddhism spreads to Japan from China, becoming Shingon and Tendai traditions.

800s–900s. *Kaula-Jñāna-Nirṇaya* of Matsyendranātha presents a six-chakra system, with centers for the first time identified as *cakra* (wheels) in their familiar locations; also introduces the notion of subtle body "sites" (*sthāna*, sometimes a synonym for *cakra*) with "spokes, leaves, and petals,"[11] as well as the practice of locating phonemes of the Sanskrit alphabet in "knots" (*granthi*, sometimes a synonym for *cakra*). *Netra Tantra* also presents a six-chakra system, using the word *cakra*, but with eccentric names and locations. Notion of *kuṇḍalinī* energy developing (as *kuṇḍalī*, "ring-shaped") in *Tantrasadbhāva Tantra*.

800s–1200s. Flourishing of Siddha cult ("perfected beings" who attempt to achieve bodily and spiritual perfection and powers—*siddhi*—by meditative and alchemical processes), as well as Śaktism (worship of the goddess Śakti—Śiva's consort), Kaulism (initiatory, clan-based form of Tantra), and Kashmiri Śaivism. *Haṭha* yoga developing.

900s. *Kālacakra Tantra* (Buddhist) teaches a six-chakra system.[12]

900s–1000s. Earliest known use of the word *kuṇḍalinī* in *Jayadrathayāmala* in Hindu Tantra. *Kubjikāmata* presents a seven-chakra system (though not identified with the word *cakra*)—not only with familiar locations, but also with familiar names and links to goddesses (Ḍākinī, Rākiṇī, Lākinī, etc.). *Tantrāloka* of Abhinavagupta (fl. 975–1025), a foundational text of Kashmiri Śaivism that codifies teachings from earlier schools, uses a five-chakra system (with the first two chakras combined) and develops the notion of circulation of kundalini ("the descent of transcendent consciousness into the human microcosm [body], and the return of human consciousness toward its source").[13]

1100s. Muslim invasions of Indian subcontinent begin; destruction of Nālandā University.

1100s–1200s. Gorakṣanātha codifies principles of hatha yoga and founds Nāth Siddha (Perfected Lords) monastic order. *Gorakṣa Paddhati* teaches six-chakra system with standard names and numbers of lotus petals; *iḍā* and *piṅgalā* named as left and right channels; kundalini mentioned, as well as the "great lotus" at the crown of the head (*sahasrāra*, what we now call the seventh chakra); but elements are distributed in five centers at heart, throat, root of the palate, brow, and crown.[14]

1200s. Buddhism virtually extinct in India.

1290. *Jñāneśvarī* (also known as *Bhāvārtha-Dīpikā*) of Jñānadeva (1275–96; also known as Jñāneśvar and Dnyāneshwar), a commentary in verse on the *Bhagavad Gītā* in the Nāth tradition, contains an account of awakening kundalini, calling it the "mother of the world"—a frequently used epithet (6.14).

1200s–1300s. *Śāradā-Tilaka Tantra* of Lakṣmana Deśikendra, a manual of *mantra* (words of power) yoga, correlates fifty letters of the Sanskrit alphabet with the petals of the six chakras and teaches a technique of visualizing and dissolving them; the twenty-fifth chapter details the practice of yoga, mentioning that opinions differ on the number of chakras (called *ādhāra*, "support"). *Rudrayāmala* not only links letters with petals in each chakra, but also links goddesses with gods (Brahmā, Viṣṇu, Rudra, Īśvara, Sadāśiva, and Paraśiva); early use of term *sahasrāra* ("thousand-fold"—the seventh chakra); *svayambhū-liṅga* ("self-existent mark"; phallic symbol of Śiva, around which the kundalini is coiled) is linked with root chakra and *bāna-liṅga* (bow mark) with heart chakra.[15] *Ṭoḍala Tantra* describes the practice of kundalini yoga, linking realms of the cosmos with chakras; mentions seed-syllable mantras of the elements and *nyāsa* (visualizing Sanskrit phonemes in various parts of the body, possibly a precursor to associating them with the chakras).[16]

1300s–1400s. Yoga Upanishads emerging—seven-chakra system (or "six plus one," as David Gordon White calls it[17]) fully established, with sahasrara as the seventh (though one text adds three further chakras); each element has its *yantra* (symbol), color, and associated realm, but elements are not yet identified with the chakras (e.g., earth is feet to knees; water, knees to thighs; fire, thighs to navel; air, navel to nose; akasha, nose to crown).[18] *Haṭha-Yoga-Pradīpikā* of Svātmarāma provides practices for purifying the nadis and meditations singling out the fourth and sixth chakras.

1500s. Mughal Empire established—the height of Muslim rule in Indian subcontinent (1526–1707). *Śiva Saṃhitā* explains a more or less standardized six-plus-one chakra system, mentioning a third *liṅgam* (mark) in the brow chakra and detailing the psychic powers associated with each chakra.[19]

1577. *Ṣaṭ-Cakra-Nirūpaṇa* of Pūrṇānanda Giri (active 1523–77)—each chakra now has a fully developed *maṇḍala* (circle), including petals with Sanskrit phonemes and pericarp associated with an element, yantra, color, animal, *bīja* (seed-syllable) mantra, god, and goddess;[20] *itara-liṅga* (other mark) associated with brow chakra.[21] This is the root text (as translated by Sir John Woodroffe in *The Serpent Power*, 1919) from which much of the Western chakra system developed.

Part 1
East Is East and West Is West

Chapter 1
The Mysterious Maps of Bipin Behari Shom

In India in the late 1840s, two mysterious maps of the human body came into the hands of a young man of Calcutta (now Kolkata). Both showed the outlines of a naked, mustachioed man with upraised arms, palms facing outward. The torso of one displayed a series of six stars with differing numbers of rays—four at the crotch, six at the belly, ten at the base of the breastbone, twelve at the heart, sixteen at the throat, and eight at the forehead.[1] Squiggling spiral lines in the belly connected several of the stars, suggesting to those trained in Western science poorly understood or inadequately rendered intestinal coils. However, those trained in Eastern esoteric science would have recognized these lines as *nāḍī* (Sanskrit: "channels"), subtle-body conduits of vital energy running between the *cakra* (wheels)—centers of this energy whose activation would result in a seven-step process of consciousness expansion leading to enlightenment.

The torso in the other map was replaced by a cryptogram consisting of a table with eleven columns and eight rows. The head, arms, and legs sprouted from this table. Most of the table's eighty-eight slots contained numbers, though a few were empty. The central column contained not only numbers, but also a sequence of eleven images squeezed into eight rows, ranging from a tortoise and a cobra with flaring hood at the bottom, through a series of multirayed stars (or perhaps flowers with differing numbers of petals), to a goose at the forehead and a pair of superposed circles at the crown. A "key" to the numbers, ranging from one to eighty-eight, provided an apparently random list of gods, elements, alphabet letters, behaviors, conditions of human existence, and states of consciousness, as in the following sequence:

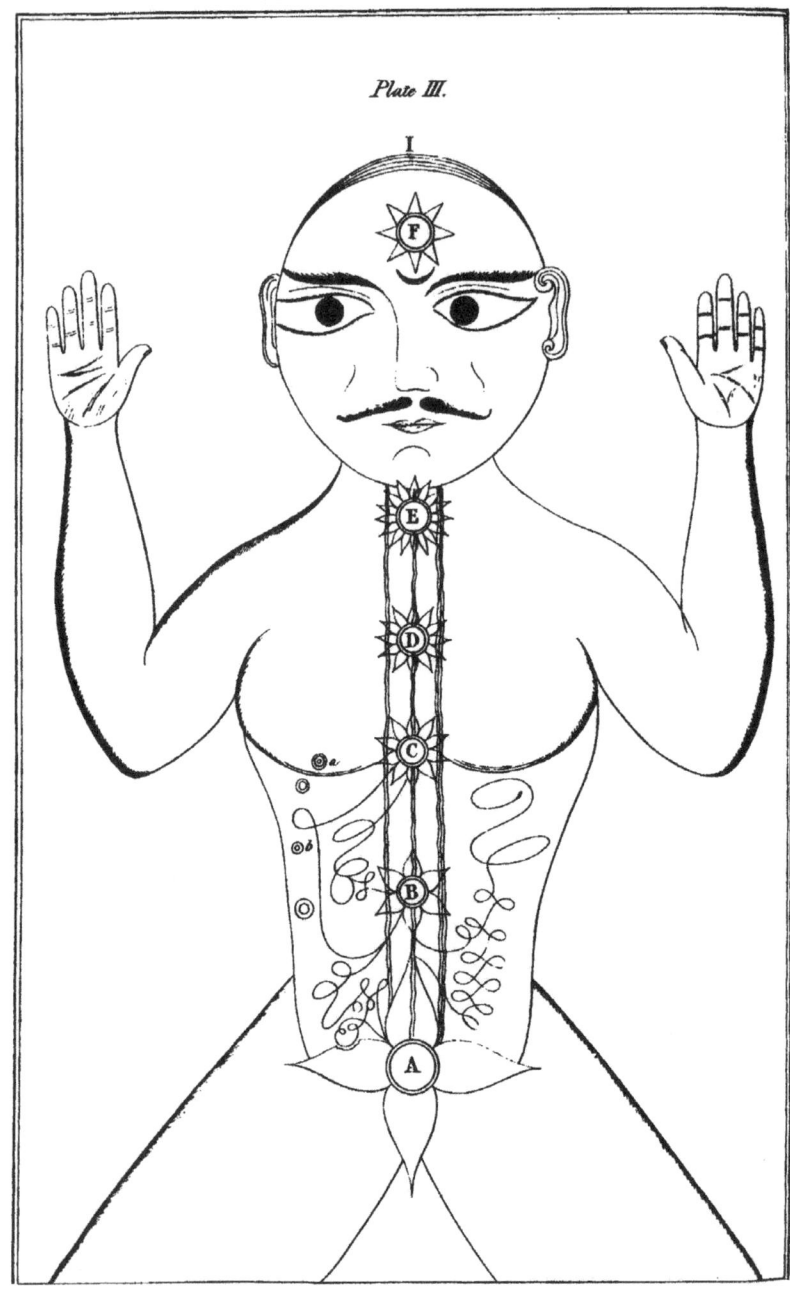

Figure 1. Mysterious Map A (reprinted from Bipin Behari Shom, "Physical Errors of Hinduism," in *The Sessional Papers Printed by the House of Lords,* 1853)[3]

The Mysterious Maps of Bipin Behari Shom 35

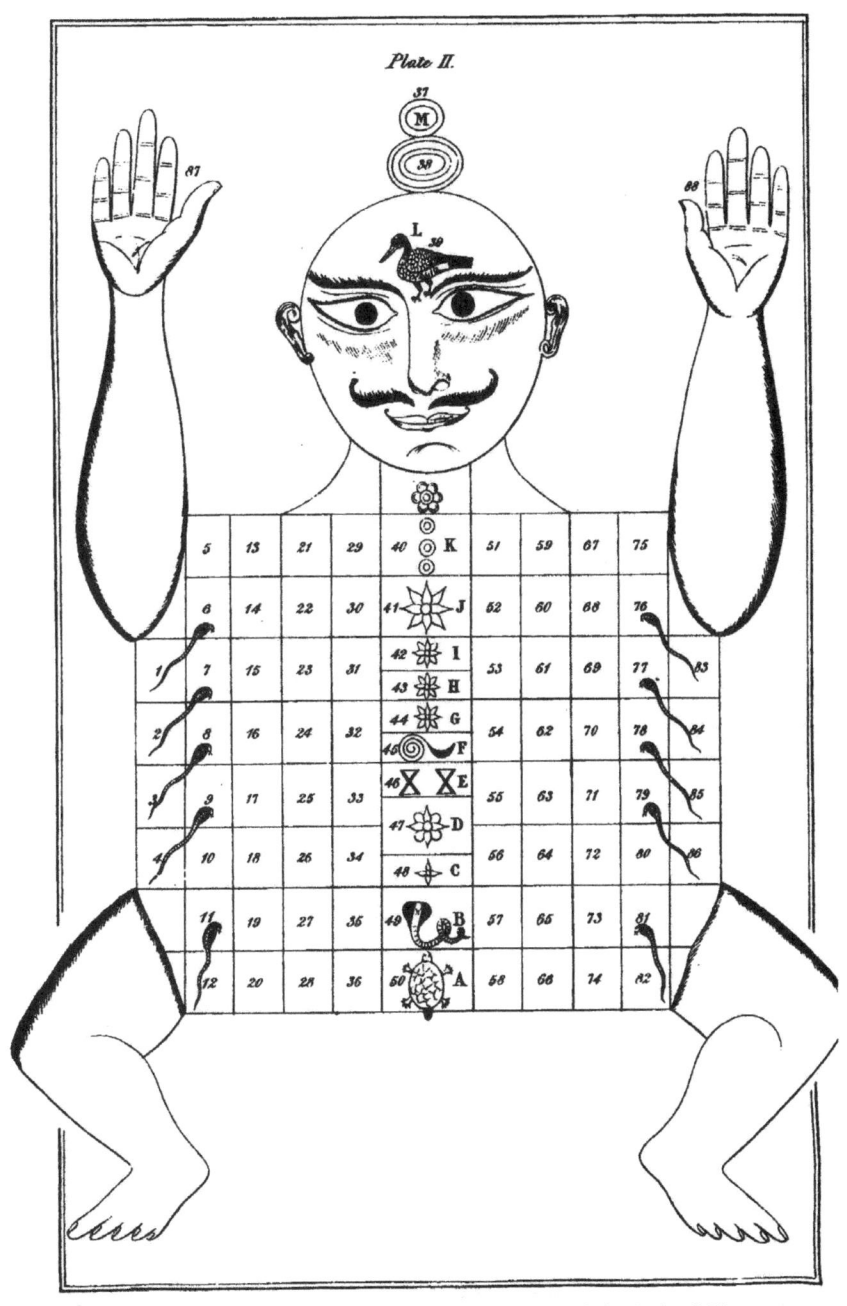

Figure 2. Mysterious Map B (reprinted from Bipin Behari Shom, "Physical Errors of Hinduism," in *The Sessional Papers Printed by the House of Lords,* 1853)

11. Religious penance
12. Anger
13. The dreaming state
14. Goodness
15. The vowel *a*
16. Brahma
17. Pedantry
18. Intelligence
19. The place of the mind
20. Fire[2]

The loss of the original Sanskrit words makes any attempt to decode this cryptogram speculative at best. However, parallelisms between the horizontal rows suggest that the words in the key need to be rearranged in the order of these rows from left to right and bottom to top, possibly resulting in a series of aphorisms on meditative methods of raising *kuṇḍalinī*, the "serpent power" coiled at the base of the spine, whose awakening is said to confer godlike spiritual powers on the practitioner and lead to enlightenment.

"Errors" of Hinduism

The name of the young man who discovered and described these two maps of the human body was Bipin Behari Shom. He was a graduate of the Free Church Institution in Calcutta (founded 1843; now Scottish Church College). The institution's founder was Alexander Duff, a Scottish missionary who came to India in 1830 with the intention of establishing an educational institution for Indians, with instruction delivered in English and Bengali instead of the vernacular-only education favored by the contemporary Anglo-Indian government. Though the Christian Bible was part of the curriculum, conversion to Christianity was not a requirement for attendance.[4]

Our young scholar was a Hindu of the Śūdra caste, the lowest of the four primary castes in the Hindu social system—the workers. Though educated from boyhood in the Free Church Institution and later employed there as an instructor, he had not converted to Christianity.⁵ We know of him because of the prize-winning essay he wrote for a competition sponsored by the *Calcutta Review* (founded and edited by Duff) on the theme "Physical Errors of Hinduism." This essay, published in 1849, included engravings of the two maps—possibly the first graphic illustrations (as opposed to purely verbal descriptions) of the chakra system in an English publication intended for a nonscholarly Western audience.⁶

Shom's essay attempted to demolish the validity of the Hindu religion on the basis of comparing Western scientific knowledge with literal interpretations of traditional Hindu knowledge on such subjects as "geography, astronomy, chemistry, botany, and physiology."⁷ However, the mysterious maps referred to a category of esoteric knowledge expounded in the Tantras, texts "containing rites of a most secret nature, some of which are exceedingly impure, by which a man is said to become a *siddha*, or supernaturally gifted." The Tantras "are also the great source from which are drawn almost all the *mantras* by which the different manifestations of Shiva and Shakti are worshiped."⁸

Whereas the Vedas, the foundational texts of Hinduism, are said to be thousands of years old, the Tantras are a relatively recent development, whose written form dates back to about the eighth century CE. Yoga scholar Georg Feuerstein translates the Sanskrit word *Tantra* as "loom, web." Traditionally, the word meant "that by which knowledge is expanded." Tantric texts "specialize in esoteric or occult matters," including *mantra* (thought or intention expressed as sound)—sacred Sanskrit syllables, words, or phrases chanted outwardly or inwardly to achieve particular spiritual or magical ends. Tantric masters are called Siddhas ("perfected ones" or "adepts").⁹

Śiva, the "Destroyer," is one of the three main Gods of Hinduism. In the tantric tradition, Śakti is one of many names for his consort. One form of religious practice based on Tantra involves rituals that partake of five things forbidden to orthodox Hindus: drinking wine; eating meat, fish, and parched grain; and engaging in extramarital sexual intercourse—in which the participants are said to enact the union of Śiva and Śakti. These are the "exceedingly impure" secret rites mentioned by Shom. They are traditionally referred to as the "left-hand path" (*vāma-mārga*), which is sometimes associated with sorcery. Forms of Tantra that avoid such excesses are referred to as the "right-hand path" (*dakṣina-mārga*).[10]

As Shom told the tale, the mysterious maps came to him in the following way: A wealthy Brahmin (highest caste; the teachers) by the name of Gunga Gobinda Singha, who lived near the city of Murshidabad in what is now West Bengal, "spent the greater part of his fortune in making researches into the Hindu Shastras [textbooks]." He exhausted the knowledge of the local pandits (Brahmin experts on Hindu texts and traditions). So he moved to Nadia, a town some seventy miles away, where there was an ancient and renowned Sanskrit college. There, his teachers enabled him "to drink deep at the foundation of Sanskrit lore." Not satisfied, Singha "invited several pandits from the upper provinces"—the foothills of the Himalayas. They were "known by the name of Daudus," and the maps came from them.[11]

Shom was probably referring to Dadus, followers of a sixteenth-century Hindu saint, Dadu Dayal (1544–1603), an ecstatic poet. David Lorenzen links Dadu to the influence of the monastic Nāth tradition of Hindu Tantra—within which *haṭha* (forceful) yoga developed. The form of yoga taught today in popular Western yoga classes evolved from principles of hatha yoga.[12]

According to Shom:

> The pandits of our country are for the most part either ignorant of this department of Hinduism altogether or they observe that secrecy which its doctrines require of them. Hence, we have been enabled to do nothing more than to collect the leading points of two great theories of the human frame from the two annexed maps, with the assistance of a learned pandit. These theories, as exemplified by the maps, are as famous for their novelty as for their extravagance.[13]

At the death of Singha, these maps "fell into the hands of a native gentleman of our quarter [of Calcutta] . . . who gave them to us for inspection." Before publishing the maps in the *Calcutta Review*, Shom was assured of their scarcity by several Sanskrit scholars, who were "startled at the sight." They exclaimed, "We have never seen such things before—better keep them to yourself, and do not show them to the public." Because Shom was of a lower caste, he was told not to try to pronounce the incantations (mantras) associated with the maps—a right reserved for Brahmins.[14]

What are the "two theories of the human frame" to which Shom refers? With sarcasm, perhaps born equally of personal scorn toward elitist Brahmin pandits for their condescension and of the religious scorn of his Scots mentor toward Hinduism, Shom replied:

> Do they treat of the bones, muscles, arteries, veins, nerves, and ligaments? Do they describe the several organs of the human body, external and internal, such as the eye, the ear, the nose, the lungs, the stomach, the liver, the intestines, et cetera? No! These are commonplace things, and therefore they are left to the observation of the vulgar. The tantric theory on which the well-known *yoga* called *Shat-chakra-bheda* [Piercing of the six wheels] is founded, supposes the existence of six main internal organs called *chakras* or *padmas* [lotuses], all having a general resemblance to that famous flower, the lotus.[15]

Thus was the notion of the chakras first introduced by a native Indian to the English-speaking world.[16] Shom could scarcely conceal his disdain: "With regard to the chakras or padmas, it should be remarked that they are even to this day believed really to exist within the body of every individual. What then are we to think of those who could believe such absurdities?" Furthermore, "even when we show them by actual dissection the nonexistence of the imaginary chakras in the human body, they will rather have recourse to excuses revolting to common sense than acknowledge the evidence of their own eyes." Even worse, "They say, with a shamelessness unparalleled, that these *padmas* exist as long as a man lives, but disappear the moment he dies." Never mind that tantric teachings located the chakras in a subtle body surrounding the physical body like an invisible sheath. This subtle body could not be dissected, therefore it had no existence for Western science.[17]

Shom's impression of the second map was that it had something to do with "anatomy and phrenology," a popular nineteenth-century practice of reading people's character by noting the location of bumps on their heads—except the *torso* was the object of examination in this case. This map was a demonstration of what he called a second "great theory" about the human body, that

> the seats of all mental faculties, passions, and feelings are within the great trunk of the body; and that each of the faculties and passions has its respective material organ [i.e., chakra], by which its function is carried on—so that the brain, which is the real seat of all the mental functions, is altogether put out of the question.[18]

Well, perhaps not entirely—ever since the publication of these maps more than a century and a half ago, the brains of Easterners and Westerners alike have been exercised in attempting to decipher the meaning of tantric teachings about the chakras. The maps themselves were forgotten, replaced by others of a similar nature brought to the attention of Western esotericists and scholars decades later. As ancient texts explaining the theory and practice of activating the chakras came to light and were translated into modern languages, these teachings were gradually disseminated throughout the world. The result was a proliferation of scholarly studies, psychological speculations, mythological interpretations, clairvoyant investigations, channeled explanations, and myriad applications, from promoting physical vitality and health to achieving psychic powers and transcendental states of consciousness. The notion of the chakra system had begun its journey from the ancient East to the modern West.

East and West

The British colonial poet Rudyard Kipling famously wrote that "East is East and West is West and never the twain shall meet."[19] In discussions of spiritual belief and practice, the terms *East* and *West*, usually referring to Asia versus Europe and America, have a long but suspect history. In India, this history reflects in part the contact of indigenous (especially Hindu) philosophy and religion with European rational philosophy and Christian religion (in the form of proselytizing Catholic and Protestant missions). It also reflects European (especially English) colonialism and racism—exploitative attempts to civilize the "savages" of a so-called darker race while draining their home of its wealth.

Yet, aside from issues of historicity, the distinction between East and West has an intuitive appeal, similar to that between Aristotelian and Platonic thinking. The former mode of thought, based on sensory observation of particulars and deductive reasoning, leads to rational thinking that foregrounds an empirical world of concrete facts; the latter, based on mental contemplation of generalities and inductive reasoning, leads to mystical thinking that foregrounds a theoretical world of abstract ideals. Aristotelian thinking set the stage for the Western tendency to prioritize the so-called objective world, observable by the five senses and measurable by mathematics and the instruments of science, over the so-called subjective world of feelings, thoughts, and states of consciousness. However, Hindu thinking prioritizes states of consciousness, seeing them as steps in a process of discerning ultimate truth, while calling the objective world an illusion.

For the purposes of this book, I make a distinction between an indigenous "Eastern" chakra system that originated in India about a thousand years ago and a highly modified "Western" chakra system that developed from the former over a period of roughly a century, beginning around 1880—and that is now so divergent from its roots that it might as well have been invented without them. Yet the stages of this development may have served deep cultural and spiritual needs, despite the apparently justifiable accusation of cultural misappropriation.

I feel emboldened to retain the opposable categories of East and West by remarks made some years ago by Sudhir Kakar, an Indian writer trained as a Western psychoanalyst. Kakar became interested in exploring traditional methods of healing psychological and spiritual ills in various parts of India in the 1980s—before accusations of colonial thinking and cultural misappropriation became as shrill as they are now in American academia. The result was *Shamans, Mystics and Doctors*—a wonderful mix of philosophical and psychological speculation and soul-searching with anthropological research and personal memoir. In concluding his book, Kakar makes a distinction between Eastern and Western thinking that seems not only plausible, but also usable, without favoring one over the other as colonial thinking does so blithely:

> Human freedom in the traditional Indian context . . . seems to imply an increase in the potential to experience different inner states while limiting action in the outer world to stereotypes and unquestioning adaptation. The Indian emphasis has been on the pursuit of an inner differentiation while keeping the outer world constant. In contrast, the notion of freedom in the West is related to an increase in the potential for acting in the outer world and enlarging the sphere of choices, while keeping the inner state constant to that of a rational, waking consciousness from which other modes of inner experience have been excluded as deviations.[20]

Thus Eastern thinking prioritizes "inner states" over "outer action," whereas Western thinking does the opposite. Placed in relation to the chakra system, this distinction means the Eastern version is about passing through inwardly experienced states of consciousness, each more expansive than the last, until the ultimate "freedom"—liberation from the limitations of self—has been achieved.

However, the Western version is about developing the human potential for happiness in the outer world through actions taken in any of seven categories, ranging from physical and emotional to intellectual and spiritual. For the individual seeker, whether Eastern or Western, these approaches may not be mutually exclusive. But for Eastern or Western culture, they seem to reflect widely held but apparently contradictory notions of self-realization.

Without being smug about spiritual teachings that differentiate between a limited self, to which the notion of worldly happiness is appealing, and a transcendent self that has achieved supreme bliss, let us adopt these opposing notions of self-realization as the starting point for our inquiry into the evolution of the Western chakra system.

Chapter 2
The Universe according to Tantra

Starting who knows precisely where and when, the spiritual movement called Tantra began to sweep through Asia, probably originating in northwest India a few hundred years after the beginning of the Common Era. Over several centuries, this movement spread throughout the whole of India, deeply affecting the practice of Hinduism and of Buddhism. It crossed cultural, linguistic, and regional boundaries, including the Himalayas, to become established in Tibet and China. It even passed over the seas into Japan and Malaysia (Bali). Aspects of this movement survive to the present day in India (where it is still called Tantra), Tibet (Vajrayāna), China (Mìzōng/Esoteric School), and Japan (Tendai and Shingon). From about 1880, Tantra began to be transmitted to the West, where it has had a profound influence on European and American culture, especially since the influx of teachers of Tantra from India and Tibet in the 1960s.

Westerners who have heard the word *Tantra* tend to associate it with flamboyant gurus of the 1960s and 1970s who preached a gospel of free love and sex as a pathway to god consciousness, such as Bhagwan Shree Rajneesh (now known as Osho). However, practices taught in contemporary yoga classes, as well as teachings associated with the New Age chakra system, also have their roots in Tantra, which comprises a much larger field of spiritual theory and practice than that embraced by what we now call sacred sexuality.

Because of its wide historical and geographic spread, Tantra is difficult to define. Here is an attempt by Anagarika Govinda, a twentieth-century, German-born scholar and practitioner of tantric Buddhism:

> The word *"tantra"* is related to the concept of weaving and its derivatives (thread, web, fabric, etc.), hinting at the interwovenness of things and actions, the interdepen-

dence of all that exists, the continuity in the interaction of causes and effects, as well as in spiritual and traditional development, which like a thread weaves its way through the fabric of history and of individual lives. The scriptures which in Buddhism go under the name of *Tantra* (Tib. *rgyud*) are invariably of a mystic nature, i.e., trying to establish the *inner* relationship of things: the parallelism of microcosm and macrocosm, mind and universe, ritual and reality, the world of matter and the world of the spirit.[1]

More recently, David Gordon White, an American scholar of South Asian religion, developed the following frequently cited "working definition" of the term:

Tantra is that Asian body of beliefs and practices which, working from the principle that the universe we experience is nothing other than the concrete manifestation of the divine energy of the godhead that creates and maintains the universe, seeks to ritually appropriate and channel that energy, within the human microcosm, in creative and emancipatory ways.[2]

In another context, White fleshed out this definition with a number of adjectives intended to describe what he called the "tantric universe," portrayed in ancient texts and contemporary teachings as follows:

1. "*divine*, world-affirming"—"the field upon which the godhead fully realizes itself, and offers realization to those humans who propitiate it" [i.e., those who place themselves in a favorable relationship with it, as through contemplation, devotion, worship, sacrifice]
2. "*anthropic*"—"seemingly created for human self-realization, with man the measure of all things and that creature

who is specifically adapted to plumbing the depths of its mysteries"
3. "*pulsating, vibratory*"—"matter, souls, and sound are the stuff of the outpouring of godhead into manifestation"
4. "*bipolar, sexualized*"—"all change and transformation are viewed as so many instances of an interpenetration of male and female principles" [i.e., Śiva and "his self-manifestation or self-reflection" as Śakti] and "metaphysical categories, animals, plants, and minerals all being possessed of a gender marking"
5. "*hierarchized*"—"that which is highest, closer to the source of all manifestation, is subtler and capable of encompassing, penetrating into, and reabsorbing into itself that which is lower on the great chain of being"
6. "*radiating*"—"with the source of the manifest world being located in the center of a vast network of metaphysical categories, divinities, phonemes, etc., all of which are interconnected through a complex interplay of correspondences"
7. "*emancipating*"—"born of the boundless playing out of divine consciousness, its every constituent part, including the human body and spirit, as well as brute manifestations, are intrinsically free"; thus "bodily, practical, concrete experience . . . in conjunction with knowledge, is liberating"[3]

Though White pans New Age appropriations of tantric theory and practice, this list demonstrates why New Agers have found the tantric worldview appealing.[4] Contemporary Wiccan, pagan, and westernized shamanistic practices derive from principles similar to those in the first point. All forms of Western esotericism relate to the second and sixth points—especially the notion of correspondences, by which the chakras are frequently linked to planets (astrology), metals (alchemy), planes of existence (occultism), the Tree of Life (Kabbalism), and so on. The third point is the basis for sound healing and the fourth, for sacred sexuality. The seventh point could be said to underlie *any* modern spiritual belief or practice that seeks transcendence of conditioned existence and its attendant suffering without denying the body's and the self's capacity for joy, bliss, or ecstasy.

The Eastern Chakra System

The form of the Eastern system most familiar in the West first appeared in *The Serpent Power*, a 1919 publication by Sir John Woodroffe (1865–1936), a British judge on the high court of Calcutta. A student of Tantra, Woodroffe wrote under the name Arthur Avalon, apparently to protect himself and his Indian coauthors and cotranslators—in particular Atal Bihari Ghose (1864–1936)—from exposure during a period when Tantra was vilified by Indians and European-Indian residents alike.[5] However, for simplicity's sake, I refer to Avalon as Woodroffe throughout this book.

The Serpent Power was an exposition of Tantra as it related to the chakras, including an annotated translation of *Ṣaṭ-Cakra-Nirūpaṇa* (Description of the six centers), a famous Bengali treatise in Sanskrit from 1577 that included a verbal description of each chakra as a *maṇḍala* (circle) to be drawn or painted and used as a focal point for meditation. For the purposes of this book, I will consider this treatise as the end point of the development of the Eastern system and the starting point for the development of the Western system.[6]

As presented in *The Serpent Power*, the Eastern system consisted of three primary nadis. As we have seen, the nadis are "channels" conducting *prāṇa* (vital force) in the subtle body. They are somewhat akin to nerves or arteries in the physical body. Ancient texts differ on the number of nadis—some say 72,000, others greatly magnify that number, and still others state that only a dozen are important. In most Western texts that reference the Eastern system, just three are mentioned: *iḍā* (comforting), *piṅgalā* (tawny), and *suṣumṇā* (gracious).

Ida is on the left of the central channel, which runs along the spine. Ida is associated with the moon, which in Hindu mythology

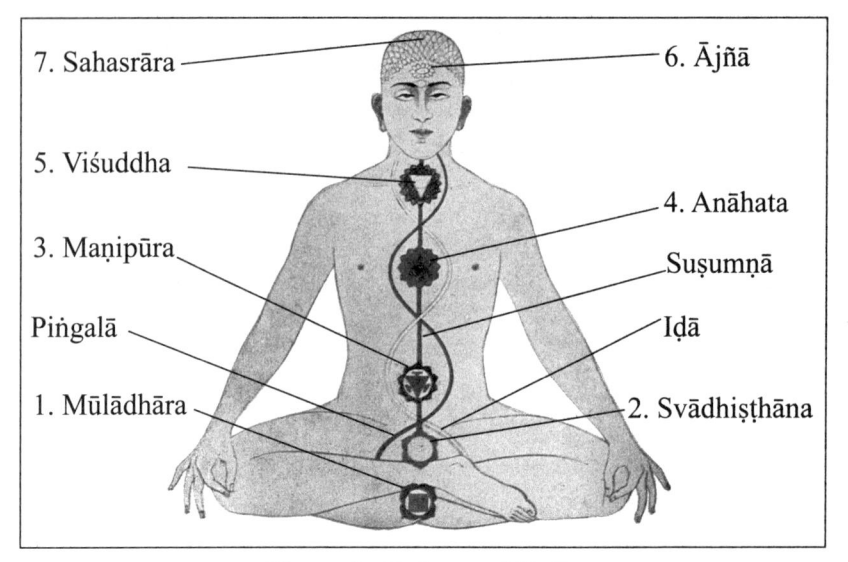

Figure 3. Chakras and Nadis
(adapted from John Woodroffe, *The Serpent Power*, 1919/1986)

is considered to be male. It begins at the base of the torso and ends at the left nostril. In some versions of the chakra system, ida runs parallel to the central channel. In others, it crosses and recrosses the central channel, and the chakras form at each crossing. It is presumably called comforting because *prāṇāyāma* (breath control) techniques that focus on the left channel and nostril are said to be cooling in the hot Indian climate.[7]

Pingala is on the right of the central channel. It is associated with the sun, which is female. It begins at the base of the torso and ends at the right nostril. Like ida, it either runs alongside the central channel or crosses and recrosses it. Pranayama techniques that focus on pingala are said to heat the body.[8] Tawny is a brown or reddish-orange color, that of dried earth on a hot summer day.

Sushumna starts at the base of the torso and extends to a point at the crown of the head called *brahmarandhra* (aperture of the god Brahma), from which the soul is said to exit at death—a very ancient belief in Hinduism, long predating the chakra system.

Sushumna is gracious, perhaps, in the sense of bestowing grace or liberation.

The chronology demonstrates that the central channel was the first nadi identified with a function, even before it had its present name. The names for ida and pingala seem to have developed as much as a thousand years later.

Along the central channel are six chakras, psychoenergetic centers typically located at the base of the spine, the genitals, the navel or solar plexus, the heart, the throat, and the forehead (at the point between the eyebrows where the nose begins). The standard names for these are as follows:

- *Mūlādhāra* (root-support); also called *guda* (rectal) chakra. Older texts sometimes label all the chakras with the term *ādhāra* (support).
- *Svādhiṣṭhāna* (own place); also called *meḍhra* (genital) chakra. There are varying explanations of the meaning of *svādhiṣṭhāna*: perhaps "private" or "secret"; or "her own place," when referring to the dwelling place of *kuṇḍalinī-śakti* ("serpent power," said to be female), which is the force that activates or pierces the chakras;[9] or "place where the breath arises," as one text explains.[10] Older texts sometimes label all the chakras with the term *sthāna* (place).
- *Maṇipūra*, sometimes *maṇipūraka* (jeweled city); also called *nābhī* (navel) chakra. Older texts sometimes use the word *pīṭha* (seat) for the chakras—a word that means "pilgrimage site." These sites were mapped not only geographically (e.g., the holy city of Benares, now called Varanasi, is a pitha), but also within the body. The use of the word *pūra* (city) in the name of this chakra may be a remnant of this tradition.[11]
- *Anāhata* (unstruck sound); also called *hṛdaya* (heart) chakra. Certain types of yoga involve focusing on subtle sounds that become audible when one meditates on the heart center.

Such sounds are considered to be modifications of a universal sound current (*śabda*) set in motion by the Absolute (Brahman) when the manifest universe was created. This is the unstruck sound, often identified with the syllable *oṃ*. Alternately, a sound heard inwardly rather than with the ears is an unstruck sound. In *nāda* (sound) yoga, there is a series of such sounds that become increasingly subtle as the meditator progresses, ranging from thunder to the tinkle of a bell. A minor chakra named *hṛt* (heart) is sometimes depicted below anahata. It has eight petals and portrays the celestial wish-fulfilling tree.

- *Viśuddha* (purifying); also called *kaṇṭha* (throat) chakra. In a practice called *bhūta-śuddhi* (purification of the elements), the five chakras described thus far are each associated with an element (*bhūta*): earth, water, fire, air, and akasha (*ākāśa*; "radiance," "space," or "ether"). A preparatory practice for raising the kundalini involves meditating on each in turn, from the bottom up, then dissolving earth into water, water into fire, fire into air, and air into akasha. The name of this chakra may refer to this practice (though other forms of purification are also described in connection with the chakras, such as *nāḍī-śuddhi*, "purification of the nadis," a form of pranayama).

- *Ājñā* (command); also called *bhrūmadhya* (brow) chakra. It is said that this is the chakra through which the commands of the guru come. Alternatively, it represents *manas* (mind) and its mastery indicates that the mind is under the practitioner's command.

- *Sahasrāra* (thousand-fold); sometimes referred to by its location: *mūrdhan* ("head," or, as David Gordon White translates it, "cranial vault"). *Sahasrāra* is actually an abbreviation for *sahasrāra-dala* (thousand-fold petals) or *sahasrāra-kamala* or *sahasrāra-padma* (each meaning "thousand-fold lotus"). Thus the usual English translation is "thousand-petaled lotus." In many texts, the chakras are referred to collectively or individually as *padma* (lotus), which may be the more ancient term. This chakra is located at the crown of the head, either at the brahmarandhra or just above it. The lotus is usually turned downward.

The Eastern system seems to be a curious mix of terms referring to supports, sites, seats, wheels, and lotuses. Why not use just one term specifying the location, as in the case of the nabhi, hridaya, and kantha chakras? This hash may be a result of the system's having originated in many traditions, such that each chakra name reflects one of the currents that poured into it. Alternatively, the names may have been purposely adopted, each to indicate a function or practice involved in raising the kundalini—for example, breath in the second chakra, an inner pilgrimage in the third, the yoga of subtle sounds in the fourth, and the purification of elements in the fifth. Thus the names would be a mnemonic system for recalling such practices, as well as an indication of function, such as achieving a solid base (posture) for meditation in the first or command of mind in the sixth.

The term *padma* has special relevance to the chakra system. In graphic representations of the seven chakras as mandalas, each is portrayed as a multicolored lotus. One color is for the petals, another for the pericarp (center), and a third for an area within the pericarp dedicated to a particular element.

The chakras have varying numbers of petals, distributed as follows: 4, 6, 10, 12, 16, 2, 1000. Each set of petals carries a selection of the fifty letters (phonemes) of the Sanskrit alphabet. The number of petals in the first six chakras equals fifty and the number in the seventh equals twenty times fifty—for twenty repetitions of the alphabet. Within each set of petals, the letters themselves have a unique color. For example, the painting of the anahata chakra mandala reproduced in *The Serpent Power* has sixteen vermilion petals with deep red letters, as well as a red pericarp, and a smoky central region for the element air.[12]

In the pericarp of each chakra lotus except the seventh, several images appear:

- *Yantra* (device)—a colored symbol of the element (earth, water, fire, air, akasha, mind) associated with that chakra, as a focal point for visualization
- *Bīja* (seed syllable)—a colored phoneme associated with that element and chakra, to be used for both visual and auditory meditation practice
- *Vahana* (carrier)—an animal acting as the bearer of the bija, again associated with an element
- *Devāta* (god)—usually with consort, corresponding to various manifestations of Śiva and Śakti

For example, in figure 4 and plate 1A, the pericarp of the anahata lotus carries these images: two interlaced triangles, one pointing upward, the other downward (yantra); the Devānagarī character for the Sanskrit phoneme *yam* (bija); an antelope as bearer of the bija (vahana); and the god Īśa and his consort Kākinī (devatas).

The tripartite vertical line in this figure and plate is intended to represent sushumna. Note that its interruption in the center of the pericarp is an attempt at perspective. The lotus is supposed to be oriented on a horizontal plane, facing upward, in imitation of a real lotus floating on water. In present-day portrayals of the chakra mandalas, the vertical line (if present) may stop at the top of the lotus and resume at the bottom, as if the lotus were hanging in midair, facing us, like a sunflower.

The distinction is important. Eastern teachings on the chakras correlate them with discrete planes of being (*loka*, "realms") and states of consciousness, with the most material plane at the bottom (*bhū-loka*, "earth realm") and the most spiritual plane at the top (*satya-loka*, "realm of truth"). However, Western teachings favor an evolutionary or progressive interpretation in which the chakras are arranged along a continuum of human potential from

The Universe according to Tantra 53

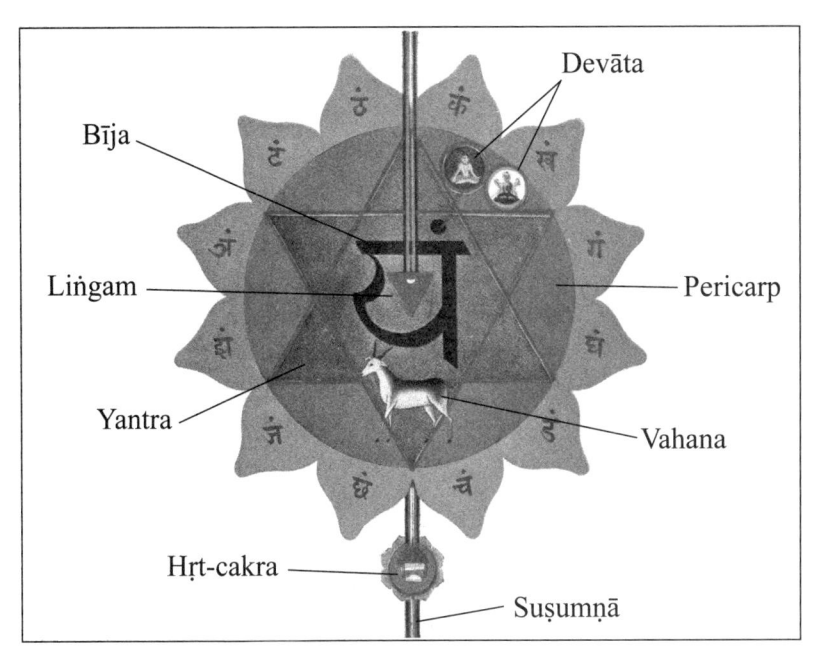

Figure 4. *Anāhata-cakra*
(adapted from John Woodroffe, *The Serpent Power*, 1919/1986)

the entirely material first chakra (survival) to the entirely spiritual seventh (enlightenment). The shift from portraying the chakras as vertical, discontinuous layers to horizontal medallions strung along sushumna nadi seems to reflect this reinterpretation.

Returning to our discussion of the Eastern system, three chakras (first, fourth, and sixth) carry one further image not present in the others—that of a *liṅgam* (mark). The meanings of the term and its visual representation run from graphic (the phallus of Śiva) to abstract ("mark" or "characteristic") and may include the subtle body (*liṅga-śarīra*). Illustrations of the chakras usually depict the lingam abstractly, as a colored column of light with rounded edges. Sometimes a serpent is coiled three times around the lingam in the first chakra to represent kundalini, the serpent power in its quiescent state (before it has arisen to activate or pierce the chakras). A twentieth-century Indian spiritual teacher links the three lingams with the development of the subtle body. He also adds a fourth lingam in the seventh chakra, to represent the final stage. The radiant *jyotir-liṅgam* (light-mark) represents the state of enlightenment.[13]

The Sanskrit names of the other lingams need not concern us. However, the locations correspond to another factor of traditional chakra lore—that of *granthi* (knots). Ancient texts used the term as a general name for the chakras, like *adhara*, *shthana*, *padma*, and so on. The chakras were said to knot the physical and subtle aspects of the body together. These knots must be dissolved for the practitioner to achieve liberation. In some traditions, the knots are located in the first, fourth, and sixth chakras, just as are the lingams. In others, they are associated with the fourth, fifth, and sixth chakras.

I do not list the colors, letters, yantras, bijas, gods and goddesses, and so on for all seven chakras because little of this information has been carried over into the Western chakra system. Western depictions are often greatly simplified, including only the rainbow colors and petals. The Western lotuses generally have but one color apiece, and the color scheme bears no relation either to the petal or yantra colors in the Eastern system. Only the number of petals is shared between systems—as in the case of plate 1, which shows Eastern and Western images of the heart chakra.

Explanatory texts on the Eastern system often include correspondences that are not depicted in graphic representations. Just as the first six chakras correspond to the elements, so are they often linked to minerals, metals, planets, spiritual powers, states of consciousness, and realms of existence. Ancient and modern writers on the chakras, Eastern as well as Western, share a mania for creating correspondences between the seven chakras and groups of seven of just about anything. These lists do not line up cross-culturally, except perhaps in one case—that of the seven lokas, which bear a close relation to the seven planes of existence outlined in Theosophical literature.

Because of reciprocal influences between Indian spiritual teachers and the Theosophical Society in India, some modern chakra systems in both East and West agree on the importance of linking the chakras with realms, planes, and a variety of subtle bodies. But these linkages have not been carried over into popular Western presentations of the chakra system. They subsist in esoteric discussions of the system by practitioners who are focused on the development of spiritual powers. The strongest resonances between East and West occur in such discussions because the motivation is identical—the desire of Eastern tantric practitioners and Western esotericists for mastery of self and universe by means of spiritual powers acquired through meditation and ritual.

Chapter 3
Reversing Creation: Yoga and the Chakras

The word *yoga* means "union." The Hindu tantric vision of union with godhead is symbolized by ecstatic sexual intercourse between a male god (often represented as one of many forms of Śiva) and a female goddess (often represented as one of many forms of Śakti). In this polarity, the male component represents a static or passive transcendent reality and the female an active, dynamic creative force. Their coupling generates the phenomenal universe in several stages. Each stage involves the ecstatic union of lesser representatives of Śiva and Śakti associated with increasingly dense levels of reality.

In the tradition of Kashmiri Śaivism, this cosmic coupling produces thirty-six stages of creation called *tattva* ("categories," i.e., cosmic principles) between the transcendent godhead and the densest level of matter (there are only twenty-five tattvas in the earlier Sāṃkhya philosophy that underlies the *Yoga Sūtra* of Patañjali). The names and order of these stages need not concern us at the moment. Suffice it to say that the first fifteen stages and their tattvas produce *manas* (mind). Mind produces four further sets of tattvas, including five organs of sensation or cognition (*jñānendriya*) and five organs of action (*karmendriya*), collectively called *indriya* (faculties), to be enumerated later. Then come five subtle elements (*tanmātra*), called sound, touch, form, taste, and smell; and five gross elements (*mahā-bhūta* or *bhūta*), akasha, air, fire, water, and earth. Note that the order of elements in Western esotericism, based on ancient Greek teachings, reverses the positions of air and fire. The tantric order is usually presented in Western books on the chakras.

Mind is associated with the sixth chakra. The subtle and gross elements are associated with the fifth through first chakras and are represented symbolically in the chakra mandalas of each. The gross elements appear as the yantra and the subtle elements as the color of the area that contains the yantra. The indriyas are associated with the chakras by implication but are not graphically portrayed in the mandalas.

From the standpoint of the tantric practitioner, each chakra represents an ever-more-subtle series of parallels, both "horizontally" (as in the case of the first chakra's set of four tattvas: earth, smell, generation/procreation, and smelling) and "vertically" (in rising from one chakra to the next).[1] Such practitioners seek to *reverse* the process of creation to achieve liberation from the laws of the phenomenal universe and experience godlike omniscience and power. The method is to recreate the union of god and goddess on each level of reality and transcend it, resulting in what David Gordon White calls the sequential "absorption" or "implosion" of earth into water, water into fire, fire into air, air into ether, ether into mind, and mind into transcendent consciousness.[2] This process may be enacted in several ways:

- Ritual sexual intercourse in the physical body with a partner who represents and embodies the god or goddess of the opposite gender
- Detailed visualization of such a union in a solo meditation practice
- Direct contact with the targeted states of consciousness, and their associated beings and powers through the use of symbolic diagrams (mandalas or yantras) or sounds (mantras)—practices I explain later

Ancient tantric texts are often unclear about the degree to which their instructions are to be taken literally. Should they be acted on physically, with a partner; or taken allegorically or symbolically and acted on imaginarily, during meditation? For example, Hindu tantric texts dealing with the first form of enactment, ritual sexual intercourse, are often explicit about partner (not necessarily one's spouse); setting (usually a group led by a guru); procedure (which may involve a ceremonial feast in which substances normally forbidden in orthodox Hinduism—wine, beef, fish, and so on—are consumed); and the production, combination, and shared oral consumption of sexual fluids, especially semen and menstrual blood. Buddhist tantric texts and later Hindu texts tend to internalize such processes, often along the lines of the second and third forms of enactment.

The problem of literal versus allegorical interpretation led to an early twentieth-century scholarly debate over whether the literal sexual practices of Hindu Tantra were a degenerate version of original tantric teachings, supposedly preserved in Vajrayāna Buddhism, or whether Vajrayāna represents a later, sublimated version of Hindu tantric sexual ritual. Probably, the three forms of enactment existed simultaneously in both Hindu and Buddhist forms, reflecting three levels of skill in tantric practitioners—something like the inferior, middling, and superior categories mentioned in early (nontantric) Buddhist teachings. Indeed, one form of Tantra delineates similar categories: *paśu* ("brutes," i.e., those overcome by lust in sexual rituals), *vīra* ("heroes," i.e., those able to endure the rites in the proper frame of mind), and *divya* ("divines," for those who do not need such rites to achieve oneness with godhead).

Another means of differentiating between tantric practitioners involves the right-hand and left-hand paths. Though both paths are largely carried out in secret, the right-hand path offers few challenges to orthodox Hinduism. For example, the sexual partner is usually one's spouse. However, the left-hand path is antinomian, contravening social convention by partaking of forbidden substances and sexual intercourse with low-caste women or prostitutes rather than one's wife. As in the black mass of Western magic, which similarly contravenes the conventions of the Catholic mass, power is invoked through the breaking of social, sexual, and spiritual taboos.

The terms *right-hand path* and *left-hand path* are often encountered in Theosophical writings as synonyms for *white magic* and *black magic*—the latter viewed pejoratively. David Gordon White has noted certain practices of tantric sorcery designed to enhance the power of the (usually male) magician through invoking and controlling fearsome female spirits called *yoginī* and to have deleterious effects on enemies.[3] Such practices might legitimately be labeled as black magic, which could be defined as exerting spiritual power to subvert the sovereign will of another. However, it may not be legitimate to assume that all practitioners of the left-hand path are so-called black magicians (no reference to race).

One modern British esotericist attempts to diminish the oppositional rhetoric in Western views of these paths by stating that in right-hand practice, the woman (ostensibly one's spouse) sits on the right of the man and in left-hand practice she (someone other than one's wife) sits on the left.[4] But I have also seen references to meditative concentration on the right channel of the chakra system to acquire personally beneficial spiritual powers and concentration on the left channel to acquire socially negative powers over others. The latter are called the "six actions" (*ṣaṭ-karman*) and are associated with sorcery or black magic.[5]

Without drawing attention to the fact, White treats the right-hand and left-hand paths with the respect due to any body of sincerely cultivated spiritual beliefs and practices, while referring to magical uses of tantric ritual as sorcery. This strikes me as a useful methodology, which I will adopt on the rare occasions when I need to refer to these terms.

Though the chakras themselves may play a part in Western tantric sexual practices, such practices no longer play a part in Western usage of the chakra system—beyond earmarking the "sexual" second chakra and the "heart-opening" fourth chakra as keys to more satisfying romantic relationships, as mentioned in the introduction.

Hatha Yoga

During the twelfth century, two legendary figures named Matsyendranātha and Gorakṣanātha, purportedly teacher and student, began to reform and codify aspects of tantric practice into what we now know as hatha yoga—including early attempts to collate or formulate teachings on the chakras. The hatha yoga of that time likely bore little relation to what goes by this name today. *Hatha* is usually translated as "forceful," suggesting not only that the desired state of union with god consciousness was achieved in a more active and dynamic way than through passive meditation, but also that this was a challenging spiritual path, requiring fortitude. According to White, hatha yoga developed from the Siddha cult, which involved the pursuit of bodily perfection, longevity, eternal youthfulness, and the aspiration to achieve "embodied enlightenment" (*jīvanmukta*), in which one lived as a physical being with the omniscience and superpowers of a god.

As taught today, hatha yoga usually consists of "eight limbs" (*aṣṭāṅga*). The terms for these are derived from the *Yoga Sūtra* of Patañjali, composed in the first half of the first century CE (thought they may have originated elsewhere). The Sanskrit and English terms are so well-known to yoga teachers and serious students that they scarcely bear repeating. However, the following alternative translations may suggest why this yoga is called forceful: (1) moral mastery; (2) ethical mastery; (3) postural mastery; (4) respiratory mastery (pranayama); (5) sensory mastery; (6) concentrative mastery; (7) meditative mastery; and (8) liberative mastery (*samādhi*, "ecstasy").

An old Eastern esoteric explanation of the term hatha divides it into *ha* and *ṭha*, claiming that the former represents the sun and the latter, the moon.[6] Hence, hatha yoga is the practice of integrating the solar and lunar polarities, usually through pranayama practices such as alternate nostril breathing, thus stimulating pingala and ida. The goal is to cause the kundalini to rise up through sushumna from the root chakra to the thousand-petaled lotus, resulting in the liberated state of oneness with godhead and/or freedom from the endless cycle of rebirth.

Attendees of Western yoga classes are usually exposed to just the postural aspect of yoga, perhaps with a few minutes of pranayama at the beginning. The postural practice may be utterly unrelated to that of the yogis of seven or eight hundred years ago. Present-day yoga scholars, such as Mark Singleton, are of the opinion that most so-called ancient postural practices originated within the last hundred years—with contributions from Swedish gymnastics, as well as other ancient and modern Eastern sources.[7] This is not to denigrate the value or authenticity of modern postural practice. However, it is to anticipate the theme of the present book: a similar hybridization of ancient and modern sources, both Eastern and Western, resulted in the Western chakra system.

More traditional pranayama and posture practices for the development of the chakras often involve breath retention (*kumbhaka*), muscular "locks" (*bandha*), hand positions (*mudrā*), and acts of physical purification (*śuddhi*). These possess a genuinely ancient hatha yoga pedigree—though they may have been revived and modernized during the last hundred years after centuries of neglect. One of these revivers and modernizers was Swami Sivananda Saraswati (1887–1963), first in the twentieth century to apply the term *kundalini yoga* to his reformulation of ancient and modern teachings (some originating within the Theosophical movement) in a 1935 publication of that name. Further research must be done to determine to what extent such teachings are genuinely traditional or are relatively recent innovations that have ricocheted between East and West before being absorbed into contemporary yoga practice and claimed as traditional.

Though some popular Western books, such as Anodea Judith's *Wheels of Life*, link the development of the chakras with certain yoga postures, I make no attempt to trace the origins of these correspondences, which are often derived from some relatively modern teacher. As we shall see, adaptations of pranayama played an important role in the early development of the Western chakra system—though these experimental traditions have been largely forgotten now. As for the rest of the eight limbs, many Western books on the chakras trot them out, but such information has little relevance to the uses to which we Westerners put the system.

Writers on the chakras may perhaps be accused less of *guilt* by association, than of an attempt to create *authenticity* by association. However, what we have made of the chakra system may also derive from another order of authenticity—as a reflection or measure of how we in the West think about and experience the process of spiritual development.

Mantra Yoga

One branch of hatha yoga is mantra yoga, a set of practices integral to raising the kundalini and directing it through the chakras from lowest to highest. However, mantra yoga is not limited to this application. According to Feuerstein, the word derives "from the root *man* 'to think' and the suffix *tra*, suggesting instrumentality." He defines it as "thought or intention expressed as sound."[8] Here is my definition: a mantra is any phoneme (letter of the Sanskrit alphabet), syllable, word, name, phrase, sentence, scriptural passage, song/poem, or prayer, with or without linguistic meaning in any of its parts, chanted outwardly (vocalized) or inwardly (silently) to achieve an end, such as the following:

- Quieting the mind as a basis for meditation
- Aiding concentration in meditation
- Achieving a desired (specific, targeted) altered state of consciousness
- Either invoking and controlling or worshiping and becoming one with a god, goddess, or some other supernatural being
- Mastering various spiritual powers (*siddhi*), including those associated with chakras, subtle bodies, and higher or lower realms of being[9]
- Effecting change in the outer universe, such as healing self or others; controlling the thoughts, feelings, or actions of others; or modifying conditions or situations favorably (for self or others) or unfavorably (for others)[10]
- Liberating oneself from physical phenomena and their noumenal causes (i.e., the elements of earth, water, fire, air, and

ether/akasha) to become like a god (while living) and/or to free oneself from the endless cycle of rebirth (after death)[11]

The effectiveness of a mantra lies in correctly matching the purpose for which it was created with the intention for which it is to be used, pronouncing it faultlessly, and having it activated or empowered by transmission from a qualified spiritual teacher or guru.

As noted, each chakra is associated with a "seed syllable" or bija mantra. Western books on the chakras dutifully list them. However, they seem to play no part in Western chakra practice. Only *om*, the mantra of the sixth chakra, is in use in Western yoga practice, but usually in contexts unrelated to the chakras (e.g., chanted at the beginning and end of a postural yoga class).

Mantras are often used in Eastern meditation practices adapted for Westerners to achieve the first three effects listed. The principle behind the use of mantras as aids in quieting the mind, praying, or worshiping have cognates in other religions, for example in the use of the prayer beginning "Hail Mary" in the Catholic church. Some Western magical practices use words or phrases of power, with or without linguistic meaning, for purposes three through six and perhaps seven. Eastern teachings that filtered through Theosophy into the practices of the Golden Dawn—a secret order organized in the late nineteenth century to develop meditational and ritualistic methods of ceremonial magic—resulted in experiments with the seventh purpose, though these were based more on visualization than on outward or inward chanting.[12]

Nada Yoga

As noted, the traditional name for the fourth chakra is *anāhata*, "unstruck sound." In one tradition of hatha yoga, meditators focus on the heart chakra in an attempt to hear a series of inner sounds. In the *Haṭha-Yoga-Pradīpikā* of Svātmarāma, dating from the fourteenth or fifteenth century, these sounds are listed in several stages, as follows: ocean, thunder, deep- and middle-voiced drums; blown conch shell, gong, and horn; tinkling bells, flute, vina (a soft-toned, sweet, bowed string instrument), and the humming of bees (4.85–86). Following the progression of these sounds from loudest to softest, or least to most subtle, provides a path to oneness with the Absolute, *śabda-brahman* (the Absolute as sound). This path is called *nāda* (inner sound) yoga. Detailed instructions for the practice of nada yoga are given in 4.65–102.

As we shall see, the concept of nada yoga played an important role in the transmission of the chakra system from East to West, via the Theosophical Society. The linking of sound to the chakras also played a vital role in the development of Western sound healing, especially since the 1970s.

As shabda yoga, the "yoga of the sound current," nada yoga became the focal point for a new religious movement originating in India in the mid-nineteenth century. Called Radhasoami or Sant Mat (Path of the Saints), this movement linked inner sounds with chakras, states of consciousness, and realms of being. It developed alongside the Theosophical Society, and there seems to have been a reciprocal influence between Sant Mat and Theosophical teachings. This relationship has been suspected by scholars for decades, but has been largely unstudied. Sant Mat has had a profound but nearly invisible effect on the development of the Western chakra system.

Laya Yoga

Another branch of hatha yoga involves meditation on visual images rather than on sounds generated externally or internally, as in the cases of mantra and nada yoga. Laya yoga is said to be the "yoga of meditative absorption," but the word *laya* itself means "dissolution." In some Hindu traditions, the outbreath of godhead creates the phenomenal universe, whereas the inbreath (taking place millions of years later) reabsorbs and dissolves the universe, resulting in an equally lengthy state of quiescence called *pralaya*. Laya yoga seems to be based on a similar principle operating within the consciousness of a human being who aspires to become a god or merge with godhead.

In laya yoga, a simple or complex visual image is drawn outwardly and used as a focal point for meditation. After concentration on this image with eyes open, the eyes are closed and the image is reconstructed internally in every detail. The external image is dispensed with when the internal image can be reproduced in every detail. Once the internal image has been built up, it is gradually dissolved, piece by piece, in imitation of godhead's dissolving of the universe.

In connection with the chakras, two types of images are used: the simple yantra and the complex mandala. As indicated, just as each chakra has a seed syllable, so does it have a yantra, a simple symbol that represents it as a focal point for concentration. These yantras are associated with the elements—so traditional lists include only five. In order from bottom to top, these are:

1. Inverted triangle within a square (or just a square), representing earth
2. Upwardly turned crescent moon, representing water
3. Inverted triangle with T-bar handles on each side, representing fire
4. Six-pointed star made of two superimposed triangles, one pointing up, the other pointing down, representing air
5. Circle, representing akasha

Some twentieth-century Indian teachers, such as Satyananda Saraswati (1923–2009; a student of Sivananda), have completed the series by adding yantras for the remaining chakras:

6. Inverted triangle within a circle, representing mind
7. Jyotir-lingam, a "self-illuminated" column or phallic symbol representing Śiva, or oneness with godhead[13]

A mandala is a complex, usually circular, meditation diagram intended to represent the cosmos, like a map. Thus, in some Tibetan Buddhist mandalas, five Buddhas or bodhisattvas (enlightened beings) are represented at top, bottom, left, right, and center. Each is associated with a cosmic realm or state of consciousness placed in one of the four cardinal directions, with the being in the center representing the realm or state of consciousness from which the others emanate (or originate). The mandalas of the chakras could also be considered maps of the cosmos—but each represents a single plane of being or state of consciousness associated with a particular element.

As indicated, traditional diagrams of the chakra mandalas visually encode information about the planes or states of consciousness they represent, some within the pericarp, some within the petals. The Sanskrit letters inscribed on the petals of each chakra represent particular creative forces (*mātṛkā*; "matrices"). These matrices generate reality at the levels of mind, akasha, air, fire, water, and earth—the elements associated with the sixth through first chakras. When the petals and letters of a particular chakra are perfectly visualized and dissolved in the practice of laya yoga, the intended result is mastery and transcendence of the associated matrika forces and the element from which they derive.

As noted, within the central circle of each chakra is the image of its yantra, the Devānagarī character for its bija, the vahana animal, and the representation of Śiva and Śakti appropriate to its element. In another stage of meditative practice, the god and the goddess are to be brought together in ecstatic union, then dissolved—once again to represent the mastery and transcendence of the realm and state of consciousness associated with a particular chakra.

The words *yantra* and *mandala* are often used interchangeably, as if they were synonyms—perhaps because their function as aids to concentration during meditation is similar. However, there are reasons to maintain a clear distinction between these terms in connection with the chakra system. First, the visualization and dissolving of the yantra representing a chakra and its element is a much simpler practice than working with a mandala. It could be considered a beginner's practice—laya yoga with training wheels.

Second, the yantra provides a symbolic point of reference for distinguishing between the elements and the realms and states of consciousness they represent. Each could be used as a focal point for meditation to place practitioners en rapport with a chakra's realm or state of consciousness, allowing for exploration. Once practitioners have familiarized themselves with that realm and state of consciousness, visualizing the yantra becomes a convenient means of instantly summoning them as needed. Thus I use the word *yantra* to refer only to the simple symbols of the elements that act as shorthand references to the more complex mandalas with their petals, pericarps, bijas, animals, and gods and goddesses.

Many books on the Western chakra system dutifully provide graphic images and verbal descriptions of the chakra mandalas. But few demonstrate an understanding of their purpose—and almost none make practical use of them or any of their parts. *These mandalas are visually encoded meditation manuals with instruction geared toward any level of ability on any of several yogic paths.* Thus, if you are a beginner in laya yoga, here are the yantras to use for placing yourself en rapport with the realms and states of consciousness associated with each chakra and element. To go further, you could use the animals as symbols of the spiritual powers available at each level. To go further still, visualize and dissolve the ecstatic union of each level's god and goddess.

You could also use the colors of the chakras as a means of placing yourself en rapport with them, their states of consciousness, and their realms of being. But in the Eastern tradition, the lotus of each chakra has several colors, not one as in the West. The primary colors are those for the petals and the yantras. These color associations are given in one book as follows: (1) red/yellow, (2) orange (or vermilion) / white, (3) green / flame red, (4) orange (or vermilion) / smoky blue, (5) purple / etheric blue (or white); (6) white /

Table 1
The Sanskrit Alphabet

16 VOWELS							
अ a 5.1	आ ā 5.2	इ i 5.3	ई ī 5.4	उ u 5.5	ऊ ū 5.6	ऋ ṛi 5.7	ॠ ṝī 5.8
ऌ l̥i 5.9	ॡ l̥ī 5.10	ए e 5.11	ऐ ai 5.12	ओ o 5.13	औ au 5.14	अं [ṃ] 5.15	अः [ḥ] 5.16

33 CONSONANTS (+ 1 CONJUNCT)					
Gutturals	क ka 4.1	ख kha 4.2	ग ga 4.3	घ gha 4.4	ङ na 4.5
Palatals	च ca 4.6	छ cha 4.7	ज ja 4.8	झ jha 4.9	ञ ña 4.10
Cerebrals	ट ṭa 4.11	ठ ṭha 4.12	ड ḍa 3.1	ढ ḍha 3.2	ण ṇa 3.3
Dentals	त ta 3.4	थ tha 3.5	द da 3.6	ध dha 3.7	न na 3.8
Labials	प pa 3.9	फ pha 3.10	ब ba 2.1	भ bha 2.2	म ma 2.3
Semi-vowels	य ya 2.4	र ra 2.5	ल la 2.6	व va 1.1	
Sibilants	श śa 1.2	ष ṣa 1.3	स sa 1.4		
Aspirant + Conjunct	ह ha 6.1	क्ष [kṣa] 6.2			

violet (or white).¹⁴ Thus the means of visualization would be to see a bicolored lotus in the location of each chakra.

In a later stage of building up visualizations of the chakras, you could add the correct number of petals for each, then add the characters for the Sanskrit phonemes on each petal and dissolve them one by one. You would start with four (first chakra) and build up to sixteen (fifth chakra) stages in this process, ending with the two petals of the sixth chakra, suggesting the dissolving of mind and the experience of duality—resulting in liberation.

In table 1, the order of the alphabet is traditional:

- Sixteen vowels—though present-day academic scholarship recognizes only thirteen
- Thirty-three consonants
- A final conjunct, blending two previously listed consonants—also not recognized by scholars as part of the alphabet

The vowels *a*, *i*, and *e* represent the first three of the thirty-six tattvas. The remaining vowels develop from them and are arranged in pairs to represent various creative manifestations of Śiva and Śakti, all existing beyond space and time. The final two vowels symbolize the creation of our universe of space and time by the gathering up and breathing out of Śiva's power. The thirty-three consonants each represent a tattva, including the two sets of senses, subtle elements, and gross elements mentioned previously. This conjunct portrays the union of Śiva and Śakti that is present even in the most material level of our universe.¹⁵

In this table, the numbers indicate, first, the chakra, second, the petal of that chakra to which the letter corresponds. Thus *5.4* indicates the fourth petal of the fifth chakra. I have noted scholarly quibbles by placing unrecognized sounds in brackets.

The manner in which the chakra petals are mapped into the alphabet suggests that the practitioner starts from the bottom of the table—the end of the alphabet—by applying *mind* (the element of the sixth chakra) to the problem of transcending the forces that make up our universe of illusion. The meditator then runs through the alphabet backwards, ascending through the chakras, to dissolve the elements and the powers (matrika) that sustain these elements from last to first. Once the first letter, *a*, is dissolved, all that is left to overcome is the duality of mind itself, represented by Śiva and Śakti—the two petals of the sixth chakra and their associated phonemes.

It is possible that the twenty repetitions of the Sanskrit alphabet associated with sahasrara, the thousand-petaled lotus, are related to the four sets of five tattvas ($4 \times 5 = 20$). The five gross elements could be dissolved one at a time, moving backward through the alphabet once each for earth, water, fire, air, and ether. The dissolving of duality at each level, represented by the sixth chakra, leads to the next. Then the process moves on to the five subtle elements (smellables, tastables, viewables, touchables, audibles),[16] the five organs of action (genital/procreation, anus/digestion, foot/locomotion, hand/manipulation, mouth/communication), and the five organs of sensation or cognition (olfactory, gustatory, visual, tactile, auditory).

If enlightenment has not yet been achieved through this comprehensive process of breaking the ties that bind us to our universe of illusion, it could be repeated for the next five tattvas, in ascending order: *manas* (mind), *ahaṃkāra* (ego), *buddhi* (intuitive understanding), *prakṛti* (created reality), and *puruṣa* (transcendent self). This would complete the cycle of imploding the twenty-five tattvas of Sāṃkhya. However, in Kashmiri Śaivism, as noted, there are eleven more tattvas, for a total of thirty-six.

A further five repetitions of dissolving the alphabet could result in the dissolution of the next five tattvas, called the five *kañcuka* (coverings) that create *māyā* (illusion): *niyati* (necessity), *kāla* (time), *rāga* (attachment), *vidyā* (limited knowledge), and *kalā* (separation into parts). Perhaps the tattva of maya itself represents the sixth chakra in this sequence, as did that of mind in the lower tattvas.

The final cycle of five represents an ascension through levels of godhead: *sad-vidyā* (omniscience), *īśvara* (omnipotence), *sādākhya* (all-being), *śakti* (all-power), and *śiva* (all-in-all). The last two tattvas are not the gods themselves, but their powers within conditioned reality. Beyond the thirty-six tattvas is *Parama-śiva*, ultimate reality, without conditions—understood as the eternal union of Śiva and Śakti (as gods).[17]

Yet another means of liberation encoded into the chakra mandalas is the devotional path of Śaktism (a still extant tantric goddess cult dating back to the ninth or tenth century CE). Thus there are images of the god and goddess, Śiva and Śakti, to be worshiped on each level, to be brought into relationship with each other and oneself. Each image of Śakti represents a generative power of creation in the phenomenal universe at the level of a particular element and state of consciousness. In meditation, or in practice with a partner, the task is to become one with this power as you allow Śiva and Śakti to achieve ecstatic union with each other and yourself. Dissolve yourself into them and their images into you to achieve the goal of absorbing and transcending the element, state of consciousness, and realm of being they represent.

If you are a beginner in mantra yoga, there are the seed syllable mantras to use for the purpose of placing yourself en rapport with each chakra, element, realm, and state of consciousness. There also are the phonemes transcribed on each petal of a chakra's lotus, whose sounds represent specific generative powers in the universe. Use these sounds to place yourself en rapport with all the powers that relate to a particular element and level of the universe. If you are an advanced practitioner, visualize these petals and letters and dissolve them as you follow outer chanting into inner chanting into the progression of sounds heard in nada yoga and their resolving into silence to transcend each element and level of being.

In comparison, the Western chakra system, with its focus on developing the chakras in order to achieve a better, happier, or more fulfilled life along physical, emotional, mental, and spiritual lines seems rather wimpy. No wonder the original yogis called their spiritual practice of mastery and transcendence hatha, or forceful, yoga.

Chapter 4
The Western Chakra System

Whereas the Eastern chakra system evolved for a thousand years before its pieces came together in the sophisticated system presented in *Ṣaṭ-Cakra-Nirūpaṇa*, the Western system required a little more than a century to develop into the form that is ubiquitous today. Just as there are a multitude of variations of the Eastern system with differing numbers of chakras, locations, and functions, so there are variations of the Western chakra system. However, in the case of both East and West, there is one model of the chakras that has become traditional, a standard of comparison for others, past and present, and the template from which further systems evolve.

But what is this so-called Western system? To my knowledge, the term has not previously been used, except informally, to differentiate versions of the chakras evolved in metaphysical circles in the West from their Hindu forebears. Here are the salient features, listed in the chronological order in which the Western chakra system's components were recognized, schematized, and adopted:

- A seven-chakra base (1880s)
- Association of each chakra with a nerve plexus (1880s)
- A list of vernacular (non-Sanskrit) names (1920s)
- Association of each chakra with a gland of the endocrine system, with minor variations from system to system, especially with regard to the pituitary and pineal glands (1920s)
- Single colors attributed to each chakra in order of the spectrum—either seven colors, including indigo, or six colors plus white (1930s)
- An evolutionary scale of psychological and spiritual attributes, functions, or qualities assigned to each chakra, eventually becoming the familiar single-word list seen in the introduction (1970s)

The Western Chakra System

To this listing may be added a number of less common attributes (in alphabetical order):

- Associations with layers of the aura, subtle bodies, and planes
- Developmental stages in the evolution of humanity
- Developmental stages in the evolution of the individual
- Diseases of mind or body associated with each chakra
- Elements, in the form of westernized interpretations of the tattvas
- Positive and negative emotions for each chakra
- States of consciousness and psychic powers

Beyond these categories, there is an endless number of correspondences based on Western esotericism or alternative healing practices, including but not limited to the following:

- Alchemical metals
- Astrological signs and planets
- Foods and herbs
- Gemstones and minerals
- Homeopathic remedies
- Kabbalistic sephiroth (spheres) pertaining to various aspects of creation
- Musical notes
- Shamanistic totem animals
- Tarot cards

Most of these sets of correspondences are unique to a particular teacher and often are not carried forward from one generation of teachers and books to the next. There is so much variation in these lists that it would be useless to catalog them or attempt to trace their sources.

Differences in lists of correspondences tend to develop along the lines of writers' interest in and use of the chakra system—their motivations. I have seen the following approaches:

- Acquisition of psychic or spiritual powers, such as seeing auras or experiencing astral projection
- Application to postural yoga practice, in which the chakras are used to enhance the effects of the postures or postures are used to activate the chakras
- Esoteric theorizing, such as absorbing the chakras into an existing Western esoteric system (e.g., astrology, Kabbalah, magic, or tarot) or using the chakras as a template to explain or synthesize other esoteric systems (as did Caroline Myss 1997 *Anatomy of the Spirit: The Seven Stages of Power and Healing*, which absorbed kabbalistic teachings into the chakra system)
- Healing of physical, emotional, or psychological disease through alternative modalities such as acupuncture, homeopathy, massage, Polarity Therapy, Reiki, shamanism, and sound healing
- Intuitive diagnosis of physical, emotional, psychological, or spiritual problems in self or others
- Scientific validation of the existence of the chakras and their use in therapeutic settings
- Self-help in achieving balanced personal development and greater satisfaction and happiness (becoming a better person)
- Self-realization through tapping unrecognized or underdeveloped human potential (becoming a better human being)
- Self-transcendence through achieving spiritual liberation or enlightenment (becoming a fully realized spiritual being)

These are not mutually exclusive categories. Writers on the chakras may develop their material along several lines at once.

Apparently hybrid systems, in which Western writers adopt Sanskrit terms and Eastern chakra descriptions, such as the numbers of lotus petals assigned to each chakra in *Ṣaṭ-Cakra-Nirūpaṇa*, should be identified as Western on the basis of their inclusion of any of the above-listed components, correspondences, or motivations.

Thus a Western scholar of comparative religion, such as Mircea Eliade (*Yoga: Immortality and Freedom*, 1958), may legitimately write about the Eastern chakra system. An Indian writer, such as Harish Johari (*Chakras: Energy Centers of Transformation*, 1987), may develop a new set of painted images based on imagery from Ṣaṭ-Cakra-Nirūpaṇa and write a book on the chakras that appeals to Western audiences yet remains firmly rooted in the Eastern tantric tradition. A Western student of an Indian spiritual master, such as Sivananda Radha (*Kundalini Yoga for the West*, 1978), may seek to explain Eastern teachings for Western minds and yet remain in the Eastern tantric tradition. Furthermore, an Indian spiritual master, such as Satyananda Saraswati (*Kundalini Tantra*, 1984), may absorb Theosophical teachings into an explanation of the chakras yet still present an Eastern system.

However, a Western author, such as Anodea Judith (*Wheels of Life*, 1987), may use the Sanskrit names of the chakras, the number of their petals, their seed syllables and deities, and so on—but if these are associated with the rainbow colors, the endocrine glands, and psychological qualities (not to mention gemstones, planets, and so on), this is a Western system. Furthermore, a Western student initiated into a tantric lineage, such as Jonn Mumford (who studied with Satyananda Saraswati), may present a Tantra-based system with left-hand-path motivations that are equally present in East and West, such as the desire for increased sexual satisfaction, development of psychic powers, and influencing people and circumstances through sex magic (*Psychosomatic Yoga*, 1962; *Sexual Occultism*, 1975; *A Chakra and Kundalini Workbook*, 1994)—yet without referencing the rainbow colors and chakra qualities of most Western systems. This would be a truly hybrid East/West chakra system—in my experience, a rarity.

For the purposes of this book, I adopt Judith's *Wheels of Life* as a standard model of the Western chakra system (even though she identifies the pineal gland with the sixth chakra and the pituitary with the seventh—a controversial choice as we shall see). I likewise adopt Satyananda's *Kundalini Tantra* as a standard model of the modern Eastern system. I could have made other choices, yet both books were published in the 1980s, a period of consolidation of teachings on the chakras in East and West in an attempt to resolve discrepancies within their respective lineages. Neither book represents a final stage in continuously evolving teachings about the chakras, but each represents a comprehensive synthesis of then-current teachings in America and India.

Typology of Expounders and Systems

It may be helpful to develop a classification system for clarifying roles and functions in the evolution of the chakra systems, East and West. I suggest four possible roles for the expounders of such systems:

- **Innovators**—generate a new system or add new components (including new chakras or correspondences) to an existing system
- **Consolidators**—collect and correlate information from a variety of chakra systems and synthesize them into a coherent whole
- **Disseminators**—pass on consolidated chakra systems to later generations without adding new material
- **Validators**—provide evidence for the existence and functions of the chakras based on personal, professional, or group experience or on scientific experiment (or both)

In the development of the Eastern chakra system, the unknown originators of four-, five-, and six-chakra systems during the first millennium of the Common Era were innovators. In the early centuries of the second millennium, the writers or compilers of the Yoga Upanishads and other fundamental treatises on yoga, such as the *Haṭha-Yoga-Pradīpikā*, were consolidators. The same would be true of the author of *Ṣaṭ-Cakra-Nirūpaṇa* in the seventeenth century. Sir John Woodroffe, in translating this text in *The Serpent*

Power, was a disseminator. The nineteenth-century Indian saint Sri Ramakrishna, a tantric initiate who described personal experience of states of consciousness associated with the chakras, as recorded in *The Gospel of Sri Ramakrishna* (1942), was a validator.

It may also be useful to classify chakra systems into the following related categories:

- **Formative**—the product of an innovator, a body of speculative associations and correspondences, often unsystematic and sometimes chaotic and self-contradictory
- **Interpretive**—the product of a consolidator, often the result of mining the work of previous innovators and multiple systems, producing an orderly and systematic presentation through the discovery of underlying principles and the resolution of contradictions
- **Explanatory**—the product of a disseminator whose object is to transmit an existing system as clearly and concisely as possible, usually without adding anything new
- **Experiential**—the product of a validator whose object is to describe a chakra system as actually experienced by self or others in experimental, therapeutic, or spiritual practice

In the evolution of the Western chakra system, the great formative systems are those of H. P. Blavatsky, founder of the Theosophical Society, and a principle channel for the transmission of Eastern notions of the chakras to the West; and Alice Bailey, a third-generation Theosophist and channeler who was a deep student of Blavatsky's writings. The British Theosophist and clairvoyant Charles W. Leadbeater, briefly an informal student of Blavatsky's, produced an influential work that has been continuously in print for some ninety years—*The Chakras*—yet his system is more interpretive than formative, despite his innovation of perceiving the chakras clairvoyantly.

The teachers I have chosen as standards of comparison for Eastern and Western chakra systems, Satyananda Saraswati and

Anodea Judith, may be classified as consolidators and their systems as interpretive. To the extent these systems have become standard references for students of the chakras, they may be considered authoritative. But that does not mean they cannot be superseded by further innovation and consolidation.

Explanatory books on the chakras are legion and have little relevance to the evolution of the Western chakra system—except that versions of the system disseminated by such books compete with each other and may lead to the dominance of a single system, recognized as traditional or authoritative. Thus is it possible to speak of *a* Western chakra system, understood as the combination of locations, names, gland associations, rainbow colors, and functions or qualities described earlier. One such book can represent the class: *The Chakras: A Beginner's Guide* (1999) by Naomi Ozaniec.

Experiential chakra systems may involve information about how validators developed awareness of the chakras and practices for readers or workshop participants to use to do the same. In the case of scientific research, such systems may include information about tools and research methods, experimental design, and charts or tables of results.

One such system is that of William Brugh Joy (1939–2010), author of *Joy's Way: A Map for the Transformational Journey* (1979). Joy was a medical doctor who discovered he had clairvoyant and channeling abilities and quit the medical profession to become a spiritual teacher and healer. His book was in print for more than ten years and workshops based on it were popular.

Joy claimed to have discovered and mapped the chakras clairvoyantly in 1973. His system had sixteen chakras, including a "Transpersonal Point" above the head and additional chakras in "knees, hands, feet, elbows and shoulder."[1] He taught a complicated series of physical practices for activation, development, healing, and balancing the chakras, based on guidance from what he called his Inner Teacher:

If some of this material sounds familiar, especially to one who has read Alice Bailey, I make no apology. Whoever and whatever my Inner Teacher is, it is obviously familiar with the concepts channeled not only by Alice Bailey but by Rudolf Steiner, Edgar Cayce and others, as well. I was amazed when in January 1977 I read Alice Bailey's book *Esoteric Healing* and found in it many concepts that I had received from my Inner Teacher and had already been teaching.[2]

I call *Joy's Way* an experiential chakra system because it is based on the personal testimony of a validator—even if some readers may not be convinced of the validity of what the author describes. The work of validators is often received skeptically by Westerners, especially when the descriptions of experiential systems involve clairvoyant information or experimental data that might not pass a rigorously scientific peer review.

Systems may also be mixtures of the above—as in the case of Leadbeater's clairvoyant illustrations of the chakras. As we shall see, *The Chakras* is both interpretative *and* experientially descriptive—so Leadbeater is both a consolidator and a validator. *Kundalini Tantra* and *Wheels of Life* also involve experiential components, so their authors are not only consolidators, but also validators.

Source Amnesia

As the Eastern system evolved over many centuries, attribution of its components to particular tantric teachers, lineages, or scriptures was not a general practice. Some powerful teachers, such as Matsyendranātha and Gorakṣanātha—traditionally seen as the originators of yoga practice—may have left their mark on the chakra system, but only in a general way. No specific component can be traced directly to either. Indeed, their very existence is legendary due to the lack of reliable historical records. By the time of *Ṣaṭ-*

Cakra-Nirūpaṇa, such components had become so thoroughly traditional and were so thoroughly synthesized in this new presentation that connections to previous sources were lost. Even today, the name of the author of this treatise, Swami Pūrṇānanda, is rarely recalled. Despite the brilliance and concision of his synthesis, his work too has become part of nameless tradition.

Olav Hammer, a Swedish historian of religions, has noted a similar phenomenon in the evolution of New Age beliefs. He calls it *source amnesia*: "In psychology, the term refers to the not uncommon fact that one may remember a piece of information but forget where one learnt of it." Furthermore, "source amnesia typically takes place when a general term used in connection with an older tradition becomes associated with specific, modern reinterpretations." Gradually, "a chain of transmission is built up, in which the latest spokespersons may have a horizon in time that stretches no more than twenty or thirty years back, and in which anything older than this is considered to belong to a diffuse, ancient past."[3]

In researching this history of the development of the Western chakra system, I have seen many cases of source amnesia. In fact, this book would not exist were it not for my attempt to track current beliefs about the chakras to their origins in the writings of the esotericists, clairvoyants, scholars, psychologists, yogis, and energy healers whose unintentional collaboration created the Western system. What took hundreds of years to transmit in ancient India, whether orally or in the form of palm-leaf manuscripts, now takes twenty or thirty years in print media. Internet use has likely contracted this time frame even more.

In the process of reconnecting so-called traditional teachings on the chakras to their relatively recent sources, I have concluded there are several reasons for source amnesia. The following list is not intended to be exhaustive:

- **Unintentional vagueness**: The writer has forgotten where source material came from or is relying on memory or notes

of oral dissemination, as in workshops or informal conversation, or on handouts whose sources are unknown or undocumented.
- **Intentional vagueness**: The writer wishes to project a sense of autonomous authority to impress publisher and readers or is concerned about being accused of stealing material borrowed from others or of having nothing new to say.
- **Careless scholarship**: The writer or publisher does not understand the importance of documenting and citing source material, does not know how to format notes and bibliography, or feels no need to do so due to projected audience or considerations of length and format.
- **Original synthesis**: The writer has assembled material from diverse sources in a new way, providing fresh understandings and insights, and believes either that these innovations do not violate copyright law (i.e., they deal with ideas or principles rather than exact words) or that they represent a new revelation of spiritual or religious doctrine or practice that supplants whatever came before.
- **"Justifiable" appropriation**: The writer believes in an ageless wisdom that is perennially expressed in ancient and modern spiritual and religious doctrines and practices, whether as irruptions from a collective unconscious or as teachings from an everlasting lineage of mortal or immortal, incarnate or discarnate (i.e., channeled), human or extra-planetary spiritual masters, thereby nullifying the notion of intellectual property rights.
- **Broken transmission**: Due to source amnesia or misattribution practiced by previous authors, the writer is unable to ascertain the true origins of teachings that are increasingly perceived as traditional (i.e., sourceless).

Ironically, even Hammer was a victim of source amnesia:

The association between the chakras and the colors of the spectrum appears to have originated with the American [*sic*; British] esotericist Christopher Hills. . . . Hills' metaphysical system is partly based on an interpretation of the symbolism of colors first presented in his book *Nuclear Evolution: A Guide to Cosmic Enlightenment*, published in 1968. A complete system of correspondences with the chakras was probably worked out some time during the seventies, and appeared in print in the sequel *Nuclear Evolution: [Discovery of] The Rainbow Body* (1977). Basically, all subsequent New Age authors base their theories on Leadbeater's concepts as revised by Hills. Source amnesia is once again in operation here, since Hills' ideas are adopted without any reference to the fact that the rainbow model of the chakras is an innovation.[4]

As we shall see, the chakra and color associations Hammer attributes to Hills were probably derived from books of the 1950s on color therapy by S. G. J. Ouseley (not cited by Hills), which were widely available in England while Hills was living there. In turn, Ouseley's books were derived from writings published in the 1930s and 1940s by American clairvoyant Ivah Bergh Whitten and her British student Roland Hunt (not cited by Ouseley). Whitten herself drew upon the teachings of Leadbeater (also without acknowledgment).

Occult Correspondences

The eighteenth-century Swedish scientist and mystic Emanuel Swedenborg (1688–1772) stated a law of correspondences that brought into relation everything we might experience at any level of being, from material to spiritual to divine. Here is how he explained this law in his most popular book, *Heaven and Hell* (1758):

Absolutely everything in nature, from the smallest to the greatest, is a correspondence. The reason correspondences occur is that the natural world, including everything in it, arises and is sustained from the spiritual world, and both worlds from the Divine.[5]

Among such correspondences, Swedenborg listed animals, plants, and minerals ("metals noble and base, stones precious and common"). He also added "foods of all kinds."[6] Other correspondences included: sun, moon, and stars; and seasons and times of day ("morning, noon, evening, night").[7] Furthermore, "all things of man's body [including "members, organs, and viscera"] correspond to all things of heaven"—"for man's interiors [inner senses] are what receive heaven, while his exteriors [outer senses] receive the world."[8]

Swedenborg went on to say that "no one can know about the spiritual things in heaven to which natural things in the world correspond except from heaven"—i.e., by illumination.[9] Such illumination is acquired by perceiving that "the correspondence of natural things with spiritual things, or of the world with heaven, is through uses [functions or purposes] and the form[s] in which uses are clothed are correspondences."[10] Thus the outer form of anything in the material world is a symbol of that thing's use, function, or purpose in the spiritual world, which itself is a reflection of its ultimate end in the divine world, or mind of God:

> The universe has been so created and formed by the Divine that functions can clothe themselves in materials that enable them to present themselves in act [causes] or in results [effects], first in heaven and then in this world, and so step by step all the way to the lowest things in nature.[11]

With these ideas in mind, it becomes possible to understand why a physical endocrine gland (Swedenborg's "external form") is said to correspond to a subtle-body chakra ("internal form"), a layer of the aura and its associated nonphysical body ("spiritual things"), a higher plane of existence ("the world of heaven"), and a state of consciousness in an ascending hierarchy of such states—at the summit of which is cosmic consciousness ("the Divine"). It is also possible to see how elements, metals, gemstones, totem animals, foods—even days of the week—could become attached to the chakras as correspondences.

Swedenborg's writings were widely disseminated and highly influential during the nineteenth and early twentieth centuries, the formative years of the Spiritualist and Theosophical movements. Their impact on the development of Western occultism and the chakra system has been enormous, if largely unrecognized (perhaps as a result of source amnesia).

Yet the notion of occult correspondences through multiple levels of being has an ancient heritage. It could be traced back at least to pagan beliefs from before and after the beginning of the Common Era. Such beliefs stated that during its descent into incarnation, the human soul passed through seven levels of being, each corresponding with a planet, an archon (ruler), and an ability, temperament, or aspect of the self that together determined the expression of one's personality and the shape of one's fate.[12]

Over time, these planetary levels of being became correlated with magical gemstones and alchemical metals, thus building up tables of correspondences that would form the basis of Western esotericism. Early examples of such tables appeared in *Three Works of Occult Philosophy* (1531) by Cornelius Agrippa (1486–1535). Thus there is nothing new about Swedenborg's law of correspondences except the phrasing. Yet, because of the popularity of Swedenborg's *Heaven and Hell* during the late nineteenth and early twentieth centuries, this phrasing would have been familiar to early formulators, consolidators, disseminators, and validators of the Western chakra system.[13]

As noted, the Western chakra system embraces a multitude of occult correspondences. I am tempted to add Leland's Law as a corollary of Swedenborg's: "If you encounter or can think of seven of anything, they must refer to the chakras." So it could be said there are two basic classes of correspondences: discovered and developed.

Writers on the chakras who *discover* the Sufi notions of seven subtle organs of perception—Persian, *lataif* (plural); usually encountered in New Age books as *latifah* (singular)—seven planes of being, and seven colored lights associated with higher states of consciousness, immediately link them to the chakras. Never mind that, in one tradition, the lataif are layers ("envelopes") of increasing subtlety that develop a "man of light" through stages correlated with seven "prophets of your being" from Adam to Muhammad.[14] In another, there are only five lataif, corresponding to the solar plexus, the heart (left side, right side, and center), and the head.[15] Clearly, we need to exercise cultural sensitivity (not to mention deeper scholarship) before allowing centuried Sufi mystical beliefs to validate the far-from-ancient Western chakra system. The same thing would apply to recent attempts to fold Native American beliefs into the Western system.

Writers who *develop* lists of chakra correspondences may feel they are making intuitive or psychic discoveries, justified perhaps by channeling, clairvoyance, muscle testing, or use of a pendulum. However, these correspondences vary to such an extent that there is no universally accepted list—except in the case of the defining characteristics of the Western system: locations, names, gland associations, colors, and qualities.

I assume that if these correspondences were illuminative in the Swedenborgian sense, they would have some universality, at least within Western culture. Yet certain *principles* governing the assembly of such lists have emerged and are almost universally practiced. For example, once the color yellow became associated with the third chakra, writers who dealt with the subject of food generally identified yellow foods as stimulating to the third chakra. Lemons and yellow bell peppers might appear on the list. But there would often be little agreement between such lists. Most of these lists disappear when the books containing them go out of print. This is why I have largely left occult correspondences out of account in the present book.

Researcher or Investigator?–My Position

I write this book primarily as a researcher of esoteric history. Yet I do so also as an investigator of obscure possibilities of consciousness, such as astral projection. My approach is analogous to that of a twentieth-century Italian writer on Tantra and the chakras, Julius Evola, who sought "to *interpret* esoteric knowledge" through substantiating "some elements" because of an "ability to read between the lines of the texts, my personal experiences, and the comparisons I have established with parallel teachings in other esoteric traditions." As a "guiding principle," Evola chose "to maintain the same distance both from the two-dimensional, specialized findings typical of university-level and academic orientalism and from the digressions of our contemporary 'spiritualists' and 'occultists.'"[16] However, as my book demonstrates, some of these so-called digressions play a vital role in the development of the Western chakra system.

I make a distinction between exoteric science and esoteric science, such as the many types of yoga. Exoteric science attempts to describe phenomena experienced in physical reality on the basis of objective observation by the senses and scientific instruments (such as microscopes and telescopes), to derive principles and laws from such observations, and to demonstrate theories about them through the use of mathematics—or to confirm with observation what mathematics suggests, as in the case of theoretical and quantum physics. Whatever cannot be observed or demonstrated on these bases does not exist for exoteric science.

Esoteric science attempts to describe apparently nonphysical phenomena on the basis of subjective observation by inner or intuitive senses, using only the mind or consciousness of the perceiver as the instrument and spiritual practices such as meditation as a means of directing that instrument. Allegory and symbolism are used to describe the results of such subjective observation, which often require representation in imagery derived from physical sense impressions in order to be collected, understood, and communicated—perhaps to be compared with the observations of others for verification and codification. Such descriptions may be bound by cultural and personal symbol systems, which in turn can influence how people exposed to those symbol systems perceive, describe, and relate further observations or inner-sense impressions of similar subjective phenomena. Thus does a spiritual tradition—such as that associated with Tantra, kundalini, and the chakras—develop and evolve. Similar principles operate in Western esotericism.

Many ancient and modern spiritual, mystical, and religious traditions throughout the world posit the existence of one or more subtle (nonphysical) bodies, perceivable to the inner senses, containing various "anatomical" parts, and serving various functions. Because of their universality, such notions could be considered "facts" of human consciousness, even if they cannot be observed, described, or demonstrated by materialistic science. Such facts may be described in different ways by different individuals and cultures and may not be recognizable when compared with one another—unless we dig beneath the surface-level differences produced by cultural and personal symbol systems to see an underlying similarity of function.

Thus, a center of vital energy clairvoyantly perceived as a portion of the human subtle body might appear like an opening flower, pink in color, to one individual or cultural group and like a circular vortex of violet-colored electricity to another. These observations do not necessarily invalidate each other. We might have to look into cultural or individual meanings of pink versus violet and flower versus electricity to understand any similarity of function underlying these observations.

In tracing the transmission and transformation of the chakra system from East to West, we must be sensitive to cultural context—what was transmitted from one side carried with it cultural significances (allegories and symbols) that were received on the other in barely recognizable ways. Yet underlying similarities of use, function, or purpose may have remained unchanged. Even so, the development of the Western chakra system has been defined as much by what did not get carried over from the Eastern original as by what did. It has also been defined by what was added in the Western system that had no homologues in the original.

For example, crystals and gemstones corresponding to the prismatic colors of the Western system do not correspond to anything in the Eastern system. However, the principle of associating bija mantras with states of consciousness and chakras may have a similar function—as a means of placing a practitioner en rapport with the level of being or consciousness represented by a particular chakra. Thus a yoga practitioner's chanting of the bija mantra for the third chakra would correspond with an esotericist's placing of a yellow gemstone on an altar for magical or meditative purposes—even though the characteristics of the third chakra in the Eastern and Western systems may be radically different.

As for the distinction between exoteric and esoteric, I see each as a "view" (darshana) that provides a different perspective on reality—one pertaining to the so-called outer universe, the other to the inner. On the surface, each view may seem to be mutually exclusive; yet each may provide valuable assistance in understanding aspects of our experience when appropriately applied. I see all such views as valid to the extent that they are useful to us, rather than true in any absolute sense. Thus, for me, "reality" consists in as many views of it as I have tolerance for.

It is conceivable that the list of evolutionary qualities in the Western chakra system refers to an ascending hierarchy of ever-more-synchronized brain functions. These levels may be achievable through meditative and other practices designed to get various parts of the brain to interact ever more cooperatively and efficiently. In that case, there would be no chakras or subtle bodies as such. But these constructs could be useful ways of organizing thoughts about, and experiences of, achieving nonordinary brain states. Such states—which experiencers might describe as self-transcending, ecstatic, liberated, or enlightened—could refer to the so-called cosmic consciousness associated with the seventh chakra.

Satyananda Saraswati hinted at such a possibility more than thirty years ago when he linked the first two chakras to primitive instincts and the reptilian brain; the third and fourth chakras with emotions, the mammalian brain, and the limbic system; and the fifth and sixth chakras with higher brain functions and the neocortex. Saraswati believed that the seventh chakra existed in a subtle (nonphysical) body and was located above the crown of the head. In my analogy with hierarchies of brain functioning, this chakra would represent a transcendent working together of all the lower levels.[17]

But I now lay aside the investigator's theorizing of possibilities of consciousness for the fact-marshalling role of historian of Western esoteric beliefs. Nobel-prize-winning German author Hermann Hesse wrote a book called *The Journey to the East*, which became a classic for spiritual seekers in America in the 1960s and 1970s—the period during which the Western chakra system as we know it came together. Thus equipped with definitions of the Eastern and Western chakra systems and the roles of contributors to each, let us pursue a journey in the opposite direction, tracking the movement of the chakras from East to West.

Part 2
Esoteric Matrix:
The Chakra Teachings of
H. P. Blavatsky
(1879-91)

Chapter 5
Journey to the West

Little did the founders of the Theosophical Society, Madame Helena Petrovna Blavatsky and Colonel Henry Steel Olcott, anticipate the welcome they would receive in India when they arrived in Bombay on February 16, 1879.[1] Blavatsky (1831–1891) had been born into an aristocratic family in Russia and spent many years traveling the world seeking metaphysical knowledge from obscure books and remote spiritual teachers. Olcott (1832–1907), a practicing New York lawyer and specialist in agriculture reform, had served as an investigator of fraud in suppliers to the army and navy during the Civil War (hence his title) and on a fact-finding committee appointed to look into the assassination of President Abraham Lincoln. Blavatsky and Olcott shared an interest in Spiritualism. They had met in 1874 at a Vermont homestead where Olcott was performing a journalistic investigation of a pair of mediums, the Eddy brothers.

Blavatsky had only recently arrived in America from Paris. She had read Olcott's articles and wanted to meet the writer and join the investigation. Her own metaphysical explorations had allowed her to develop theories of mediumistic phenomena that went beyond what she felt were the relatively simplistic explanations of contemporary Spiritualists—that such phenomena were produced by the action of deceased humans, often the relatives of those in the audience, working through the physical mechanism of the medium.

Blavatsky called her body of theories occultism, claiming she had learned them during her world travels and through her association with spiritual Adepts or Masters, with whom she was constantly in touch through the exercise of her own spiritual abilities. She and Olcott became fast friends and were practically inseparable after they returned to New York. They conducted regular salons for other spiritual seekers, which resulted in the founding of the Theosophical Society (TS) in 1875. In 1877, Blavatsky published her first book, *Isis Unveiled: A Master Key to the Mysteries of Ancient and Modern Science and Theology*, about which a prepublication reader of the manuscript said that it had "a revolution in it."[2] Much of the book was received by means of dictation from Blavatsky's Masters, written down by her and edited by Olcott.

Under guidance from the Masters, the pair pulled up their roots in America (Blavatsky had recently become an American citizen) and headed by boat to India via England, France, and Egypt. They believed that the source of the teachings they called occultism lay in the traditions of ancient India and that an unbroken line of spiritual Masters had passed those teachings down through generations to the present time. They wanted to place themselves in relation to such teachers—Olcott especially, since Blavatsky already had her contacts.

After setting up house in Bombay, the TS founders established a monthly journal, the *Theosophist*, still published today. All TS proceedings, including this journal, were conducted on the basis of three objects, of which the universal brotherhood of humanity was foremost. The second object underlined the importance of studying the ancient wisdom of the Hindus as contained in known texts, such as the Vedas and the Upanishads, and ones yet to be discovered, preserved, and translated. The third object involved the investigation of unexplained laws of nature and unknown powers latent in humanity.[3]

Everywhere the founders went, they were mobbed by hundreds—sometimes thousands—of native-born Hindus (in India) or Buddhists (in Ceylon, now Sri Lanka), who were overjoyed at encountering Westerners interested in meeting them on their own terms rather than exploiting them or denigrating them, as did the representatives of the British Raj and the Christian missionaries from England and America. As editors, the founders welcomed submissions to the *Theosophist* from Indian writers, who were finally able to express their religious and metaphysical views freely to the West, without being ignored or put down by the biased views of the Anglo-Indian Christian press.[4] Despite what Kipling said about

East and West never meeting, they did in fact meet in the pages of the *Theosophist*, thus beginning the journey of the chakra system from East to West.[5]

Glimpses of Tantric Occultism

Within a year of their arrival, the founders began to receive letters and articles about the esoteric teachings of Tantra, representing the second stage of transmission of these ideas to the West, after Shom's *Calcutta Review* article published thirty years earlier. For example, in the January 1890 issue, an anonymous letter signed "Truth Seeker" drew attention to an unsigned series of articles entitled "The Dream of Ravan: A Mystery," a retelling of episodes from the *Rāmāyana* published in 1853–54 in the *Dublin University Magazine*. "Truth Seeker" quoted from a footnote in the fourth installment:

> This extraordinary power, who is termed elsewhere the "World Mother"—the "Casket of Supreme Spirit," is technically called kundalini, which may be rendered serpentine, or annular. Some things related of it would make one imagine it to be electricity personified.[6]

According to Karl Baier, this statement in the *Theosophist* represented "the first appearance of the famous serpent power on the stage of Theosophy. From here its career in modern popular religion starts."[7] It is likely that the 1854 *Dublin University Magazine* footnote represented the earliest appearance of the word *kundalini* in a nontechnical public forum.

"Truth Seeker" ended his letter with an impassioned plea for more information from "correspondents of the Theosophist": "We Western Theosophists earnestly desire information as to all the best modes of soul-emancipation and will-culture, and turn to the East for light."[8] As Baier indicates, "This letter brought about a series of answers in the following issues of the *Theosophist*," including several articles on "Tantrism and tantric yoga"—one of which dealt with the chakras.[9] The *Theosophist*'s subscription list included Americans, Britons, Anglo-Indians, and native Indians and quickly grew to include other European and Australasian nations. Thus did the worldwide dissemination of teachings on kundalini and the chakras begin.

Little is known about the author of the articles on tantric yoga beyond his name, Baradakanta Majumdar, his caste (Brahmin), and his location at the time of writing (Rajshahi, then in Bengal, now in Bangladesh). He appears to have been a writer of novels, tales, and philosophical works in Bengali and the publisher of a Bengali children's magazine based in Calcutta.[10] As an authority on Tantra, he collaborated with Woodroffe some thirty years later on *Principles of Tantra* (1913), where he is described as being "an old man" and having been "English-educated."[11] Majumdar provided the long introduction to volume two of Woodroffe's work.

Majumdar's contributions to the *Theosophist* were modest, amounting to just a few pages. The first appeared in the issue for April 1880: "Tantric Philosophy." Here is the opening:

> It is deeply to be regretted that the Tantras have not found favor with some scholars and truth-seekers of this country. People generally feel as if an intuitive repugnance at the very name of Tantra, which seems to associate with it all that is impure, ignoble, and immoral; but yet there are many Tantras hiding in their neglected pages golden keys which may well open the sealed gates of mysterious nature.[12]

Majumdar claimed there were more than one hundred sixty Tantras, mostly written in Bengali. "The Tantriks like the Freemasons and Rosicrucians studiously hide their books and secrets from the outside world"[13]—which makes me wonder whether they used their reputation for impurity as a means of ensuring their secrets would remain hidden, at least from the conventional majority.

Majumdar explains the noble conception of godhead revealed in the Tantras, with scriptural references, to demonstrate his point about golden keys. However, the only value of the article for our purposes is that it represents another early use of the word *kundalini*, defined as "the grand pristine force which underlies organic and inorganic matter," a manifestation of "the one great primeval force or power which created the universe."[14]

Majumdar's next contribution to the *Theosophist* was a two-part article, "A Glimpse of Tantric Occultism," which appeared in the issues for July and October 1880. It represented the first appearance in English of extracts and summaries from *Ṣaṭ-Cakra-Nirūpaṇa*. Majumdar calls the text *Ṣaṭ-Cakra-Bheda* (Piercing of the six chakras), which is actually the name of a tantric practice rather than the title of the text.[15] However, readers familiar with Woodroffe's 1919 translation of *Ṣaṭ-Cakra-Nirūpaṇa* in *The Serpent Power* will recognize identical descriptions of the chakras.

Considering Woodroffe's 1913 collaboration with Majumdar, I think it probable that the latter was responsible for introducing Woodroffe to *Ṣaṭ-Cakra-Nirūpaṇa*. Though scholarly and popular books trace the transmission of the chakra system from East to West to *The Serpent Power*, the first appearance in English of the *Ṣaṭ-Cakra-Nirūpaṇa*'s concatenation of colors, lotus petals, Sanskrit letters, elements, and so on, occurred nearly forty years earlier.

Olcott provided the following editorial note for the first part of the article:

> The fondness of the Asiatic mind for allegory and parable is well illustrated in this paper on tantric occultism. To a Western man who cannot read the meaning between the lines, it will very likely seem void of sense. . . . The significant feature of the present essay is that the tantric yogi from whose work the extracts are translated, knew the great and mysterious law that there are within the human body a series of centers of force-evolution, the location of which becomes known to the ascetic in the course of his

physical self-development, as well as the means which must be resorted to to bring the activities at these centers under the control of the will. To employ the oriental figurative method, these points are so many outworks to be captured in succession before the very citadel can be taken.[16]

This statement sums up key points in the transmission of the notion of the chakras from East to West:

- We cannot take their descriptions in Hindu books (and portrayals) literally.
- They deal with hidden energies of nature.
- They are force centers involved in an evolutionary process.
- They remain unknown until we reach a certain stage of self-development.
- Their action must be brought under the control of the will.

Already the Western mind has begun the process of assimilating, if not appropriating, the schema of the chakras. The notions of hidden forces, evolution, and control by the will are well-documented in Blavatsky's writings of that time and thus formed the interpretive lens through which the Eastern chakra system was viewed.[17] The notion of force centers appeared perhaps for the first time here. Subsequent Western writings on the chakras, with the exception of those designed to place tantric texts in their proper cultural context, usually exhibit one or more of the key points just listed—especially those of force or energy centers and evolution.

Blavatsky first mentioned the chakras two years later—though without using the word. In the August 1882 issue of the *Theosophist*, she referred to "the series of six centers of force in the human body (fed at the inexhaustible source of the seventh or the Unity, as the sum total of all)"—thus reinforcing the tendency for later writers, including Annie Besant, Charles W. Leadbeater, and Alice

Bailey, to use the terms *chakra* and *force center* more or less interchangeably.¹⁸ Blavatsky's addition of a seventh center of force also initiated the Western practice of numbering seven chakras rather than the six described in Majumdar's article and the *Ṣaṭ-Cakra-Nirūpaṇa*, in which the thousand-petaled lotus at the top of the head was not labeled as a chakra.

Tantric Anatomy

The next installment of the East/West transmission of the notion of the chakras appeared in the March 1888 issue of the *Theosophist*: "The Anatomy of the Tantras," signed by "B. B." These are the initials of Baman Das Basu (1867–1930), identified by yoga scholar Mark Singleton as the author of this article.¹⁹ Cited by the *Oxford English Dictionary* as its earliest noted usage of the word *chakra*, "The Anatomy of the Tantras" served several purposes, among them, to bash Bipin Behari Shom, called "a Hindu renegade," for his *Calcutta Review* article (though that article was unsigned—Basu may not have known who wrote it);²⁰ and to identify the esoteric anatomy of the nadis and chakras with the nervous system of the physical body, perhaps for the first time. (See the following tables; tabular presentations of the chakras in this book are to be read from the bottom up, duplicating their order from the base of the spine to the crown of the head.)

Basu's identification of the seventh chakra with the medulla oblongata, at the base of the brain, would place it below the sixth chakra instead of at the crown of the head. This chakra is usually not identified with a nerve plexus but rather with the brahmarandhra, or anterior fontanel.

Blavatsky relied on this list for her Esoteric Instructions (to be discussed in the following chapter). Leadbeater, a member of the TS since 1883, may have read Basu's article when it came out—though he slightly modified Basu's correspondences in *The Chakras*: coccygeal (related to the sacral plexus), splenic, solar, cardiac, pharyngeal, carotid (related to the cavernous plexus).²⁷

Table 2
Basu's Tantric Anatomy (1888)

Sanskrit Names[21]	English Names	Locations
Suṣumṇā (gracious)	Central channel	Spinal cord
Iḍā (comforting)	Left channel	Left sympathetic cord
Piṅgalā (tawny)	Right channel	Right sympathetic cord
Citra (shining)[22]	...	Gray matter in spinal cord
Brahmadaṇḍa (staff of Brahma)[23]	...	Central canal of spinal cord
Triveṇī (triple braid)[24]	...	Medulla oblongata (where the sympathetic cords meet)
Kailāsa (Mount Kailash)[25]	...	Brain

Table 3
Basu's Chakras (1888)

Chakras	Eastern Names	Later Western Names	Locations
Seventh	Sahasrāra	Crown	Medulla oblongata
Sixth	Ājñā	Brow	Cavernous plexus
Fifth	Viśuddha	Throat	Laryngeal/pharyngeal plexus
Fourth	Anāhata	Heart	Cardiac plexus
Third	Maṇipūra	Navel / Solar plexus	Epigastric (solar) plexus
Second	Svādhiṣṭhāna	Genital	Prostatic plexus[26]
First	Mūlādhāra	Root	Sacral plexus

The term *laryngeal plexus* is medically obsolete, referring to the meeting point of two laryngeal nerves in the area of the thyroid gland. The term *cavernous plexus*, probably referring to nerves passing through the cavernous sinus, has also fallen out of use. Internet searches for these terms yield references not only to nineteenth- and early twentieth-century medical texts, but also to twenty-first-century websites that continue to associate the throat chakra with a laryngeal plexus and the brow chakra with a cavernous plexus—thus demonstrating the persistence over time of Basu's identification of plexuses and chakras.

Scholarly books that attempt to trace the source of correlations between the chakras and nerve plexuses often attribute them to an Indian medical doctor, Vasant G. Rele, who published his own slightly different list in *The Mysterious Kundalini* forty years after Basu's *Theosophist* article. Rele's book came out in 1927—the same year that Leadbeater published *The Chakras*—and has been continuously in print ever since,[28] whereas Basu's article was largely forgotten, a victim of source amnesia. Most New Age books on the chakras, including Judith's *Wheels of Life*, borrow their anatomical correspondences for nadis and chakras from Leadbeater.[29]

Following Blavatsky's assertion of seven force centers, Basu's 1888 association of the chakras with nerve plexuses was the first component of the Western chakra system to fall into place.

Chapter 6
Madame Blavatsky's Esoteric Instructions

The notion of the chakras did not play a significant role in Blavatsky's teachings or writings until the last years of her life, when, in England, she established the Esoteric School of Theosophy (also known as the Eastern School of Theosophy and the Esoteric Section of the TS). The program was for Blavatsky to teach a specially pledged group of twelve personal students, six male and six female, on a weekly basis—the so-called Inner Group. This group would take notes, compare them, and assemble a transcript, which would be edited for publication as an Esoteric Instruction. Blavatsky would supervise the editing. These instructions would circulate privately to members pledged to secrecy throughout the world.[1]

Two such instructions were produced according to the program. The third was issued after Blavatsky died in 1891, supposedly edited by her. Two further instructions were issued under the joint editorship of Annie Besant (1847–1933), an Inner Group member, and William Q. Judge (1851–1896), a founding member of the TS who headed the American Section, headquartered in New York. After Blavatsky's death, Besant and Judge were joint heads of the Esoteric School (ES). After Judge reformed the American Section as an independent body in 1894–95, he issued a sixth such instruction.

In 1897, Besant published the first three instructions, plus notes of oral teachings given during the Inner Group sessions, as part of a third volume of Blavatsky's 1888 two-volume occult masterwork, *The Secret Doctrine: The Synthesis of Science, Religion, and Philosophy*. Blavatsky had promised to release a third and fourth volume of *The Secret Doctrine*, claiming they were nearly complete. However, no trace of these volumes could be found after her death. Thus Besant assembled various unpublished papers of Blavatsky's to make up the promised third volume and padded them with the Esoteric Instructions. The move was controversial, since these teachings were supposed to be kept secret.[2] Despite ill will generated by those who felt that Besant had violated a sacred pledge when she published these writings, as well as aspersions cast on her organization and editing of the material, this so-called third volume of *The Secret Doctrine* assumed canonical status for many Theosophists, such as Leadbeater and Bailey, who drew heavily on its contents in their explorations and expositions of Theosophical tenets—including the chakra system.[3]

Blavatsky discussed the chakras in Esoteric Instruction No. 3. Several things she said play key roles in later Western teachings about the chakras. But, because of her highly condensed presentation, the length of her sentences and paragraphs, and her nineteenth-century habit of frequent emphasis of important words with italicization or capitalization—not just first letters, but sometimes whole words—it is not easy to perceive the contemporary relevance of these teachings. I propose to break them down into brief numbered passages and provide commentary between them. For further ease of reading, I have modernized the English and simplified the Sanskrit.[4]

Hatha versus Raja Yoga

1. He who has studied both systems, the hatha and raja yoga, finds an enormous difference between the two: one is purely psycho-physiological, the other purely psycho-spiritual.

Hatha yoga focuses on the mastery of the physical body as a road to mastery of the mind and ultimately to enlightenment. Hence it is physiologically based, as in the practices of postures (*āsana*) and breath control (pranayama), but psychically oriented (toward the psyche as mind or soul). *Rāja* (kingly) yoga focuses on the mastery of the mind as a road to enlightenment and is directed toward spiritual dimensions beyond even the soul, using meditation as its means.

In Blavatsky's terminology, based on Sanskrit words, there are seven principles of consciousness, which are created by seven hierarchies of divine spiritual beings—the so-called deva kingdom (*deva* means "shining ones," i.e., gods or angels). These principles and hierarchies correlate with seven planes of existence and seven layers of the aura:

- First: Dense body (*sthūla*)
- Second (sometimes third): Subtle body (*liṅga*—often called etheric double or etheric body by later Theosophists)
- Third (sometimes second): Vitality or life force (*prāṇa*)
- Fourth: Desire (*kāma*; sometimes called *kāma-rūpa*, "desire body")
- Fifth: Mind (*manas*; sometimes divided into lower mind, or *kāma-manas*, and higher mind, or *buddhi-manas*)
- Sixth: Spiritual intelligence (*buddhi*, sometimes called intuition)
- Seventh: Divine nature, encapsulating the other principles like an envelope or "auric egg" (*ātman*; sometimes called monad when compounded with buddhi or buddhi-manas)[5]

The first four principles are called the lower quaternary and the remaining three the higher triad (sometimes called the monad). According to Blavatsky, hatha yoga attempts to master the lower quaternary—body, subtle body, vitality, and desire—to achieve the fifth principle of mind; whereas raja yoga attempts to master the fifth principle to achieve the spiritual sixth and seventh principles—hence oneness with the divine. Thus the seven principles imply a continuum from most to least physical or least to most spiritual. As we shall see, the Western chakra system was woven on the loom of these principles, even though this framework gradually disappeared from view during the century between Madame Blavatsky's death and Shirley MacLaine's 1990 appearance on the *Tonight Show*, when the chakras went mainstream.

2. The Tantrists do not seem to go higher than the six visible and known plexuses, with each of which they connect the *tattvas*; and the great stress they lay on the chief of these, the *muladhara* chakra (the sacral plexus), shows the material and selfish bent of their efforts toward the acquisition of powers. Their five breaths and five tattvas are chiefly concerned with the prostatic, epigastric, cardiac, and laryngeal plexuses. Almost ignoring the agneya [ajna], they are positively ignorant of the synthesizing pharyngeal plexus.

Since hatha yoga is an outgrowth of Tantra, it may seem as if Blavatsky is still talking about the practice of hatha yoga. However, yoga practitioners called Tantrikas were said to follow the left-hand path of developing psychic powers for selfish purposes. Blavatsky considered them "black magicians" (sorcerers—again, no reference to race).

As noted, the seventh chakra in Basu's *Theosophist* article, "The Anatomy of the Tantras," was not associated with a "visible and known" nerve plexus. The tattvas are the elements described earlier: earth, water, fire, air, and akasha. Blavatsky called the tattvas "forces of nature" and enumerated seven, correlating them with the seven principles.[6]

The muladhara (root) chakra is the seat of the kundalini, hence the "great stress" placed upon it by practitioners of Tantra. Western writers tend to see this chakra as the most materially focused of the seven, equating it with matter. They correlate the seventh, or crown, chakra with spirit and perceive the remaining five chakras as a continuum of diminishing materiality and increasing spirituality.

The five breaths (*prāṇa-vāyu*) are related to the way vitality or life force circulates through the subtle (etheric) body nerves (nadis). These also are correlated with elements and colors. Their names and functions need not concern us. They were a focus of Leadbeater's clairvoyant investigations of the chakras, to be discussed later.

It is probable that Blavatsky was striking out against a book by Rāma Prasād, *The Science of Breath and Philosophy of the Tattwas,* popularly known as *Nature's Finer Forces,* published by the TS in 1890. Earlier in this instruction, she had mentioned the book disparagingly because "it recommends black magic of the worst kind."[7] I deal with *Nature's Finer Forces* in chapter 10.

Most Eastern and Western books on the chakras locate the throat chakra in the area of the laryngeal *and* pharyngeal plexuses. However, as the next passage makes clear, Blavatsky associated the pituitary body with the pharynx, and by implication with ajna, the sixth chakra.

> 3. But with the followers of the old school it is different. We begin with the mastery of that organ which is situated at the base of the brain, in the pharynx, and called by Western anatomists the pituitary body. . . . The arousing and awakening of the third eye [pineal gland] must be performed by that vascular organ, that insignificant little body, of which, once again, physiology knows nothing at all. The one is the energizer of will [pituitary], the other that of clairvoyant perception [pineal].

Again Blavatsky distinguished between practitioners of Tantra, who begin with the first chakra, and practitioners of raja yoga, who begin with the sixth.

The Pineal Gland

> 4. The pineal gland is that which the Eastern occultist calls *devaksha,* the "divine eye," or the "third eye." To this day, it is the chief and foremost organ of spirituality in the human brain, the seat of genius, the magical "Sesame" uttered by the purified will of the mystic, which opens all the avenues of truth for him who knows how to use it.[8]

Blavatsky is the likely source for all later references to a correspondence between the pineal gland and the esotericists' third eye. She devoted a section of the second volume of *The Secret Doctrine*, "The Races with the 'Third Eye,'"[9] to connections between the pineal gland; a vestigial third eye in certain reptiles, as noted by contemporary biologists; ancient Greek myths of the Cyclops; the spiritual powers of occultism; and Indian depictions of the eye of Śiva as a third eye on the forehead, which she called "an exoteric license."[10]

Some later esotericists—apparently with Bailey as the first—took this license literally and correlated the brow (sixth) chakra with the pineal gland and the notion of the third eye. However, the seventeenth-century French philosopher René Descartes called the pineal the "seat of the soul" (in a letter of January 29, 1640).[11] This fact was also mentioned by Blavatsky in *The Secret Doctrine*[12] and became the basis for the pineal's correlation with the seventh chakra, via Esoteric Instruction No. 3, in Leadbeater's *The Chakras* and later Western systems influenced by his book.

> 5. When a man is in his normal condition, the introspective Adept can see the golden aura pulsating in both the glands, a pulsation like that of the heart, never ceasing throughout life. This motion, however, under the abnormal condition of effort to develop clairvoyant faculties, becomes intensified, and the aura takes on a stronger vibratory and pulsating or swinging action. The arc (of the pituitary gland) mounts upward, more and more, toward the pineal gland, until finally, the current striking it—just as when the electric current strikes some solid object—the dormant organ is awakened and set all aglowing with the pure akashic fire.

These words graphically describe the passage of the kundalini (here called "pure akashic fire") from the sixth to the seventh chakra.

6. This is the psycho-physiological illustration of two organs on the physical plane which are the concrete symbols of, and represent respectively, the metaphysical concepts called manas and buddhi. The latter [buddhi], in order to become conscious on this plane, needs the more differentiated fire of manas. But *once the sixth sense has awakened the seventh*, the light which radiates from it illuminates the fields of infinitude: for a brief space of time, man becomes omniscient. The past and the future, space and time, disappear and become for him the present. [Original emphasis.]

It seems that the principle of spiritual intelligence (buddhi) is ordinarily not available to us on the physical plane and that it must be made to work through a physical organ—the pineal gland—before we can experience or perceive through this principle. However, we do have access to the principle of mind (manas), acting through the pituitary body. Blavatsky indicates that under "abnormal condition of effort to develop clairvoyant faculties" (probably the word *abnormal* here means only that it is unusual for so-called normal human beings to engage in such pursuits), the pituitary/mind connection can be made to activate the pineal / spiritual intelligence connection.

The sixth sense is said to be "the psychic sense of color" (the clairvoyant ability to perceive color on planes other than the physical, as in the case of aura perception), and the seventh is "spiritual sound."[13] In Hindu philosophy, shabda-brahman (sound as the Absolute) is the spiritual substratum of the manifested universe—sound, or vibration, is the first created thing that generates all else.[14] Thus activation of the seventh sense, associated with the pineal gland and spiritual intelligence, allows us to perceive the sonic/spiritual substratum of the universe—with effects such as omniscience in space and time.

Chakras in the Head

7. Our seven chakras are all situated in the head, and it is these master chakras which govern and rule the seven (for there are seven) principal plexuses in the body, and the forty-two minor ones to which physiology refuses that name.... And if the term *plexus*, in this application, does not represent to the Western mind the idea conveyed by the term of the anatomist, then call them chakras or padmas, or the wheels, the lotus hearts and petals.

The notion of there being forty-nine plexuses—and by implication forty-nine major and minor chakras—may seem like a pat application of the esoteric principle of grouping everything visible and invisible into categories based on the number seven. However, in *The Serpent Power*, Woodroffe cites an ancient manuscript that lists the Sanskrit names of the seven major chakras and forty-two minor ones, for a total of forty-nine.[15]

A twentieth-century Indian author, Shyam Sundar Goswami, compiled an exhaustive study of references to the chakras from nearly one hundred fifty Upanishads, Tantras, Puranas, and related texts spanning almost the entire history of the development of Hinduism and yoga. The system he presented comprises thirteen chakras, seven of which are in the head. The sixth chakra (ajna) doubles as the first of the head chakras and there is an additional chakra (hrit) between the third (manipura) and fourth (anahata).[16]

The critical thing to notice about this passage is that there are now seven chakras in the body, associated with nerve plexuses, and seven higher chakras in the head. Here we see the beginning of a tradition of multiple chakra systems that surfaces from time to time during the evolution of the Western chakra system, usually in esoteric rather than popular presentations.

Path of the Saints

The names of the seven chakras in the head do not concern us, since they were never mentioned by Blavatsky. The source of her information may have been a twelve-chakra system in use by the Radhasoami faith (also called *Sant Mat*, "Path of the Saints"), a sect combining elements of Sikhism and the Nāth Siddhas (a monastic order of "perfected lords" founded in the twelfth or thirteen century, within which the principles of hatha yoga evolved). This sect was established not long before Blavatsky's arrival in India and grew alongside the TS. Reciprocal influence between the organizations has been suspected by scholars but has not been sufficiently studied.[17]

The founder of the Radhasoami faith was Seth Shiv Dayal Singh (1818–78), known as Soami Ji (Beloved Teacher). An account of his teachings is given in *Sar Bachan* (True words), which refers to the six chakras of the physical body, each of which is considered to be a state of consciousness or realm of reality in addition to having a location in the body. The *sahasdal kamal* ("thousand-petaled lotus," a synonym for sahasrara, or crown, chakra) is considered to be the first of six further chakras, associated with higher states of consciousness and heavenly realms. These chakras are not located in the physical body but are accessed by meditation on the thousand-petaled lotus—especially on the "sound current" (*surat shabda*) perceivable there.[18]

Soami Ji's successor was Salig Ram (also Saligram; 1829–98), also known as Huzur Maharaj, a high-ranking official in the Indian postal service—and therefore fluent in English. He became a disciple of Soami Ji in 1858 and helped to found the Radhasoami Satsang (community) in Agra in 1861. Saligram touched the TS at several points during the 1880s and 1890s. Not only was he a subscriber to the *Theosophist* as early as 1882,[19] but also he garnered a reference in one of the Mahatma (Great Soul) letters, communications from the two Masters behind the founding of the TS. In this letter, received in 1881, Saligram is identified as

"Suby Ram." The letter's recipient was A. P. (Alfred Percy) Sinnett (1840–1921)—a friend of Blavatsky's and editor of an influential Anglo-Indian Newspaper, the *Pioneer*. The Mahatma informed him that "no harm" would come from joining Saligram's group as long as Sinnett refrained from becoming too deeply involved (presumably by being initiated).[20] Sinnett himself referred to Saligram as "a cultivated and highly respected native Government official" who had informed Sinnett about his guru, Soami Ji.[21]

In the 1890s, Olcott and Besant visited the group and met Huzur Maharaj. A brief account of this meeting occurs in a talk given by Babuji Maharaj (Madhav Prasad Sinha, 1861–1949), the fifth Agra guru, some forty years later, on March 25, 1931. Babuji had been living at the Agra ashram since 1873—so this was probably a firsthand account. However, he attributed Sinnett's position as editor of the *Pioneer* to Olcott—perhaps conflating Sinnett's earlier involvement with Saligram with Besant and Olcott's visit.[22] Though Olcott and Besant stopped in Agra for a few days during Besant's first lecture tour of India, on February 7–9, 1894, Olcott's published reminiscences do not mention a side trip to hear Huzur Maharaj speak.[23]

A two-part article on Radhasoami beliefs appeared in the June and August 1895 issues of the *Theosophist*, with an editorial note saying that they were written by someone who had been a devotee, they were based on Saligram's own words, and they had been sent to Saligram for revision.[24] The second part of this article posited not twelve but fourteen chakras: the seven of the body, including the thousand-petaled lotus; and seven beyond that, accessible through meditation on the thousand-petaled lotus.

A 1909 publication by the third Agra guru, Brahm Shankar Mishra (1861–1907, known as Maharaj Saheb), claimed six chakras in the "material-spiritual realm," represented by the physical body; six above that in the "spiritual-material realm," represented by the gray matter of the brain; and a further six in the "purely spiritual" realm, represented by the white matter of the brain.[25] This triple division reflects traditional Hindu teachings about the existence of three bodies: physical (*sthūla-śarīra*), subtle (*liṅga-śarīra* or *sūkṣma-śarīra*), and causal (*kāraṇa-śarīra*). Though the implication that each body has its own set of chakras does not occur in Radhasoami teachings, Besant and Leadbeater's notion of multiple subtle bodies, each with its own chakra system, may have originated from it.

It is difficult to determine the extent to which the Radhasoami sect and the TS influenced each other's teachings on subtle bodies, planes, and chakras during this early phase of contact between the organizations. Yet Radhasoami teachings intersect the history of the Western chakra system several times—including an indirect reference by Leadbeater in *The Chakras* to a "school" in India that "makes free use of the chakras" and has sixteen thousand members "spread over a large area."[26]

As we shall see, Radhasoami teachings may be the source of later writings on the Western chakra system that link the pineal gland to the *sixth* chakra rather than the seventh.[27]

The Seven Rays

Blavatsky continues her discussion of the chakras:

> 8. When the time comes, [ES] members . . . will be given the minute details about the master chakras and taught to use them. Till then, less difficult subjects have to be learned. If asked whether the seven plexuses . . . are the centers where the seven rays of the Logos vibrate, I answer in the affirmative.

In Theosophical literature, the Logos (Greek for "word") refers to the great consciousness that created the cosmos, or a somewhat lesser being who created our portion of it, including the physical earth and its associated nonphysical planes—what I like to call our reality/learning system, to avoid confusion between scientific and

Theosophical references to our solar system. In science, the term *solar system* refers only to the physical sun and planets. Theosophical teachings add a spiritual dimension, including the planes and the notion that the sun and planets are great conscious beings. The universal Logos is identified with the "central sun" of the cosmos, and the so-called Solar Logos with the sun of our system.

Just as a ray of light divides into seven beams or rays of color, so the light of the universal Logos divides into seven rays representing specific functions, qualities, or departments. Every lower entity involved in the creation and sustaining of the cosmos or in the evolutionary process of returning to oneness with this Source of all being may be classified by its ray—from divine beings to humans, animals, plants, and minerals. The concept is frequently alluded to in Blavatsky's writings but rarely developed beyond cryptic hints.[28] She made a start in the Esoteric Instructions, but these teachings were systematized and developed by later Theosophists.

Perhaps the clearest early statement of the notion of seven rays occurs in an article by Blavatsky's Indian friend and colleague T. Subba Row (1856–90): "as seven distinct rays radiate from the 'central spiritual sun,' all Adepts and Dhyan Chohans are divisible into seven classes, each of which is guided, controlled and overshadowed by one of seven forms or manifestations of the divine wisdom," experienced as "the spiritual light which radiates from one's own Logos."[29] Here, the term *Logos* refers to a human being's *monad*, the highest self, beyond even the soul. There are said to be seven types of monads, corresponding with the seven rays. The term *Dhyan Chohan* appears to be a Blavatskyean coinage from the Sanskrit word for meditation (*dhyāna*) and a Tibetan word meaning lord (probably derived from Mongolian *khaan*, "king of kings"[30]). In Theosophical literature, *Dhyani-Chohan* refers to the highest devas and human Adepts.

In another passage in *The Secret Doctrine*, Blavatsky makes clear that the notion of the seven rays originated in the oldest Hindu scripture, the *Ṛg Veda*:

> This verse in the Veda (10.5.6), "The seven wise ones [rays of wisdom, Dhyanis] fashion seven paths [or lines, as also *races* in another sense]. To one of these may the distressed mortal come" . . . is one of the most pregnant in occult meaning. The "paths" may mean lines . . . , but they are primarily beams of light falling on the paths leading to wisdom. (See *Ṛg Veda 4.5.13*) . . . They are, in short, the seven rays which fall free from the macrocosmic center, the seven principles in the metaphysical, the seven races in the physical sense.[31]

This passage makes clear that there are correspondences not only between the chakras, nerve plexuses, and rays, but also between these categories and the seven principles. Alice Bailey further developed the connections between the seven rays, principles, and races and the seven chakras.

The Aura

> 9. Not only Adepts and advanced chelas [disciples], but also the lower order of psychics, such as clairvoyants and psychometrists, can perceive a psychic aura of various colors around every individual, corresponding to the temperament of the person within it. . . . Every human passion, every thought and quality, is indicated in the aura by corresponding colors and shades of color, and certain of these are sensed and felt rather than perceived.

Although Blavatsky does not mention a connection between the chakras and the aura, most Western writers assume these elements of esoteric anatomy are related. The Upanishads speak of several "sheaths" (*kośa*) that surround the supreme Self at the core of our being.[32] But these seem to imply an inward movement from less to more subtle. I have not seen pre-Theosophical Indian references to these sheaths' being perceptible beyond the confines of the body—as is the aura—or to their colors.[33] Thus it seems that the pairing of chakras and auras is a uniquely Western contribution to chakra lore. The process of assimilating these notions into the Western chakra system has its roots in this passage and the next.

> 10. As a string vibrates and gives forth an audible note, so the nerves of the human body vibrate and thrill in correspondence with various emotions under the general impulse of the circulating vitality of prana, thus producing undulations in the psychic aura of the person which results in chromatic effects.

Leadbeater's clairvoyant investigations of the chakra system originated in this passage. In a subsequent chapter, I discuss his system for describing the circulation of prana through the etheric body in terms of colored rays passing through the chakras. Late twentieth-century developments along the lines of pranic healing, such as those of Choa Kuk Sui, can thus be traced back to Blavatsky through Leadbeater.[34]

Although the connection between aura, chakras, colors, and sounds is not made explicit in this passage, the principle that color and sound are related lies behind certain twentieth-century developments in color therapy and sound healing that use the notion of the chakras as a base. Thus many Western chakra systems list not only color correlations for the chakras, but also sound correlations (usually the seven notes of the diatonic scale).

As demonstrated by these ten passages from Esoteric Instruction No. 3, Blavatsky was responsible for the following contributions—direct and implied—to the development of the Western chakra system:

- Laying the basis for a seven-chakra system by means of the seven principles

- Linking the process of activating the third eye to the head chakras
- Correlating the pituitary with the sixth chakra and will and the pineal with the seventh chakra and clairvoyant perception—thus allowing two of seven endocrine gland associations to fall into place
- Indicating correlations between chakras, plexuses, elements (tattvas), and pranas
- Hinting at a correlation between chakras and rays
- Linking pranic circulation and colors in the aura
- Implying correlations between planes, colors, sounds, layers of the aura, and chakras

Clearly, Blavatsky was an innovator in the evolution of the Western chakra system. As with others of this type, such as Alice Bailey, her contribution was somewhat jumbled and chaotic (or at least not described in systematic terms). But it provided a rich vein of esoteric material for later innovators and synthesizers to mine. I would be leery of calling her system formative—it is not a system at all, merely a collection of hints that barely mentions the chakras. Yet this set of hints is the matrix from which the Western chakra system emerges over the next one hundred years.

Chapter 7
Inner Group Teachings

Much of the material in the Esoteric Instructions, especially the one I have been quoting, was derived from a meditation practice given to Blavatsky's Inner Group. The practice was designed to raise the kundalini. Clues about it are scattered throughout transcripts of the first several meetings of the group. The Esoteric Instructions contained background material designed to explain every element of this practice to ES members without ever mentioning it, except in the cited remark that members eventually would "be given the minute details about the master chakras and taught to use them."[1]

The theoretical basis of the practice is summarized in the following statement, in which Blavatsky comments on the power of chanting AUM (*om*):

> Esoteric Science teaches that every sound in the visible world awakens its corresponding sound in the invisible realms, and arouses to action some force or other on the occult side of nature. Moreover, every sound corresponds to a color and a number (a potency spiritual, psychic or physical) and to a sensation on some plane. All these find an echo in every one of the so far developed elements and even on the terrestrial plane, in the lives that swarm in the terrene atmosphere, thus prompting them to action.[2]

In Blavatsky's teachings, sound is spiritual, color is psychic, and number is physical—as in the vibrational frequencies of sound and light that produce musical notes and prismatic colors. By *sensation on some plane*, Blavatsky means that sound, color, and number also correspond to the seven principles of consciousness, each of which is correlated with a particular plane of existence. The "so far developed elements" refer to the five elements (out of seven—

two are as yet unmanifested in our world): earth, water, fire, air, and ether (akasha). The phrase *swarming lives* refers to elementals (conscious beings associated with the elements, such as earth/gnomes, water/undines, fire/salamanders, and air/sylphs), nature spirits, and devas/angels. Thus the Esoteric Instructions contain diagrams that demonstrate correlations between seven planes, principles, and elements; seven colors and musical notes; and seven elements, planets, metals, and days of the week (see figure 5 for an example).

The chakras themselves are never mentioned by name in these diagrams and rarely in accompanying discussion. Yet they will eventually replace the seven principles as the source of each layer of the aura, in the mid-twentieth century—while keeping the connection with rainbow colors and musical notes established in the following chart.

In the Inner Group teachings, Blavatsky referred to the chakras as nadis:

> [She] believed that the nadis correspond to the divisions of the [spinal] cord known to anatomists. There are thus six or seven nadis—or plexuses—along the spinal cord. The term however is not technical but general, and is applied to any knot, center or ganglia. The sacred nadis are those which run along or above sushumna. Six are known to science and one (near the atlas) [remains] unknown.[3]

Here, again, we see that the seven plexuses of the human nervous system connected with the chakras in Basu's 1888 *Theosophist* article can be correlated to the principles and colors listed in diagrams in the Esoteric Instructions.[4] According to Blavatsky, "these seven principles are derived from the seven great hierarchies of angels or Dhyani-Chohans, which are, in their turn, associated with colors and sounds, and form collectively the manifested Logos."[5] Blavatsky spoke of these seven hierarchies of angels as seven rays, each of which corresponds to one of "the seven colors of the solar spectrum." Also, "each hierarchy furnishes the aura of

							SOUND	
These Correspondences are from the Objective, Terrestrial Plane.	ĀTMAN is no Number, and corresponds to no visible Planet, for it proceeds from the Spiritual Sun; nor does	ĀTMĀ	it bear any relation either to Sound, Colour, or the rest, for it includes them all.			As the Human Principles have no Numbers *per se*, but only correspond to Numbers, Sounds, Colours, etc., they are not enumerated here in the order used for exoteric purposes.		
NUMBERS	METALS	PLANETS	THE HUMAN PRINCIPLES	DAYS OF THE WEEK	COLOURS	MUSICAL SCALE		
						Sanskrit Gamut	Italian Gamut	
1 AND 10 Physical Man's Key-note	IRON	MARS The Planet of Generation	KĀMA RŪPA The vehicle or seat of the Animal Instincts and Passions	TUESDAY *Dies Martis*, or Tiw	1. RED	SA	DO	
2 Life Spiritual and Life Physical	GOLD	THE SUN The Giver of Life physically. Spiritually and esoterically the substitute for the inter-Mercurial Planet, a sacred and secret planet with the ancients	PRĀNA OR JĪVA Life	SUNDAY *Dies Solis*, or Sun	2. ORANGE	RI	RE	
3 Because BUDDHI is (so to speak) between ĀTMĀ and MANAS, and forms with the seventh, or AURIC ENVELOPE, the Devachanic Triad	MERCURY Mixes with Sulphur, as BUDDHI is mixed with the Flame of Spirit (See Alchemical Definitions)	MERCURY The Messenger and the Interpreter of the Gods	BUDDHI Spiritual Soul, or Ātmic Ray; vehicle of Ātmā	WEDNESDAY *Dies Mercurii*, or Woden. Day of Buddha in the South, and of Woden in the North—Gods of Wisdom.	3. YELLOW	GA	MI	
4 The middle principle—between the purely material and purely spiritual triads. The conscious part of *animal* man.	LEAD	SATURN	KĀMA MANAS The Lower Mind, or Animal Soul	SATURDAY *Dies Saturni*, or Saturn	4. GREEN	MA	FA	
5	TIN	JUPITER	AURIC ENVELOPE	THURSDAY *Dies Jovis*, or Thor	5. BLUE	PA	SOL	
6	COPPER When alloyed becomes Bronze (the *dual* principle)	VENUS The Morning and the Evening Star	MANAS The Higher Mind, of Human Soul	FRIDAY *Dies Veneris*, or Frige	6. INDIGO OR DARK BLUE	DA	LA	
7 Contains in itself the reflection of Septenary Man	SILVER	THE MOON The Parent of the Earth	LINGA SHARIRA The Astral Double of Man; the Parent of the Physical Man	MONDAY *Dies Lunae*, or Moon	7. VIOLET	NI	SI	

Figure 5. Correspondences from Blavatsky's Esoteric Instruction No. 1 (reprinted from H. P. Blavatsky, *The Secret Doctrine*, vol. 5: *Occultism*, 1897/1938/1947)

one of the seven principles in man" (see figure 21).[6] Yet, as noted, we each are specially linked to *one* of these seven primordial rays. Thus, in the practice to be described, colors are used to meditate on the principles—but the color of our personal ray is the primary one to focus on.

The Inner Group practice is an early (if not the first) Western adaptation of tantric principles of meditation for raising the kundalini. In the Tantras, the technique is called *nyāsa* (placing). Feuerstein defines it as "an esoteric means of distributing psychospiritual power (*shakti* [kundalini]) in the body and thereby creating a new inner and outer reality for oneself."[7] White goes further, describing it as "the cosmologization or divinization of the body (or of an object), effected by touching its various parts and depositing corresponding deities or energies into them, usually through the use of bīja-mantras."[8] Often the visualization of letters of the Sanskrit alphabet in various body parts is involved. In Blavatsky's practice, the body parts are segments of the spine and portions of the brain, the substitutes for Sanskrit letters are colors, the corresponding energies are those of the seven principles, the yantra is a triangle, and the mantra is AUM.

The practice as a whole was probably taught in stages, but there are few indications of what those stages were. Furthermore, precise instructions were not passed on in publically available teachings. Though there are admonitions to pronounce AUM in a certain way, only a living teacher could demonstrate it.[9] Also, the determination of a student's ray may have depended on Blavatsky's interpretation of the results of a particular meditation experiment or her clairvoyant observation of the student's aura.

Finally, not only is some essential information missing from the Inner Group transcripts, but also the tables of correspondences in the Esoteric Instructions appear to contradict each other. Careful reading and deep study may reveal subtle shades of difference in Blavatsky's approach to these tables, in which case the contradictions are merely apparent. However, some may be what Blavatsky called "esoteric blinds"—information intended to mislead people who have not been given the key by the teacher of the system. The purpose of such blinds is to protect people from the dangers of misapplying the system through ignorance or misguided intentions to gain personal power or harm or control others.[10]

We must keep these considerations in mind when perusing the practice as I have reconstructed it from the transcripts. (All page references are to Henk J. Spierenburg, *The Inner Group Teachings of H. P. Blavatsky*.)

Table 4
Blavatsky's Kundalini Practice Correspondences (1891)

Principles	Colors	Plexuses (Physical)[15]	Brain Locations (Superphysical)[16]
Auric egg (as atman)	Prismatic; blue (when perceived in aura)	Atlas / Foramen magnum	Skull filled with akasha (light)
Buddhi	Yellow	Pharyngeal	Pineal
Higher manas	Indigo	Laryngeal	Third ventricle [or pituitary]
Lower manas	Green	Cardiac	Pituitary [or corpora quadri-gemina[17]]
Kama	Red	Epigastric (solar plexus)	Cerebellum
Prana	Orange	Prostatic	[Pons]
Linga	Violet	Sacral	[Medulla oblongata]
Auric egg (stand-in for sthula)	Blue	Coccygeal	[Atlas / Foramen magnum]

The Kundalini Practice

The correspondences in table 4 have been deduced from the Inner Group teachings and Esoteric Instructions in support of Blavatsky's kundalini practice. There are eight stages in the table because Blavatsky noted that the auric egg and color could be taken as first or seventh in the sequence. Only by including the auric egg in this table as the final stage was it possible to make the following connections: the pituitary is the fourth stage and correlates with kama; there are three stages (inclusive) between that and the pineal; and the final stage is that of the skull filled with akasha (light).[14] The practice proceeds as follows:

- Shut out "all worldly thoughts and troubles" (4).
- "There are three vital airs" (4), which are expressions of akasha moving through the three primary channels (sushumna, ida, and pingala). A current may be raised in these channels by means of will or desire. If the channels are not pure, energizing them with will or desire may result in black magic—"This is the reason why all sexual intercourse is forbidden in practical occultism" (5). Once this current has been established, it will pass from the central canal "into the whole body" (5) and circulate throughout the auric egg (the constantly shifting layers of principles that surround the human body and that are enclosed by the highest principle, atman; partially visible to clairvoyant vision as the human aura).[11]
- To raise the current, visualize a screen of colored light at each of seven stages along the spine, from the sacrum to the atlas or from the lowest lumbar to the foramen magnum. The color changes with each stage, according to which of the seven principles is under contemplation (4, 95).
- Within the screen of colored light, visualize an equilateral triangle representing the monad (highest self, called *ātma-buddhi-manas*), with atman at the apex and buddhi and

manas at the two lower angles. This triangle must be considered not only as a geometrical form but also as a representation of the monad (11, 13). Focus on the triangle rather than lose yourself in the colored light (12). At some point, the triangle form will disappear, leaving only the direct experience of what it represents (11).
- Stop at the first sign of discomfort (4).
- AUM may be chanted aloud at each stage on the note representing your ray, once you have determined it (11).
- Your ray can be determined by identifying the color in the aura at the back of the neck (11); or by tying a piece of wool to the ring finger of the left hand, using a different color for each day of the week, then meditating and noting the results (5).
- When you have discovered your color, "the day of that color should be chosen as the day for special effort, and a ring of the metal of the day worn on the 4th finger of the left hand. When the dominant color is found, it alone should be used and the seven colors abandoned" (10).
- The stages along the spine represent the physical plane. To go on to the superphysical planes—"psychic, spiritual, and divine" (4)—repeat the process in seven stages using the seven "master chakras" in the brain.[12]
- During this phase, the colors "are not to be thought of so much as physical colors, but as the essence of color, the pure bright hues seen in the sky [as in a rainbow]" (4).
- In the third stage, corresponding to yellow, there are three degrees: yellow, yellow-orange, and red-orange (10).
- At the fourth stage, corresponding with the pituitary, cease visualizing color: "Only the pulsating of the interblended essence of color should be thought" (4).
- There may come a point when the colors turn into sounds, indicating that you have passed from the psychic to the spiritual planes; in the meantime, "try to obtain colored sounds" (17).[13]

- Do not force the current beyond the atlas. After that point, "the current will go on by itself." If it does not do so, reverse the process by bringing the current down again, stage by stage. Then "make a fresh effort" (17).
- Beyond the foramen magnum, "watch the colors changing like a rainbow" as the current moves you through the stages—but always be thinking of the color of your ray (17).
- The kundalini awakens when a vibrational connection is established between the pituitary body and the pineal gland (4), resulting in the experience of waves of light (12), the opening of the third eye (15), and a moment of omniscience, "enclosing the past and the future in the present" (11). Focus on the light, not the third eye (12).
- The plane reached (psychic, spiritual, divine) "depends on the intensity of the thought, the purity and sublimity of the aspiration" (4).

In the Inner Group Teachings and in Esoteric Instruction No. 4, a master table of correspondences appears, listing seven items in each of the following categories:

- Elements (bhutas)
- Divine lokas [realms] and states
- Infernal (or terrestrial) lokas and states
- Planes of corresponding hierarchies
- Principles
- Senses (tanmatras)
- Colors
- Consciousness
- Organs of cognition or sensation (jnanendriyas)
- Organs of action (karmendriyas)
- Corresponding spiritual organs and seats of sensation in the physical body[18]

Impressive yet mysterious—and too large to reproduce here—this table may be Blavatsky's most important contribution to the transmission of the chakra system from East to West. However, its influence has been indirect—probably because only Inner Group members were aware of its true purpose as a support for the practice outlined in this chapter. Later esotericists—especially Leadbeater and Bailey—mined it for information to support their versions of the chakra system. After them, it was largely forgotten. Yet it represents a more refined version of the matrix from which the seven-chakra Western system was derived than the textual excerpts discussed in the previous chapter.

The Eastern contribution to this table includes the bhutas, tanmatras, jnanendriyas, and karmendriyas. These are tattvas of Sāṃkhya philosophy. Ordinarily, there are five tattvas in each category—but Blavatsky expands the number to seven and assigns a principle to each. Of the remaining tattvas listed in the twenty-five-tattva Sāṃkhya system, three appear among the principles themselves: atman (divine self) as a substitute for purusha (divine person), buddhi (spiritual intelligence; sometimes called *mahat*, higher mind), and manas (mind).

There is no need to go into detail about these correspondences, except to note the expansion of tattvas from five to seven in each category. We have seen how the original five gross and subtle elements of the Eastern chakra system were mapped into the first five chakras, with mind correlated to the sixth chakra. In *Ṣaṭ-Cakra-Nirūpaṇa*, the template from which the Western chakra system arose, the thousand-petaled lotus was not considered to be a chakra and had no element assigned to it, thus creating what David Gordon White called a "six plus one" system.[19]

The unnoticed innovation in Blavatsky's table of correspondences is that it laid the groundwork for the Western seven-chakra system—on the basis of the seven principles. The chakras have not yet been directly named in conjunction with the principles. However, their locations are implied in the column of "spiritual corresponding organs and centers of sensation," which includes the pineal gland (seventh or crown chakra); "root of nose, between eyebrows" (sixth or brow chakra); throat and heart (fifth and fourth chakras—but both assigned to a single principle); "spleen and liver" (the source of Leadbeater's spleen chakra, which he sometimes identified as the third chakra and sometimes as the second); and the "region of the umbilical cord" (the navel chakra, which Leadbeater sometimes identified as the second chakra and sometimes as the third).

There is no equivalent in this column for the root chakra. However, there is an entry for "the akasha that fills the skull"—presumably a duplication for the function of the crown chakra. There is also one for the stomach, which appears to duplicate the location of spleen and liver and umbilical cord or navel. In Eastern teachings on the chakras, the third chakra is often associated with "digestive fire" in the belly.[20] Western teachings have followed suit and linked the stomach to the third, or solar plexus, chakra.[21]

Perhaps the least explored and most confusing aspect of Blavatsky's table is the correlation of divine and infernal realms and states of consciousness with "planes of corresponding hierarchies." In the meetings of the Inner Group during which the components of this table emerged, and in the Esoteric Instruction derived from these meetings, Blavatsky was developing a comprehensive system of states of consciousness correlated with the microcosmic human planes and the macrocosmic divine planes she called "kosmic."

The basis for this aspect of the system was the Hindu notion of seven heavenly realms (loka, as listed in *Viṣṇu Purāṇa* 2.7) and seven infernal realms (*tala*, as listed in *Viṣṇu Purāṇa* 2.5). In the Yoga Upanishads, there was an attempt to map the seven lokas onto the subtle body, beginning with the feet and knees and thighs. The four remaining lokas correspond with the locations of the four chakras from navel to brow (*Nāda-Bindu Upaniṣad* 1–4). In another of these texts, the seven talas are located from the sole of the foot to the hips and the lokas from the navel to the crown, skipping the first two chakras and adding locations at the belly and upper heart (*Śāṇḍilya Upaniṣad* 7.44). English translations of the Yoga Upanishads were not available in Blavatsky's time, but her table of correspondences displays a similar intention—mapping realms of existence or planes onto the subtle body by means of the seven principles and implying a correlation between their locations and the chakras.

The missing key to the correspondence of the items in this table to the chakras is that the talas, as terrestrial lokas and states, correspond to the seven stages of the spine in the kundalini practice, and the divine lokas and states correspond to the seven master chakras in the brain. I feel confident in making this assertion on the basis of Radhasoami teachings about the chakras in the body, reflecting terrestrial concerns, to be transcended by meditating on those in the head, reflecting divine states and realms.[22]

The column representing "planes of corresponding hierarchies" condenses and collates material in *Viṣṇu Purāṇa* 2.7 on the inhabitants of the heavenly lokas with material from Blavatsky's writings on postmortem states and the hierarchy of Dhyani-Chohans, from elementals and nature spirits to the highest devas.[23] This column is the template from which Besant and Leadbeater developed and consolidated their system of planes and inhabitants, through clairvoyant investigations undertaken after Blavatsky's death.

To conclude this pair of chapters on Blavatsky's contributions to the Western chakra system, let us add several further points to the list of such contributions at the end of the previous chapter:

- Early, if not the earliest, Western tables of occult correspondences connected to the chakras
- Early, if not the earliest, Western practice for raising the kundalini to achieve higher states of consciousness
- Establishing the matrix from which the Western system of seven chakras evolved and laying the groundwork for their correlation to subtle planes and bodies

Part 3
Whirling Wheels:
Theosophical Clairvoyance
(1890s–1920s)

Chapter 8
Annie Besant and the Higher Planes

Blavatsky's premature death in 1891, a few months before her sixtieth birthday, marks the end of the first phase of transmission of the chakra system from East to West. The publication of *A Working Glossary for Students of Theosophical Literature* in 1890 indicates that tantric terms such as *chakra* (defined therein as "center of psychic energy"), *kundalini-shakti* ("the serpentine force"), *ida*, *pingala*, *sushumna*, and *brahmarandhra* were already current in America by then—four years before Swami Vivekananda's appearance at the World Parliament of Religions in 1893 and six years before the publication of his book *Raja Yoga*, which discussed these terms.[1] As we shall see, contemporary yoga scholars often cite this book as a benchmark in the dissemination of yogic teachings in America, apparently unaware of the groundwork already laid by the TS for the reception of such teachings.

Some scholars of the Theosophical movement are disdainful of Theosophical teachers and teachings developed after Blavatsky's death, calling the teachers second- or third-generation Theosophists and the teachings neo- or even pseudo-Theosophy. Such distinctions do not matter in the history of the Western chakra system, which assimilated information from any apparently reliable source.

In this book, I consider the contributions of two lifelong Theosophists, Annie Besant and Charles W. Leadbeater, and two founders of related movements who began as Theosophists, Rudolf Steiner and Alice Bailey—all major figures in the history of early twentieth-century occultism and mysticism. Besant's and Steiner's impact on the evolution of the Western chakra system is not as noticeable as Leadbeater's and Bailey's. Without the latter two, the Western system is virtually inconceivable. We will also examine the contribution of several less-well-known figures who were Theosophists or were influenced by Theosophical teachings.

Annie Besant, the estranged wife of an Anglican clergyman with a violent temper, left the church when she left her husband. She successively became an atheist, an advocate of Free Thought (working to ensure that dissenters from Church of England views were heard in public and political forums), a member of the National Secular Society (advocating separation of church and state), a socialist, and finally a Theosophist. She also campaigned against vivisection (scientific experimentation on animals) and for the rights of laborers and women, as well as public education and free meals for indigent children.

In 1888, she was sent *The Secret Doctrine* to review, requested to meet the author, and was sufficiently impressed to join the Theosophical Society. For the next forty-five years, she traveled the world lecturing and publishing articles and books on Theosophy as applied to every area of human life from politics to psychic and spiritual development. In 1907, after the death of Olcott, she became the second president of the TS.[2]

As a personal student of Blavatsky, Besant took up many hints provided in the Esoteric Instructions and Inner Group teachings, using logic and intuition to fill them out in plausible and practically useful ways. Having met Leadbeater in England in 1890, Besant developed her own style of clairvoyance in 1895, at his suggestion. The two often collaborated on clairvoyant research, including investigation of higher planes, human evolution, the life of Jesus, and the makeup of the atom. Besant specialized in the theoretical overview of whatever they turned their attention to, while Leadbeater specialized in graphically described details. She renounced these clairvoyant investigations in 1913, turned her attention to Indian politics, and campaigned for India's independence from British rule.[3]

Besant often mentioned the chakras (centers) in her pre-1913 lectures and writings, but never gave a detailed description of each. Her earliest contributions to the subject were several manuals written in the 1890s to promote Blavatsky's teachings in a popular, less technical form. In *The Seven Principles of Man* (1892) and *Man and His Bodies* (1896), she defined and explained the following points:

- There are seven planes of existence, ranging in a continuum of increasing subtlety from wholly material to wholly spiritual.
- On each of these planes, we have a body—sometimes more than one—suited to perceive and interact with it.
- We cannot interact with these planes unless we develop the sense organs of their respective bodies.
- These sense organs are called the chakras (centers).

Besant struggled for years to find a suitable terminology to describe the planes and bodies, preferring English words to the Sanskrit terms for the seven principles employed by Blavatsky. In table 5, the columns for planes and bodies derive from Besant's *Theosophy* (1912). The column for principles derives from the revised edition of *The Seven Principles of Man* (1897). The columns are arranged from highest to lowest, but numbered in reverse order. Some later writers correlate principles, chakras, bodies, and planes, so this order will facilitate comprehension when I discuss such correspondences.[4]

The physical, etheric, astral, and mental bodies and their corresponding principles make up the *personality*. The causal body is the reincarnating *individuality*. As with Blavatsky, the principles of atma, buddhi, and manas (the higher triad) make up the monad. Though the monadic body and plane are virtually inaccessible (unmanifested), the principle of mind can become increasingly illumined by buddhi, then atma, resulting in the elevation of the individuality to the status of a god—a Master, who functions in the nirvanic or atmic body.

Only in later writings did Besant provide names for the sixth and seventh planes. In earlier books, she indicated that these planes are not manifested during our evolutionary cycle. Thus, in the second and third columns, there are seven bodies and principles spread over five manifested planes. I have added the names of the two highest bodies in brackets, since they can be inferred from their associated planes. I have also added *Brahman* and *paramātman* to the third column. Though these terms are not numbered among the seven principles, they correlate with Hindu teachings about levels beyond atman—thus there is a parallel with Besant's monadic and divine planes.

Table 5
Planes, Bodies, and Principles according to Besant (1897–1912)

Planes		Bodies	Principles
7. Divine (unmanifested)		[Divine]	[Brahman (Absolute)]
6. Monadic (unmanifested)		[Monadic]	[Paramatman (supreme self)]
5. Nirvanic/Atmic/Spiritual[5]		7. Nirvanic/Atmic/ Spiritual	7. Atman (highest self)
4. Buddhic/Intuitional		6. Buddhic/Intuitional	6. Buddhi (spiritual intelligence)
3. Mental	Upper sub-planes	5. Causal	5. Buddhi-manas (higher mind)
	Lower sub-planes	4. Mental	4. Kama-manas (lower mind)
2. Astral/Emotional		3. Astral	3. Kama (desire)
1. Physical	Upper sub-planes	2. Etheric	2. Prana (vitality) or Linga (subtle body)[6]
	Lower sub-planes	1. Physical	1. Sthula (dense body)

In *The Seven Principles of Man*, Besant explained how the sense organs of the physical body function—in esoteric terms. A physical sense impression received through the eyes, ears, nose, tongue, or skin is passed through the equivalent sense organs (etheric-body chakras) in the etheric body and received by an astral-body center of sensation (astral-body chakra)—whereupon it becomes an experience of seeing, hearing, smelling, tasting, or touching. This sensation is then passed to the equivalent centers in the mental body (mental-body chakras), whereupon it becomes a perception. Once the mental body has registered this perception, a response is sent back through the astral and etheric bodies and the perception is now fully apparent to our physical brain.[7]

For Besant, this model explained how most people receive and interpret sense impressions derived from physical experience. Only five senses and centers of sensation or perception are normally active in the physical, etheric, astral, and mental bodies.

To register and remember experience on the astral plane, we must develop astral-body centers of sensation into astral sense organs—which is to say, we must activate, develop, and coordinate the astral-body chakras, adding the sixth and seventh. The same would be true of experiences in the mental body on the mental plane. However, none of these astral or mental plane experiences can be recalled unless there are links from these bodies back to the physical brain—through the chakras of the etheric body. The more developed these links are, the more we remember of experiences on the astral or mental plane.[8]

Some people rarely remember their dreams, which are said to take place on the astral plane. The reason *may* be that they have not yet developed the astral body—but it is more likely that the links from the astral body through the etheric-body chakras to the physical plane consciousness are insufficiently developed. Individuals who have a highly developed astral body may cruise the astral plane every night, as what Besant and Leadbeater called invisible helpers—those who provide aid, comfort, and direction to suffering dreamers and the recently deceased. But if the links in the etheric body are not sufficiently developed, these experiences will not register in the physical brain upon awakening.⁹

It can be inferred from these ideas that if the etheric, astral, and mental bodies have chakra systems, then the higher bodies (causal, buddhic, nirvanic) must also have them. Yet I have seen only a single reference in Theosophical literature to causal-body chakras, in which the author admitted that "no information is available" about them.¹⁰

Astral Projection

Besant's contributions to the knowledge of the chakra system were not carried forward by later writers, partly because of their complexity and partly because they would be of use only to astral projectors. However, astral projection played a key role in the early days of the TS, as evidenced by the organization's third object, letters of Blavatsky about experiments along these lines, and other records from before Blavatsky and Olcott relocated to India.¹¹

After the move, Olcott's interest in the subject persisted. For example, in a lecture of 1882, he spoke of a connection between the chakras and astral projection, as taught by a Madrasi swami by the name of Sabhapaty (1840–?), whom he had met in Lahore in 1880.¹² Showing his audience an illustration from a publication by one of the swami's students, Olcott noted "a series of lines and circles [traced] on the naked body of a man" in lotus posture. Then he described the "triple line," representing ida, pingala, and sushumna, which "passes down the front of the head and body, making the circles at center points." There was also a "line up the spine, and over the cerebellum and cerebrum," which then "unites with the front line."¹³

Olcott continued:

> This is the line traveled by the will of the yogi in his process of psychic development. He, as it were, visits each of the centers of vital force in turn and subjugates them

to dependence upon the will. The circles are chakras, or centers of vital forces, and when he has traversed the entire circuit of his corporal kingdom, he will have perfectly evolved his inner self—disengaged it from its natural commixture with the outer shell, or physical self. His next step is to project this "double" outside the body, transferring to it his complete consciousness, and then, having passed the threshold of his carnal prison-house, into the world of psychic freedom, his powers of sight, hearing, and the other senses are indefinitely increased, and his movements are no longer trammeled by the obstacles which impede those of the external man.[14]

Sabhapaty Swami called his teachings "Vedantic Raj Yoga." Olcott understood that Sabhapaty was teaching the system of Patañjali, which can indeed be interpreted in terms of astral projection.[15] For example, *Yoga Sūtra* 3.43 specifically mentions astral projection as *ākāśa-gamanam* (passage through space), achieved through meditating on becoming "as light as cotton down."[16]

Some modern Hindu teachers carry forward the connection of chakras to astral projection. For example, Satyananda Saraswati identifies a power of the root chakra as "astral levitation" (probably with reference to *Yoga Sūtra* 3.43);[17] and a power of the brow chakra as the ability of the mind "to manifest actively without the aid of the physical body," which is "the faculty of astral projection" (this is his interpretation of *mahāvideha*—"great state without the body"—a term used in *Yoga Sūtra* 3.44).[18] Furthermore, the lingams in the first, fourth, sixth, and (in Saraswati's system) seventh chakras represent states of development and clarification of the astral body from vague dusky outlines to resplendent luminosity.[19]

However, Sabhapaty's teachings were perhaps more influenced by Tantra than by Patañjali. In *Esoteric Cosmic Yogi Science, or Works of the World Teacher*, a collection of Sabhapaty's teachings published in 1929 by William McKinley Estep (1896–1967), there is a brief mention of the eight limbs of yoga taught in the *Yoga*

Sūtra. But the majority of the book deals with principles of laya yoga designed to dissolve the powers of creation.[20]

As indicated by the numbers in plate 2, Sabhapaty used a twelve-chakra system, not unlike that taught in the Radhasoami movement. But his locations for the six lower chakras were unconventional (see below) and the six additional chakras were located much more specifically in the head than they are in Radhasoami. Karl Baier believes Sabhapaty's system was the origin of Blavatsky's notion of seven master chakras in the head.[21]

In plate 2, the upper chakras are numbered 7–12, with 7 being the uppermost; the lower chakras are numbered 13–18, with 18 being muladhara. The remaining numbers refer to various channels and states of consciousness. In one phase of Sabhapaty's teachings, the twelve centers are called faculties and kingdoms, possibly meaning realms or planes—i.e., lokas. In *Om: A Treatise on Vedantic Raj Yoga Philosophy*, the faculties associated with the chakras (called *kamala*, "lotuses") are arranged in a continuum from spirit to matter, in the order in which they were emanated by "Infinite Spirit":

1. **Wisdom**—twelfth chakra in the center of the skull (presumably the crown); called *dvadaśānta* (beyond the twelve) or *parātpara* (supreme of supremes)
2. **Wit/Intelligence**—eleventh, at the top of the brain; called brahmarandhra or *para* (greater supreme)
3. **Knowledge**—tenth, in the middle of the brain; called *tatpara* (lesser supreme)
4. **Prudence**—ninth, at the bottom of the brain; called sahasrara or *kalā* (division/parts)
5. **Memory**—eighth, in the center of the forehead; called *nāda* (sound)
6. **Muse** (fancy or imagination)—seventh, between the eyebrows; called *bindu* (point)
7. **Ambition**—sixth, at the tip of the nose; called ajna

8. **Conscience**—fifth, in the center of the tongue; called vishuddha
9. **Intellect**—fourth, in the throat; called anahata
10. **Passions/Notions/States of mind**—third, in the heart; called manipura
11. **Senses**—second, in the navel; called svadhishthana
12. **Nature/Elements**—first, at the base of the penis; called muladhara[22]

To achieve oneness with Infinite Spirit, each of these faculties must be purified with mantras and dissolved, starting at the end of this list and proceeding upward in the order of the chakras. If the swami's intention had been for us to enhance rather than transcend the faculties described in his system, this list would have represented the first instance of a chakra system as a continuum of human potential—the basis of the Western chakra system.[23]

References to Sabhapaty's teachings virtually disappeared from Theosophical literature in the mid-1880s, several years before Besant joined the TS.[24] However, it is clear that she was interested in the theory and practice of astral projection, not only from descriptions of personal experiences, as recorded by Leadbeater in *Invisible Helpers*,[25] but also from references throughout her lectures and books to the processes by which subtle bodies develop—from *Man and His Bodies* to *Invisible Worlds*.

As Besant's collaborator, Leadbeater shared this preoccupation with astral projection and encoded it into his version of the chakra system, thus providing a Theosophical equivalent of tantric traditions that link the development of the chakras to the acquisition of spiritual powers. Such connections are infrequently encountered in later popularizations of the chakra system, which deal more with physical, emotional, mental, and spiritual fulfillment on the physical plane. Yet they do sometimes occur in books by Western esotericists and writers on psychic development. I return to the subject of astral projection and the chakras in the final chapter.

Besant was a consolidator of information about the chakras, bodies, and planes rather than an innovator. She mined Blavatsky's work for information on these subjects to develop a coherent synthesis from fragments and hints. Above all, she wanted to make Blavatsky's work accessible and comprehensible to the public, placing equal weight on esoteric theory and safe and intelligent practical application. However, Besant never generated an interpretive or explanatory chakra system. After sifting through hundreds of her books, pamphlets, and articles, I have yet to discover a single list of the seven chakras by name and function. When discussing the chakras, Besant always referred to them in general terms as a whole system rather than focusing on parts.

Yet Besant's most significant contribution to the Western chakra system may have been the notion that each subtle body had its own set of chakras—a notion suggested not only by Blavatsky's seven chakras along the spine followed by seven more in the head, but also by the Radhasoami teachings to which Besant was exposed when she first came to India in the early 1890s. As noted, by 1909, these teachings included three sets of chakras, one for the physical realm, one for the physical/spiritual realm, and one for the purely spiritual realm. Besant would have identified these realms with the physical, astral, and mental planes. The implications of this notion of multiple chakras systems would not be explored until the late 1980s in the work of Barbara Brennan.

Chapter 9
The Lotus Petals of Rudolf Steiner

Known as the founder of the Anthroposophical Society and the originator of ideas that led to the development of the Waldorf School model of education and agricultural techniques called biodynamic farming, Rudolf Steiner (1861–1925) began his public career as a scholar lecturing and writing on German philosophy and literature. He shifted his attention to esoteric subjects around the turn of the century and became head of the German Section of the Theosophical Society in 1902. Steiner was popular and prolific. Due to differences of opinion with Annie Besant after she became president of the TS in 1907, Steiner broke away from the TS during the last weeks of 1912 and the first of 1913, taking most of the German Section with him and restructuring it into the Anthroposophical Society.[1]

Initiation and Its Results

Before the break, Steiner produced several highly regarded books that were translated from German into English and brought out by Theosophical publishing companies in England and America—in particular, *The Way of Initiation, or How to Attain Knowledge of Higher Worlds* (1908) and *Initiation and Its Results: A Sequel to "The Way of Initiation"* (1909)—and in Germany in 1909 as a single volume under the title *Wie erlangt man Erkenntnisse der höheren Welten?* (*How does one attain knowledge of higher worlds?*). Extensively revised by Steiner in 1918 and retranslated in English several times, the book is now known as *How to Know Higher Worlds*.[2] I prefer the earliest German and English versions, which use Theosophical terminology such as *etheric body* (*Ätherleib/Ätherkörper*) and *astral body* (*Astralleib/Astralkörper*), rather than the awkward and less clear revisions and translations *ether body* (*Ätherleib*) and *soul body* (*Seelenleib*).

Corresponding to a sequence of five articles in *Lucifer-Gnosis* with the subheading "Über einige Wirkungen der Einweihung" (On some results of initiation), the first four chapters of *Initiation and Its Results* dealt with the chakras, providing one of the earliest manuals of chakra development published in the West. Steiner was the first Theosophical writer to describe clairvoyant visions of the chakras in detail and arguably the second (after Blavatsky) to publish a system for developing them. I say "arguably" because Blavatsky's Inner Group Teachings and Esoteric Instructions referred indirectly to the chakras, whereas Steiner deals with them directly.

Steiner describes five chakras, ignoring the first and seventh—perhaps following the Buddhist Tantras, which combine those at the forehead/crown and genitals/anus, resulting in a five-chakra system. He calls them wheels (*Räder*), lotus flowers (*Lotusblumen*), centers (*Mittelpunkte*), and sense organs of the soul (*Sinnesorgane der Seele*).[3] He numbers them from the top down instead of from the bottom up and identifies them with the number of petals in each and their approximate locations in the physical body, never using the Sanskrit names. Just as mastery of each chakra in the Eastern system confers certain spiritual powers, so each of Steiner's chakras is associated with a type of clairvoyance.

Steiner's approach is based on what appears to be a radical reinterpretation of the purpose of the lotus petals. As we have seen in tantric teachings, the petals of the six chakras from root to brow are assigned letters of the Sanskrit alphabet. However, Steiner assigned specific spiritual qualities to these petals. In this, he was following the tantric tradition in which *vṛtti* (modes of conduct) are assigned to the petals of the chakras.[5]

According to Steiner, before development, the chakras appear dark in color and "without movement—inert." When development begins, they appear "lucent." As this development progresses, they not only glow but also begin to revolve—at which point clairvoyance becomes possible.[6]

In the throat chakra, eight of the sixteen petals "were developed already in an earlier stage of human evolution, in the remote

Table 6
Chakras according to Steiner[4]

Usual Numbers	Locations	Petals	Types of Clairvoyance	Steiner's Numbers
Sixth	Between eyes	Two	Connection with superhuman entities; perception of higher worlds	First
Fifth	Larynx	Sixteen	Thoughts of others; insight into laws of natural phenomena	Second
Fourth	Heart	Twelve	Feelings of others; observation of powers in animals and plants	Third
Third	Solar plexus	Ten	Capacities/talents of others; how all parts of nature work together	Fourth
Second	Abdomen	Six	Communication with higher beings (in the astral world)	Fifth
First	Abdomen	Four	. . .	Sixth

past" but are presently inactive. The other eight "can be developed by a person's conscious practice."[7] At some stage in this process, the previously developed petals are reactivated. Steiner gives eight "functions" (*Seelenvorgänge*; "soul processes" in the most recent translation) that are necessary for the development of the throat chakra petals[8]—based on Steiner's interpretation of the eightfold path of Buddhism (right ideas, resolutions, speech, and actions, and right management of life, endeavor, learning, and introspection).[9]

Of the heart chakra's twelve petals, six also were developed long ago and remain quiescent until the other six develop. The achievement of six "requirements" (*Eigenschaften*[10]) allows us to develop this chakra: control of thoughts, control of actions, perseverance, tolerance, impartiality, and equanimity.[11] These requirements derive from Theosophical teachings about preparation for the tutelage of a Master—a stage called the Probationary Path. The Theosophical teachings themselves were derived from *Viveka-Cūḍāmaṇi*, verses 16–34, by ninth-century mystic and spiritual preceptor Śaṅkara. They are explained in Besant's *The Ancient Wisdom* (1896; *Die Uralte Weisheit*, 1898), where they are called mental *attributes* (a better translation than "requirements" for *Eigenschaften*).[12] The ten petals of the solar-plexus chakra do not follow the pattern of the throat and heart chakras. Nothing is said about half the petals having been developed in earlier ages. There is no list of five attributes or functions to be developed. Instead, instructions on meditation are given, similar to those expounded in Besant's *Thought Power* (1901; *Das Denkvermögen*, 1902).[13]

Steiner notes that the development of the third chakra is more difficult than that of the throat and heart. The development of the six petals of the second chakra, which Steiner vaguely locates "in the center of the body," is even more difficult. As with the third chakra, there is no division into previously and yet to be developed petals and no indication of three things to be accomplished. According to Steiner: "The functions of the body, the inclinations and passions of the soul, the thoughts and ideas of the spirit must be brought into complete union with each other" in order to produce "complete mastery of the whole personality by means of self-consciousness, so that the body, soul, and spirit make but one harmony." The key word seems to be *purification (geläutert werden)*.¹⁴

In a lecture of 1902, "The Higher Life," Besant speaks in similar terms of the purification of the bodies—physical, astral, and mental—that compose the personality. Perhaps the three things to be accomplished with respect to the six-petaled lotus are the purification of actions, feelings, and thoughts.¹⁵

The development of what we call the sixth chakra comes later. Steiner's words on the subject are cryptic:

> This is the moment when the two-petaled lotus in the region of the eyes is required. If this begins to stir, the individual attains the power of setting his higher ego in connection with spiritual, superhuman entities. The currents which flow from this lotus move so toward these higher entities that [these] movements . . . are fully apparent to [*völlig bewußt sind*—"are fully cognizable by"] the individual. Just as the light makes physical objects visible to the eyes, these currents reveal the spiritual things of the higher worlds. Through sinking himself into [i.e., meditative absorption in] certain ideas which the teacher imparts to the pupil [individually] . . . the latter learns to set in motion, and then to direct the currents proceeding from this lotus-flower of the eyes.¹⁶

This passage may be explained through reference to Besant's *Thought Power*, by way of the *Yoga Sūtra* of Patañjali. In the latter, there are three higher stages of training the mind: *dhāraṇā* (concentration), *dhyāna* (meditation), and samadhi ("contemplation"; more often "absorption" or "ecstasy"). In *Thought Power*, Besant defines *concentration* as "one-pointedness of mind," such that the mind is "an instrument that can be used at the will of the owner," utterly without distraction. She defines *meditation* as the steady direction "to any object, with the object of piercing the veil, and reaching the life [essential beingness behind the form], and drawing that life into union with the life to which the mind belongs [essential beingness of the meditator]."[17] Contemplation, or absorption, occurs as a natural development from the other two stages:

> When the mind is well-trained in concentrating on an object, and can maintain its one-pointedness—as this state is called—for some little time, the next stage is to drop the object, and to maintain the mind in this attitude of fixed attention *without the attention being directed to anything*.[18]

The results of such a state are these:

- The mental body is stilled.
- Consciousness escapes from the mental body and passes into the causal body.
- There is a momentary swoon or lapse in consciousness.
- Objects of consciousness of the lower worlds are replaced by those of the higher.
- The higher self (which Besant calls "ego") can now mold the mental body into its own shape, passing on to it "high visions of the planes beyond [its] own."[19]

As noted, Steiner did not deal with the four-petaled root chakra. However, in the Theosophical teachings of his time, there were four primary "qualifications" or "attributes" (*Eigenschaften*) required for probation and discipleship, again derived from Śaṅkara. Steiner lists them as the following:

- "Discrimination between the eternal and the temporal" or "between the true and false"
- "Right estimate of the eternal and the true as opposed to the perishable and the illusory" (in Śaṅkara, desirelessness; which is to say, desiring only the eternal and the true)

- "Six qualities" (identical to the "requirements" described in conjunction with the heart chakra)
- "Longing for freedom" (liberation—in Śaṅkara, from the round of earthly incarnations; in Steiner, from the "limits of [one's] narrow self" or personality)[20]

Steiner distributes the attainment of these four qualifications throughout the stages of the practice he describes, dealing with them primarily in conjunction with the development of the etheric body from the astral body. I am tempted to correlate them with the four petals of the root chakra because they form the basis of the whole program. If I am right, then in Steiner's system the development of the root chakra comes last and is never attempted directly, resulting organically from the development of the astral and etheric bodies.[21]

It is now possible to make several observations about Steiner's approach to the chakras:

- Numbering from the top down indicates not only a preferred direction of practice, but also an increasing order of difficulty of development.[22]
- Delineation of the stages of chakra development (inert, glowing, revolving) allows students' progress to be tracked by teachers with clairvoyant vision.
- Assigning stages in the training of those on the Probationary Path to specific chakras and petals acts not only as a mnemonic device for trainees but also as a means for clairvoyant teachers to determine which aspects of this path are as yet undeveloped and to suggest remedies (for example, when the petal of the heart chakra connected to tolerance is absent, dark, or dim).
- Linking types of clairvoyance to the development of particular chakras provides not only a means for students to measure their own progress but also an incentive for the safe development of such powers by sticking to the program out-

lined for each (Steiner makes many remarks, not included here, on reliable and unreliable types of clairvoyance and safe and dangerous methods of clairvoyant development).

From his exposition of the astral-body chakras, Steiner proceeds to the development of the etheric body. A maxim of Theosophical teaching at this time was that each lower body should be developed by the body above it.[23] Thus we must have developed the astral body chakras before we should undertake the development of the etheric body. From Steiner's description, it appears that the etheric body provides us with vitality involuntarily. It functions without direction from our will. We have to stake out the territory, first by creating a "preliminary center" (*vorläufiger Mittelpunkt*; I prefer "provisional center")[24] in the head to serve in place of a sixth chakra (or to connect the etheric body to the brow chakra of the astral body). This achievement allows one to "determine for himself the position of his etheric body" (*die Lage seines Ätherkörpers selbst zu bestimmen*), so as to "direct the etheric body to all sides" (*den Ätherkörper nach allen Seiten zu drehen*).[25] Steiner's phrasing is obscure—I suspect he means directing our attention through the etheric body as if it were an instrument of observation, so we can point it in any direction we wish to investigate.

With further development, we can move that provisional center into the area of the throat, thereby connecting the etheric body with the throat chakra of the astral body. At this point, we are able to create a "skin" (*Häutchen*; I prefer "membrane") that allows the etheric body to register sensations from the etheric level of being (the upper subplanes of the physical plane).[26]

Once we are able to move the provisional center into the area of the heart in the physical body and connect it to the heart chakra of the astral body, we have achieved our goal. (Apparently, we do not need to move the temporary center into locations in the etheric body that correspond with the lower three chakras.) According to Steiner, the result is:

a most complicated structure, a really wonderful organ. It glows and shimmers with all kinds of color and displays forms of the greatest symmetry—forms which are capable of transformation with astonishing speed. Other forms and outrayings of color proceed from this organ to the other parts of the [physical] body, as also to those of the astral body, which they entirely pervade and illumine. The most important of these rays move, however, toward the lotus-flowers. They pervade each petal and regulate its revolutions. Then, streaming out at the points of the petals, they lose themselves in the surrounding space. The more evolved a person may be, the greater becomes the circumference to which these rays extend.[27]

This "most complicated structure" or "wonderful organ" has functions similar to those of the spleen chakra described in Leadbeater's *The Hidden Side of Things*, published four years later. It may be that Leadbeater followed up on Steiner's hints and, by means of clairvoyant investigation, produced a detailed schema of how this "wonderful organ" supplies rays of different colors to the organs of the physical body and the chakras of the etheric body. The question of who came first would be difficult to answer—especially since the functions of Leadbeater's spleen chakra are detailed in Blavatsky's Esoteric Instructions. I deal further with the spleen chakra in chapter 12.

Throughout his teachings on the chakras, Steiner insists on the vital importance of developing the twelve-petaled lotus associated with the heart. He even claims that the fire of kundalini is manufactured in this "organ at the heart," though it must be "fanned into life" as a result of occult training that cannot be openly spoken about.[28] When activated, the kundalini not only "streams in luminous loveliness through the self-moving [*sich bewegenden*, i.e., revolving] lotus-flowers and the other canals [*Kanäle*; nadis as channels?] of the evolved etheric body," but also "radiates outward on the surrounding spiritual world and makes it spiritually visible, just as the sunshine falling upon the surrounding objects makes visible the physical world."[29] Furthermore, "the spiritual world becomes plainly perceptible as composed of objects and beings only for the individual who . . . can send the fire of the kundalini through his etheric body and into the outer world, so that its objects are illuminated by it."[30]

Though Steiner was an innovator and validator, his teachings on the chakras had little impact on the development of the Western chakra system.

Chapter 10
The Law of Breath and the Tree of Life

As noted, one of the objects of the Theosophical Society has been to investigate unknown laws of nature and latent powers in humanity. The implication is that a relationship exists between these laws and powers, such that an understanding of laws and an application of powers would result in apparently magical or miraculous events. I say "apparently" because, in Theosophical teachings, no event that occurs under natural laws could properly be called a miracle. Blavatsky made explicit statements to this effect to counter Roman Catholic beliefs that God was capable of abrogating physical laws to produce miracles—an "unphilosophical" view, in her opinion.[1]

This object of the TS provided shared ground between Western and Eastern esotericism—especially Tantra and related yogas, which posited a correspondence between the universe (macrocosm) and the human body (microcosm). As noted, tantric practitioners sought to achieve oneness with the divine powers that permeate the universe (Śiva and Śakti, for example) to acquire supernatural powers, such as god-like omniscience and omnipotence. This shared ground was the channel of transmission of esoteric ideas between East and West, funneling the Eastern chakra system to Europe and America and Theosophical notions of planes, bodies, and related phenomena back to India.

Subtle Forces (Rāma Prasād)

Blavatsky's books, especially *The Secret Doctrine* (1888), were early instances of such transactions. Another was *Nature's Finer Forces* by Rāma Prasād, an Indian member of the TS. The "finer forces" of the title are those that link unknown laws of nature with unknown powers in humanity—forces that operate on the subtle (hence "finer") planes and manifest themselves through the subtle bodies.

I have not been able to determine Prasād's birth and death dates. He was active in the TS in India from 1883 (he is mentioned in Olcott's reminiscences) to 1908 (when the last of his numerous articles for the *Theosophist* was published).[2] He was university educated, had achieved a master's degree, and worked as a lawyer. He was president of the Meerut Theosophical Society.[3]

Nature's Finer Forces was first published in 1884 in Lahore as *Occult Science: The Science of Breath*, under the authorship of Pandit Ram Prasād Kasyapa. The book was a translation, with commentary, of a Sanskrit manual of breath control (pranayama). Prasād proceeded to publish a series of essays called "Nature's Finer Forces: Their Influence on Human Health and Destiny" in the *Theosophist*, from 1887 to 1889. In 1890, a book combining these essays with the translation from *Occult Science* was published by the Theosophical Publishing Society as *The Science of Breath and the Philosophy of the Tattwas: Translated from the Sanskrit with Fifteen Introductory and Explanatory Essays on Nature's Finer Forces*—usually cited as *Nature's Finer Forces*.

A second edition, revised and corrected by George Robert Stowe Mead (1863–1933)—a member of Blavatsky's Inner Group—was brought out in 1894. Third and fourth editions followed, keeping the book in print for some sixty years. It has been called "the *first* [book in English] 'to explain and advocate the practice of yoga.'"[4] The yoga it explained is now called *svara* (breath sound) yoga.

The manuscript Prasād translated is identified as the eighth chapter of *Śivagama*, the rest of which the translator presumed to be lost.[5] Either the text was defective or the translator misunderstood what he read. Agamas are a category of tantric scriptures, many of which involve a dialogue between Śiva and his consort Pārvatī, as does this text. The true source is *Śiva-Svarodaya* (Śiva on the sound of breath), the date of which is unknown—probably after the fifteenth- or sixteenth-century *Haṭha-Yoga-Pradīpikā*, since it references pranayama techniques from this text without explanation, as if they were common knowledge.

Prasād's manuscript was also defective (or expurgated—see below) in that it contained only 335 verses—61 fewer than the version generally in use. Furthermore, Prasād counted some verses but left them untranslated, while Mead excised others in the second edition. These omissions occurred in a section entitled "How to Produce Sexual Attachment," including information on seduction and on conception of children—presumably considered unfit for Victorian and Theosophical audiences.[6]

Prasād's essays in *Nature's Finer Forces* cover such topics as prana, nadis, lotuses (chakras), the centers in heart and head, and subtle bodies (koshas). They mention *Ṣaṭ-Cakra-Nirūpaṇa* and provide Prasād's translations of long excerpts from *Praśna Upaniṣad*. There is also a discussion of Patañjali's *Yoga Sūtra*. But the main focus is on the tattvas (elements). The *Śiva-Svarodaya* gives colors and symbols for each:

- Earth—yellow square
- Water—white crescent moon
- Fire—red triangle
- Air—green circle
- Akasha—every color, with the "shape of an ear" (in practice, a dark blue ovoid)[7]

The majority of the book deals with an elaborate system of Hindu chronological divisions related to solar and lunar cycles, breath control, the Vedic zodiac and planets, and correlations with the elements. The purpose is to determine the ideal moment when the macrocosmic (celestial) and microcosmic (human) *tides* of prana are aligned to produce personal or collective misery or good fortune, disease or health, as well as wealth, victory in battle, and prediction of death. Essays and text each contain instructions for meditation on the tattvas using breath, color, symbol, and bija mantras.

Nature's Finer Forces appears to have been immensely popular in Western esoteric circles as a manual of occult development.[8] However, in itself, it contributed little to the understanding of the chakras. As we shall see, the ways later writers used the book represented further steps in the transmission of the chakra system from East to West.

Kingly Yoga (Swami Vivekananda)

The first Indian yogi to garner national attention in the United States was Swami Vivekananda (1863–1902), who traveled from India to Chicago to attend the World Parliament of Religions in 1893. Vivekananda was a disciple of a tantric yogi in India, Sri Ramakrishna. He was a charismatic speaker and American audiences were so enthusiastic about his teachings that he remained until 1895. He toured England and Europe from 1895 to 1897. After a brief sojourn in India, he came back to America for a second stay from 1899 to 1902, returning to India in the year of his death. While in America, he founded the Vedanta Society of New York (1894), which is still in existence.[9]

Yoga scholars are virtually unanimous in citing Vivekananda's US tours as the birth of yoga in America. In 1896, the swami published *Yoga Philosophy: Lectures Delivered in New York, Winter of 1895–96, on Rāja Yoga, or Conquering the Internal Nature*. The term *raja yoga* is often associated with the meditation practices of Patañjali's *Yoga Sūtra*. Now known simply as *Raja Yoga*, Vivekananda's book achieved great popularity and is considered a classic by students of yoga for its translation of and commentary on the *Yoga Sūtra*. Scholars point to *Raja Yoga* as a benchmark in the transmission of Eastern teachings on yoga to the West.[10]

The chapters that deal with pranayama ("Prana," "The Psychic Prana," and "The Control of the Psychic Prana") provide a

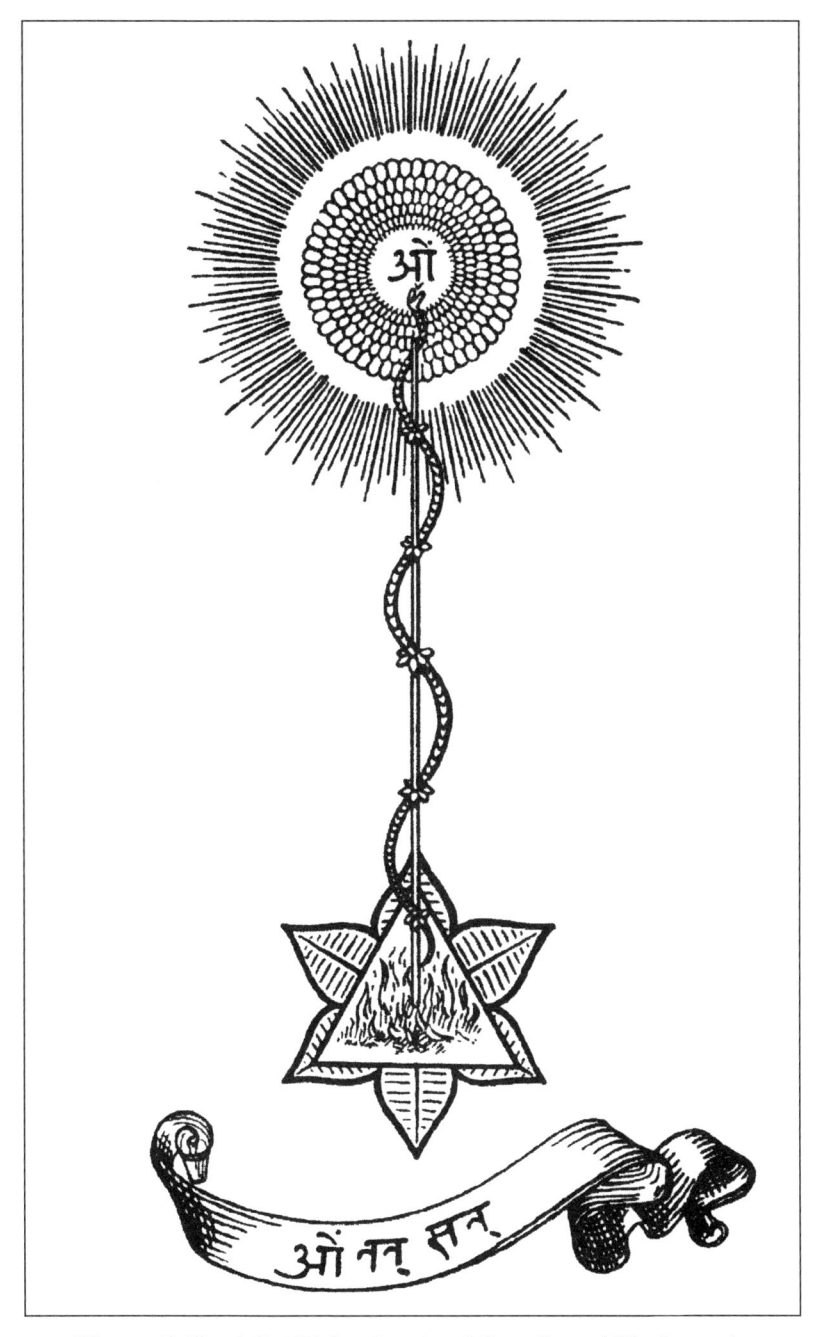

Figure 6. Kundalini Rising (reprinted from Swami Vivekananda, *Yoga Philosophy*, 1896)

short course in what we now call kundalini yoga. Vivekananda briefly deals with all the components of the Eastern chakra system: prana, kundalini, the three major nadis, and the seven chakras. The chakras are given their Sanskrit names—possibly the first appearance of these names on American soil.

Author Stefanie Syman claims that Vivekananda "ended his series of classes [on which *Raja Yoga* was based] on a vivid note, depicting the sushumna as a brilliant thread, strung with six lotuses."[11] Another first was the publication of this image (figure 6), which was embossed on the cover of the first edition and printed as a frontispiece in several later ones.[12]

The Sanskrit legend is the mantra *Oṃ tat sat* (Eternal supreme truth) and *om* is repeated within the radiating structure at the top, representing the thousand-petaled lotus. Further examination of the diagram reveals several irregularities. The kundalini-shakti arises, as in some tantric traditions, from the six-petaled lotus—svadhishthana, the *second* chakra. But the presence of five further small lotuses between this chakra and the thousand-petaled lotus at the top indicates that the six-petaled lotus is intended as the first. Furthermore, the triangle in the six-petaled lotus is the yantra of the third chakra, which tradition links with the element fire and a lotus with ten petals.

Vivekananda's chapters on kundalini yoga contain nothing that a present-day yoga student has not already encountered in multiple contemporary sources—yet his explanations are clear and concise. Several exercises in breath control are provided. There is no mention of the colors and chakra qualities that play such an important role in the later Western system, since these had not yet been developed. Indeed, there is no mention of powers attributed to the chakras. Yet these chapters of *Raja Yoga* may be the first manual of chakra development written and published in England and America by an Indian teacher.[13]

The Human Aura (Auguste Jean-Baptiste Marques)

As noted, Madame Blavatsky discussed the human aura in Esoteric Instruction No. 3. An earlier instruction, No. 2, included a colored plate of the human aura—perhaps one of the earliest attempts to portray the colors of the aura. Blavatsky's colors were linked with the seven principles, but there was no sign of colored layers.[14] Another plate in this instruction implied the existence of seven concentric rings associated with the principles but did not show them surrounding the human form.[15]

In the 1890s, after Blavatsky's death, the aura became the subject of widespread speculation and clairvoyant investigation within the TS—primarily, but not exclusively, within the London Lodge. A. P. Sinnett, who had returned to London from India in the mid-1880s, was president of the lodge and supervised such research, presenting a paper on the subject in 1893.[16] This paper was followed by Charles W. Leadbeater's first appearance in print, "The Aura," an article in the *Theosophist* (1895). This article included what may be the earliest material on the meanings of colors in the aura—certainly, within the TS; possibly, in Western esotericism.

There had been a longstanding disagreement between Blavatsky and Sinnett about the names and ordering of the principles. Both described them in terms of a continuum from lowest material to highest spiritual. However, Blavatsky insisted that the principles appeared as layers in the aura in an order unique to each person, based on that person's level of spiritual evolution, whereas Sinnett described the layers of the aura as a continuum, with the denser ("lower," more material) layers lying closer to the physical body and the increasingly ethereal ("higher," more spiritual) layers extending ever farther away.[17]

Leadbeater participated in clairvoyant investigations connected to the London Lodge, yet Besant had been a member of Blavatsky's Inner Group. After they began their joint investigations in 1895, Besant and Leadbeater distanced themselves from Sinnett's position by retaining the notion of increasingly ethereal layers of the aura extending outward from the physical body, but without identifying them with the principles.[18] By 1896, in *Man and His Bodies*, Besant was referring to layers of the aura in terms of subtle bodies rather than principles. The more subtle the body, the farther out it extended from the physical body. Thus the outer edges of these subtle bodies were progressively arranged around the physical body like nested dolls. The core of each subtle body was obscured by the physical body, but the outer edges could be perceived by clairvoyants as the etheric-, astral-, mental-, and causal-body layers of the aura—and, more rarely, layers associated with the buddhic and nirvanic bodies.[19]

Also in 1896, a French physician and diplomat living in Hawaii, where he was active in Theosophical circles, entered this discussion by providing the first graphic illustration of the human aura, in color, with the layers and principles clearly identified—Auguste Jean-Baptiste Marques (1841–1929). His small book, *The Human Aura*, is valuable for its citations and bibliography of sources documenting the early history of the notion of the aura in the TS prior to the publication of Leadbeater's *Man: Visible and Invisible* (1902), a standard reference on the subject. Furthermore, he worked with his own clairvoyant investigators, providing clarification, correction, and amplification of the work of the London Lodge—especially in the area of the effects on the aura of constant changes in pranic tides and their dominant tattvas, as discussed by Prasād in *Nature's Finer Forces*. (See plate 3.[20])

The importance of Marques in the history of the Western chakra system is that he made explicit a connection between the principles and layers of the aura that was implied in Besant's and Leadbeater's later writings on the subject but was occulted by their desire not to appear in conflict with Blavatsky's teachings. Though nearly forgotten today, Marques's book was widely known and cited by writers outside the TS (such as Ella Adelia Fletcher—discussed in the next section). It formed an essential link between the chakras and the layers of the aura, via Blavatsky's principles. This link was carried forward by a few writers on these subjects, reappearing from time to time, like the esoteric shadow of the developing Western chakra system, until it became explicit in the 1980s in the work of Rosalyn Bruyere and Barbara Brennan.

Rhythmic Breathing (Ella Adelia Fletcher)

Nature's Finer Forces was popular enough at the turn of the twentieth century that it might as well have been the first yoga manual in English. Similarly, for most yoga practitioners, *Raja Yoga* was the first manual of chakra development. What would happen if someone brought the two together—and added the substratum of the Western chakra system present in the writings of Blavatsky? Improbable as the combination may sound, these elements were fused in a virtually forgotten book published in the United States in 1908: *The Law of the Rhythmic Breath: Teaching the Generation, Conservation, and Control of Vital Force* by Ella Adelia Fletcher (1846–1934).[21] The book's importance lies in its setting the precedent for all future presentations of the Western chakra system. It synthesized teachings from ancient Indian scriptures and contemporary Indian teachers; from Western esoteric systems, such as astrology and Theosophy; from Western scientific studies of human physiology; and from the latest alternative healing modalities. Thus *The Law of the Rhythmic Breath* was the *Wheels of Life* of 1908.

Fletcher had a brilliant fifteen-year career as a journalist and author. She first emerged into the public eye in 1893 as E. A. Fletcher, her byline in *Demorest Family Magazine*, a popular woman's journal, for which she was the health and beauty editor.[22] When the magazine folded in 1899,[23] Fletcher published a widely and favorably reviewed book, *The Woman Beautiful: A Practical Treatise on the Development and Preservation of Woman's Health and Beauty, and the Principles of Taste in Dress* (1899). Based on the book's success, she contributed a syndicated weekly Sunday column on health, fitness, and beauty to the New York *Herald* in 1902 and 1903, where she covered such subjects as weight loss through exercise, stretch breaks for "brain workers," facial massage to remove wrinkles—even fencing—in half-page spreads illustrated with photographs. She also answered readers' questions and included recipes for homemade herbal cosmetics.

Fletcher was adopted by the New Thought movement—a form of healing that used auto-suggestion through positive affirmations to develop and maintain perfect health. She contributed to *Nautilus Magazine*, edited by Elizabeth Towne (1865–1960), a prolific author of what we now call self-help books. Indeed, the slogan of *Nautilus* was "Self-Help through Self-Knowledge."

The Law of the Rhythmic Breath was serialized monthly in *Nautilus* for several years before it was published in book form, starting in December 1905. Towne wrote that "Miss Fletcher is a deep student of occultism, a daring but careful investigator and an original woman and writer. She is past mistress of yoga lore, theoretical and practical."[24] Fletcher retired to Honolulu, Hawaii, after a 1909 visit and lived there with her sister for the rest of her life, producing no further books.

The Law of the Rhythmic Breath extracts the principles and techniques of svara yoga from their original cultural environment and transplants them into the New Thought culture of early twentieth century. Fletcher cites Blavatsky's major books, from *Isis Unveiled* to *The Voice of the Silence*, especially the Esoteric Instructions in the third volume of *The Secret Doctrine*. Vivekananda's *Raja Yoga* makes several appearances, rubbing shoulders with contemporary scientific thinking on the brain and nervous system. The bibliography references English translations of half a dozen ancient Hindu and Buddhist scriptures; seven books of Besant; clairvoyant investigations of the aura by several authors, including Marques and Leadbeater; books on astrology and New Thought; and an 1878 Spiritualist text by Edwin Dwight Babbitt, *Principles of Light and Color*, that became the basis not only for Besant and Leadbeater's investigations of what they called occult chemistry but also for the practice of color healing to be discussed in the next part of this book.

The Law of the Rhythmic Breath went one step beyond *Nature's Finer Forces* by conjoining breath control and the aura (human microcosm) with the tattvas and astrology (celestial macrocosm) by means of the seven principles. The functions of sushumna and the "vital centers" (such as the solar plexus) were treated in several chapters, but she mentioned only one chakra by its Sanskrit name (muladhara) and one by its English translation (thousand-petaled lotus).[25] Thus the connection between principles and chakras that was implied in Blavatsky's Esoteric Instructions became a tad more explicit—another stage in consolidating the groundwork for the Western chakra system.

Fletcher was a consolidator. Synthesizing material from Blavatsky's Esoteric Instructions, she created a list of color correspondences to the seven principles, describing them in quasi-rainbow order. However, she placed the fourth principle, kama, in relation to red; gave three versions, or levels, of manas; and left out prana. Atman was linked with white, resulting in a sequence of eight colors:

1. **Red**—kama (desire)
2. **Orange**—sthula (gross body)
3. **Yellow**—linga (subtle body or etheric double)
4. **Green**—lower manas (kama-manas; lower mind)
5. **Blue**—manas (mind)
6. **Indigo**—higher manas (buddhi-manas; higher mind)
7. **Violet**—buddhi (spiritual intelligence)
8. **White** (or transcendent blue)—atman (highest self)[26]

It would be a quarter century before the rainbow and the chakras were linked in the spectral order we are now familiar with—and by that time the connection with the principles would be lost.

Flying Rolls (Golden Dawn)

Nature's Finer Forces also played an important role in the development of ceremonial magic in the 1890s, in what is now called the Golden Dawn tradition, which dates back to the founding of the Hermetic Order of the Golden Dawn in 1888. One of the founders, Samuel Liddell MacGregor Mathers (1854–1918), who was a Freemason, a Rosicrucian, and a member of the Theosophical Society, began experimenting with Prasād's information on pranic/tattvic tides. The project was to develop a means of relating the celestial macrocosm to the human microcosm, to determine when the forces of the elements were ideally aligned for magical work. Breath control, external concentration, and internal visualization were each employed—and the focal point was a set of tattva cards that illustrated the symbols and colors provided in Prasād's translation of *Śiva-Svarodaya*.

Fellow members participated in these experiments, and the results were written up and distributed to other members for study as "Flying Rolls."[27] Some of these papers involved experiments in astral projection through what we now call active imagination or creative visualization—hence, perhaps, the reference to flight. A paper entitled "On the Tattwas of the Eastern School," attributed to Mathers, explains the procedure in detail—effectively transplanting the principles of *Śiva-Svarodaya* into the soil of Western occultism. These experiments did not directly involve the chakras, only the elements with which they are associated, so I will not describe them.[28]

Spheres, Pillars, and Paths (Kabbalah)

In the Flying Rolls of the 1890s, Golden Dawn members speculated not only on the tattvas' possible role in ceremonial magic but also on their connections to the Tree of Life from the kabbalistic tradition of Jewish mysticism. The tree is defined as "a set of symbols used since ancient times to study the Universe . . . a geometrical arrangement of ten sephiroth, or spheres, each of which is associated with a different archetypal idea."[29] Given the correspondence of the chakras to the tattvas, it was inevitable that these speculations would eventually correlate the chakra system and the Tree of Life. Despite the similarity of purpose—each system describes the creation or emanation of lower levels of being from higher ones, starting with the most spiritual and ending with the most physical—the functions of the seven chakras and those of the ten sephiroth do not line up well.

The Tree has three pillars: left, right, and middle. These are assumed to correlate with ida, pingala, and sushumna. There are three pairs of sephiroth distributed along the left and right pillars, each pair linked horizontally along the same plane. There are also four sephiroth along the middle pillar (sometimes five, when "a mysterious 'invisible' *sephirah* [singular of sephiroth]" named Daath [knowledge] is included[30]), each on its own plane.

In 1896, Marques published a "Human Aura Diagram of Concordances [correspondences]," which brought into relation HPB's seven principles, the seven layers of the aura, and the ten sephiroth—but without mentioning the chakras.[31] The earliest instance of a correlation between sephiroth, principles, and chakras occurred more than a decade later, in *Liber 777*, a 1909 private publication by former Golden Dawn member Aleister Crowley (1875–1947), who is said to have studied with Sabhapaty Swami.[32]

Crowley juxtaposed a list of the seven principles labeled "The Soul (Hindu)," with a list he called "The Chakkras [*sic*] or Centers of Prana (Hinduism)"—thus making the connection between principles and chakras implied in Blavatsky's Esoteric Instructions fully explicit for the first time.[33]

To bring the seven principles and chakras into alignment with the ten sephiroth (listed by number rather than name), Crowley divided manas into two parts, higher and lower, and split lower manas into three further subdivisions. In the chakras column, he assigned the three subdivisions of lower manas to Tiphereth (beauty) and the fourth chakra, but left out Malkuth (kingdom)—possibly because *muladhara* means "root-support" and thus naturally fell into line with Yesod (foundation).[35]

The following year, Crowley elaborated on the connection between chakras and the sephiroth in his magazine *Equinox: The Review of Scientific Illuminism*. Called "The Temple of Solomon the King" and running through several issues of *Equinox*, this book-length series of articles fleshed out the lists of correspondences from *Liber 777* in the context of an instructional and semiautobiographical account of the initiatory progress of one Frater Perdurabo. The section on the chakras drew heavily on *The Esoteric Science and Philosophy of the Tantras* by Sris Chandra Basu, the first English

Table 7
Crowley's Chakra Correlations (1909)

Principles	Sephiroth	Chakras
7. Atman	1. Kether (Crown)	7. Sahasrara (Crown)
6. Buddhi	2. Chokmah (Wisdom)	6. Ajna (Brow)
5. Higher manas (Buddhi-manas)	3. Binah (Understanding)	5. Vishuddha (Throat)
4c. Lower manas (Kama-manas)	4. Chesed (Mercy)	4c. Anahata (Heart)
4b. Lower manas (Kama-manas)	5. Geburah (Severity)	4b. Anahata (Heart)
4a. Lower manas (Kama-manas)	6. Tiphereth (Beauty)	4a. Anahata (Heart)
3. Kama	7. Netzach (Victory)	3. Manipura (Navel)
2. Prana	8. Hod (Glory)	2. Svadhishthana (Genital)
1. Linga	9. Yesod (Foundation)	1. Muladhara (Root)
0. Sthula[34]	10. Malkuth (Kingdom)	. . .

translation of the *Śiva Saṃhitā*, published in 1887 (uncited, with minor changes in phrasing).[36] Within this section, a diagram of the chakras appears—perhaps the first to be published by a Westerner using the now familiar image of the meditating yogi to show their location in the body.

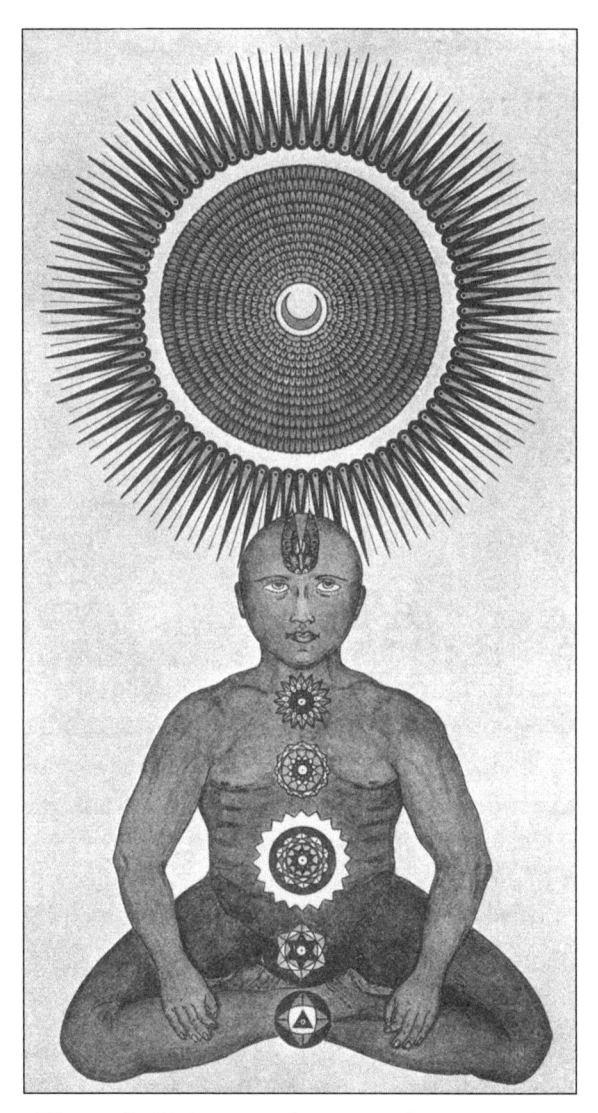

Figure 7. Chakra Locations according to Crowley (reprinted from *Equinox*, 1910/1972)

I have not been able to trace an earlier source of this diagram, so I do not know whether it is traditional or has been adapted from a traditional source. Note the similarity of presentation of sahasrara to Vivekananda's in figure 6 in the present book. The chakras are given the correct number of petals. The sunburst surrounding the third chakra reflects verses in the *Śiva Saṃhitā* (2.32–34) that deal with a health-giving solar digestive fire in the belly. The image for the sixth chakra is decidedly westernized, turning its two petals into the wings of a dove.[37]

Other correlations of the chakras and the Tree of Life followed in the 1930s: *A Garden of Pomegranates* (1932) by Israel Regardie (1907–85), who, following in the footsteps of Crowley, codified the teachings of the Golden Dawn into workable system of ceremonial magic;[38] and *The Mystical Qabalah* (1935) by Dione Fortune (Violet Mary Firth, 1890–1946).[39] Both Regardie and Fortune studied the Golden Dawn tradition in groups that developed after the original Hermetic Order of the Golden Dawn split into rival factions around 1900.

Reasons for differences between Crowley's, Regardie's, and Fortune's correlations of the sephiroth and the chakras require a fuller explanation of Kabbalah than I am able present here. Suffice it to say that there is practically no resemblance to the current New Age consensus as presented in *Wheels of Life* and other books, such as Caroline Myss *Anatomy of the Spirit*. Such books usually eschew Daath and attempt to link the qualities of the Western chakra system with the functions of the sephiroth (see figure 8, left side).

The New Age mapping proceeds as follows:

- The first sephirah on the middle pillar (Kether/Crown) goes with the seventh chakra (not a bad correlation, since each is at the top of its system and in its way represents the Absolute from which the other "lower" sephiroth and chakras emanate).
- The first pair below the crown (Chokmah/Wisdom and Binah/Understanding) goes with the brow chakra (not a bad

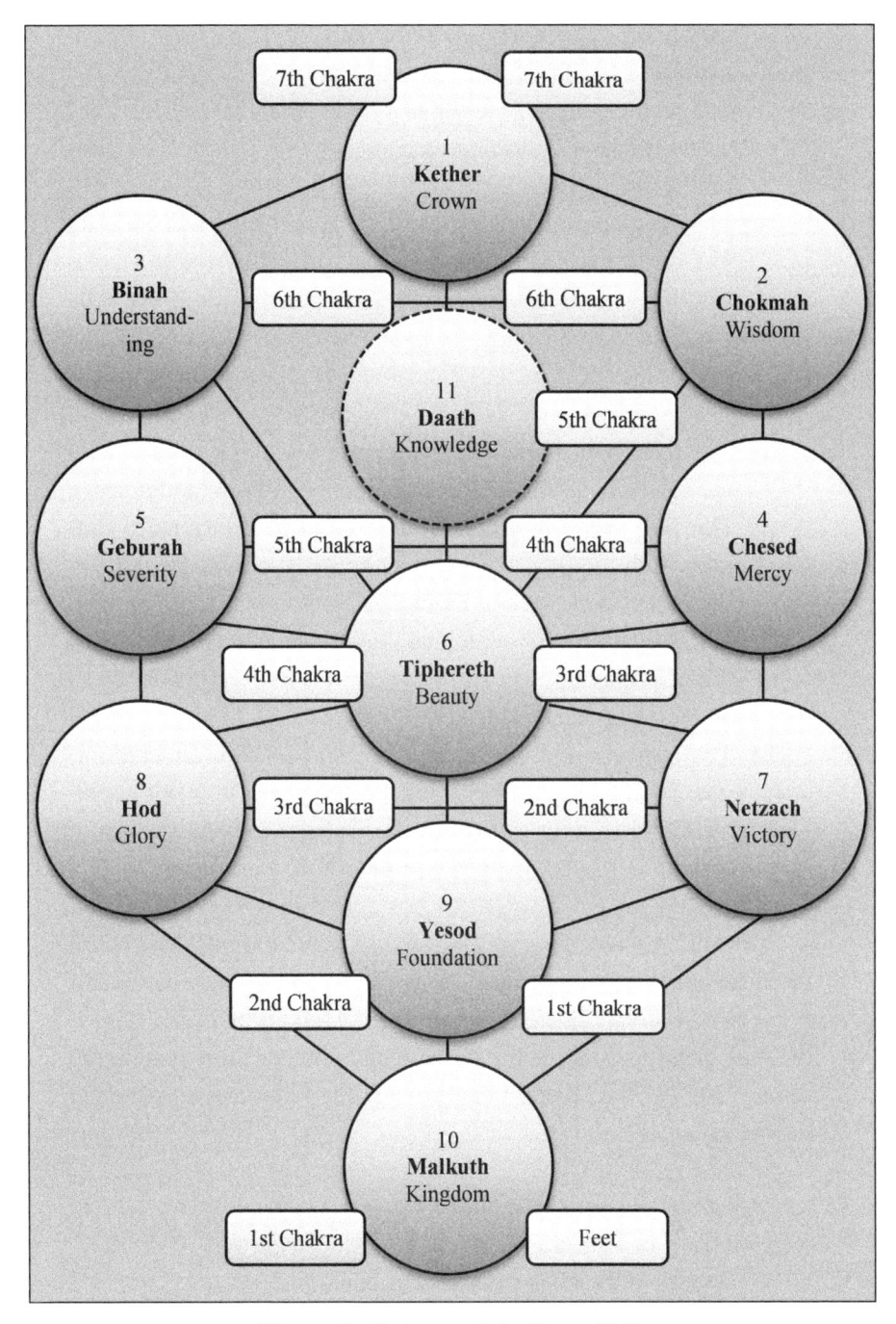

Figure 8. Chakras and the Tree of Life

match for the element of mind and the "insightful" third-eye).
- The second pair (Chesed/Mercy and Geburah/Severity) goes with the throat chakra (not a good match for akasha, or communication/expression).
- The next sephirah along the middle pillar (Tiphereth/Beauty) goes with the heart chakra (not a bad match for love/relationships—until one is tasked with understanding what the latter have to do with the kabbalistic interpretation of this sephirah as "the 'place of incarnation'; the mystery of sacrifice"; the relevance to air is not clear).
- The third pair (Netzach/Victory and Hod/Glory) goes with the solar-plexus chakra (not a bad match for fire and power).
- The next sephirah on the middle pillar (Yesod/Foundation) goes with the genital chakra (seems like a better match for the root chakra, though Francis King links this sephirah with "formative forces," which could perhaps be associated with the generative power of the sexual chakra; the reference to water is not clear).
- The last sephirah on the middle pillar (Malkuth/Kingdom) goes with the root chakra (not a bad match, since this sephirah is linked with earth and "the physical universe; solidity; rigidity").[40]

The alternative mapping (left side of figure 8) links Daath with the throat chakra, which means that the fourth, third, second, and first chakras are all shifted up one level. Malkuth is placed below the feet. The functions of the seventh and sixth chakras remain the same.[41] Adding the Western chakra qualities, we now we have the following:

- Knowledge linked with the fifth chakra of communication
- Mercy and severity in the airy heart chakra of love
- Beauty in the fiery solar-plexus chakra of power

- Glory and victory in the watery genital chakra of sexuality
- Earthy foundation in the grounding base chakra

A true kabbalist would call the links in each of these approaches superficial, if not ignorant, since the sephiroth deal with powers of creation, not personal happiness, as in the Western chakra system. Furthermore, each sephirah is said to emanate from the last in a ten-stage process whose progress between the pillars is more complex than the simple downward direction of evolving elements in the chakra system. Finally, the twenty-two paths that link the sephiroth with each other provide the Tree of Life diagram with its richness as a spiritual teaching tool—but have no correlation in the chakra system.

It could be argued that Crowley, Regardie, and Fortune had an easier time finding meaningful correlations between the sephiroth, chakras, and tattvas than did later writers simply because the Western chakra system was still in the process of formation and the now traditional chakra qualities had not yet developed. It could also be argued that, as with the chakras and the lataif of the Sufis, the chakras and the sephiroth are culturally incompatible systems and cannot be mapped into each other without confusion. Be that as it may, New Age books on the chakras tend to list the sephiroth among their correspondences without going into detail, simply passing on the constantly developing body of Western chakra lore.

Chapter 11
Chakras of the Apocalypse (James Morgan Pryse)

The chakras have been connected not only to Jewish mysticism but also to Christian mysticism. While researching this book, I came across an odd illustration in Mark Singleton's *Yoga Body: The Origins of Modern Posture Practice*. This illustration, from 1928, paired the chakras with non-Eastern images, such as a horseman carrying a bow in the first chakra, a seven-headed serpent in the second, and a hanging balance in the third. More bizarre was the account given by Singleton of the book from which the illustration came—it "locates the key to the ultimate spiritual truth of yoga—and also, disconcertingly, of the biblical Apocalypse—in the individual body."[1]

The author of the book was a mysterious American yoga teacher, Cajzoran Ali, whom I discuss in a later chapter. Ali used an odd Greek term, *speirema*, as a substitute for the phrase *serpent power*—an important clue. It led me to a student of Blavatsky, James Morgan Pryse (1859–1942), who had previously used this word in *The Apocalypse Unsealed* (1910).

Pryse was born in the American Midwest of Welsh parents. His father was a Presbyterian minister, who taught him how to read Greek. As an adult, in the middle 1880s, he joined the Theosophical Society and settled for a few years in Los Angeles, where he began studying Sanskrit. He had set up and sold several print shops by this time. In 1889, William Q. Judge, president of the American section of the TS and vice-president of the international organization, asked Pryse to help him set up a printing press in New York for the publication of Blavatsky's Esoteric Instructions for distribution to American members of the Esoteric School. Blavatsky then requested that he do the same for her in London on behalf of the European members of the ES. Thus Pryse was in near daily contact with Blavatsky during her last year. Pryse returned to America in

1895, eventually resettling in the Los Angeles area, where he spent the rest of his life.[2]

The Apocalypse Unsealed was an "esoteric interpretation" of the Revelation of St. John, with translation and commentary. It remained in print through four editions until the early 1930s. Pryse believed that Revelation was "a manual of spiritual development and not, as conventionally interpreted, a cryptic history of prophecy." As such, he referred to Revelation as the "*initiation* of Ioannes," using the Greek form of the saint's name.[3] To explain the stages in this initiation, Pryse drew on his understanding of Platonic philosophy and the Greek mysteries, the Jewish Bible and Christian gospels, the Upanishads, Western astrology, the Eastern chakra system—and Blavatsky's Esoteric Instructions. His synthesis of such disparate materials is impressive, supported by diagrams, tables, and the solution of "a series of elaborate puzzles, some of which are based upon the numerical values of Greek words."[4]

Though Pryse was not a part of Blavatsky's Inner Group, his understanding of the Esoteric Instructions was so profound that he either intuited or revealed the ultimate purpose of her kundalini practice. It is possible that, in consulting with Blavatsky about the printing of the Instructions, he received information that allowed him to penetrate more deeply into their meaning than other writers before or since. Regardless of whether *Apocalypse Unsealed* sheds light on Revelation, it certainly illuminates the Esoteric Instructions. Whether or not it is useful as a manual for raising the kundalini and awakening the chakras, it creates a plausible plotline for the unfolding of stages in Blavatsky's kundalini practice, laying out the course and markers by which experimenters might chart their progress.

Pryse lists the chakras using their Sanskrit names, linking each with a nerve ganglion (plexus). Other by-now-familiar aspects of tantric anatomy are referenced, such as ida, pingala, and sushumna. As noted, Pryse provides a Greek equivalent for kundalini, which he calls the "serpent coil"—speirema. He also suggests that the brahmarandhra (which he translates as "door of Brahma") was referred to "in early Christian mysticism" as the "door of Iesous [Jesus]."⁵

Pryse links seven signs of the zodiac with Blavatsky's seven tattvas and the chakras. He relates the remaining signs to the five prana-vayus, currents of vitality that circulate through the body performing various functions essential to life. He also provides a circular diagram of the zodiac, within which a human form is curled, head at Aries, foot at Pisces, front facing outward, to show how the chakras line up, top to bottom, from Cancer to Capricorn.⁶

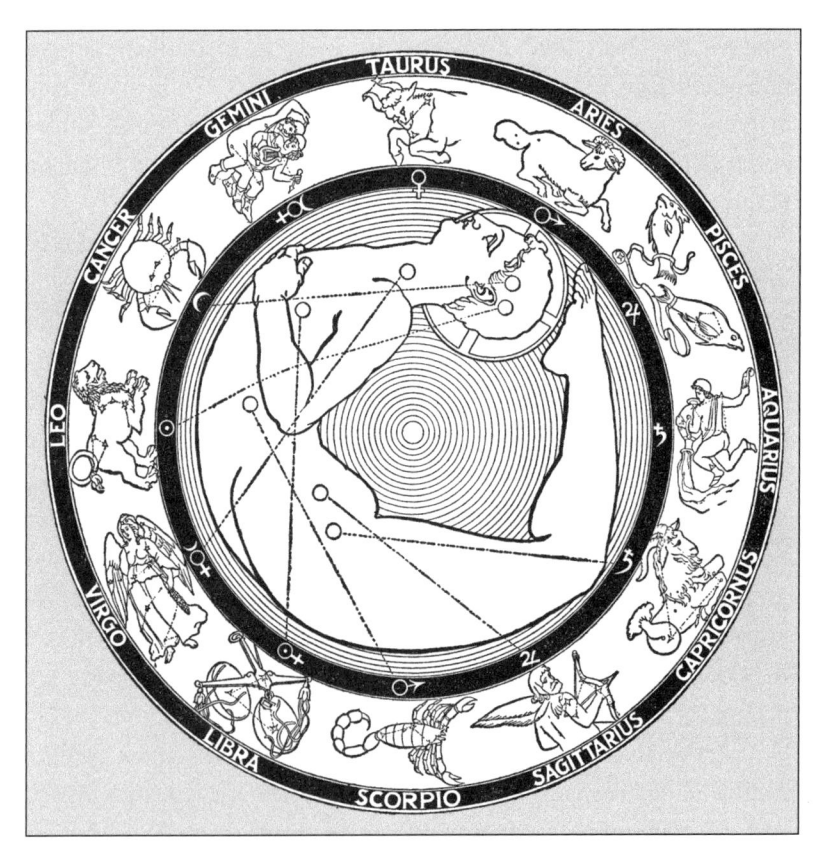

Figure 9. Pryse's Chakras, Planets, and Signs
(reprinted from James M. Pryse, *The Apocalypse Unsealed*, 1910)

Pryse connects the seven churches in Asia (Rev. 1:11) with the seven chakras in the body, and the stars associated with these churches (Rev. 1:20) with Blavatsky's seven rays. He also links the chakras with the seven seals of the Book of Life (Rev. 5:1). These seals must be broken, just as the chakras must be pierced by the kundalini, in the following order: second, third, fourth, fifth, sixth, first, seventh.[7]

Pryse refers to Blavatsky's seven chakras in the brain and mentions the sounds associated with them. He claims that, in Revelation, these sounds are represented by the seven trumpets (Rev. 8:6).[8] There are two more sets of seven chakras to be conquered before the initiation is complete. One is associated with the heart—three angels having to do with Babylon's fall and four with the harvesting of the earth (Rev. 14). The last set of chakras has to do with the generative organs—the seven angels bringing golden vials of plagues, which Pryse calls scourges (Rev. 15:6–7).

The Kundalini Practice Revisited

Here is Pryse's blow-by-blow account of Blavatsky's kundalini practice. Blavatsky's version, as given in chapter seven, provides clearer instructions on what practitioners are supposed to do, but Pryse's more definitely articulates the stages:[9]

- Kundalini is aroused "by conscious effort in meditation," ignoring sushumna and concentrating instead on ida and pingala to form "a positive and a negative current along the spinal cord."
- "On reaching the sixth chakra," these currents "radiate to the right and left, along the line of the eyebrows."
- Kundalini, "starting at the base [lower end] of the spinal cord, proceeds along the spinal marrow [central canal], its passage through each section thereof corresponding to a sympathetic ganglion being accompanied by a violent shock, or rushing sensation."

- When "it reaches the conarium [pineal gland]," it "passes outward through the *brahmarandhra*, the three currents thus forming a cross in the brain."[10]
- "In the initial stage the seven psychic colors are seen."
- When kundalini passing through sushumna "impinges on the brain there follows the lofty consciousness of the seer, whose mystic 'third eye' now becomes, as it has been poetically suggested, 'a window into space.'"
- "The brain-centers are successively 'raised from the dead' by the serpent-force."
- "In the next stage, the seven 'spiritual sounds' are heard in the tense and vibrant aura of the seer."
- "Sight and hearing become blended into a single sense, by which colors are heard, and sounds are seen—or, to word it differently, color and sound become one, and are perceived by a sense that is neither sight nor hearing but both."
- "The psychic senses of taste and smell become unified."
- "The two senses thus merged from the four are merged in the interior, intimate sense of touch."
- Touch "vanishes into the epistemonic faculty [manas/mind], the gnostic power of the seer—exalted above all-sense perception—to cognize eternal realities."
- "This is the sacred trance called in Sanskrit *samadhi*."

Further stages lead to "rebirth in the imperishable solar body"—presumably the higher principles of atman (self), buddhi (spiritual intuition), and manas (intelligence), which combine to make up the monad.[11] Pryse claims that the entire process, from awakening of the kundalini to rebirth in the solar body—is laid out in Revelation.[12]

Multiple Chakra Systems

Pryse also provides a key to a mysterious passage in the Inner Group Teachings in which Blavatsky speaks of a seven-stage process undergone on the physical plane, followed by either seven stages distributed among the "psychic, spiritual, and divine" planes or sets of seven stages undertaken in each of these planes.[13] Pryse opts for the second interpretation but subdivides the psychic plane into two parts, for a total of five planes. These planes are called *physical*, *phantasmal* (presumably astral), *psychic* (presumably mental), *spiritual* (buddhic), and *aura* (Blavatsky's auric envelope, correlated to atman—presumably her "divine" plane). They are linked to the five elements, as in the Eastern chakra system (though Pryse swaps the places of fire and water). Chakra systems associated with the first four planes must be mastered and transcended in the following order to produce the solar body:[14]

1. "The opening of the seven seals, the conquest of the seven principal centers of the sympathetic nervous system" (correlated with the "region of the navel," the "passional nature," and "emotions, appetites, and passions"; linked in diagrams with "animal-psychic forces" and the "psychic" centers of the "phantasmal world"—presumably kama and Besant's astral body)
2. "The sounding of the seven trumpets, the conquest of the seven centers in the brain, or cerebro-spinal system" (correlated with the "region of the head, or brain"; linked with the "noetic forces" and centers of the "spiritual world"— presumably buddhi-manas, the higher mind, and Besant's causal body)
3. "The harvesting of the earth and its vine, the conquest of the seven cardiac centers" (correlated with the "region of the heart, including all the organs above the diaphragm" as "seat of the lower mind" and "including the psychic nature"; linked with "psycho-mental forces" and the "phrenic" centers of the "psychic world"—presumably kama-manas, the lower mind, and Besant's mental body)
4. "The outpouring of the seven scourges, the conquest of the generative centers" (correlated with the "procreative"

region; linked with "vital forces" and the "creative centers" of the "physical world"—presumably *prāṇa-liṅga-sthūla*, the combination of vitality, etheric form, and dense form that Besant identifies as the physical body.)

I am not aware of teachings by Blavatsky on cardiac and generative chakras, though she does say: "There are three principal centers in man: heart, head, and navel," and "There are seven brains [centers?] in the heart"—thus covering the locations of three of Pryse's sets of centers.[15] However, Pryse justifies his system by correlating each plane with a zodiac. We have seen how he assigns seven signs to the chakras and the remaining five signs to other forces. Four times twelve is forty-eight—which, plus the sun at the center, makes forty-nine: the number of chakras posited by Blavatsky in the Esoteric Instructions.[16]

Despite indications that Pryse was possibly giving forth teachings privately passed on to him by Blavatsky and linking the Esoteric Instructions with *The Voice of the Silence*, I do not find this example of numerological play persuasive. If the head, heart, belly, and generative organs can each have a set of seven chakras, and each of these areas is itself associated with a chakra, then there could be seven chakras in the root, throat, and brow centers as well, thus making up the total of forty-nine. The idea that there may be seven chakras (or layers) within each chakra is sometimes encountered in later writers and will be dealt with in the final chapter of this book.

The Snake and the Cross

Pryse included a diagram of the location of the nerve plexuses, or ganglions, in his book (see figure 10). As noted, this aspect of the chakra system was the first to click into place, in Basu's 1888 *Theosophist* article, as recounted in chapter 5. The diagram in *Apocalypse Unsealed*, published twenty-two years later, indicates how firmly ingrained this set of correlations had become. Though Pryse does not list the chakras on the diagram, in context this image may be the first graphic representation of the locations of the chakras in the physical body—seventeen years before Rele's *The Mysterious Kundalini*, which yoga historians usually credit as first.

A subsequent diagram (see figure 11) makes the connection of the chakras to ganglia clearer—and adds an early list of westernized chakra functions. This diagram may be the first visual representation of the chakra system published by a Western (or at least American) author, fifteen years after Vivekananda's. The four circles represent the four planes (physical, phantasmal, psychic, and spiritual), indicating that certain chakras belong to each. The uppermost phrase, "The Conqueror," the eighth in the sequence from bottom to top, represents the final outcome of having mastered the seven chakras.

The mystical numbers associated with the chakras in this "Gnostic Chart" are derived from the numerological equivalents of the letters in the Greek words Pryse used to define the chakra functions. Obviously synthetic, these numbers and names were not carried forward into later versions of the Western chakra system—though the attempt to develop a list of unique chakra functions became a major preoccupation for writers on the chakras for the next seventy years.

With figures 10 and 11 in mind, it becomes clear that the frontispiece of *Apocalypse Unsealed* (plate 4) also is a representation of the chakra system. Note that the functions of the chakras are placed to reflect the positions of the chakras illustrated in figure 11. Furthermore, in plate 4, the cross entwined with a serpent portrays the initials of the Theosophical Society. A similar insignia appears on the cover of the first edition of Blavatsky's *The Secret Doctrine* (and many subsequent reprints)—but as a T-cross, with the serpent's head drooping over the right bar of the *T* rather than erect above the Christian cross, as here. Pryse's modified TS insignia portrays the rising of the kundalini serpent from foot (base) to head (crown) of a human form with outstretched arms. Read in this way, the crux of the cross would correspond to the location of the

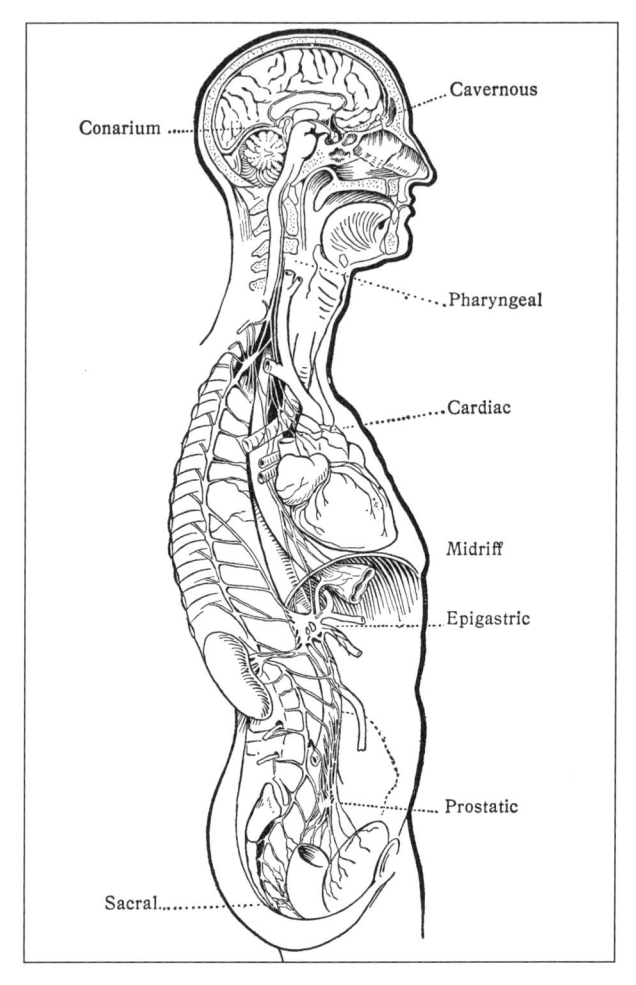

Figure 10. Chakra Locations according to Pryse (reprinted from James M. Pryse, *The Apocalypse Unsealed*, 1910)

throat chakra—which is why the word *cross* figures at this level of the enrobed human form. This form represents not only the Conqueror—presumably a Master—but also a being described in Rev. 1:12–15:

> I saw seven golden candlesticks; and in the midst of the seven candlesticks one like unto the Son of man, clothed

Chakras of the Apocalypse (James Morgan Pryse)

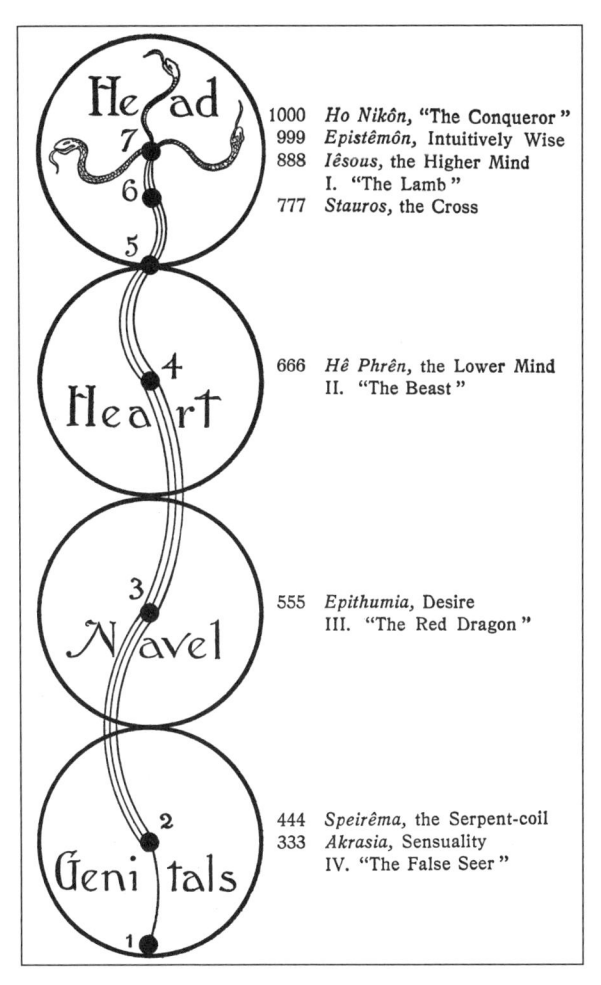

1000	*Ho Nikôn,* "The Conqueror"
999	*Epistêmôn,* Intuitively Wise
888	*Iêsous,* the Higher Mind
	I. "The Lamb"
777	*Stauros,* the Cross
666	*Hê Phrên,* the Lower Mind
	II. "The Beast"
555	*Epithumia,* Desire
	III. "The Red Dragon"
444	*Speirêma,* the Serpent-coil
333	*Akrasia,* Sensuality
	IV. "The False Seer"

Figure 11. Chakra Functions according to Pryse (reprinted from James M. Pryse, *The Apocalypse Unsealed*, 1910

with a garment down to the foot, and girt about the paps with a golden girdle. His head and his hairs were white like wool, as white as snow; and his eyes were as a flame of fire; and his feet like unto fine brass, as if they burned in a furnace; and his voice as the sound of many waters.

The message of plate 4, perhaps, is that for Pryse, the meaning and purpose of the TS is to evolve ordinary humans into superhuman Masters by means of an initiatory path involving kundalini and the chakras (seven candlesticks)—in other words, the kundalini practice taught by Blavatsky to her private students and the resulting activation and mastery of the seven principles.

In this plate, the phrases *lower mind* and *higher mind* refer respectively to kama-manas and buddhi-manas and *intuitively wise* to buddhi. Thus the Conqueror is the seventh principle, or atman. Having perceived these clues, we can correlate the other levels of plate 4 with their principles, as in table 8.

Blavatsky insisted in the Esoteric Instructions that sthula, the physical body, was not itself a principle.[17] Linga, the first genuine principle, has multiple meanings in Sanskrit, among them "mark" or "sign," "subtle body," and "phallus." Pryse probably had the last of these meanings in mind in assigning linga to the sacral plexus and linking it with sensuality. Prana is associated with vitality, hence its connection with the serpent power. The *antaḥkaraṇa* (inner instrument), defined by Blavatsky as the link that must be developed between lower and higher mind for spiritual progress to occur, is also not a principle.[18] Thus, though there are eight levels in the plate 4, it nevertheless remains true to the notion of seven principles.[19]

Though Pryse's melding of Eastern liberation and Western eschatology is striking, I consider him more a consolidator than an innovator. He added no new material to the Western chakra system. Rather, he synthesized disparate materials to outline a coherent system of spiritual practice based on Blavatsky's fragmentary late teachings. This interpretive synthesis influenced a number of esotericists in the first half of the twentieth century, including Alice Bailey, Cajzoran Ali, Ivah Bergh Whitten, and Edgar Cayce. Yet Pryse's contribution was forgotten in the latter half of the century, and the seven seals of Revelation are no longer cited in most versions of the Western chakra system.

Nevertheless, Pryse's synthesis marked a vitally important stage in the development of the Western chakra system. As noted,

Table 8
Chakras according to Pryse

Chakras	Plexuses	Seals	Planets	Signs	Functions	Principles
...	...	...	...	...	Conqueror	Atman
Sahasrara	Conarium [pineal]	Seventh	Sun	Leo	Intuitively wise	Buddhi
Ajna	Cavernous	Fifth	Moon	Cancer	Higher mind	Buddhi-manas
Vishuddha	Pharyngeal	Fourth	Mercury	Virgo	The Cross	Antahkarana
Anahata	Cardiac	Third	Venus	Libra	Lower mind	Kama-manas
Manipura	Epigastric [solar plexus]	Second	Mars	Scorpio	Desire	Kama
Svadhishthana	Prostatic	First	Jupiter	Sagittarius	Serpent-coil [kundalini]	Prana
Muladhara	Sacral	Sixth	Saturn	Capricorn	Sensuality	Linga (sthula)

Crowley was the first to link the principles and chakras explicitly in 1909. Just one year later, Pryse placed this correspondence into an evolutionary context—symbolized by the progression of numbers in figures 11 and plate 4 (333, 444, etc.). Thus the chakras became a continuum of human evolutionary potential, ranging from purely material to purely spiritual, as represented by the seven principles. Every subsequent step in the development of the Western chakra system elaborated and refined this continuum of human potential.

Chapter 12
Charles W. Leadbeater and the Serpent Fire

Interested in Spiritualism, trained as an Anglican clergyman, the young Charles Webster Leadbeater (1854–1934) joined the Theosophical Society in December 1883. He met Madame Blavatsky in England when she was briefly in Europe, in 1884. Inspired by the recent publication of Sinnett's *The Occult World* (1881) and *Esoteric Buddhism* (1883), based on teachings received as letters from spiritual Masters in Tibet, Leadbeater wrote to the Masters in late October and received a reply directing him to go to India with Blavatsky on her return trip. He quickly arranged his affairs and joined her in Egypt a few weeks later, arriving at the TS headquarters in Adyar on December 21.[1]

In his memoir, *How Theosophy Came to Me*, Leadbeater describes how he developed clairvoyant abilities in 1885. He was at Adyar. Mired in controversy over having allegedly produced fraudulent psychic phenomena, Blavatsky had permanently returned to Europe. Olcott was away on tour. Leadbeater claimed to have been visited by one of the Theosophical Masters, who suggested "a certain kind of meditation connected with the development of a mysterious power called *kundalini*." He had "heard of that power, but knew very little about it" and "supposed it to be absolutely out of reach for Western people." The Master advised him to "make a few efforts along certain lines, which he pledged me never to divulge to anyone else except with his direct authorization, and told me that he would himself watch over those efforts to see that no danger ensued."

Leadbeater "took the hint" and worked diligently for some forty days, during which "certain channels [nadis] had to be opened and certain partitions broken down [by either piercing the chakras or dissolving the knots (granthis) between certain chakras]." After the Master enabled a breakthrough allowing Leadbeater to use his astral sight whether awake or asleep, his training continued under the guidance of several Masters (probably visiting him in astral form). He was further instructed by a physically embodied teacher, a Madras lawyer deeply involved in Theosophical work and a frequent contributor to the *Theosophist*, T. Subba Row.[2]

Subba Row had been influential in getting the founders of the TS to move their headquarters from Bombay to Adyar in 1882. Blavatsky considered him to be a "great occultist" and an authority on Indian esoteric philosophy. However, he was not known to his family for having such interests or knowledge. According to Olcott,

> While he was obedient as a child to his mother in worldly affairs, he was strangely reticent to her, as he was to all his relatives and ordinary acquaintances, about spiritual matters. His constant answer to her importunities for occult instruction was that he "dared not reveal any of the secrets entrusted to him by his Guru."[3]

Blavatsky claimed that Subba Row had the same Master she did—Morya (also known as Master M). Most Theosophists assume that Subba Row's instruction came from that source. However, I suspect that Subba Row was a practitioner of Tantra. He would have maintained secrecy to his friends and family about his association with Tantra because of the bad reputation of such teachings in conventional Hindu society.

Indeed, according to Olcott, Subba Row claimed that "'one-third of his life is passed in a world of which his own mother has no idea.'" Olcott assumed he meant "transcorporeal [astral body] activities," but I wonder whether this was a reference to his tantric involvement.[4] How else to explain his sudden access to what Olcott called "a storehouse of occult experience" and "stored up knowledge of Sanskrit literature," which Olcott assumed to have arisen from a past life.[5] Subba Row's association with the TS gave him an opportunity to bring out the knowledge he had acquired as a tantric practitioner under the auspices of an organization that had so far made a favorable impression on the Indian people.

Leadbeater said he had "heard of" kundalini—which makes me think that Subba Row may have been partially responsible for what Leadbeater knew of it. At any rate, Subba Row often drove by carriage from Madras to Adyar "to take part in the instruction and testing" involved in the development of Leadbeater's clairvoyance. Leadbeater reports that this instruction required "a year of the hardest work I had ever known." He kept his pledge, so the exact nature of this instruction was never revealed.[6]

The first fruits of Leadbeater's training developed about ten years later, when he was living in London, where he clairvoyantly investigated, lectured about, and published articles, pamphlets, and books on subjects such as the human aura, the astral plane, and past lives. His 1895 article in the *Theosophist*, "The Aura," later published as a pamphlet, provided a comprehensive list of colors in the aura and their meanings and briefly mentioned the chakras (using an alternative spelling common at that time). Leadbeater spoke of the challenges of reading an aura "perfectly": "the general brilliancy of the aura, the comparative definiteness or indefiniteness of its outline, and the relative brightness of the *chakrams* or centers of force . . . have to be taken into consideration."[7]

Leadbeater expanded material from the article/pamphlet into a book, *Man Visible and Invisible*, in which he mentioned the chakras only to say they were not illustrated in the color plates depicting various states of the aura. However, he made an important point that we will examine in the final chapter, that the "seven chakras or centers of force . . . exist in all the vehicles [of consciousness—i.e., subtle bodies]."[8]

Leadbeater's first substantial reference to the chakras occurs in 1898, in his answer to a question submitted to the *Vahan*, a Theosophical journal founded by Blavatsky just before she died. The question concerned the existence of organs in the astral body. This passage summarizes and extends what we learned from Besant's approach to the chakras:

> Theosophical students are familiar with the idea of the existence in both the astral and the etheric bodies of man of certain centers, sometimes called chakras, which have to be vivified in turn by the sacred serpent-fire as the man advances in evolution. Though these cannot be described as organs in the ordinary sense of the word—since it is not through them that the man sees or hears, as he does here through eyes and ears—yet it is apparently very largely upon their vivification that the power of exercising these astral senses depends, each of them as it is developed giving to the whole astral body the power of response to a new set of vibrations. . . .
>
> They are . . . points, perhaps, at which the higher force from planes above impinges upon the astral body. . . . They are in reality four-dimensional vortices, so that the force which comes through them and is the cause of their existence seems to well up from nowhere.[9]

Leadbeater uses what became the preferred Theosophical translation of the tantric term *kundalini-shakti* ("serpent fire"; in non-Theosophical contexts, "serpent power"). The reference to the fourth dimension reflects contemporary scientific and mathematical speculation, providing a useful way to support the esoteric notion of subtle bodies and planes for inquiring readers. Thus this passage provides an early instance of appealing to science for validation of clairvoyantly perceived information—a tendency demonstrated by most Western books on the chakras and by some written by modern Eastern teachers, such as Satyananda.

The passage contains a largely unnoticed innovation, perhaps concealed by the phrase *well up*. In the Eastern system, the energy that awakens the chakras either rises from the lowest chakra, descends from the highest chakra, or circulates in both directions—in all cases traveling along the spine. However, in Leadbeater's system, the vortices form along the *outer* edge of the astral and etheric bodies, absorbing forces from their respective planes and channeling them into the core of each body along a whirling, drain-like funnel (a lesser known meaning of *cakra* is "whirlpool"). Each funnel converges on an astral or etheric *center* correlated to some physical organ or nerve plexus, usually located along the spine. Just as the layers of the aura, as subtle bodies, are arranged around the physical body like nested dolls increasing in size, so the organ or nerve plexus is surrounded by its rarified etheric center, a more expansive and rarified astral center, and an even more expansive and rarified mental center.

Astral energy entering the vortex of each astral chakra carries information about the astral plane down the funnel to the corresponding astral center along the spine. This information is registered by the astral center along the line of that center's function—for example, the fifth (throat) center's function is clairaudience, so the information registered by that center corresponds to sound or speech on the astral plane. Astral energy and information may then pass through the etheric equivalent of the astral center and thence to the physical organ or nerve plexus. If the corresponding etheric center is sufficiently developed, this information can be received by the nervous system and recalled by the physical brain. A similar pattern holds true for the mental body and the etheric body, whose chakras and centers are attuned to their own levels of being—respectively, the lower mental plane and the etheric subplanes of the physical plane.

In this model, undeveloped chakras have no stems or funnels and no flowerlike openings to the outer edge of a subtle body. They have no means of accessing information from the plane on which that body operates. Developed chakras have not only a center along the spine, but also a stem or funnel and an opening in the surface of the etheric, astral, or mental body. These structures of centers, stems, and flowers provide what Besant and Leadbeater call the sense *organs* of the etheric, astral, or mental bodies.[10]

The exact dates of Leadbeater's clairvoyant investigations of the chakras are not known. I suspect they occurred in the latter half of the 1890s, perhaps in conjunction with Annie Besant. According to TS historian (and later international president) C. Jinarājadāsa, Besant and Leadbeater undertook several periods of joint investigation from 1895 to 1898, but he makes no mention of when they might have explored the aura and the chakras.[11]

In 1897, Besant used magic lantern slides of the paintings of the aura later published in *Man Visible and Invisible* to illustrate her lectures during a seven-month tour in America. In 1905, Besant and Leadbeater copublished *Thought-Forms*, which dealt with how thoughts and feelings are perceived by clairvoyant vision. The book included plates made from the originals of other magic lantern slides used during Besant's 1897 tour, whereas the text was based on an 1896 article by Besant in *Lucifer* (yet another journal founded by Blavatsky).[12] These details, as well as Leadbeater's reference to the chakras in the *Vahan*, noted above, suggest 1895–98 as the period during which his teachings on the chakras evolved, perhaps followed up in later years by ad hoc investigation to fill in details.

The Inner Life

Following his own lecture tours in America from 1900 to 1901 and 1902 to 1905, Leadbeater faced accusations of sexual improprieties with young boys. He resigned from membership in the TS in 1906 after an internal investigation in which he denied wrongdoing but admitted having taught them to masturbate to relieve sexual frustration as a matter of psychological and spiritual health. However, he resumed clairvoyant investigations with Besant in 1907, the year she was elected as the second president of the TS. Amid controversy, she reinstated Leadbeater in 1909 and invited him to live and work at the TS International Headquarters in Adyar, India.[13]

During his extended residency at Adyar (1909–14), Leadbeater gave regular evening talks to resident workers on the rooftop of the compound's central building, publishing two series of them in 1910 and 1911 in separate volumes, under the collective title *The Inner Life*.[14] Volume 1 provided details of his clairvoyant investigations of the chakras in chapters on "Force-Centers" and "The

Serpent-Fire." Here is a summary of what he observed during these investigations:

- **Appearance**: "saucer-like depressions in the surface" of the etheric body
- **Motion**: vortices "in rapid rotation"; "sluggish" or "glowing and pulsating with living light"
- **Petals**: actually spokes resulting from wavelike "undulations" as forces "rush round in the vortex"
- **Color**: a "shimmering, iridescent effect like mother-of-pearl," yet each has "its own predominant color"
- **Size**: two inches across (when undeveloped) and dull in color to saucer-sized (four to six inches) and "blazing and coruscating like miniature suns" (when developed)
- **Function**: bringing "the Divine Life [vitality] into the physical body"[15]

When fully awakened, the etheric-body chakras "bring down into physical consciousness" the characteristics of their associated astral centers. According to Leadbeater, this "is the only way in which the dense body can be brought to share all [the] advantages" (powers) associated with the astral centers. Thus the etheric-body chakras become "gates of connection between the physical and astral bodies."[16]

Leadbeater also perceived a protective web between each etheric-body chakra and its astral counterpart: "This web is the natural protection provided by nature to prevent a premature opening up of communication between the planes—a development which could lead to nothing but injury." Using alcohol, drugs, and tobacco, as well as becoming the victim of physical accident or emotional trauma engendered by terror or rage (including one's own) can damage or destroy this web.[17] The result is undesirable exposure to astral influences and beings—what contemporary astral projectors call negative entities.[18]

Leadbeater did away with the genital chakra, moved the navel chakra into its place, and added a spleen chakra—which, being on the left side of the body, was out of alignment with the spine. I return to the spleen chakra momentarily and deal with possible reasons for these changes in the next chapter.

Concerning correspondences, Leadbeater referred to a table in Blavatsky's Esoteric Instructions, stating: "These seven [chakras] are often described as corresponding to the seven colors and to the notes of the musical scale."[19] He also commented on Rudolf Steiner's recently published account of the chakras, examined earlier:

> I have heard it suggested that each of the different petals of these force-centers represents a moral quality, and that the development of that quality brings the center into activity. I have not yet met with any facts which confirm this, nor am I able to see exactly how it can be, because the appearance is produced by certain quite definite and easily recognizable forces, and the petals in any particular center are either active or not active according as these forces have or have not been aroused, and their development seems to me to have no more connection with morality than has the development of the biceps.[20]

Following in the footsteps of the Tantras, Leadbeater assigned spiritual powers to the chakras in a typically Western way, as a continuum of human potential. As we shall see, it is difficult to deduce the rationale determining which powers get assigned to which chakras in the Tantras. Leadbeater's presentation is orderly and progressive, implying that, as the kundalini rises through each chakra of the astral body, that body's development is enhanced until it becomes completely formed and functional, able to operate without hindrance on the astral plane. However, fully developed etheric-body chakras allow memories of experiences on higher planes to become to our ordinary waking consciousness on the physical plane. The result is a state of "continuous consciousness," in which the experiencer is simultaneously aware of happenings on the physical and astral planes whether the physical body is awake (active) or asleep (resting).

Pryse and Leadbeater appear to have come up with their respective arrangements of the chakras as a continuum of human potential at about the same time. The preface of *Apocalypse Unsealed* is signed September 1910. Leadbeater's chapters on the chakras in *The Inner Life* were first published as an article in the *Theosophist* in May of that year.[21] However, Leadbeater's version makes no mention of the principles; it describes, in fact, two separate but related continuums, one for the astral body and one for the etheric.

Table 9 lists Leadbeater's descriptions of the colors and powers associated with the astral and etheric-body chakras. The powers associated with the latter are essentially the same as with the former. They allow not only full perception and recall of astral experiences in ordinary waking consciousness, but also perception on the etheric level of being—which may include seeing, hearing, or experiencing the feelings of etheric beings such as nature spirits (elves, gnomes, fairies, etc.). I have added a column listing Blavatsky's color associations for comparison.

The Hidden Side of Things

In 1913, Leadbeater published another two-volume series of rooftop talks, *The Hidden Side of Things*. The fourth chapter of volume 1 dealt with "How We Are Influenced by the Sun." Several sections of this chapter detailed Leadbeater's clairvoyant investigations of the chakras of the etheric body (or etheric double, as he called it) in relation to "vitality"—Leadbeater's name for prana.[23] Having introduced the spleen chakra in *The Inner Life*, Leadbeater proceeded to clarify its function. It draws in vitality from sunlight and breaks it down into five colored energies, or rays, which are then distributed throughout the chakra system. Each chakra specializes in a particular ray, absorbing it and passing it on to vivify other etheric-body chakras and the physical nerves and organs associated with them.

There is no need to summarize this complex material here. It is

Table 9
Leadbeater's Colors and Powers (1910)

Locations	Colors (Leadbeater)	Colors (Blavatsky)[22]	Astral Body Powers	Etheric Body Powers
7. Crown	Prismatic with gold and white center	Prismatic/blue	Perfection of faculties	Continuous consciousness between waking and sleep
6. Between eyebrows	Half rose-yellow / half purplish-blue	Yellow	Astral sight	Waking visions / clairvoyance
5. Throat	Silvery blue	Indigo	Hearing astral beings	Clairaudience
4. Heart	Golden	Green or yellow	Comprehension of feelings of astral beings	Awareness of joys and sorrows of others
3. Spleen	Sun-like	Red or green	Astral travel	Recall in physical body of astral journeys
2. Navel or solar plexus	Red and green	Violet or red	Power of feeling / sensitivity to astral influences	Consciousness of astral influences
1. Base of spine	Orange-red	Orange-red	Awakening of kundalini	Awakening of kundalini

perhaps better presented visually than verbally. In 1925, just before Leadbeater released *The Chakras*, such a visual portrayal was produced by a resident worker at Adyar, Canadian Lieutenant Colonel Arthur E. Powell (1882–1969): *The Etheric Double: The Health Aura*. Powell compiled everything Leadbeater had previously written on the chakras and illustrated it with diagrams of individual chakras and of the system as a whole.

Figure 12 depicts the absorption of so-called vitality globules from the sun by the spleen chakra and their differentiation into colored pranas with various functions that are then distributed to the chakras. The chakras are identified not only by location and number of petals but also by the psychic powers that develop when the kundalini is awakened in the "base of spine" chakra and rises through each in turn to the "top of the head" chakra. As noted, this list of psychic powers represents Leadbeater's attempt to rationalize the apparently random catalog of such abilities in Eastern teachings. These abilities are listed in the *Śiva Saṃhitā* as follows:

1. **Muladhara**—levitation, "brilliancy of the body," freedom from disease; cleverness, omniscience; mastery "of unheard of sciences together with their mysteries" (5.64–66)
2. **Svadhishthana**—adoration by "all beautiful goddesses," freedom from disease and death; "moves throughout the universe fearlessly"; fearless recitation of Shastras and "sciences unknown" (5.76–78)
3. **Manipura**—"destroys sorrows and diseases, cheats death, can enter the body of another"; perceives adepts, discovers medicines and hidden treasures (5.81–82)
4. **Anahata**—clairvoyance, clairaudience, and astral travel ("power to walk in the air") (5.86)
5. **Vishuddha**—wisdom, instant understanding of the mysteries of the Vedas; adamantine strength "for a thousand years" (5.91, 94)
6. **Ajna**—salvation, destruction of karma (5.99, 111)

7. **Sahasrara**—knowledge of Brahman, liberation from rebirth (5.125)[24]

This catalog appears chaotic to the Western mind because there does not seem to be a discernible progression from lower to higher chakras. However, Leadbeater's list does imply such a progression. Though supplanted in many popular books on the chakras (it does not appear in Judith's *Wheels of Life*), this list did not entirely vanish from Western teachings that correlate the chakras with psychic development, such as *The Psychic Healing Book* by Amy Wallace and Bill Henkin (1978).[25] I return to Leadbeater's list of chakra functions in the final chapter.

In *The Hidden Side of Things*, Leadbeater was drawing on ancient Hindu teachings on the five prana-vayus. The *Chāndogya Upaniṣad*, dating to around the sixth century BCE, speaks of channels of the heart with five colors (brown, white, blue, yellow, and red) that are the same as the colors of the sun (8.6.1). By the time of the fourteenth- or fifteenth-century-CE Yoga Upanishads, the prana-vayus are identified with names, functions, colors, elements, bijas, and locations in the body (rectum, navel, heart, throat, and the whole body—thus suggesting a relation to at least four chakras).[26]

As noted, several years before the publication of *The Inner Life* and *The Hidden Side of Things*, Steiner described a "wonderful organ" in the area of the heart with functions similar to those of the spleen chakra described by Leadbeater. Steiner's association of the heart with this organ corresponds to the passage from the *Chāndogya Upaniṣad*. However, Blavatsky had stated in one of the Esoteric Instructions that "the spleen acts as the center of prana in the body, from which the life is pumped out and circulated"[27]—and Leadbeater went with her.

Perhaps to avoid burdening his English listeners and readers with Sanskrit words (a policy also adopted by Besant when speaking outside India), Leadbeater did not mention the names of the five prana-vayus in *The Hidden Side of Things*. A table in *The Chakras* restored this missing information, citing the *Gheraṇḍa*

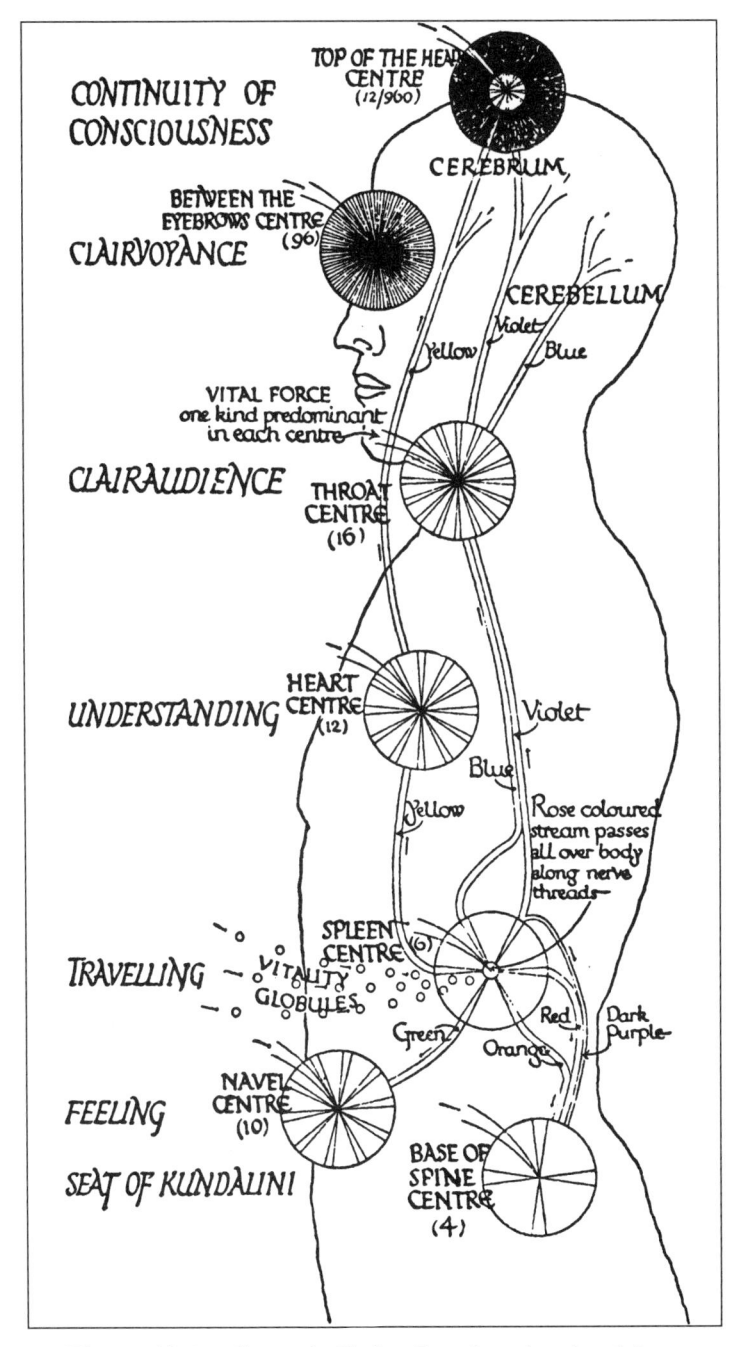

Figure 12. Leadbeater's Chakra Functions (reprinted from
A. E. Powell, *The Etheric Double*, 1925)

Saṃhitā and making it appear that "the five airs as thus described seem to agree fairly well with the five divisions of vitality which we have observed,"[28] as if these correlations confirmed Leadbeater's clairvoyant observations rather than inspired or influenced them. The colors, of course, are different. Leadbeater's system does not use brown or white, as mentioned in the *Chāndogya Upaniṣad*. He retains blue, yellow, and red, while adding green and rose and changing red to orange-red and blue to blue-violet. Thus all seven colors of light in Sir Isaac Newton's division of the spectrum are represented (plus rose, which lies outside that spectrum).

The prana-vayus play little or no role in the evolution of the Western chakra system until the development of a popular system of pranic healing by Chinese-Philippine businessman and occultist Choa Kok Sui in the 1980s. Nevertheless, Leadbeater has taken an important East/West step by bringing the chakras and the rainbow colors into association with each other more explicitly than did Blavatsky in the Esoteric Instructions. It would be some years yet before correspondences between the chakras and the spectrum would sort themselves into the root to crown, red to violet pattern we are familiar with today.

Chapter 13
The Duel of Leadbeater and Woodroffe

There are two radically different photographs of Sir John Woodroffe—who, as noted, wrote under the pseudonym Arthur Avalon. One shows a scholarly British man in middle age, seated with book in hand, a thoughtful expression. He wears a tie and jacket. Behind him books rise row upon row. That is clearly Sir John, trained in the law at Oxford University and employed in the high court of Calcutta, first as an advocate, then as a judge, finally as chief justice. He was also a professor of law at Calcutta University and later at Oxford University in England.

The other photograph shows him in a guise that few Brits of his generation would have condoned. He is barefoot, wearing a thin Indian tunic, and standing in front of an ancient Indian temple. That would be Arthur Avalon, the writer and lecturer on Tantra. He was a scholar in that field as well, having translated numerous tantric texts from Sanskrit into English. But he was also the disciple of a tantric guru, whose teachings he presented in *Principles of Tantra*, mentioned in chapter 5. Woodroffe was bucking against not only the conventions of Anglo-Indian society, but also those of Hindu society, since he was explaining and defending the philosophy and mysticism of Tantra, ignored by scholars as unimportant and shunned by orthodox Hindus as morally repugnant.[1]

As noted by his biographer, Kathleen Taylor, the name Woodroffe chose for his alter ego, Arthur Avalon, suggests the quest for the Holy Grail in Western myth and mysticism.[2] Perhaps for him the salvation sought by King Arthur's knights corresponded to the salvation sought by Indian practitioners of Tantra.

The Serpent Power

Woodroffe's *The Serpent Power*, first published in 1919, played a vital role in transmitting Indian teachings on kundalini and the chakras from East to West. For decades, *The Serpent Power* and

Leadbeater's *The Chakras* were among the few sources of such information available in the West, the former more Eastern than Western, vice versa for the latter.

Because of the impeccable scholarship evinced in *The Serpent Power*, this book had an impact not only on Western esotericists but also on Western scholars and psychologists, such as Carl Jung. Its publication marked a new epoch in the development of the Western chakra system. The first epoch was represented by the introduction of tantric teachings on kundalini and the chakras to the West via the Theosophical Society. These teachings were first presented by Indians and then interpreted in terms of Western esotericism by Blavatsky. Clairvoyant investigations by Steiner and Leadbeater ensued. *The Serpent Power* and *The Chakras* became the primary Western authorities on the topic. Alice Bailey, the subject of the next chapter, acknowledged her debt to both sources.[3]

Woodroffe was aware of Leadbeater's *The Inner Life*. In the introduction to *The Serpent Power*, he took Leadbeater to task for how little his clairvoyant observations tallied with tantric tradition. There is no need to enumerate Woodroffe's gripes. To do so would merely summarize material already presented in the first three chapters of this book and lay it side by side with that presented in the previous chapter. However, there are three points to comment on.

First, Woodroffe was unable to countenance Leadbeater's alarm over "phallic sorcery"—sorcery undertaken in connection with the sexual center. Woodroffe's Indian informants seemed "in general unaware" of such subjects.[4] However, he admitted in a footnote that there were tantric practitioners who sought sexual "commerce with female spirits and the like," but the text translated in *The Serpent Power* had "nothing to do with sexual black magic"; instead it dealt with liberation.[5]

In *Kiss of the Yoginī*, David Gordon White lays bare the sexual substratum of tantric ritual, especially that of the left-hand path. Sorcery involving sexual commerce with the terrifying goddesses called yogini appears as the subject of some of the earliest tantric texts.[6] Other forms of sorcery, such as the "six actions," which involve control of victims and destruction of enemies, recur in these texts over hundreds of years.[7] One senses that Woodroffe was whitewashing (or at least trying to avoid triggering cultural prejudice against Tantra) and Leadbeater was right on this count.

Second, Woodroffe pointed out that Leadbeater altered the number of spokes in sahasrara from 1000 to 960. In a footnote, Woodroffe indicated that the number 1000 is merely "symbolic of magnitude," though it also reflects twenty repetitions of the fifty letters of the Sanskrit alphabet. Thus Leadbeater dropped twenty repetitions of two of these letters to come up with 960. Perhaps 960 spokes was simply what he *saw* during clairvoyant observations and, without realizing the rationale of the petal/letter linkages in the Eastern system, he felt he was correcting an error. However, I suspect he was proceeding along tried-and-true Western esoteric lines—through numerology.

In *The Inner Life*, the numbers of petals or spokes are given as 4, 6, 10, 12, 16, 96, and 960, with the sixth chakra having two petal-like halves, each with 48 spokes. These numbers yield the following numerological derivations:

- $4 + 2 = 6$ (first and sixth chakras to get second)
- $4 + 6 = 10$ (first and second to get third)
- $4 + 6 + 2 = 12$ (first, second, and sixth to get fourth)
- $4 + 10 + 2 = 16$ (first, third, and sixth to get fifth)
- $4 + 12 = 16$ (first and fourth to get fifth)
- $6 + 10 = 16$ (second and third to get fifth)
- $4 \times 12 = 48$ (first and fourth to get half of sixth)
- $6 \times 16 = 96$ (second and fifth to get sixth)
- $6 \times 10 \times 16 = 960$ (second, third, and fifth to get seventh)
- $10 \times 96 = 960$ (fifth and sixth to get seventh)
- $4 \times 12 \times 10 \times 2 = 960$ (first, fourth, and fifth times two petals of sixth to get seventh)

Leadbeater also mentioned a "subsidiary whirlpool" within sahasrara that generates twelve additional spokes—perhaps referring to the guru chakra mentioned in *Gheraṇḍa Saṃhitā* 6.10, which is situated at the top of the head and has twelve petals.

Third, Woodroffe described in detail the experience of an unnamed European friend who had read some English translations of tantric texts and who "believed he had roused [kundalini] by meditative processes alone"—that is, without a guru. His friend wrote to him in vivid detail about the sights, sounds, and other sensations that accompanied his experiments. The most dramatic result was the rising of the kundalini in a spiraling motion that wove back and forth between the left and right channels, crossing the central channel. When it reached the head, the kundalini spread out like wings, reminding this friend of the caduceus (wand) of the god Mercury.[8]

This story is the likely source of an illustration of the movements of kundalini forming a caduceus that first appeared in Leadbeater's *The Hidden Life in Freemasonry* (1926) and a year later was carried over into *The Chakras*.[9] Graphic portrayals of the caduceus/chakra correlation are a staple of New Age books on the chakras and pop up frequently on the Internet. Such illustrations dramatically demonstrate the grafting of Western cultural symbols

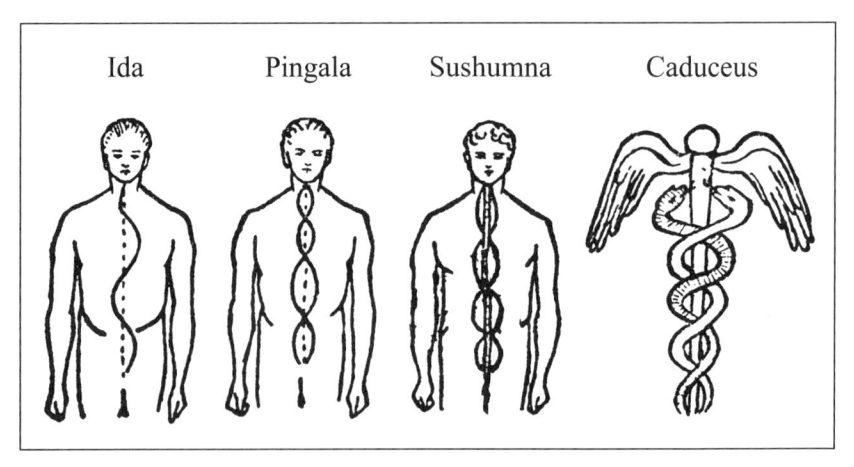

Figure 13. Nadis and Caduceus (adapted from C. W. Leadbeater, *The Hidden Life in Freemasonry*, 1926)

and ideas onto Eastern tantric roots—a project Woodroffe was denigrating in Leadbeater, but of which he became an unwitting agent.

The Chakras

Seventeen years after the publication of *The Inner Life*, Leadbeater produced what may be his best-known work, *The Chakras: A Monograph*, which has sold hundreds of thousands of copies since it came out in 1927.[10] Though present-day readers already exposed to the Western chakra system find the book confusing, it nevertheless represents an important stage in the splitting away of the Western system from the Eastern one.

When I edited and annotated Leadbeater's book, I identified how the material on this subject from *The Inner Life* and *The Hidden Side of Things* was cut and pasted, rearranged, and modified. I noted what was omitted or added and how certain elements were changed. In an appendix, I included changed and omitted passages, as well as supplementary material from another book. Assuming an audience of well-read Theosophists, Leadbeater used obscure technical terms that would frustrate beginners or send them to other books, now unavailable. I created a stand-alone version of *The Chakras* so readers would not have to go elsewhere to find what they needed to understand it.[11]

The most noticeable additions made to *The Chakras* were the dozens of references to Sanskrit texts. These references were supplied by Leadbeater's literary assistant, Ernest Egerton Wood (1883–1965), who came to live and work at Adyar in 1908, just before Leadbeater's reinstatement and return. Wood became interested in learning Sanskrit some years earlier and continued to study for the rest of his life, publishing translations of several classics.[12]

As Wood reported in his autobiography, Leadbeater was living in Sydney, Australia, in 1926, when *The Chakras* was written. He was now a bishop in the Liberal Catholic Church—a reinvention of Catholicism along Theosophical lines, for which he had laid the groundwork during the war years, through clairvoyant investigations of the sacraments. Wood rejoined him there after a stay at Adyar, describing his role in the production of the book as follows:

> I placed before Bishop Leadbeater all the information on the subject available in Sanskrit works known to me. This book lagged for a long time, so I tried to make some investigations myself. Concentrating on the chakra between the eyebrows, I became aware of a double rotation like that of two plates revolving in opposite directions. I put this idea before Bishop Leadbeater. For several weeks he told me that he could not find it, but at last he did find such a double rotation in all the chakras, and explained it in his book.[13]

The Chakras cited many texts mentioned in this book, including the *Bhagavad Gītā*, *Garuḍa Purāṇa*, *Gheranda Saṃhitā*, *Haṭha-Yoga-Pradīpikā*, *Praśna Upaniṣad*, *Ṣaṭ-Cakra-Nirūpaṇa*, *Śiva Saṃhitā*, the Yoga Upanishads, and the *Yoga Sūtra* of Patañjali. Leadbeater also referred frequently to *The Serpent Power*. Woodroffe's eight-page discussion of the material on kundalini and the chakras in *The Inner Life* had provided Leadbeater with free advertising—why not return the favor? Since *The Serpent Power* was almost unreadable due to its compendiousness, density of language, and profusion of Sanskrit terms, Leadbeater's *The Chakras* offered a popular summary.

One important change Leadbeater made in *The Chakras* was to move the spleen chakra from third to second and the navel chakra from second to third. Now the second chakra was higher in the body than the third, as well as out of alignment with the spine. Oddly, he did not alter the order of the powers associated with the chakras he had moved. Those of the second and third chakras were now assigned to spleen and navel rather than navel and spleen.

Having discovered an 1897 French translation of a book originally published in 1723—*Theosophia Practica* by Johann Georg

Gichtel (1638–1710)—Leadbeater felt his intuitions about the existence of a spleen chakra were justified. Gichtel was a German mystic who enthusiastically studied, edited, and published the works of Jakob Böhme. His book was based on a mystical experience of 1664 that was recorded in a manuscript of 1696 and published with colored illustrations derived from descriptions in the manuscript. The mystical experience involved a serpent curled around the heart (kundalini moving through the heart chakra?). One painting highlighted seven locations in the torso and head of a human being that roughly corresponded to the locations of the chakras, including one on the left side of the body, possibly the spleen (see plate 5).[14]

Arthur Versluis argues that while this image does depict a Christian "esoteric physiology", it does not "show the exact equivalent of the *chakras*." Actually, it portrays an "unregenerate" individual, whose vital organs are under the influence of the four elements and seven astrological planets. Subsequent illustrations show the process of regeneration as a gradual elimination of these influences, which are replaced by four light-filled centers representing the Trinity (God-Jesus-Holy Spirit) plus Sophia (Wisdom). Unlike the kundalini path that runs along the spine, Gichtel's path of regeneration appears to be marked by the spiral, starting from the sun in the heart, associated with love.[15]

Leadbeater changed the chakras' color associations so that they were a closer match to those given by Blavatsky, the rose in the second chakra being akin to Blavatsky's violet (though there were still discrepancies). There was political agitation in the 1920s within the TS; hundreds of members were pushing against the policies and teachings of Besant and Leadbeater by means of a "Back to Blavatsky" movement. Perhaps Leadbeater's color changes were a sign of the times.[16]

The following table details the alterations from table 9 in the previous chapter.

Having usually encountered the rainbow system first, present-day students of the chakras find Leadbeater's colors confusing. Let us examine some possible reasons for the issues of the spleen

Table 10
Leadbeater's Colors and Powers (1927)

Names	Colors (Leadbeater)	Colors (Blavatsky)[17]	Astral Body Powers	Etheric Body Powers
7. Crown	Violet	Prismatic/blue	Perfection of faculties	Continuous consciousness between waking and sleep
6. Brow	Dark blue	Indigo	Astral sight	Waking visions / clairvoyance
5. Throat	Light blue	Blue	Hearing astral beings	Clairaudience
4. Heart	Yellow	Green or yellow	Comprehension of feelings of astral beings	Awareness of joys and sorrows of others
3. Navel	Green	Red or green	Astral travel	Recall in physical body of astral journeys
2. Spleen	Rose	Violet or red	Power of feeling / sensitivity to astral influences	Consciousness of astral influences
1. Root	Orange-red	Orange-red	Awakening of kundalini	Awakening of kundalini

chakra, the switched second and third chakras, and Leadbeater's color system.

As noted, the identification of the spleen as the source of the vitality of the physical body can be traced back Blavatsky's Esoteric Instructions, in which she says:

> The spleen corresponds to the linga-sharira [second principle], and serves as its dwelling-place, in which it lies curled up. As the linga-sharira is the reservoir of life for the body, the medium and vehicle of prana, the spleen acts as the center of prana in the body, from which the life is pumped out and circulated. It is consequently a very delicate organ, though the physical spleen is only the cover for the real spleen.[18]

The idea that the physical spleen is a cover for a real spleen must have given Leadbeater the impetus to consider a spleen chakra. In Blavatsky's list of the seven principles, linga was sometimes listed as the second principle, sometimes as the third—alternating with the principle of prana. This may be why the spleen chakra was listed as the third chakra in one book and the second in the other. However, there may be another reason, having to do with the absence of the genital chakra from Leadbeater's system.

As noted, in Buddhist Tantra, there are only five chakras. The sixth and seventh chakras are fused into one, located in the head; the first and second are also fused, and located below the navel. I indicated that Leadbeater seems to be following this lead by combining red-orange and blue-violet in his system of prana-vayus in relation to the chakras. By combining the root and genital chakras, Leadbeater effectively eliminated the latter, rolling its function into that of the first chakra. Thus there was little danger of its being awakened by unsuspecting aspirants, resulting in an exacerbation of distracting sensuality. Perhaps Leadbeater's Victorian upbringing was responsible for such a choice.[19]

In the later Western chakra system, red is assigned to the first chakra and orange to the second. Thus Leadbeater's combined red-orange color for the first chakra represents the fusion of these chakras. Indeed, Leadbeater claimed that "The orange-red ray flows to the base of the spine and thence to the generative organs, with which one part of its functions is closely connected."[20] Hence the sexual second chakra was not really eliminated, only hidden.

One advantage of hiding the sexual/genital chakra was that Leadbeater could add the spleen chakra to the system while maintaining the number seven, with all its occult correspondences. But the rose color of the spleen chakra was not part of the spectrum—implying that this chakra existed outside the scheme of the other chakras, just as its position was out of alignment with the spine, along which the other chakras were situated.

Now we can address the issue of Leadbeater's changing his mind about the position of the second and third chakras. By placing the spleen chakra second, as in *The Chakras*, he clearly made it a substitute for the missing sexual/genital chakra while maintaining the third chakra in the navel position, with which it was traditionally associated in the Tantras.

For present-day readers, the color issues are more complex. First, there is the expectation that illustrations of the chakras should show the chakra colors in the familiar rainbow order, one for each. But Leadbeater was investigating the ways in which vitality circulates between the chakras of the etheric body. His multicolored illustrations of the chakras reflect what he "saw" on the basis of what he was researching. Thus he was not recording "the color of each chakra" but the colors of several energies, or rays, moving through each chakra, one being predominant.

In Leadbeater's color system, the blue ray enters the throat and splits into a dark blue ray that proceeds to the brow chakra and a violet ray that proceeds to the crown chakra.[21] Thus these predominant rays correlate with the colors of the fifth, sixth, and seventh chakras as depicted in New Age books (blue, indigo or dark blue, and violet). We have seen how the orange-red ray represents the colors connected to the first and second chakras, and that the rose ray is not associated with the spectrum. That leaves only the green and yellow rays, corresponding to the third and fourth chakras, respectively.

How could Leadbeater not have taken the seemingly obvious step of building the chakra system in the order of the rainbow by linking yellow to the third chakra and green to the fourth? Maybe he was just reporting what he saw. However, he may also have hoped to discover validating correspondences between colors discussed in Blavatsky's Esoteric Instructions, those used in traditional tantric systems, and his own. It appears that Leadbeater collated several charts in the Esoteric Instructions to make the most favorable case for his observations—one result being that green was associated with the navel chakra and yellow with the heart chakra.[22]

In another table in *The Chakras*, Leadbeater compared his observations of the colors of the lotus petals in each chakra with those in three traditional tantric texts: *Ṣaṭ-Cakra-Nirūpaṇa*, *Śiva Saṃhitā* and the *Garuḍa Purāṇa*.[23] Those of the *Garuḍa Purāṇa* line up best with Leadbeater's observations—with three close correlations out of five (no color is given in the *Garuḍa Purāṇa* for the first chakra and the seventh is not mentioned in any of the texts). The "golden" heart chakra provides the most exact correspondence. Leadbeater was probably familiar with the *Garuḍa Purāṇa* when making clairvoyant observations recorded in *The Inner Life*. His assistant, Ernest Wood, began translating that ancient text in 1908, before they met, and published the translation in 1911—a year after the material on the chakras first came out.[24]

Leadbeater's Legacy

Shortly after the publication of *The Chakras*, an Indian spiritual teacher active in California, Rishi Singh Gherwal (1889–1964), published an impassioned protest against Leadbeater's work, citing "the harm to yoga philosophy that has been done by misinformation" from Leadbeater and calling him no "friend to the Hindus" and "the greatest enemy of yoga philosophy" and claiming that Leadbeater "has given a bad name to yoga." After complaining about the changes Leadbeater made to the number of petals in sahasrara and refuting his claim to have awakened the kundalini, Gherwal quoted at length from Woodroffe's critique in *The Serpent Power* of Leadbeater's teachings on the chakras from *The Inner Life*. Gherwal concluded that "it would really be a great joy to all yogis if Rev. Leadbeater will leave the yoga philosophy alone and give to the world what he wants, but by all means call it by some other name."[25]

Be that as it may, many subsequent Western accounts of the chakra system—and some Eastern accounts, such as those by Sri Chinmoy (1931–2007) and Satyananda Saraswati—owe something to Leadbeater's *The Chakras*.[26] Any system that mentions a spleen or splenic chakra bears his influence. Books that equate the spleen chakra with the third chakra derive their information from *The Inner Life* or from Powell's *The Etheric Double*. Those that equate it with the second chakra derive their information from *The Chakras*. The color system employed in *The Chakras* appears at least into the 1980s, after which it is more or less replaced by the familiar rainbow system. Any book influenced by Leadbeater is immediately identifiable by the presence of a rose-colored spleen chakra, a green third chakra, and a gold fourth chakra.

Perhaps the most notable contributions of Leadbeater's book to the Western chakra system are the *names* by which the chakras are known today: root, navel, heart, throat, brow, and crown. In this, he was following the tantric tradition of naming chakras according to their locations, as well as the policy of the TS under Besant, which was to substitute English for Sanskrit terms (mula, nabhi, hridaya, kantha, bhrumadya, and murdhan). Only the genital (medhra) chakra—also called sexual or sacral—was missing.

A subtler contribution to the evolution of the Western chakra system is Leadbeater's novel resolution of the question of the locations of the chakras. Based on his front-view diagram of these locations (see plate 6), later writers are apt to decry the fact that his spleen and heart chakras are out of alignment with the vertical center line of the body. But the side-view diagram (see plate 7), goes unnoticed, despite its complete makeover of the Eastern system.

The chakras originate in the spinal ganglia, as in Basu. However, they grow out from there toward the front of the body in a funnel-like shape that opens into a circular vortex. Thus, in the side view, each seems to have a stem and to develop into a blooming flower. They are no longer horizontally placed lotuses with their petals facing *upward*, as in *The Serpent Power*, but morning-glory-like flowers facing *outward*. After Leadbeater, Alice Bailey is almost alone among Western writers in illustrating the chakras as upward-facing lotuses.[27]

As noted in chapter 2, this shift in depicting the chakras may have reflected a move away from the Eastern notion of achieving liberation of the higher self through an ascending ladder of increasingly spiritual but discrete planes arranged horizontally. Replacing this notion was the Western motivation of achieving personal fulfillment through developing the lower self along a vertically arranged continuum of human potential stretching from physical survival to spiritual enlightenment.

Pryse and Leadbeater took the first steps in this new direction. The chromotherapists discussed in the next section carried it forward, linking the rainbow colors to the chakra system—thereby implying the vertical continuity of the Western chakra system. The psychologists and yogis discussed in part 5 added the chakra qualities, which, like the spectrum, shaded imperceptibly from physical to emotional, mental, and spiritual, thus completing the transformation of the chakra system into a continuum.

Note that in plate 7, the chakra at the base of the spine faces the back of the body, not the front. Decades later, in the 1970s and 1980s, the notion that the chakras express themselves with openings in both the front and the back of the body was developed from this hint—in the work of several authors discussed later: John Pierrakos, Barbara Brennan, and Choa Kok Sui.

Incidentally, the original plates portraying Leadbeater's clairvoyant perceptions of individual chakras, created by Alfred Edward Warner (1879–1968), a British printmaker working in Sydney, Australia,[28] were intended to suggest the perspective of looking into a deep funnel. Color variations in the plates in editions after the first tend to erase this effect, which I rediscovered by accident. Having copied an image of the heart chakra from a website that used scanned images from Leadbeater's book, I played with the contrast to bring out the color more strongly in a PowerPoint slide. After several such adjustments, the funnel effect suddenly appeared. (See plate 1B, an image from the first edition of *The Chakras*.)

Some later clairvoyants describe the chakras as circular disks, cylinders, or spheres, with or without cones projecting toward the front and back of the body. Sometimes the chakras are perceived as anchored to the spine, sometimes as organized vertically along an imaginary line running up the center of the body.[29] Thus Leadbeater's perception of a single flower-like funnel with a stem attached to the spine has apparently been improved or refined rather than replaced.

Despite the innovations mentioned, Leadbeater was primarily a consolidator and validator. He attempted to interpret and reconcile disparate teachings from Blavatsky, Steiner, and tantric scriptures on the basis of his own clairvoyant observations. The result could perhaps be called an eastward-leaning Western system. The influence of this system was so pervasive, even among Eastern teachers, that it is also possible to identify westward-leaning Eastern systems on the basis of borrowings from Leadbeater. For example, the sections of Saraswati's *Kundalini Tantra* dealing with the "psychic propensities" of the chakras combine traditional tantric teachings with the astral-body powers described by Leadbeater.[30]

From *The Inner Life* (including a pamphlet containing its sections on "force-centers" and the "serpent fire") to *The Hidden Side of Things* and *The Chakras*, Leadbeater's writings on the chakras were widely distributed in Western European languages during the twentieth century. Translations of one or more of these works appeared in Dutch, French, German, Italian, Spanish, and even Swedish. I have not seen native exploration of the chakras from esoteric or clairvoyant perspectives in these countries until the 1980s. Thus Leadbeater's visions of the chakras as colorful, whirling wheels reigned supreme in much of the Western world for more than half a century.

Part 4
Chromotherapy:
Science of Rays, Colors, and Glands
(1920s–1950s)

Chapter 14
Alice Bailey and the Seven Rays

Alice Ann Bailey (née La Trobe-Bateman; 1880–1949) was born into a wealthy British family. Estranged from her first husband, Walker Evans, she first encountered Theosophy during World War I, while living in California, where she worked in a fish-packing factory to support her two children. In 1917, the year she divorced her husband, she joined the Pacific Grove Lodge of the Theosophical Society. She also became a member of the Esoteric School of Theosophy, at that time headed by Besant, and began working at the school's center in Hollywood, called Krotona after the location in Italy of a school of philosophy founded by the ancient Greek mathematician, musician, and mystic, Pythagoras. There she met her second husband, Foster Bailey, whom she married in 1922.

In 1919, she began to receive inwardly and record in writing a series of dictations from a source of spiritual teaching who eventually came to be known as the Tibetan and was identified as the Master DK (Djwal Khul; various spellings), a disciple of the Master KH (Kuthumi; various spellings—one of the Masters involved in the founding of the TS). Some of these dictations were published under the name Alice Evans in the *Theosophist* in 1920–21. Because of their involvement in the back-to-Blavatsky movement, Alice and Foster lost their jobs at Krotona. They founded their own Arcane School, a correspondence course based on the teachings of the Tibetan. They also established a publishing company, now called Lucis Trust, to oversee the production of books of these teachings. From the first books of dictation, *Initiation: Human and Solar* and *Letters on Occult Meditation*, both published in 1922, to those published posthumously in the 1950s, the chakras (usually called centers or lotuses) were constantly under discussion.[1]

Bailey is a controversial figure in the Theosophical movement. For some, she represents the culmination of the Theosophical revelations that began with the Mahatma letters of the 1880s—just as the Upanishads were the culmination and "end" of the Vedas in Hindu tradition. Others deny she could have been channeling a Theosophical Master. Despite her own belief that her work was following up on and filling out hints provided in the works of her beloved mentor, Madame Blavatsky, purists in the Theosophical movement point out myriad inconsistencies and dismiss her teachings as third-generation Theosophy, neo-Theosophy, or pseudo-Theosophy.

Bailey's books provide a macrocosmic overview of the evolutionary process of consciousness on its journey into matter and back to unity with its individual and collective spiritual Source. Nearly everything she wrote is traceable, at least in outline, to statements made by Blavatsky, especially in *The Secret Doctrine* and the Esoteric Instructions. However, the degree of elaboration—in which mere hints by Blavatsky are magnified into vast hierarchical systems designed to explain how evolution proceeds at subhuman (mineral, vegetable, animal), human, superhuman (Masters), nonhuman (devic or angelic), and logoic (godlike or supercosmic) levels—often obscures these connections. Even the smallest portion of this macrocosmic plan, such as the subject of the psychic or spiritual centers (chakras) and human evolution, is dealt with so exhaustively that a whole book would be required simply to collate or summarize teachings scattered through the twenty-four books of the Bailey canon.

For this reason, I focus only on teachings that had a direct impact on the evolution of the Western chakra system. By *direct*, I mean that subsequent writers on the chakras carried these teachings forward, possibly without knowing their origin. Furthermore, I deal primarily with those aspects of Bailey's work that served as an inspiration for several generations of chromotherapists (color healers)—which is why I place her at the head of this section. For them, she was not the end of Blavatsky, but the beginning of something new—a body of literature providing a sketch of the theory and suggestions for the practice of esoteric healing (now called energy medicine).

Esoteric healing is but one of many focuses in the Bailey corpus. However, this focus is the matrix from which two components of the Western chakra system developed: the association of chakras with endocrine glands and with colors of the rainbow.

Initiation: Human and Solar

Bailey's first book, *Initiation: Human and Solar*, makes but one contribution to the development of the Western chakra system. This contribution, not often encountered in later books, concerns the relationship between seven planes, bodies, initiations, and chakras. For Bailey, initiations are expansions of consciousness that take place in late phases of human evolution. Each initiation requires the mastery of certain ethical and spiritual principles and their associated tasks, often involving not only life on the physical plane, but also life on higher planes. Thus every initiation requires the mastery of a particular body, such that it becomes a fully functional vehicle of consciousness on its associated plane.

The subject of initiation was a favorite of Besant and Leadbeater, who defined and explained a sequence of five such initiations that complete the human stage of evolution and usher in the superhuman stage. The fifth initiation produces a Master, who has fully functional vehicles of consciousness on five planes: physical, astral, mental, buddhic, and nirvanic. To these, Bailey added two more superhuman initiations involving the monadic and divine (in her terms, logoic) planes. As noted, there are only five manifested planes in our universe. An explanation of how the sixth and seventh initiations involve the two unmanifested planes is outside the scope of this book.

In *Initiation: Human and Solar*, Bailey made the following statements:

- "Each of the five initiations . . . affects one of the centers in man."
- At each initiation, a secret is imparted.

- "Each secret concerns one or other of the seven great planes of the solar system."
- "Each secret concerns some one ray or color and gives the number, note, and the vibration which corresponds."[2]

To a serious Bailey student, this summary will seem oversimplified. I have left out much, including the names by which the five initiations are known and the centers associated with each. Such things were not carried on by mainstream proponents of the Western chakra system, such as Anodea Judith. However, Vera Stanley Alder (1898–1984), a popularizer of Bailey's teachings, published the following statements in 1939, and this formulation of the same ideas *was* carried forward by a few later writers, both Eastern (Osho) and Western (Barbara Brennan):

- "The human being as a whole contains forty-nine centers, which correspond to the seven planes and their division into seven subplanes each; and the seven colored rays, each with their seven subdivisions."
- There are "seven major initiations" which have "each their seven subsidiary lesser initiations, making forty-nine in all."
- "These correspond or are allocated one to each of the forty-nine subplanes of the seven planes of matter."
- "Each of these subplanes has to be conquered by the aspirant, first within his own body by his mode of living, and secondly by his understanding, thus giving him power to act with and upon it."
- "At each of these conquests, one of his centers has been developed and coordinated to the point where the spiritual wisdom and force appertaining to it can gain admittance and henceforth flow uninterruptedly."
- "The inauguration of this flow constitutes an initiation."
- "When the aspirant has conquered or mastered all the subdivisions of a plane, he is ready to take the major initiation of that plane."[3]

As noted, in Hindu Tantra, the seven chakras were sometimes linked with seven heavenly realms called lokas. In Blavatsky's Esoteric Instructions, these realms were further linked with elements, planes, and principles.[4] Blavatsky described the planes without names, in terms of their inhabitants, and the chakras did not appear. Bailey's linkage of chakras and planes required the intermediary step of Besant's formulation of names for the planes. Since Bailey worked directly from Blavatsky's Esoteric Instructions, she did not need Leadbeater's intervention to link the principles and chakras—though she did use his account of the chakra system from *The Inner Life* for other purposes. Bailey's linking of seven initiations to the planes, bodies, and chakras appears to be original. However, it may reflect her exposure to teachings of the ES based on clairvoyant investigations by Besant and Leadbeater, to which the public has no access.

Letters on Occult Meditation

Bailey's second book, *Letters on Occult Meditation*, contains a section entitled "The Use of Color and Sound," which provided a powerful impetus for color healers. Although she often mentioned links between the seven colors of the spectrum and the seven rays and chakras, neither Bailey nor the Tibetan ever produced a definitive list of correspondences. Or, more accurately, they produced multiple apparently contradictory lists—especially those connecting colors and rays—to demonstrate that such correspondences depend on the aspects of microcosmic, human, superhuman, or macrocosmic evolution under consideration. Furthermore, the Tibetan explained there were cogent reasons for concealing the precise correlation of colors and rays:

> It is not yet permissible to give out the esoteric significance of these colors, nor exact information as to their order and application. The dangers are too great, for in the right understanding of the laws of color and in the

knowledge (for instance) of which color stands for a particular ray lies the power the Adept wields.[5]

Blinds were used to conceal such correlations. Conflicting lists of exoteric versus esoteric colors were given. Sometimes complementary colors (those opposite each other on the color wheel of three primary and three secondary colors: red/green, blue/orange, and yellow/violet) were substituted for each other. It is therefore impossible to summarize this material without placing it in contradiction with lists given in other Bailey books. Only the principles remain consistent from book to book. Such principles include the following:

- There are seven rays, three primary and four secondary, each named according to its function (what it contributes to all levels of being).
- The three primary "rays of aspect" are called (1) will/power; (2) love/wisdom; and (3) and activity/adaptability.[6]
- The four secondary "rays of attribute" are called (4) harmony/beauty/art/unity; (5) concrete knowledge / science; (6) idealism/devotion; and (7) ceremonial magic / law.[7]
- We are each affiliated with a monadic ray, one of the three rays of aspect, particularly influencing our mental body; an egoic, or soul, ray, which is the basis for all our incarnations during a vast evolutionary cycle of perfecting humanity, particularly influencing our astral body; and a personality ray, which changes from lifetime to lifetime,[8] particularly influencing our physical body, determining "its life trend and purpose, its appearance and occupation."[9]
- Other ray affiliations involve each of our bodies, the evolutionary phase represented by our race, and the phase represented by a particular historical period.[10]

Because all such ray affiliations may be described in terms of colors, it seems plausible that an Adept capable of perceiving such colors in people's auras would know instantly everything there is to know about them, thus being able to determine exactly where they are in their evolutionary development. Even in this early book, we glimpse the cycles of evolution in terms of constant permutations of rays or colors at multiple levels in time, space, and higher planes, progressing over millions of earth years until some final goal is reached—presumably, when every evolutionary stage will line up in the usual order of the spectrum. However, as complex, rich, and fascinating as is this material on the rays, our only concern here is with aspects connected directly with the development of the Western chakra system.

Bailey began by citing the chakra system as presented in Leadbeater's *The Inner Life* and Powell's *The Etheric Double*. Thus, in her *Letters on Occult Meditation*, there is a spleen chakra in the third position and the solar-plexus chakra is in the second position. The colors are given as in Leadbeater. Oddly, the sixth chakra is connected with the pineal gland and the seventh with the pituitary—the opposite of Blavatsky's correspondences in the Esoteric Instructions. In later books, Bailey restored Blavatsky's order, eliminated the spleen chakra (listing it among twenty-one minor chakras); and restored the sexual/genital chakra (which she called sacral) to its original position as second and the navel/solar-plexus chakra to its original position as third—thus also restoring the spinal alignment of the chakras. Many later books adopt the term *sacral* for the second chakra instead of *genital*. Bailey was apparently the first to do so.[11]

It is possible that Bailey first linked the pineal gland with the sixth, or forehead, chakra because of its association with the third eye in Blavatsky's writings. Other writers on the chakras, such as Anodea Judith, have made a similar correlation. I have not seen it in the published works of Besant or Leadbeater—despite an inaccurate statement in the Wikipedia article, "Chakra," that states: "C. W. Leadbeater associated the Ajna [sixth] chakra with the pineal gland." Curiously, the endnote for this statement links to a page in *The Chakras* where Leadbeater indicates that the pineal gland is linked with the crown (seventh) chakra. Nevertheless, the inaccurate Wikipedia statement has been duplicated on hundreds of websites, demonstrating the Internet's capacity for disseminating misinformation.

Here is the list of chakras as presented in *Letters on Occult Meditation*, which will serve as a basis of comparison for the ways in which Bailey's writings about the chakras evolved over the next twenty-five years:

1. Base of spine
2. Solar plexus
3. Spleen
4. Heart
5. Throat
6. Pineal gland
7. Pituitary body[12]

The Light of the Soul

In 1927, Bailey published a commentary on the *Yoga Sūtra* of Patañjali, *The Light of the Soul*. The book contained what could be called a transitional list between that given in *Letters on Occult Meditation* and those given in later books. In this list, the brow and crown centers are replaced by a single "head center" associated with both the pituitary and pineal glands. Bailey numbered the centers from the top down. If she had done so from the bottom up, as most authors do, this list would have generated confusion for readers used to seeing the solar plexus, heart, and throat chakras as the third, fourth, and fifth chakras, respectively:

1. **Base of spine**—"eliminative organs, kidneys, bladder"
2. **Sacral**—"generative organs"
3. **Spleen**—spleen
4. **Solar plexus**—stomach
5. **Heart**—"pericardium, ventricles, auricles with spleen affected"

6. **Throat**—"larynx, vocal cords and palate, thyroid gland"
7. **Head center**—"brain, pineal gland, and pituitary body"[13]

This schema demonstrates that Bailey had not yet developed a complete list of endocrine glands. Its importance lies in its initiation of the process of pushing the spleen center out of the chakra system. It also uncoupled the first and second centers that Leadbeater had fused, adding a sacral center and providing one of the common names for the second chakra. Finally, it posited a center higher than the spleen, in the area of the solar plexus, which would eventually replace the former association of the third center with the navel in many later versions of the Western chakra system.

The Soul and Its Mechanism

For later writers, Bailey's main contribution to the Western chakra system is the linking of endocrine glands—of which the pineal is one—to the chakras. This correlation appears for the first time in *The Soul and Its Mechanism* (1930), one of Bailey's few books not written under dictation by the Tibetan:

1. **Base of spine**—adrenals
2. **Sacral**—gonads
3. **Solar plexus**—pancreas
4. **Heart**—thymus
5. **Throat**—thyroid
6. **Between eyebrows**—pituitary
7. **Head**—pineal[14]

This list reappeared in Bailey's subsequent (dictated) books whenever the subject of the centers was discussed. With modifications, it also appears in many later Western books on the chakras, such as Judith's *Wheels of Life*—though, as noted, Judith switches the affiliations for the pituitary and pineal glands.[15] Other writers reverse the affiliations for the adrenals and gonads or replace the pancreas with the spleen.

Esoteric Healing

Bailey's most comprehensive exposition of the chakra system occurs in her posthumously published *Esoteric Healing* (1953), providing a summary of material scattered throughout many earlier books. The glandular associations are included, but not those pertaining to ray or color. There are so many lists of rays, colors, and centers scattered throughout Bailey's books that subsequent writers may pick and choose—or ignore such correspondences entirely. However, the book adds information on the "energy" that each chakra "registers," thus producing another early list of Western chakra qualities.

Table 11 provides the association of chakras and glands made by Bailey, the association of rays and chakras (though only applying to a special type of humanity, "the average [spiritual] aspirant"), one version of the variable association of colors, and the energies registered—the chakra qualities.

For those used to Leadbeater or the rainbow system, it is disconcerting to see the color violet associated with the second chakra; it is usually associated with the seventh. According to Bailey, the reason for this association is that the seventh ray is currently "in manifestation" (since 1675 CE) as an expression of larger historical cycles of evolution and "is playing through the planetary sacral center, and then through the sacral center of every human being," in order to bring about "needed changes" in "the sex life."[20] Because of the fundamental importance of this association of the seventh ray with the sacral center in Bailey's teaching (she devoted a whole section of the first volume of *Esoteric Psychology* to the discussion of the "needed changes" in this area[21]), any subsequent list of correspondences between violet, the seventh ray, and the second chakra can be traced to her influence.

In later developments of the Western chakra system, the ray and color associations in this list drop out, but the glands and several qualities remain:

Table 11
Bailey's Contributions to the Chakra System (1930–53)

Chakras (Centers)	Glands[16]	Rays[17]	Colors[18]	Energies Registered[19]
7. Head	Pineal	1. Will/power	Red	Synthesis/purpose
6. Brow	Pituitary	5. Concrete knowledge	Indigo	Intention/imagination
5. Throat	Thyroid	3. Active intelligence	Green	Creativity
4. Heart	Thymus	2. Love/wisdom	Blue	Love
3. Solar plexus	Pancreas	6. Devotion	Silvery rose	Desire
2. Sacral	Gonads	7. Ceremonial magic	Violet	Sexuality
1. Base of spine	Adrenals	4. Harmony	Yellow	Will-to-live

- In the first chakra, *will-to-live* becomes *survival*.
- *Sexuality* and *love* remain connected to the second and fourth chakras.
- *Desire* is sometimes added to the more familiar designation of the third chakra—*power*.
- *Creativity* is sometimes added to the more familiar designation of the fifth chakra—*communication* or *self-expression*.
- *Imagination* is more likely to appear in association with the sixth chakra than *intention*.
- The notions of *synthesis* and *purpose* in the seventh chakra fall away, replaced by *transcendence* or *cosmic consciousness*.

Some later sources link clairvoyance and mediumship with the solar-plexus chakra. Their source may be Bailey's *Esoteric Healing*. Bailey makes a distinction between the unreliable, astrally influenced psychic information received through this chakra and the more reliable, soul-based information received through the brow chakra.[22]

Whereas *Letters on Occult Meditation* had a powerful influence on esotericists in the thirty years after its publication in 1922, especially on color healers working with the chakra system, *Esoteric Healing* replaced it as the primary mode of transmission of Bailey's teachings on the chakras in the latter half of the twentieth century. For example, the notions of "blocked" chakras in the etheric body as a component or cause of physical illness and of chakra "balancing" as a mode of promoting healing and well-regulated self-development receive extensive treatment in *Esoteric Healing*.[23] These notions become the basis of, or are grafted onto, several approaches to energy healing that became popular in the 1970s and later, such as Polarity Therapy, Reiki, and Sui's Pranic Healing.

In her impact on the Western chakra system, Bailey was as much an innovator as was her revered Madame Blavatsky. However, Blavatsky's contribution consisted of fragmentary hints and speculations on ways the Eastern chakra system might be used by Western esotericists for spiritual development. Bailey's focus was different: to explain everything in Blavatsky's work to the nth degree. She produced a rich vein of material on the chakras for later writers, especially those interested in esoteric healing, to mine. Hence her system is more formative than interpretive.

The macrocosmic perspective of Bailey's work left plenty of opportunity for confusion for readers who wanted pat explanations rather than detailed expositions of why the colors, rays, and chakras are different under every conceivable evolutionary condition. As the Tibetan stated,

> In time and space and during the evolutionary process, it is not possible to say which center is expressing the energy of any particular ray, for there is a constant movement and activity. . . . This is apt to be confusing. The human mind seeks to make everything precise, stable, to bracket certain relations or to assign certain centers to certain ray energies. This cannot be done.[24]

For later writers, Bailey's primary contribution was the one characteristic that remained consistent in her treatment of the chakras after 1930: the list of endocrine gland correlations.

Chapter 15
Mysterious Glands

Not long after I determined that the association of endocrine glands with the chakras could be traced to Bailey's *The Soul and Its Mechanism*, published in 1930, I came across the illustration of the chakra system by Cajzoran Ali reproduced in Singleton's *Yoga Body*. I covered the "disconcerting" connection of the chakras with the Revelation of St. John in chapter 11. But there was another disconcerting feature: the illustration correlated the chakras and the endocrine glands, and the book in which it originally appeared, were published in 1928, two years before Bailey's.

Subsequent research determined that, though Bailey was likely responsible for transmitting chakra/gland correspondences to later authors, the story of how this set of correspondences was developed and passed on was more complex, involving not only Bailey, but at least five other persons:

- James Morgan Pryse, discussed in chapter 11
- Herman Harold Rubin, a medical doctor who published a side view of the human torso in 1925 in a book on the endocrine glands—not knowing that it would be snatched up as the basis for endocrine/chakra correspondences by the next three people in the lineup; discussed in the present chapter
- Bhagat Singh Thind, an early Indian teacher working on American soil, a representative of the Sant Mat tradition (first encountered in connection with Blavatsky's teachings on the chakras), who was likely the first to make the link between chakras and glands; discussed in the next chapter
- Cajzoran Ali, discussed in the present chapter
- Alice Bailey, discussed in the previous chapter
- Edgar Cayce, the famous American psychic, who was responsible for the association of a slightly altered list of

chakra/gland correspondences with the Lord's Prayer that became popular in the 1970s; discussed in chapter 16

Chemistry of the Soul (Herman Harold Rubin)

In the early years of the twentieth century, the endocrine system was beginning to reveal its secrets. The existence and functions of hormones produced by these so-called ductless glands were being discovered and described. In the 1920s, popular books on the influence of hormones on mood and personality began to surface. One such book, *Your Mysterious Glands: How Your Glands Control Your Mental and Physical Development and Your Moral Welfare*, by physician and eugenicist Herman Harold Rubin (1891–1973), made its way into the bibliography for Bailey's *The Soul and Its Mechanism* (1930). According to Rubin, "An individual is what he is solely because of his glands":

> We know that the physical appearance of the individual, his psychic traits, or what might be called the chemistry of his soul, are demonstrated in a great measure by the character and amount of the internal secretions of his various glands.[1]

A diagram entitled "Schematic Chart of the Endocrine System" showed a side view of a human torso with the endocrine glands marked (see figure 14). Anyone familiar with the chakra system would immediately perceive from this diagram that the locations of seven of these glands coincided with those of the chakras.[2] The diagram showed the pineal above the pituitary, thus supporting the trend in Theosophical writers on the chakras to assign the pineal to the seventh and the pituitary to the sixth chakra. As indicated, Bailey broke with that tradition in *Letters on Occult Meditation* (1922) but reverted to it in *The Soul and Its Mechanism*, perhaps after exposure to the Rubin diagram. Cajzoran Ali used this

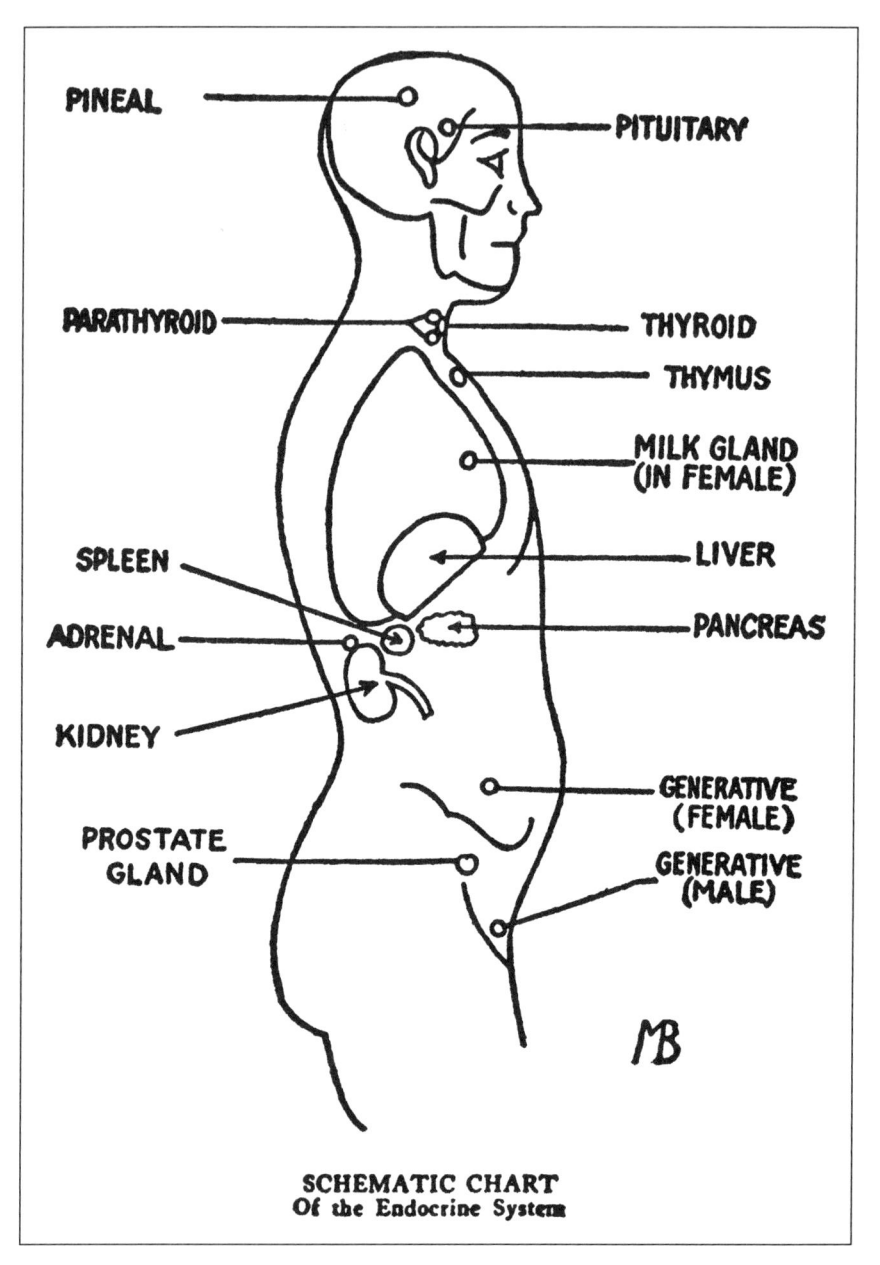

Figure 14. Endocrine Glands (reprinted from Herman H. Rubin, *Your Mysterious Glands*, 1925)

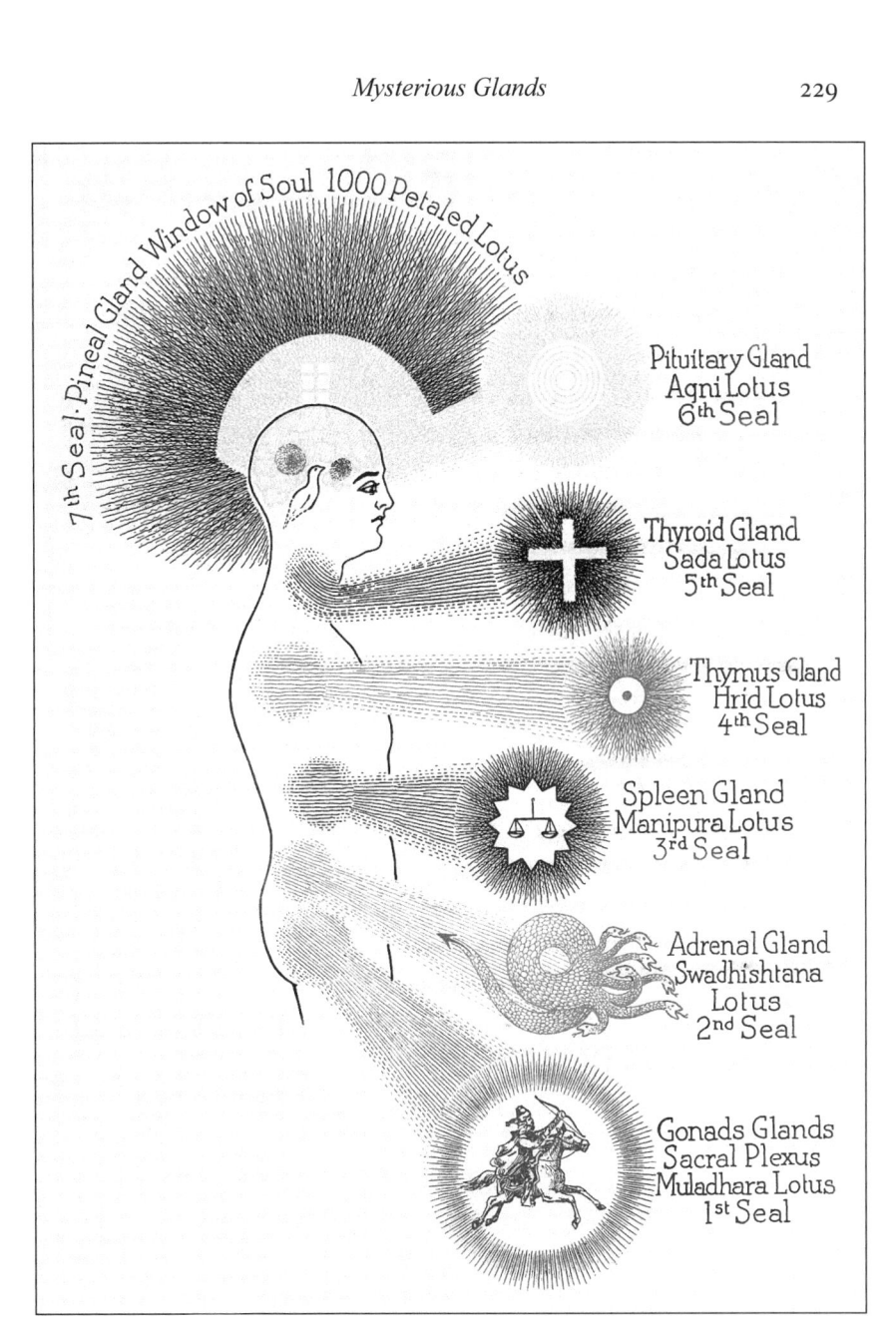

Figure 15. Ali's Chakras and Glands
(reprinted from Cajzoran Ali, *Divine Posture,* 1928)

diagram as a model for her illustration linking chakras, glands, and Revelation. (See figure 15 and plate 8; note how the ear structure in Rubin's diagram becomes a bird in Ali's.)

The Many Lives of Cajzoran Ali (Amber Steen)

Ali was unknown until recent research into the development of postural yoga practice dug her up. Her book *Divine Posture: Influence upon Endocrine Glands*, self-published in New York in 1928, was an early photographic manual of yoga postures, demonstrated by Ali herself in what must have been a risqué costume for the period—something like today's jogging bra and shorts. No one has been able to determine the identity of this mysterious "self-styled American yogini."[3] The only presumed facts of her life are that she was born in Memphis, Tennessee, in 1903 and died about 1975, in Florida.[4] Extensive research allowed me to determine the details of Ali's life—which turn out to be as disconcerting as her book.

She was born Ann Amber Steen in Pocahontas County, Iowa, January 16, 1895.[5] Often ill as a child, Steen became incapacitated from 1916 to 1917 and was operated on for a lung abscess, resulting in the removal of several ribs. After a diagnosis of tuberculosis and several further operations, she was confined to a bed or wheelchair, partially paralyzed, and sent home to her parents (then living in Harrisburg, South Dakota) to die.[6] However, she made a miraculous recovery using occult, metaphysical, and New Thought principles derived from extensive reading, including the Bible, books on health and anatomy, and "mystic astrology, divine symbolism, numerology, and tarotology." She overcame paralysis with physical exercises that eventually developed into the "divine postures" illustrated in her 1928 book.[7] During this recovery, she claimed to have been visited by a dark-skinned spiritual being (male), whom she channeled and who helped her heal. She now had a mission "to teach others to master their bodies."

She married a chiropractic student, Leonard Walter McGilvra (1897–1956) in 1919, got divorced in 1922, and went to work in

Chicago as a salesperson.[8] There she became associated with an alleged Indian Sufi teacher who called himself Hazrat Ismet Ali (also Sheikh Gulam Ismet Ali; born about 1897) and claimed to have come from Calcutta with a PhD. Perhaps because of his dark skin—did she believe this was the being who healed her?—Steen married the sheikh and traveled with him as Cajzoran Ali, teaching in several Midwestern cities and New York.[9] She published *Divine Posture* in 1928 at the height of this career, not long after the sheikh established an organization in New York for the promulgation of his teachings.

In 1929, due to an intercepted letter from Steen to her parents, the sheikh was exposed as a fraud. His real name was E. C. Williams and he was born in Trinidad, West Indies. He had gotten his start in Chicago about 1924, working as a bellhop at a Chicago men's club—though he also maintained a "Temple of Supreme Consciousness" downtown.[10] As the sheikh's confidence scheme unraveled, Steen disappeared, supposedly snatched by enemies of the cult he had established. Then the sheikh himself disappeared. The pair were arrested in Chicago and a trial ensued. The sheikh was convicted of swindling up to fifty thousand dollars from his followers and sentenced to one to five years in prison. Steen was acquitted. However, the sheikh jumped bail before his sentence began and was later apprehended in Trinidad and extradited back to the United States. In the meantime, Steen returned to New York to continue lecturing as a spiritual teacher.[11]

In the 1930s, Steen made four trips to France, traveling under her married name, Williams,[12] but calling herself Madame Zorah and claiming to be a "Zoroastrian initiate." The title may have come from Steen's association with Mazdaznan, a popular but understudied neo-Zoroastrian cult focused on health, vegetarian diet, "sun worship" (nude sunbathing), and pranayama-like spiritual practices. This cult was founded at the turn of the twentieth century by Otoman Zar-Adusht Hanish (pseudonym of Otto Hanisch; 1866–1936).[13]

Steen may have gone to India in 1934 in pursuit of initiation by a spiritual Master.¹⁴ In 1935, she published several articles in French weeklies, including illustrated translations of passages from *Divine Posture*. In 1938, she wowed the young French poet François Brousse (1913–96) with her esoteric knowledge and spent a month teaching and initiating him. Brousse published a memoir of this experience forty years later, *Isis-Uranie ou l'Initiation majeure* (Isis-Urania, or the major initiation; 1976).¹⁵

In 1939, Steen returned to the States to visit the World's Fair in New York, inviting her friend, the Russian expatriate Princess Olga Shirinsky-Shikhmatoff (1872–1963)—a linguist, concert pianist, artist, and sculptress—to join her. The two were stranded in the United States by the advent of World War II and resided in this country for the rest of their lives, remaining close friends.¹⁶

Steen remarried in 1939 or 1940. Her third husband was a Swedish-American World War I veteran, Hjalmer Agaton Ekberg (1887–1976).¹⁷ She now went under the name Amber Ann Ekberg or Mrs. H. A. Ekberg—but to her yoga associates, she was Rahanii (possibly Hindi, "living," or "experiencing").¹⁸ She lived in Homestead, Florida, near Miami, where she was active as an oil painter in a local art club.¹⁹ She may have kept a yoga studio in Coral Gables—but I have not been able to confirm this.²⁰

As Rahanii, Steen contributed a black-and-white reproduction of a Daliesque painting entitled *The Occult Anatomy of the Human Figure* to *Yoga for You* (1943) by Theosophist, architect, painter, and writer Claude Bragdon (1866–1946). She also supplied Bragdon with material for a chapter called "Occult Anatomy of the Body."²¹ It is possible that a number of passages Bragdon interpolated from channeled communications with a "Brown Brother" were provided by Rahanii/Steen. One such message declared that "the yellow and the white [races] would be the first to fuse in love and marriage and understanding" and that world peace would come with "the three hands of men: yellow, brown, and white, lying in the palm of the Aum."²² It is difficult not to read into these words something of the challenges Steen must have faced in her interracial marriage to Sheikh Ali.

I have not been able to track Steen's activities in the 1950s and 1960s, except that she cared for the princess during her final days in 1963.[23] Steen herself died in December, 1966, in Miami-Dade County.[24]

Steen's Legacy

It is difficult to dispute Singleton's contention that Steen's *Divine Posture* provided an early illustrated manual of yoga poses, some of which are similar to those encountered in today's yoga classes. Yet the true status of the book is difficult to assess. Self-published and unregistered with the copyright office (despite the statement to the contrary on the verso of the title page), the book may have had limited distribution. Worse, much of the text was plagiarized.

For example, fourteen pages of the explanatory introduction (pp. 10–27) were derived from *Health and Breath Culture according to Mazdaznan Philosophy (Sun-Worship)* (1902; 1914) by Otoman Zar-Adusht Hanish, with small omissions, interpolations, rearrangements of text, and alterations of word choice and order. The explanations of the chakras in terms of Revelation, with scriptural citations from the King James Bible, included commentary plagiarized from Pryse's *Apocalypse Unsealed*. Furthermore, "oriental interpretations" of each chakra were taken word for word from the English translation of a seventeenth-century religious travelogue called *The Dabistān*.[25] I have also detected unacknowledged passages from Woodroffe's *The Serpent Power*; Will L. Garver's *The Brother of the Third Degree* (1894), an occult novel; and Pryse's *The Restored New Testament* (1914).

With so much evidence of plagiarism, *Divine Posture* is more disconcerting than Singleton knew, especially when we consider the "Author's Note" at the end of the book:

> Unscrupulous people, who have no spiritual awakening or originality, attempt to profit by imitating the works of others. Like all good things, Divine Posture and Breath

Table 12
Cajzoran Ali on the Chakras (1928)

Lotus Names	Seals	Plexuses	Glands	Colors	Signs	Planets
1000 petaled lotus Window of soul	Seventh	Conarium	Pineal	Violet/silver/opalescent	Cancer	Moon
Agni	Sixth	Cavernous	Pituitary	Orange-yellow / golden	Virgo	Mercury
Sada	Fifth	Laryngeal	Thyroid	Dark blue / indigo	Libra	Venus
Hrid/Anahat	Fourth	Cardiac	Thymus	Green-gold	Leo	Sun
Manipura	Third	Epigastric (solar)	Spleen	Red	Scorpio	Mars
Svadhishthana	Second	Prostatic	Adrenals	Pale blue	Sagittarius	Jupiter
Muladhara	First	Sacral	Gonads	Yellow / silvery white	Capricornus	Saturn

Control, and their effect upon the endocrine glands will be imitated by those who know nothing of the true principle[s] for which they are intended. These imitators will not hesitate in giving misinformation in this great work. As they have not the real soul interest of each individual at heart, their directions in Divine Postures will be more harmful than beneficial. Therefore, in your own interests, I am urging you to guard against imitators after this book is published.[26]

Apparently, Cajzoran Ali's borrowings were *not* unscrupulous because she had "spiritual awakening" and "originality," knew the "true principles" behind what she taught, tried to see the "real soul interest" in her students, and was involved in a "great work"—which presumably exempted her from citing her sources. Here we have an egregious example of the original synthesis and "justifiable" appropriation varieties of source amnesia.

That said, the list of endocrine glands in *Divine Posture* ascends the spine in orderly fashion. Ali's list makes perfect practical sense to anyone familiar with anatomy and, as noted, was probably inspired by the illustration in Rubin's book. It was clearly *not* inspired by Alice Bailey, who placed the glands for the first three chakras in a different order: adrenals, gonads, pancreas. Anodea Judith and many later writers usually follow Bailey.

In Table 12, I include the numbers of the seals, which may seem obvious, to note a departure from Pryse, who links the second through sixth chakras with the first through fifth seals. His first chakra is the sixth seal and the seventh chakra the seventh.

In *Divine Posture*, the names of the fourth chakra, *hrid* (heart), the fifth chakra, *sada* (eternal), and sixth chakra, *agni* (fire), are unusual. They are called thus in *The Dabistān*.[27] The conarium is not a nerve plexus, but an alternative name for the pineal gland.

The colors appear to have been drawn from a foldout diagram in Blavatsky's Esoteric Instruction No. 1, where the planets and colors are associated in a similar way (the numbers indicate Ali's chakra associations): (2) Jupiter/blue; (3) Mars/red; (5) Venus/indigo; (6) Mercury/yellow; (7) Moon/violet.[28] I do not know the origin of Ali's associations of yellow and silvery white with the first chakra and Saturn, and green-gold with the fourth chakra and the Sun.

As in Pryse, the planets are associated with zodiacal signs according to traditional astrological teachings on planetary rulership. However, Ali has moved Leo and the Sun from the seventh chakra to the fourth, bumping Venus, Mercury, and the Moon and their associated signs up one chakra.

In the introductory matter to her book, Cajzoran Ali stated that God is "known as the 'Ruler Within'" and that "the center and root of all his powers and Wisdom is the Heart" (27)—which may explain why she shifted Leo and the Sun to the heart chakra. As noted, the Mazdaznan cult promoted worship of the sun as the source of health and vitality.[29]

In the early 1890s, Blavatsky's *Esoteric Instructions* provided lists of correspondences that could be interpreted as applying to the chakras, though she never used the term. In the early teen years of the twentieth century, Pryse mined these correspondences in *Apocalypse Unsealed*, added a few of his own, and clearly linked them to the chakras. In *Divine Posture*, Cajzoran Ali not only synthesized elements from Blavatsky, Pryse, Hanish, Rubin, and possibly Bhagat Singh Thind (discussed in the next chapter)—but also added postures for stimulating the endocrine glands and chakras.

Despite its limited distribution, *Divine Posture* was an early example—as was Fletcher's *The Law of the Rhythmic Breath*—of the persistent trend of Western esotericists to create original personal syntheses of existing information on the chakras and produce theoretical and practical manuals of chakra activation and development. But Fletcher's presentation was purely verbal, whereas *Divine Posture* included photographs, figures, and tabulated correspondences for each chakra. It was the *Wheels of Life* of 1928.

Chapter 16
The Sikh and the Psychic

In the latter half of the twentieth century, some people's first encounter with the chakras came not through books on yoga but through the writings of the early twentieth-century psychic and medium Edgar Cayce, which linked the seven churches in Revelation to the chakras, the endocrine system, and the Lord's Prayer (Matt. 6:9–13). In the 1960s many mass market paperbacks and booklets of Cayce's teachings were published under the editorship of his sons and the Association for Research and Enlightenment (ARE), founded by Cayce in 1931. The popularity of these books made Cayce's Christianized teachings on the chakras a factor in the evolution of the Western chakra system.

Edgar Cayce and the Glad Helpers

Born and raised in Kentucky, Edgar Cayce (1877–1944) lived in many locations, working as a professional photographer, until he settled in Virginia Beach, Virginia, where he remained for the rest of his life. He had already been doing psychic readings for twenty-five years. He discovered his mediumistic abilities during a long period of voice loss that followed an illness in 1900. He was hypnotized during a vaudeville show and regained his voice in 1901, then began experimenting with the trance state for health readings on himself and others. By the time of his death over forty years later, Cayce had done more than fourteen thousand such readings for individuals known and unknown to him and for local groups who were interested in probing him for spiritual teachings on health, meditation, the Bible, and other subjects. The personal readings were focused primarily on health, spiritual growth, and past lives.[1]

Cayce's education stopped in eighth grade. He did not read much beyond the Bible. The range and scope of the material that came through him in trance was impressive. Many of the unusual healing practices and remedies he suggested resulted in cures or remission of symptoms. Because Cayce's readings were conducted in deep trance and he remembered little or nothing of what he said, he was known as the sleeping prophet. Every reading was recorded by a stenographer, typed up, and indexed. Subsequent assessment of this material has been mixed, from the documentation of astonishing cures and accumulation of testimony on the value of Cayce's home remedies and spiritual teachings to disappointment over the large number of prophecies of earth changes and upheavals during the latter half of the twentieth century that did not occur as predicted.[2]

Two questions drove my research into the Cayce readings. First, did his attribution of endocrine glands to chakras precede and influence Cajzoran Ali's and Alice Bailey's, or the other way round—or was there some other source? Second, was Cayce's gland/chakra material spontaneously generated or produced in conjunction with questions from knowledgeable participants?

Determining the chronology of Cayce's material on the chakras from previously published books is difficult because writers, editors, or compilers usually cite the ARE's index numbers without dates. However, researchers can use a DVD-ROM published by ARE, *The Official Edgar Cayce Readings*, to determine the chronology and context of material on any subject mentioned in the readings. I gleaned the following information from this resource.

The key reading was 281–29 (October 28, 1936), part of a special series of sixty-five sessions given for a group that called itself "Glad Helpers." A dream of September 15, 1931, instructed Cayce to bring seven people together for a healing prayer group.[3] The first meeting took place on October 5, 1931, and the group met irregularly until 1944. The stated purpose of Glad Helpers was "to help individuals, physically and mentally, by attempting through meditation to awaken the divine within each."[4] The readings were primarily driven by questions ranging from personal to general to administrative. Many included healing affirmations for the use of individuals and other prayer groups sponsored by ARE members throughout the country. The practice of meditation was a recurrent theme.

An important sequence within the Glad Helpers series dealt with an interpretation of Revelation by Cayce's spiritual contacts; another dealt with functions of the endocrine glands. The reading in question (281–29) took place early in the first sequence. Group members had independently undertaken to correlate the seven centers with the seven churches in Asia (Rev. 1:11) and the seven seals on the Book of Life (Rev. 5:1). These were also coordinated with seven endocrine glands and planets. The correlations had been drawn up as a chart and Cayce's contacts were requested to assess their accuracy. All were confirmed, as given in the chart, with Cayce's contacts adding brief commentary.

A list of colors brought to Cayce included only those for the first four centers. His contacts provided two more, but the list remained incomplete. It would have been a startlingly different list from other correlations of colors and chakras, since it included black, white, and gray. However, the Glad Helpers revisited the question in reading 281–30 (February 17, 1937), in which Cayce's contacts declared that the colors of the spiritual centers "will go in the regular order of the prism."[5]

The correlation of churches with spiritual centers was identical to that in Pryse's *Apocalypse Unsealed*. Another of Pryse's books was mentioned in a memo attached to an earlier reading in the Glad Helpers series, so it is not unreasonable to assume that the makers of the chart were acquainted with *Apocalypse Unsealed*.[6] From Cayce's answers to questions from the group as the sequence on Revelation proceeded, it is clear that he had not read the book.

In reading 281–31 (March 12, 1937), a question was asked about whether the seven glandular centers were ruled by the seven angels. Cayce's contacts answered in the affirmative. The questioners continued: "Are we correct in interpreting the sounding of these seven angels as the influence of spiritual development in these other planes becoming active through the vibrating centers of the physical body during the process of purification?" An affirmative answer was given yet again, but with qualifications. It appears that this question was directly inspired by Pryse's book, since the functions of the seven angels and their trumpet calls were identical in each.

In reading 281-29, the correlation of the centers to planets appears to have been modified from that of Pryse. The latter's correlation used the seven traditional planets of ancient *astrology* (in order from first to seventh center: Saturn, Jupiter, Mars, Venus, Mercury, Moon, Sun). The Glad Helpers' list used seven planets from modern *astronomy* (Saturn, Neptune, Mars, Venus, Uranus, Mercury, Jupiter). Note that the planets for the first, third, and fourth centers are the same.

The list of glands differed from those of Ali and Bailey. The pineal and the pituitary had switched places. The pineal was now in the sixth position instead of the seventh and vice versa for the pituitary. The solar plexus was given in the third position instead of the spleen (Ali) or the pancreas (Bailey). The gonads were moved to the first center from the second. The adrenals in Ali and Bailey were dropped. The second center was assigned to the "lyden" gland—a mystery, since no such gland exists. Asking for clarity in reading 281-53 (April 2, 1941), the Glad Helpers were confirmed in their identification of *lyden* with Leydig—not a gland, but the testosterone-producing interstitial cells in the testicles (and, as one commentator adds, "their equivalent in the ovaries"), named after their nineteenth-century discoverer, Franz Leydig.[7]

In reading 281-29, Cayce was specifically asked which gland is highest, pituitary or pineal, and he answered, "The pituitary!" As mentioned, Bailey had placed the pituitary in that position in *Letters on Occult Meditation* but replaced it with the pineal in subsequent books. Later writers on the chakras who use this attribution, such as Anodea Judith, may have been influenced directly or indirectly by early Bailey, Cayce, or independent but similar reasoning based on the following fact. Since about 1932, the pituitary has been called the master gland, since it regulates the functioning of other components of the endocrine system. This would make it a natural candidate for association with the crown chakra.[8]

Eastern Wisdom for Western Minds (Bhagat Singh Thind)

I suspect a Sikh spiritual teacher working in America was the catalyst for linking the chakras and the endocrine system—having gotten information about the glands from Rubin or another source published at about the same time (perhaps from newspapers). Bhagat Singh Thind (1892–1967) was born in the state of Punjab, India, in the village of Taragarh, a little over sixty miles from Amritsar, center of the Sikh religion. He came to the United States in 1913 as a graduate from Khalsa College, Amritsar, hoping to attend an American university. He worked at first in the lumber industry in the Northwest and earned his doctoral degree in divinity at the University of California at Berkeley.

Thind served briefly in the United States Army during World War I before being honorably discharged and became something of a cause célèbre in connection with his pursuit of United States citizenship, which was granted twice (in 1918 and 1919) on the basis of his military service and was revoked twice (in 1918 and 1926) because of longstanding laws against Indian immigration, prejudice on the part of the Immigration and Naturalization Service against nonwhites, and narrow interpretations of legal precedents that would have been in Thind's favor. The case was argued before the US Supreme Court, which agreed with the Department of Immigration. Thind finally achieved citizenship in 1936.

In the 1920s, Thind began his career as an itinerant spiritual teacher, constantly crossing the country on long lecture tours—a life he pursued (in addition to marriage and raising a family) until his death. His teaching was based on the Sikh tradition and Sant Mat, the Path of the Saints, which we encountered earlier in connection with the Radhasoami movement. Thind's initiation into Radhasoami is disputed—not mentioned by his son David, who has kept Thind's teaching legacy alive; denied by Thind himself; and described ambiguously by a later Radhasoami leader. It was claimed that Thind received initiation from Baba Sawan Singh

(1858–1948) of Radhasoami Satsang Beas, who became the head of that branch in 1903.⁹ Beas is about thirty miles from Amritsar, so it is conceivable that Thind could have visited the group when he was in college. However, he may have been exposed to these teachings in other ways (books, friends, relatives, and so on) without having been initiated.

Thind's teaching was eclectic. For example, in 1927, in Cleveland, Ohio, he presented a month-long seminar, "Master Course in the Teachings of the Sikh Saviors: Sixty Free Lectures on Divine Realization." The printed program was headed, "To know, to dare, and to keep silent"—a favorite maxim of Madame Blavatsky. Furthermore, it cited the motto of the Theosophical Society: "No religion higher than truth." A lecture of March 8 was entitled "The Endochrine [sic] Glands, such as Pituitary, Pineal, Thyroid, Adrenal, Interstitial," and focused on "their uses and how to take care of them and vibrate them for long life and prosperity." Another, on March 26, called "The Philosophy and Science of Breathing," promised to treat of the "ductless glands and personality, and combination of five forces in the body [presumably the prana-vayus], and the conquest of old age." The title of the final lecture of the series, held on March 29, was "Seven Centers, Is it Dangerous to Open Them?," glossed in the program as "how to establish divine consciousness in the higher strata, compelling the lower to follow." The program also advertised, "Hindu Science of Breath and Nature Cures," free classes offered six days a week, including lessons on ten types of breath.¹⁰

Such titles demonstrate that by 1927 topics familiar to us from the Eastern chakra system and its transmittal to the West—the seven centers, the prana-vayus, the science of breath—were commingling with Western scientific knowledge concerning the endocrine system and its effects on personality. The glands mentioned have a place in Ali's, Bailey's, and Cayce's versions of the chakra system. They are listed in the order which they appeared in Cayce's system ten years later: pituitary (seventh), pineal (sixth), thyroid (fifth), adrenal (third), and interstitial (an alternative name for the cells of

Leydig; second). Only the thymus (fourth) and gonads (first) from Cayce's system are missing.

In the fall of 1927, Thind repeated this sixty-lecture program in New York City. The Alis were also there. Some issues of the *New York Times* contained ads for the lectures of Thind and those of Hazrat Ismet Ali on the same page.[11] One even placed Thind side by side with Cajzoran Ali.[12] Alice Bailey, too, was in New York, lecturing on *The Secret Doctrine* "every Saturday at 3 p.m."[13] Thus it is possible that Cajzoran or Bailey could have attended or heard reports of lectures by Thind on chakras and glands.

Thind repeated the program yet again in San Francisco in 1934. The brochure listed for sale a book entitled *Breathing and Glands*. I have not been able to examine this book, but I suspect it may have contributed to the interest within Cayce's circle on the connection between the chakras and the endocrine system.[14] The brochure also advertised a "noon hour health class" that included instruction in what it called "The Science of Breath and Nature's Finer Forces," stating that "our practice is built on the comprehension of the law of radiation, of magnetic centers, and of the psychic potencies of force centers found in all bodies and their relationship to the cosmic force centers and currents of the solar system of the universe." Thind was apparently drawing upon Prasād's *Nature's Finer Forces* and perhaps also Fletcher's *The Law of the Rhythmic Breath*.[15]

Thind made several appearances in records associated with the Cayce readings. He was brought to Cayce's attention through a letter from a regular reading recipient in 1933.[16] He was the subject of a reading on March 23, 1935, in New York City. Subsequently, he corresponded with Cayce and delivered a lecture called "Eastern Wisdom for Western Minds" at the Fourth Annual Congress of the Association for Research and Enlightenment (June 27–30, 1935).[17]

It seems probable that Thind was a catalyst for, and influence on, the Revelation/centers/ glands chart presented at the Glad Helpers reading in October 1936 (281–29). But there is no direct evidence of such a role. Although the lyden and pineal glands were mentioned in connection with psychic development as early as April 23, 1932, in a series of readings done for Cayce himself, the focus on linking glands to spiritual centers did not develop until after Thind's 1935 visit.[18]

The Lord's Prayer

The chart discussed in reading 281–29 also included correspondences between specific words of the Lord's Prayer and the seven spiritual centers and glands. All were confirmed by Cayce's contacts, as follows:

> Our Father who art in *heaven* [pituitary (7)],
> Hallowed be thy *name* [pineal (6)].
> Thy kingdom come,
> Thy *will* be done [thyroid (5)],
> On earth as it is in *heaven* [pituitary (6); later shifted to thymus (4)].
> Give us this day our daily *bread* [gonads (1)];
> And forgive us our *debts* [solar plexus; later given as adrenals (3)],
> As we also have forgiven our debtors.
> And lead us not into *temptation* [lyden/Leydig (2)],
> But deliver us from *evil* [thymus (4)].[19]

The shifts noted in brackets were made in posthumous versions, which also added the lines not present in Matthew, but familiar to most church-goers, thus creating a descending and ascending arc:

> For thine is the *kingdom* [thyroid (5)]
> And the *power* [pineal (6)]
> And the *glory*, forever. Amen [pituitary (7)].[20]

This arc is illustrated in figure 16. Just as Cayce's correlation of the chakras, churches, and seals originated in a chart of Pryse's correspondences made by the Glad Helpers, so did the correlation of the chakras and the endocrine glands with the Lord's Prayer have a precursor—a diagram from *The Rosicrucian Cosmo-Conception* (1909) by Max Heindel (1865–1919; born Carl Louis von Grasshoff). Heindel was a Danish-American Theosophist, influenced by Rudolf Steiner, who left the TS to start his own spiritual movement, the Rosicrucian Fellowship.[21] This diagram, reproduced here as figure 17, associated Heindel's version of Blavatsky's seven principles with phrases from the Lord's Prayer. Heindel's seven principles were given as follows, top to bottom (Blavatsky's follow in parentheses):

- **Introduction**—"Our father who art in heaven"
- **Divine spirit** (atman)—"Thy will be done [on earth as it is in heaven]"
- **Life spirit** (buddhi)—"Thy kingdom come"
- **Human spirit** (buddhi-manas or causal body)—"Hallowed be thy name"
- **Mind** (manas)—"[But] deliver us from evil"
- **Desire body** (kama)—"Lead us not into temptation"
- **Vital body** (prana-linga)—"Forgive us our trespasses as we forgive those who trespass against us"
- **Dense body** (sthula)—"Give us this day our daily bread"

There are two obvious clues that connect Heindel and Cayce. The first is the placement of "Give us this day our daily bread" at the bottom of figure 17—an odd choice for the first-center gonads (Cayce), but understandable as the "Prayer for the Dense Body" (Heindel), the first principle. Similarly, the association of "Deliver us from evil" with the fourth-center heart/thymus (Cayce) seems odd, but understandable as the "Prayer for the Mind," the fourth principle.

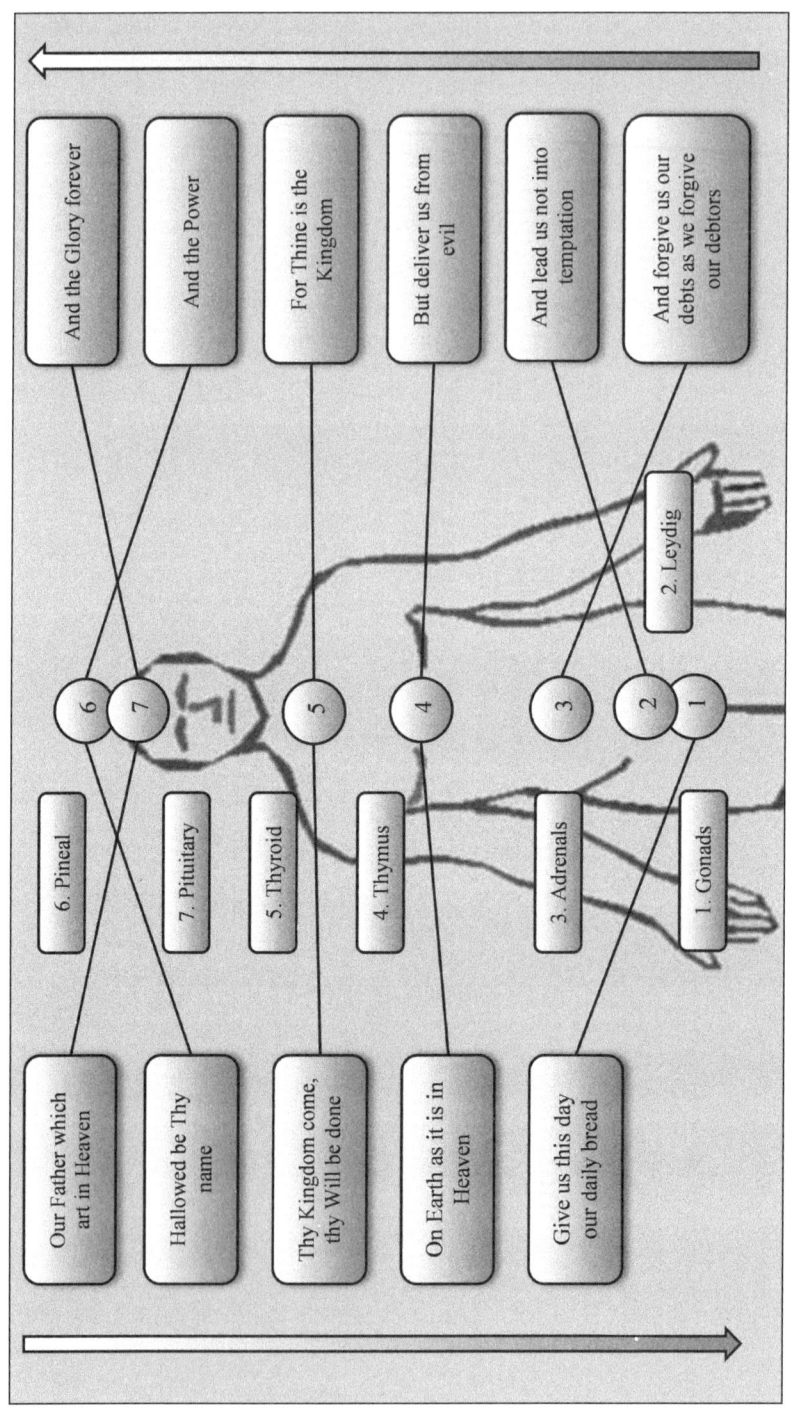

FIGURE 16. The Lord's Prayer according to Cayce (adapted from Mark Thurston and Herbert B. Puryear, *Meditation and the Mind of Man*, 1978)

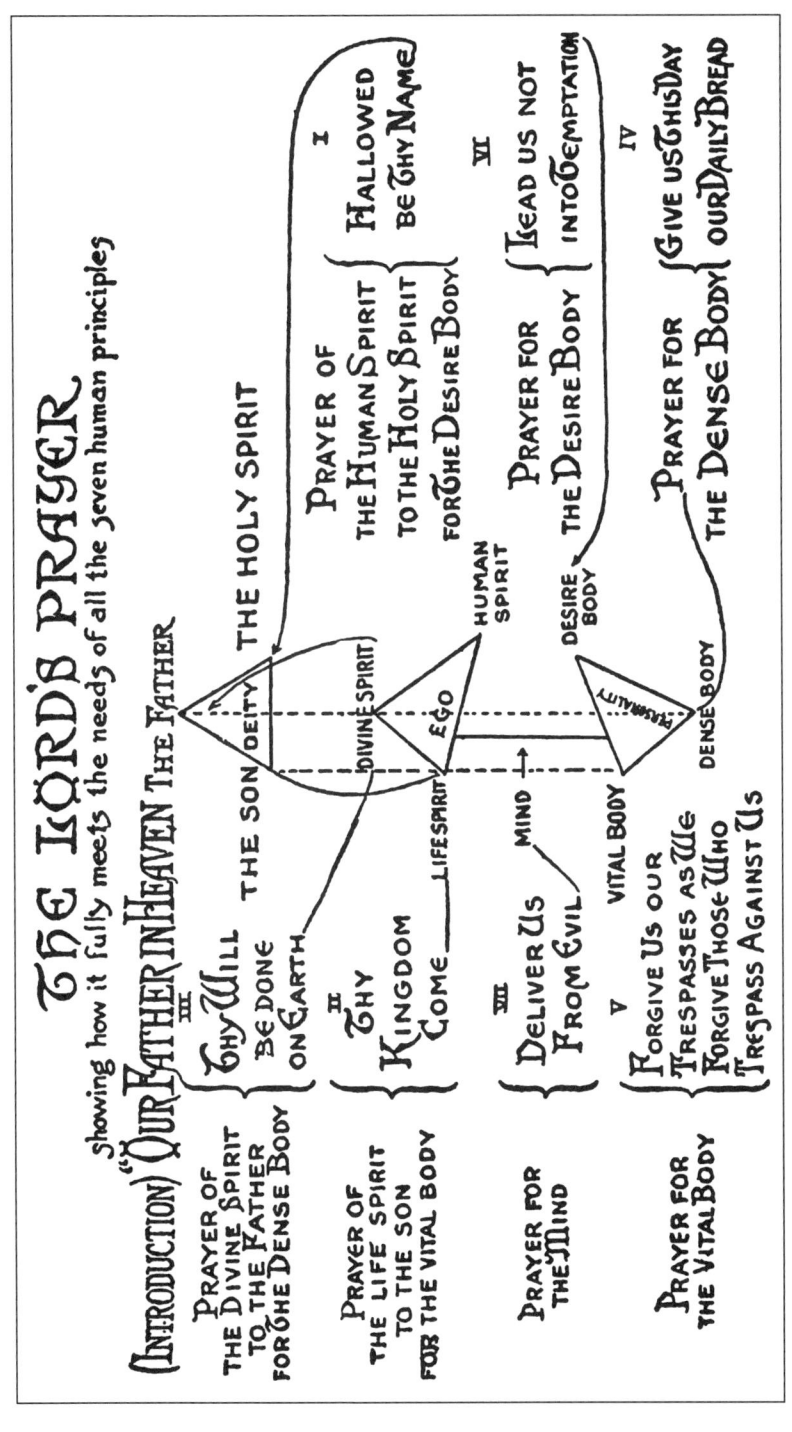

Figure 17. The Lord's Prayer according to Heindel (reprinted from Max Heindel, *The Rosicrucian Cosmo-Conception*, 1909)

As figure 16 shows, Cayce abandons Heindel's idea of an introduction and bumps the first phrase of the Lord's Prayer up a notch to his seventh center in the pituitary. Note that the Roman numerals in Heindel's version reflect the order of phrases in the prayer, not that of the principles themselves. After the introduction, the first Roman numeral (I) is assigned to "Hallowed be thy name," the "prayer of the human spirit." In Cayce's version, this phrase is linked with the sixth center, which he assigns to the pineal. Heindel's prayers of the life spirit and divine spirit (II and III) are combined and assigned to Cayce's fifth center and the thyroid. As noted, that for the mind (VII) is assigned to the fourth center and the heart/thymus. In Cayce, the prayers for the desire body (VI) and vital body (V) have been switched, probably to bring "temptation" in line with the interstitial cells of the testes and the second center. The prayer for the dense body (IV) remains in the same position in Cayce, associated with the first-center gonads.

Cayce's association of the chakras with Revelation and the Lord's Prayer first came to the attention of non-ARE members with his son Hugh Lynn Cayce's widely read *Venture Inward* (1964). A chart listed the correspondences described in the Revelation material, including the churches in Asia and their faults and virtues; the endocrine glands; the seven seals and the results of their opening; the four beasts, horsemen, and elements; and the seven planets and rainbow colors—all correlated with key words in the Lord's Prayer. This chart reproduced that developed by the Glad Helpers.[22] There was no instruction on meditating on the spiritual centers by means of the Lord's Prayer.

Not until 1975, when Herbert B. Puryear and Mark Thurston published *Meditation and the Mind of Man*, did the first public instruction on the use of the Lord's Prayer as a meditation on the centers and their glands appear. By the end of the 1980s, the Cayce Lord's Prayer meditation achieved its final form. *Awakening Your Psychic Powers: Edgar Cayce's Wisdom for the New Age* (1988) by transpersonal psychologist Henry Reed added the association of the phrase "In earth as it is in heaven" with the thymus in the prayer's initial downward pass through the chakras.[23]

Cayce's Legacy

Cayce's contribution to the Western chakra system is difficult to evaluate. He was apparently not an innovator, consolidator, or disseminator. As a medium working with spiritual contacts, he could perhaps be called a validator—which was exactly his role in relation to the lists brought to him by the Glad Helpers. The Glad Helpers themselves played the role of consolidators in their synthesis of information from Pryse and Heindel, which was innovative in its application of the endocrine glands and the chakras to the Lord's Prayer and Revelation.

Hugh Lynn Cayce stepped into the role of disseminator by publishing the Glad Helpers' chart of correlations. Others, including Puryear and Thurston, produced interpretive chakra systems based on the Cayce / Glad Helpers material. In the 1980s, Reed was primarily a disseminator. For example, in *Edgar Cayce on Channeling Your Higher Self* (1989), he published an illustration of a seated meditator with the centers marked and labeled with their connections to glands, churches, and phrases of the Lord's Prayer and indicating the order in which this prayer affects the centers—but no further explanation.[24]

Reed referred to a "Biblical theory of the chakras" encountered in Revelation,[25] which, according to Cayce, "is a symbolic description of what happens in the body of a meditator."[26] Further, Eastern traditions about the chakras have "always pointed to the endocrine glands as somehow being the physical counterparts to these psychic centers [chakras]."[27] He believed that Cayce's "interpretation of the Revelation showed that Christianity has had a secret tradition all its own concerning the psychic centers."[28] Source amnesia had obliterated not only the origins of this interpretation of Revelation in Pryse's book but also the awareness that the linking of chakras and endocrine glands had occurred a mere sixty years earlier, in America rather than the ancient East.

Nowadays, the belief in this "secret tradition" has even pushed Cayce out of the picture, allowing others to elaborate their own versions of meditating on the Lord's Prayer and the chakras. Thus

Choa Kok Sui, developer of the Pranic Healing system, produced his own version of the Lord's Prayer, using an eleven-chakra system, in *Universal and Kabbalistic Chakra Meditation* (2001). His version resolves the issue of matching up the chakras with the sephiroth on the Tree of Life by providing one chakra per sephirah (including Daath).

And there are other such correlations. Most seem to proceed in a straightforward fashion from the uppermost to the lowest chakras, without the downward and upward passes of the Cayce tradition. Thus "daily bread" becomes associated with the third chakra region of the stomach and "temptation" with the genital chakra, as in Dana Taylor's *The Lord's Prayer, the Seven Chakras, the Twelve Life Paths* (2009).

A Question of Precedence

In the association of chakras and endocrine glands, the question of precedence is not easy to settle. Thind, Ali, and Bailey each could have arrived at their lists independently, based on their exposure to Rubin's book. Or Thind could have been the catalyst for Ali and Bailey, as he later was for Cayce—perhaps in 1927, when all three were in New York. Ali could have attended Thind's breathing and meditation classes and Bailey's *Secret Doctrine* classes. Or there could have been other catalysts or a metaphysical grapevine that spread the word.

What is clear is that the order and names of the glands used in Thind's program for his 1927 Cleveland lectures are identical to Cayce's later list. Rubin's book uses the term *interstitial cells* and its equivalent, *cells of Leydig*, as in Thind and Cayce.[29] Ali's and Bailey's tabulations can both be traced to Rubin: the former through her use of Rubin's diagram for one of her own, the latter through citation in the bibliography of *The Soul and Its Mechanism*. However, Ali chose the spleen for the third center and Bailey chose the pancreas. Rubin's diagram shows the adrenals, spleen, and pancreas lying at about the same level, corresponding to the traditional position of the third chakra, which perhaps explains these differences.

It is not clear why Bailey moved the adrenals to the first chakra, thus placing the glands associated with the first chakra *above* those associated with the second. Possibly, she saw a correlation between Rubin's view of the adrenals as sources of reserve energy for physical survival and the functions of the root chakra in terms of what she called will-to-live.[30]

The following table allows us to compare chakra/gland correspondences in Thind, Ali, Bailey, and Cayce. In the absence of lecture transcripts or books by Thind that detail his teachings on these correspondences, I have assumed they are identical to Cayce's and

Table 13
Chakra/Gland Correspondences (1927–36)

Chakras	Thind (1927)	Ali (1928)	Bailey (1930)	Cayce (1936)
Seventh	Pituitary	Pineal	Pineal	Pituitary
Sixth	Pineal	Pituitary	Pituitary	Pineal
Fifth	Thyroid	Thyroid	Thyroid	Thyroid
Fourth	[Thymus?]	Thymus	Thymus	Thymus
Third	Adrenals	Spleen	Pancreas	Solar plexus or adrenals
Second	Interstitial	Adrenals	Gonads	Lyden / Cells of Leydig
First	[Gonads?]	Gonads	Adrenals	Gonads

that Cayce's were developed from the Glad Helpers' Revelation/Centers/Glands chart, which was itself derived from Thind.

Thind's source for placing the pineal in the position of the sixth chakra was probably Brahm Shankar Mishra's *Discourses on Radhasoami Faith* (1909):

> The six subdivisions of the lowest region, "'Pind" ["lowest" or "material-spiritual region"], are to be found in the human frame as the six ganglia or nervous centers commencing from the lowest in the rectum to the highest which is situated between the two eyes at the root of the nose, where the nerves from the various centers converge, and which is known as the pineal gland.[31]

Thus Cayce appears to have followed Thind, who appears to have followed Mishra. Later authors in the Cayce tradition have struggled with the issue of how to justify Cayce's correlation of the seventh chakra with the pituitary and sixth with the pineal gland. In 1973, Mary Ellen Penny Baker stated that the kundalini rises from the gonads to the pineal, then spills over into the pituitary, thus honoring the pineal's position as the highest endocrine gland in the body and Cayce's identification of the pituitary as the seventh and final center in this process.[32] In 1979, Puryear argued that the pituitary is the highest and that once the pineal is activated and linked to the pituitary, the latter is the true third eye.[33] In 2007, John Van Auken, a director of ARE, linked the pituitary with the third-eye chakra (sixth) and the pineal with the crown chakra (seventh)—thus bringing us back full circle to Blavatsky and Leadbeater.[34]

Puryear's solution hearkens back to that of Geoffrey Hodson, who resolved the pituitary/pineal controversy in an ingenious way in *The Science of Seership*. Hodson claimed that the third eye begins to function when the pituitary and pineal glands have been activated and are working in concert with each other—and both glands are associated with the brow chakra (which he called the

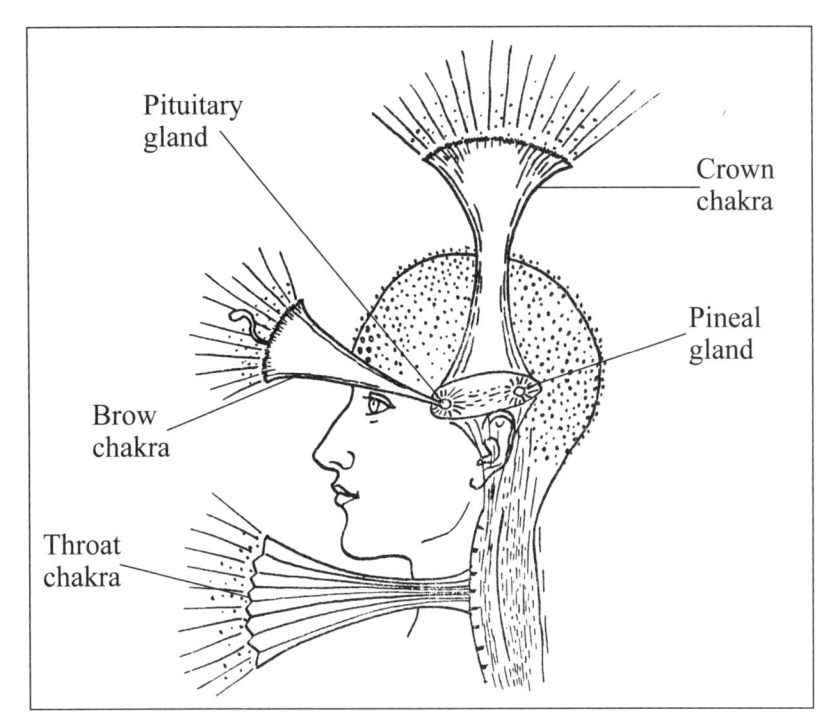

Figure 18. Head Chakras according to Hodson
(adapted from Geoffrey Hodson, *The Science of Seership*, 1929)

frontal, or ajna, chakram). "The etheric counterparts of the pituitary and pineal glands have been combined into one glowing center."[35]

This was Blavatsky's teaching in her Esoteric Instructions, as noted in chapter 6. The crown chakra (which Hodson called the coronal, or brahmarandhra, chakram) is at the top of the head, corresponding with the anterior fontanel, and does not have a gland associated with it.[36] This placement has the virtue of honoring traditional tantric teachings on the chakras, in which the seventh chakra is located at or above the crown of the head and is not considered to be a chakra at all; hence it would not be associated with a nerve plexus or endocrine gland.

Chapter 17
Lost Teachings of Cosmic Color

Where did the rainbow colors assigned to the chakras come from? We have seen that neither Blavatsky nor Leadbeater nor Bailey generated a list of color associations with the chakras in the order of the rainbow. Some Web-based commentators believe that this spectral approach cropped up in the late 1970s, when several books on the chakras featured cover illustrations with the colors in rainbow order.[1] But these covers were actually the end product of a process of transmission going back to the 1930s. The primary vector of transmission was the art/science of color healing, also called chromotherapy.

Though the idea of healing with colored gemstones has ancient roots, that of healing with colored light seems to have originated in nineteenth-century America, with Augustus James Pleasonton (1801–94), who in 1868 touted the health benefits of bathing in rays of sunlight passed through blue glass, thus instigating a "blue-glass craze." Seth Pancoast (1823–89), a physician who was an early member of the Theosophical Society and served as its vice president, studied the healing effects of light streaming through red or blue colored glass and published his findings in 1877. As noted earlier, Edwin Dwight Babbitt (1828–1905), a Spiritualist and physician published an influential book on the subject, *The Principles of Light and Color* (1878), which dealt with what he called "chromotherapeutics." Babbitt's work was carried forward by Indian-born Theosophist Dinshah P. Ghadiali (1873–1966) after his move to the United States in 1911.[2]

However, it was not until the 1922 publication of Bailey's *Letters on Occult Meditation* that the idea of forming groups for the exploration and practice of color healing was put forward as a step toward a "new school of medicine." Ideally, wrote the Tibetan, such groups should be made up of the following roles:

- Group leader, "a person with causal consciousness, who can deal with any problem in the mental body and who can study the alignment of the bodies with the Ego [higher self or soul]" (in Theosophical terms, someone far in advance of the ordinary level of human evolution, in which consciousness is focused primarily at the astral or mental level—an *Initiate* working under the direct guidance of a Master)
- Clairvoyants who can "view the subtle body of the emotions"—the aura (trained clairvoyants under the guidance of a Master; in Theosophical terms, *disciples* or higher)
- People who can "apply certain waves of color to effect certain cures" using "the power of thought" (meditators in the *probationary* stage who have trained the mental body in concentration)
- Members "of the medical profession, who will work with the physical body, under the direction of *conscious* clairvoyants" (as opposed to possibly unreliable mediums whose trance makes them completely unconscious)
- Occult meditators able to transmit "the healing forces of the higher self and of the Master" (advanced meditators who have been *accepted as pupils* by Masters)
- Transcribers for taking notes on the proceedings for "what will prove to be the literature of the new school of medicine"
- Recipients of color treatments applied not only by the "power of thought" but also by the application of "colored lights" to the physical body[3]

Masters and Rays

Bailey's tabulation of these roles was based on a Theosophical perspective on human spiritual evolution that originated in the 1880s in a series of so-called Mahatma letters, said to have been written by spiritual Masters living in the Himalayas and received by recipients in quasi-miraculous ways (controversially contested as fraudulent by contemporary critics, such as the British Society for Psychical Research). Attributed to a Master M, or Morya, and a Master KH, or Kuthumi, these teachings were developed by Madame Blavatsky, who claimed that M and KH had supported the founding of the Theosophical Society. They were elaborated by Besant and Leadbeater, who identified seven main Masters, including M, KH, Jesus, and St. Germain. And they were considerably amplified (and, in her mind, corrected) by Bailey's inner plane contact, DK, or Djwal Khul, who appeared in the original Mahatma letters as an Initiate and subsequently became a Master.[4]

By the 1920s, forty years after the receipt of the first Mahatma letters, the Theosophical perspective on human evolution entailed the following phases:

- **Unevolved people**—so-called primitives, savages, or barbarians: what civilized humans would call uncivilized; in present-day New Age parlance, infant or baby souls
- **Average people**—the ordinary level of human evolution: civilized, cultured, morally responsible, spiritually unawakened; young and mature souls
- **Evolving people**—the spiritually awakened who are "on the path" of accelerated spiritual development in order to be of service to suffering or ignorant humanity in the previous stages; old souls or spiritual seekers
- **Probationers**—spiritually talented individuals who are highly motivated to serve humanity; under observation by spiritual Masters
- **Accepted pupils**—spiritually talented and motivated individuals who are under the tutelage or guidance of a Master or the disciple of a Master
- **Chelas/Disciples**—advanced students of a Master
- **Initiates**—disciples who have successfully completed one or more of five stages in the process of becoming Masters, each stage requiring the full development of a particular vehicle of consciousness and demonstration of its skillful

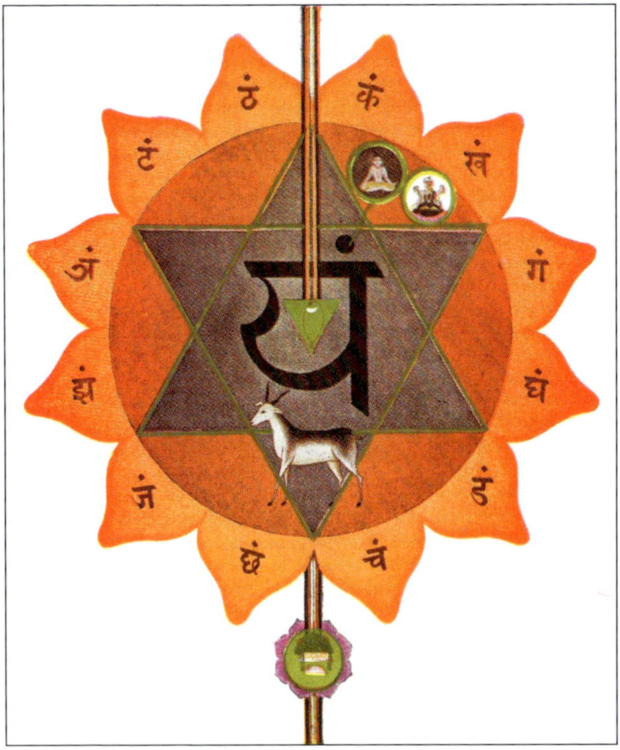

Plate 1. Chakras East and West. *A* (above), "Anāhata" (reprinted from John Woodroffe, *The Serpent Power,* 1919/1986). *B* (below), "The Heart Chakra" (reprinted from C. W. Leadbeater, *The Chakras*, 1927). The number of petals in *A* corresponds to the number of subdivisions in *B*.

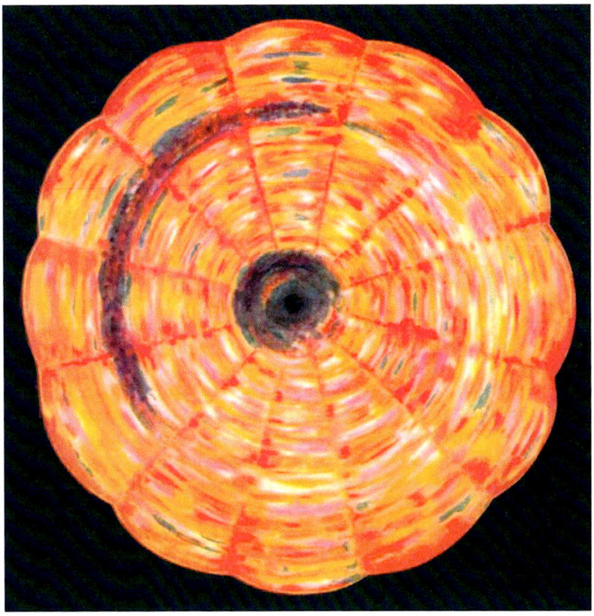

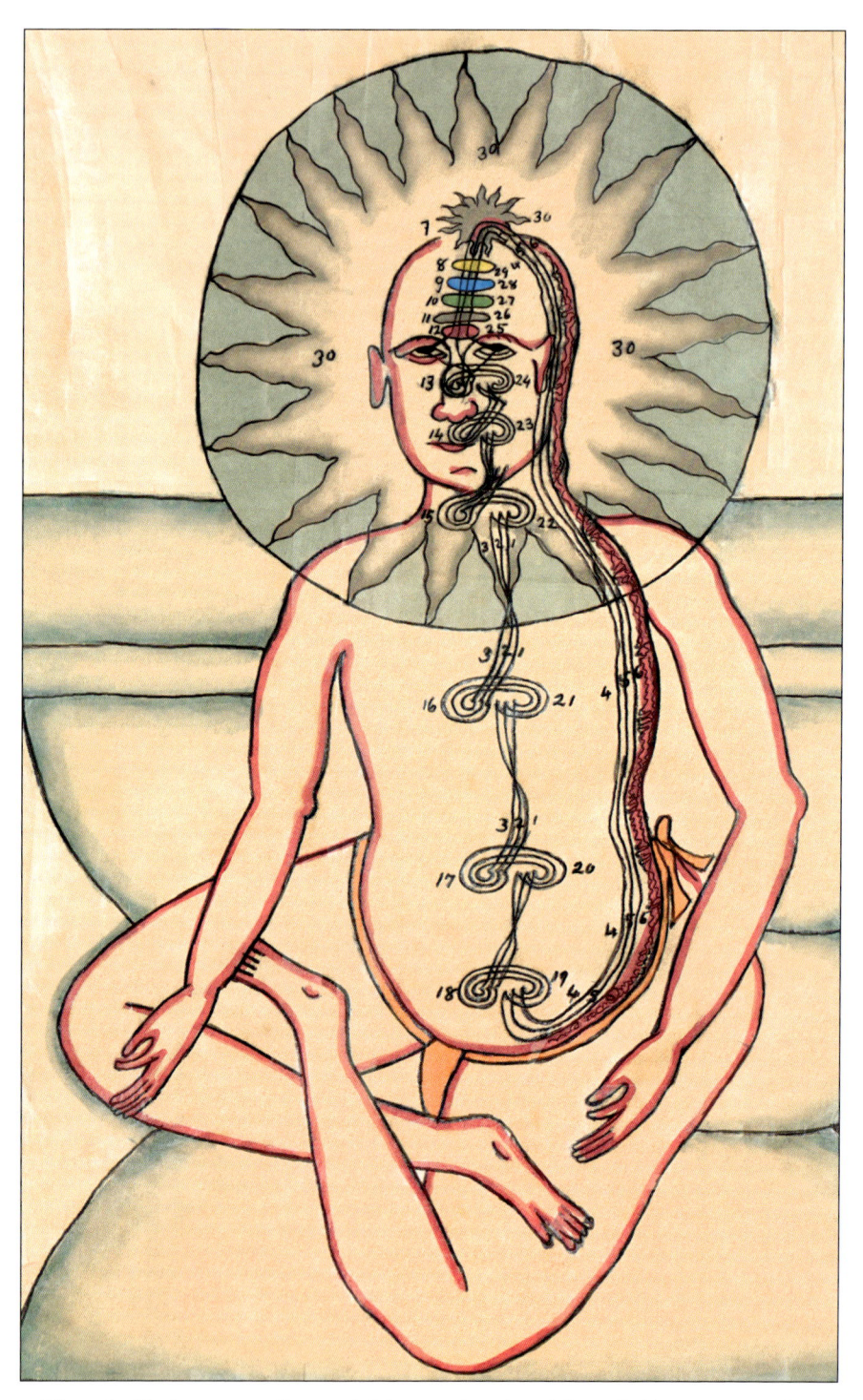

Plate 2. Chakras according to Sabhapaty (reprinted from Sabhapaty Swami, *Om: A Treatise on Vedantic Raj Yoga Philosophy*, 1880). Note chakras 7–12 in the head.

THE HUMAN AURA.

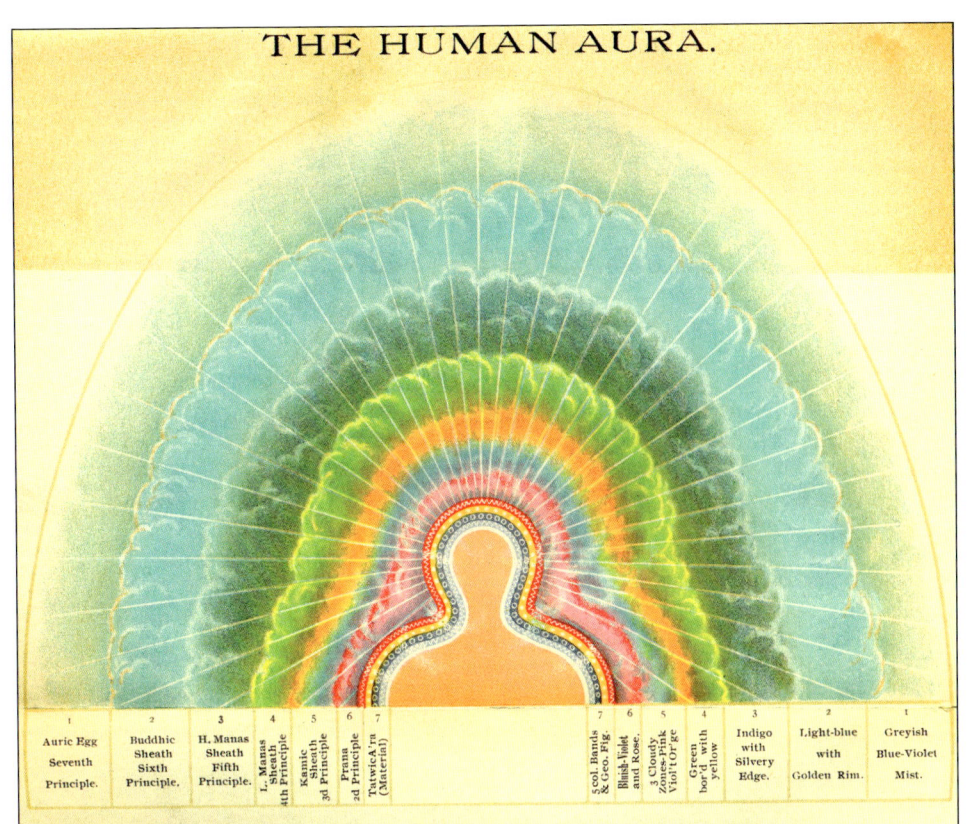

1	2	3	4	5	6	7		7	6	5	4	3	2	1
Auric Egg	Buddhic Sheath	H. Manas Sheath	Manas Sheath	Kamic Sheath	Prana Principle	Tatwic A'ra (Material)		5 col. Bands & Geo. Fig.	Bluish-Violet and Rose.	3 Cloudy Zones-Pink Viol't or'ge	Green bor'd with yellow	Indigo with Silvery Edge.	Light-blue with Golden Rim.	Greyish Blue-Violet Mist.
Seventh Principle.	Sixth Principle.	Fifth Principle.	4th Principle	3d Principle	2d Principle									

☞ The **1st Principle**, Linga, Etheric Double or Shadow Body is not indicated on plate in order not to overcrowd it.
   Of the material Emanations from the Body, only the Electric or Health Aura is indicated by the vertical lines, but the Magnetic and Caloric Emanations are not represented, as they crowd into the same space as the Pranic and Tatwic Auras, Columns 6 and 7.
   The whole drawing is not in absolute proportion, the Tatwic colored and Geometrical Emanations having been kept nearly to their natural size, in order to make them apparent, while the others, going outward, have been greatly reduced, to fit in the page.
   The natural colors are much more blended, ethereal, delicate and subdued than can possibly be reproduced.

General Perspective View of the Human Auras.

Plate 3. Aura Layers and Principles (reprinted from A. Marques, *The Human Aura*, 1896). Marques divides the most material layer of the aura into four parts: (1) a "tatwic aura" that circulates down the left side of the body and up the right side and consists of constantly shifting associations of the five shapes and colors of the tattvas (elements) described in *Nature's Finer Forces* (these "colored and geometrical emanations" depend on astrological influences that determine which tattva is in power); (2) a wave-like "magnetic aura" that pulses along the surface of the skin in the rhythm of the heartbeat and protects against germs; (3) a static, cloudlike "caloric aura" that reflects the physical body's "power of combustion" (metabolism); and (4) an outwardly radiating "electric or health aura" that indicates the overall health or vitalization of the body. (See *The Human Aura*, 18–32). The remaining layers of the aura correspond to the seven principles described by Blavatsky.

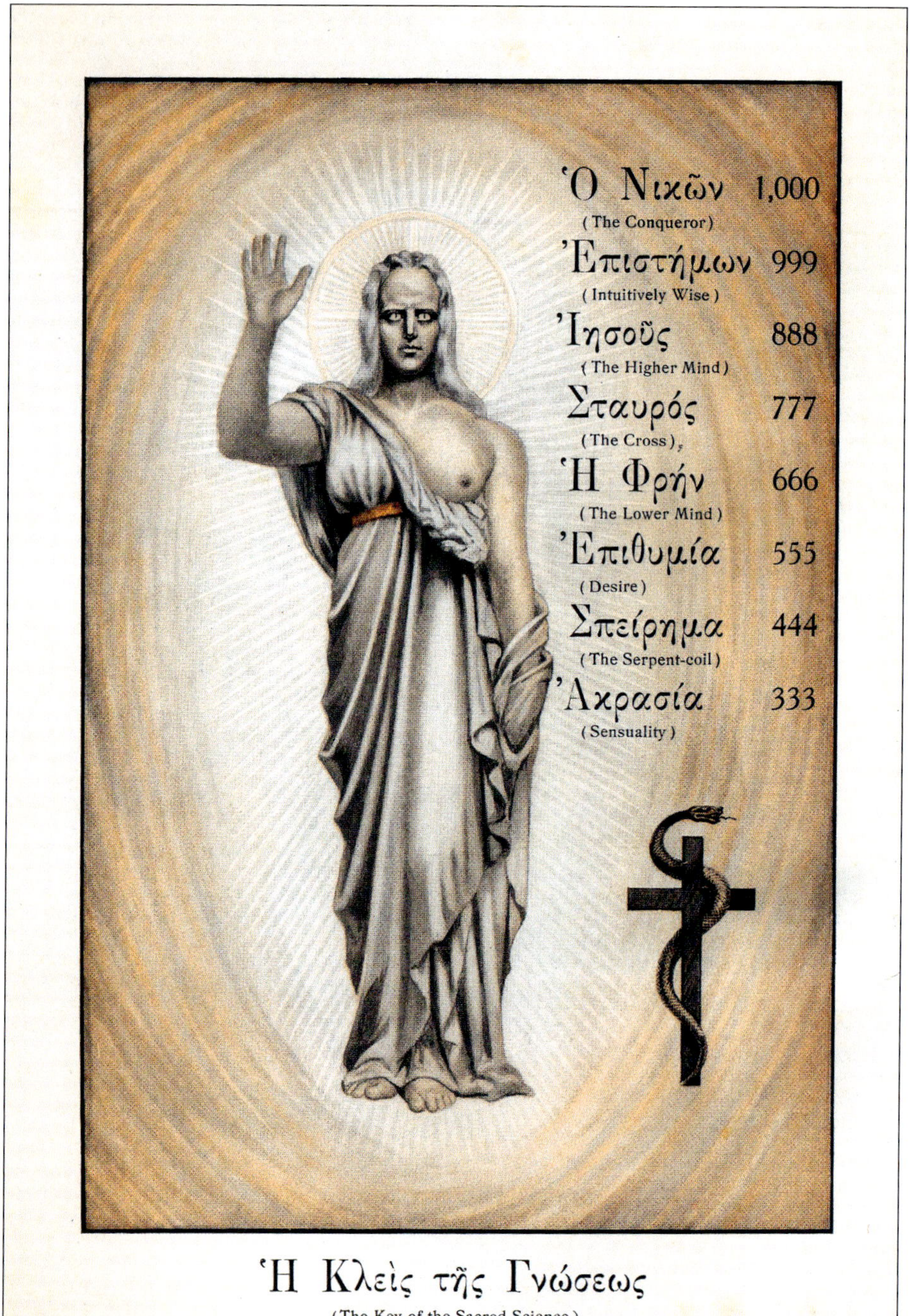

Plate 4. Pryse's Continuum of Human Potential (reprinted from James M. Pryse, *The Apocalypse Unsealed*, 1910). Each of the Greek words numbered 333 to 999 is placed at the level of one of the seven chakras in the human figure and stands for one of Blavatsky's seven principles.

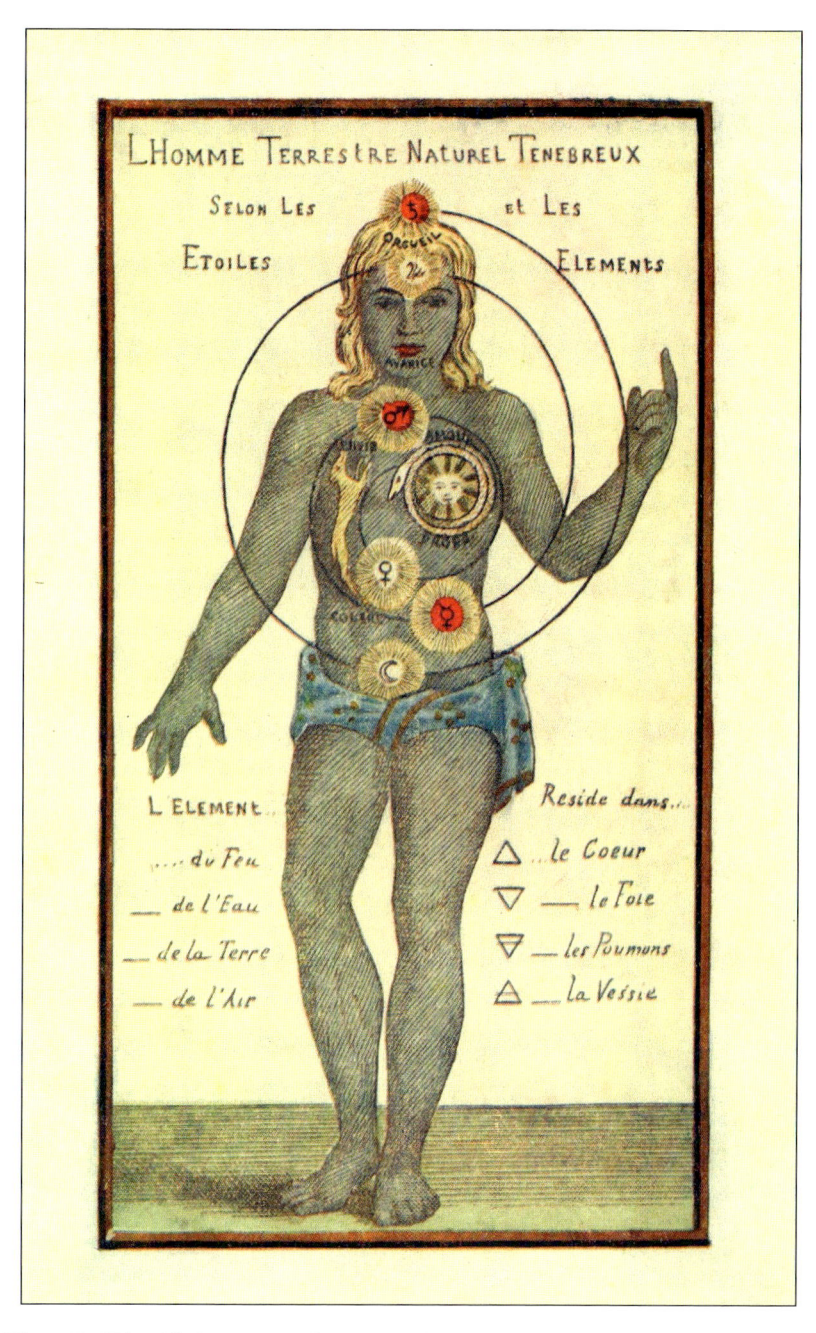

Plate 5. "The Chakras according to Gichtel" (reprinted from C. W. Leadbeater, *The Chakras*, 1927; originally from Johann Georg Gichtel, *Theosophia Practica*, 1897). The French title may be translated as follows: "Earthy, natural man in darkness according to the stars and elements." The elements of fire, water, earth, and air are paired with the following parts of the body: heart, liver, lungs, and bladder. The centers in the body are associated with faults to be overcome, such as pride in the head.

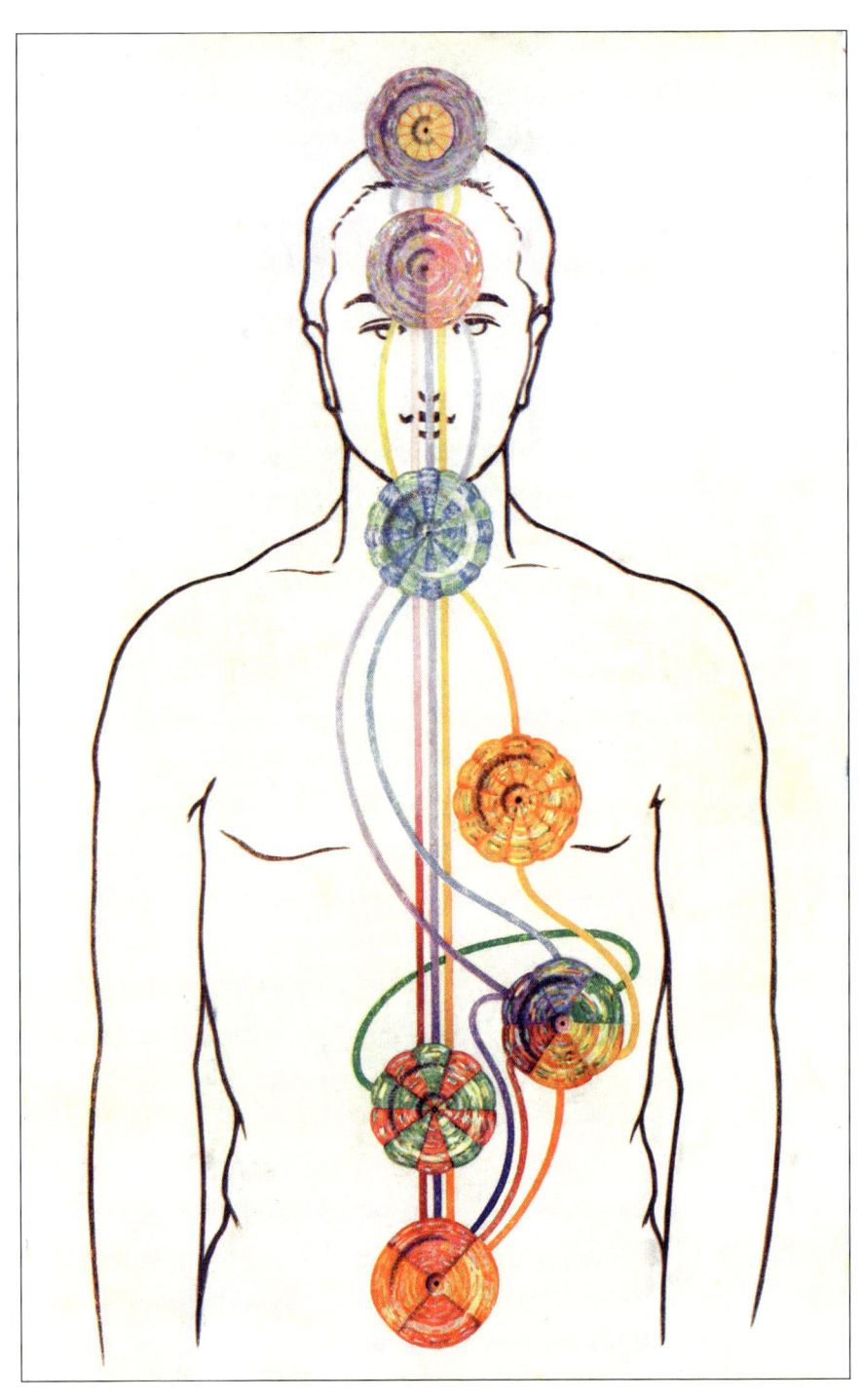

Plate 6. Leadbeater's Chakras—Front View (reprinted from C. W. Leadbeater, *The Chakras*, 1927). Note the displacement of the spleen and heart chakras from the center line of the body. The colored lines indicate various rays of vitality flowing between the chakras.

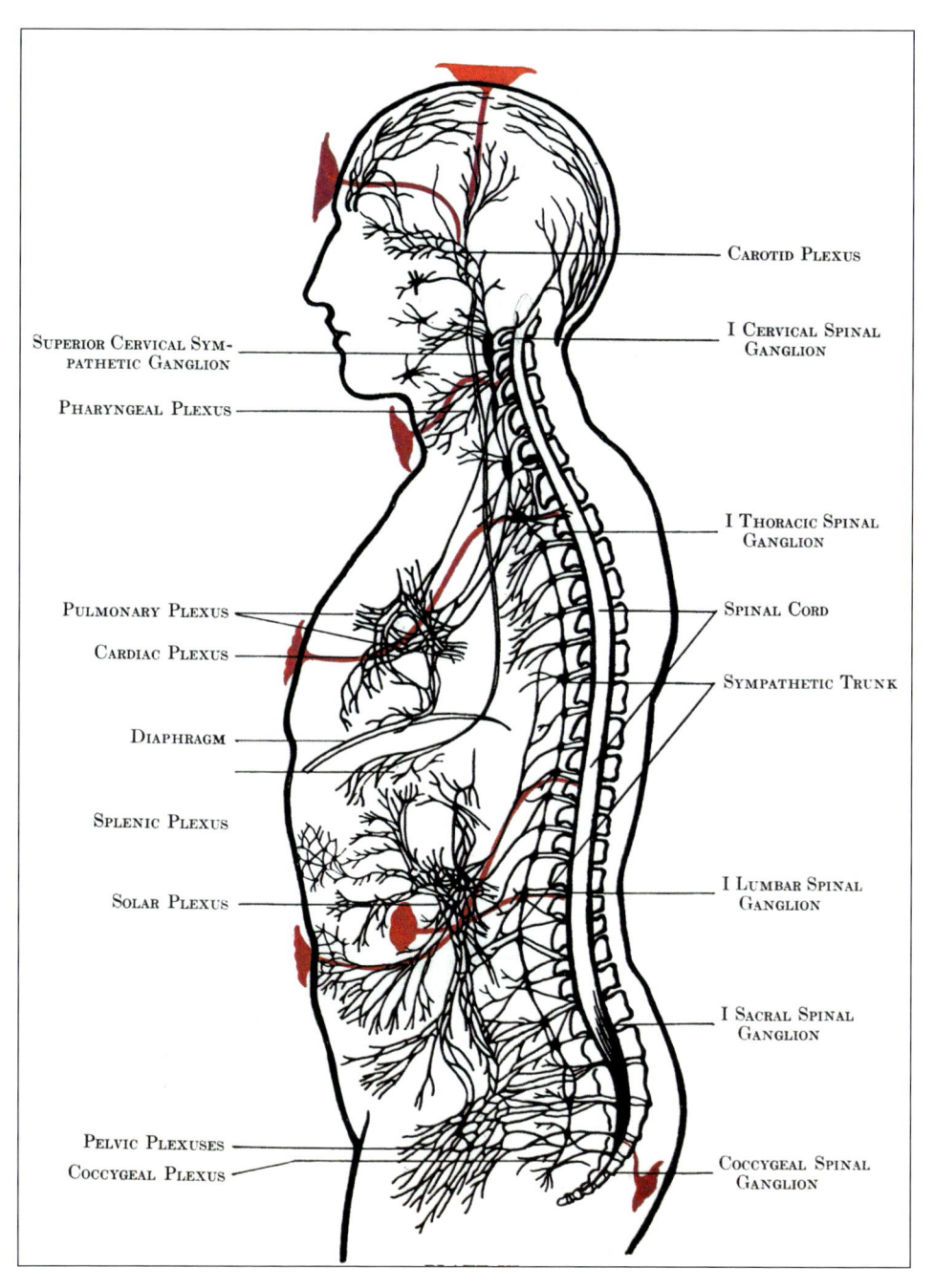

Plate 7. Leadbeater's Chakras—Side View (reprinted from C. W. Leadbeater, *The Chakras*, 1927). Note the "stems" attaching the chakras to the spine and the vortices or "flowers" showing at the front of the body.

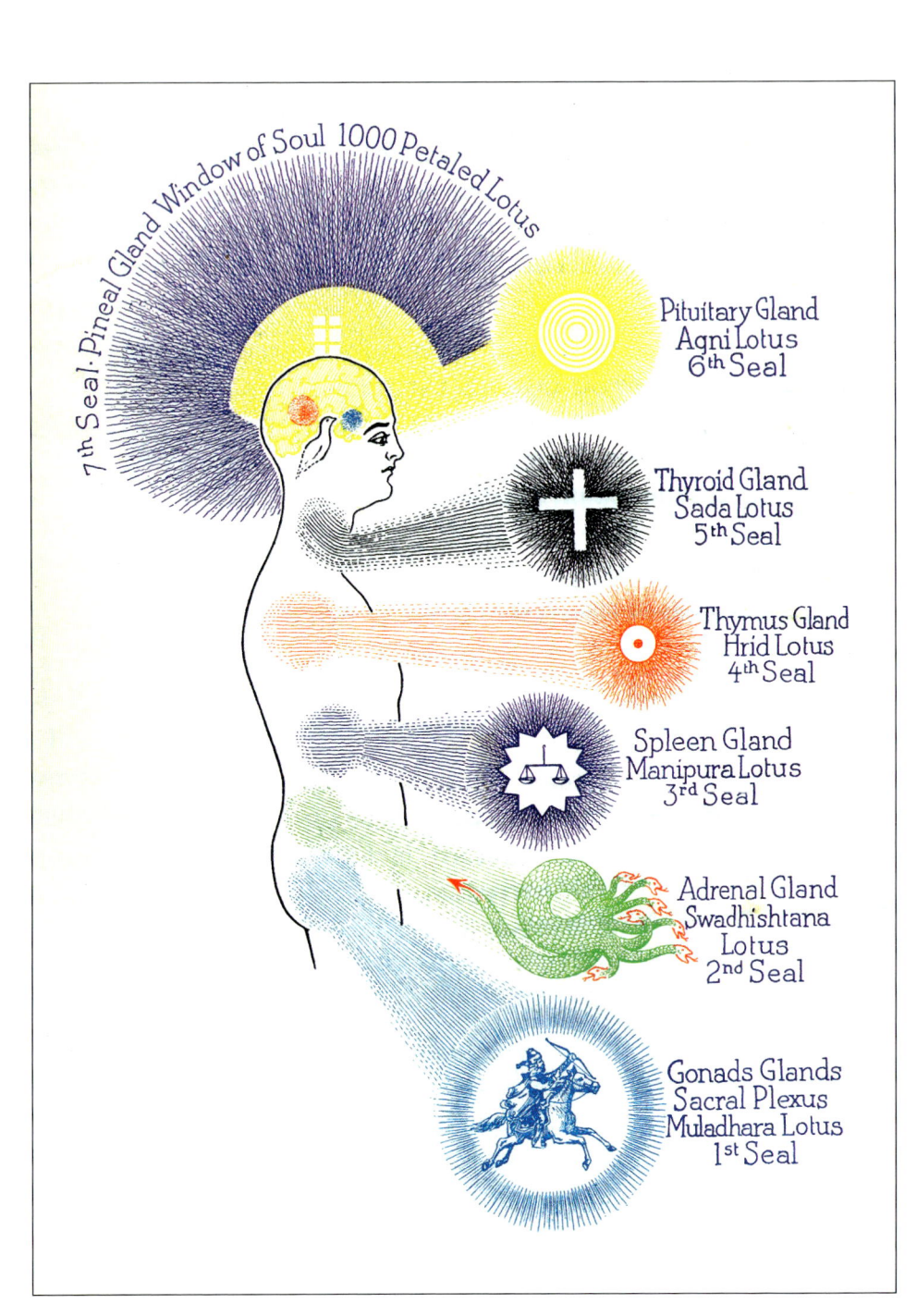

Plate 8. Ali's Chakras and Glands (reprinted from Cajzoran Ali, *Divine Posture*, 1928). The images associated with the chakras derive from the Apocalypse of St. John (also called Revelation).

use under challenging conditions (initiations) designed to test self-mastery and capacity for selfless service
- **Masters**—individuals who have successfully completed the fifth initiation and have therefore passed from the human stage of spiritual evolution to the superhuman, having godlike powers that are dedicated to the alleviation of suffering at all levels of being and to the support or acceleration of all stages in the process of spiritual evolution; roughly equivalent to the highest level of yogis and gurus in the Hindu tradition and bodhisattvas in the Mahāyāna Buddhist tradition
- **Great White Brotherhood**—the body of initiates and Masters who guide and govern the spiritual evolution of the world (no reference to race)
- **Chohan (Ray Master)**—one of seven Masters who have passed the sixth initiation and become responsible for human evolution along any of seven lines: (1) power; (2) wisdom; (3) tact, or diplomacy; (4) culture and the arts; (5) science; (6) religion; and (7) magic (work with the nonhuman devas—godlike or angelic beings responsible for creating and sustaining various levels of our reality/learning system, which includes the physical and nonphysical planes, subplanes, locations, bodies, and so on)[5]

The original Mahatma letters were first published in 1923, edited by A. Trevor Barker, who arranged them thematically to reflect some of these stages (in particular, probation and chelaship or discipleship). Other important sources of information on these stages were Bailey's *Initiation: Human and Solar* (1922) and Leadbeater's *The Masters and the Path* (1925). As noted, Bailey's later work is a comprehensive examination of how the seven rays apply to all aspects of human evolution.

One purpose of Madame Blavatsky's Esoteric School was to facilitate the process of coming under the guidance of a Master in support of one's dedication to the service of humanity. In a *Preliminary Memorandum* of 1888 concerning the purposes of the school,

Blavatsky outlined the following stages in the development of relations between probationers and Masters:

- Developing a belief in the existence of Masters
- Understanding their nature and powers
- Reverencing them in one's heart
- Drawing near to them, as much as one can
- Opening oneself up for conscious communication with them, especially a Master to whom one might dedicate one's life
- Rising to the plane where the Masters are without attempting to draw them down to one's own
- Knowing that help, instruction, and enlightenment will be given when deserved[6]

Blavatsky's Inner Group teachings, kundalini practice, and Esoteric Instructions were designed to facilitate this process. What Blavatsky called the sixth sense of spiritual color played an essential role. As noted, many pages of discussion and diagrams in the Esoteric Instructions were dedicated to the spiritual significance of color and its esoteric correlations to numbers, days of the week, musical tones, principles of consciousness, and levels of being.[7] It was within the aura, as it were, of such teachings that the association of the chakras in the order of the rainbow colors was first formulated by a little-known Theosophist who took to heart Blavatsky's color correspondences and Bailey's guidelines on groups for color healing to create a now forgotten Master movement of her own.

Ivah Bergh Whitten

A clairvoyant, aura painter, and channel who worked primarily in Los Angeles, Ivah Bergh Whitten (1873–1947; referred to throughout this chapter as Whitten despite her many changes of name) was born Ivah Chipman Richardson in Riverside, Rhode Island. She acquired the name Bergh from her first husband, prominent New York architect Louis Bergh and Whitten from her second husband,

Texas-born freelance and Western pulp fiction writer Aaron Stuart Whitten.

Whitten attended Brook Hall Seminary, a finishing school in Media, Pennsylvania. During the 1890s, she worked as a freelance writer on the arts, as editor for Lesley's News Bureau, and a contributor to several newspapers, including the *New York Herald*. In 1897, she anonymously published *Two Women Who Posed*, an expose of the New York art studio scene, under the name Facilis. For a few years at the turn of the century, Whitten had a syndicated column of humorous aphorisms called "Women's Wisdom," publishing under her maiden name, Ivah C. Richardson.[8]

Whitten dated her interest in color to 1904.[9] In 1902, Leadbeater published *Man Visible and Invisible*, which dealt with the meaning of colors in the aura. While Whitten was living in New York, Leadbeater lectured there, in April and May 1904, using stereopticon views of auras, bodies, and thought forms.[10] Besant and Leadbeater jointly issued the book *Thought-Forms* in 1905. Given Whitten's artistic leanings, it is not surprising that she may have discovered Theosophy through image- and color-based presentations of auras and moods.

Whitten was said to have "experienced a personal crisis following the death of her husband in 1907."[11] The statement is problematic. Whitten appears to have *married* Louis Bergh in 1907.[12] However, about this time, she experienced a serious illness that confined her to St. Luke's Hospital in New York City. While there, she went among the wards to cheer people up and realized the healing potential of "beautiful thoughts" on people who suffer. This realization became the basis of public work in 1907 and 1908 as a teacher of health and beauty culture, under the name Ivah de Chipenham Bergh.[13] This work took her as far afield as Chicago.[14]

Whitten's personal crisis was apparently providential and decisive:

> While recovering from a nervous breakdown she was contacted by someone she later spoke of as an Elder Brother, a member of the Great White Brotherhood. He

offered her a choice, death or a life as a lightbearer to the world. She chose the latter, soon recovered from her illness, and became an active and avid Theosophist.[15]

The Berghs had moved to Washington, DC, in November 1912 and Louis died at the end of January 1913. His health had been bad for the previous five years—the duration of their marriage.[16] It is possible that Whitten had to give up writing and teaching to care for her husband and that after his death she collapsed from shock and exhaustion.

Blavatsky also experienced the intervention of Masters in connection with serious health crises. For example, during the writing of *The Secret Doctrine*, she was offered the chance to die or recover and complete the book, and chose the latter.[17] I make the comparison not to assert special spiritual status for Whitten, but only to point to the persistence of such stories of healings by Masters with a resulting missionary call to teach. We saw something similar with Amber Steen.

Supposedly, Whitten's involvement with Theosophy led to a new career:

> Eventually she became a lecturer for the Theosophical Society on her chosen topic, the occult meaning of color. As a result of her travels, study groups formed to examine her ideas. In the late 1920s these groups organized AMICA (the Amica Master Institute of Color Awareness).[18]

Membership records at the Theosophical Society in America indicate that Whitten first joined the organization in December, 1920, in San Antonio, Texas.[19] I do not know how she got from Washington to San Antonio. Her membership in the TS was inactive from June to December, 1922. She then sponsored the membership of her second husband, Aaron Stuart Whitten (she was his third wife), in Fort Worth.[20] The Whittens took a cross-country trip from

New York to Clovis, New Mexico, and thence to San Francisco in May 1924.[21] It is possible that Whitten did some lecturing for the Theosophical Society on this trip. However, the only indication of such lecturing I have seen is an undated transcript of a lecture given at the Long Beach Lodge in California, "What Your Aura Means to You," published in *What Color Means to You*.

I have not been able to trace the Whittens' activities in the latter half of the 1920s. They next appeared in Los Angeles in the 1930 US Census, where Aaron was listed as a self-employed writer and Whitten as a teacher of color psychology.[22]

The name of the organization that developed from Ivah's teachings went through several incarnations. It began as the Aquarian *Mystical* Institute of Color Awareness. About 1939, it was renamed the Aquarian *Master* Institute of Color Awareness. The notion of a Master Institute may have developed from Russian painter and Theosophist Nicholas Roerich, who established a Master Institute of United Arts in 1921 in New York City.[23]

Whitten "began to publish her findings in the 1930s, beginning with a booklet, *What Color Means to You* (1932)," published as a limited edition under the sponsorship of Roland Thomas Hunt, a native of England who later immigrated to the United States.[24] Hunt became Whitten's most prominent student. Whitten "also developed a form of healing meditation during which a person imagines breathing in a specific color."[25] The technique was not published until after her death, in *Color Breathing: The Breath of Transmutation*, though it was mentioned in earlier publications.

Color Awareness

Whitten developed a correspondence course to promote her teachings, the Initial Course in Color Awareness, which consisted of twelve installments, one per month (later published in book form under the same title). Each installment had two parts: an inspirational opening letter dealing with generalities, asserting Whitten's authority as teacher with personal information on her occult life and successful use of the principles she taught, and providing support in the form of a pep talk for students; and a lesson dealing with technicalities, including definitions of terms, meditation practices, and explanations and lists of color correspondences. The total length of the course, as published in book form, was forty-eight pages. Thus most of the information was presented in a condensed manner as hints for students to follow up on their own with personal study.

The foreword, by Whitten's students Roland Hunt and Dorothy Agnes Bailey, informs us that the "individual lessons," as opposed to the complete course in book form, were first published in 1932.[26] This statement sets the date for the association of chakras and rainbow colors eight years earlier than the 1940 date I gave in the afterword to Leadbeater's *The Chakras*.[27] It also clarifies that Cayce's 1936 association of chakras and rainbow colors was not the earliest on record. There is evidence that Whitten's *Initial Course* was influenced by Leadbeater's book, thus setting the period for its production to the five years between 1927 and 1932.[28]

Fundamentals of Cosmic Color

Whitten's lists of correspondences in the *Initial Course* create a previously unknown bridge between Blavatsky's Esoteric Instructions of the 1890s and the Western chakra system of a century later. The following is a summary of her teachings:

Color is an emanation of God, or the Logos (the Father Principle in figure 19), whose beingness is represented by white light. On the monadic plane, the white light of the Logos splits into the seven monads, angels, or "Spirits before the Throne" (Rev. 5:6), thus creating the cosmic color rays, which are expressions of the beingness of these great entities. Each of these entities further splits into seven color rays. The great being represented by indigo, for example, will express itself as indigo-red, indigo-orange, indigo-yellow, and so on, to indigo-violet. One of these entities (the fourth) generates seven color rays that express themselves as seven Masters of the "Great White Lodge" (also called Chohans of the Rays in

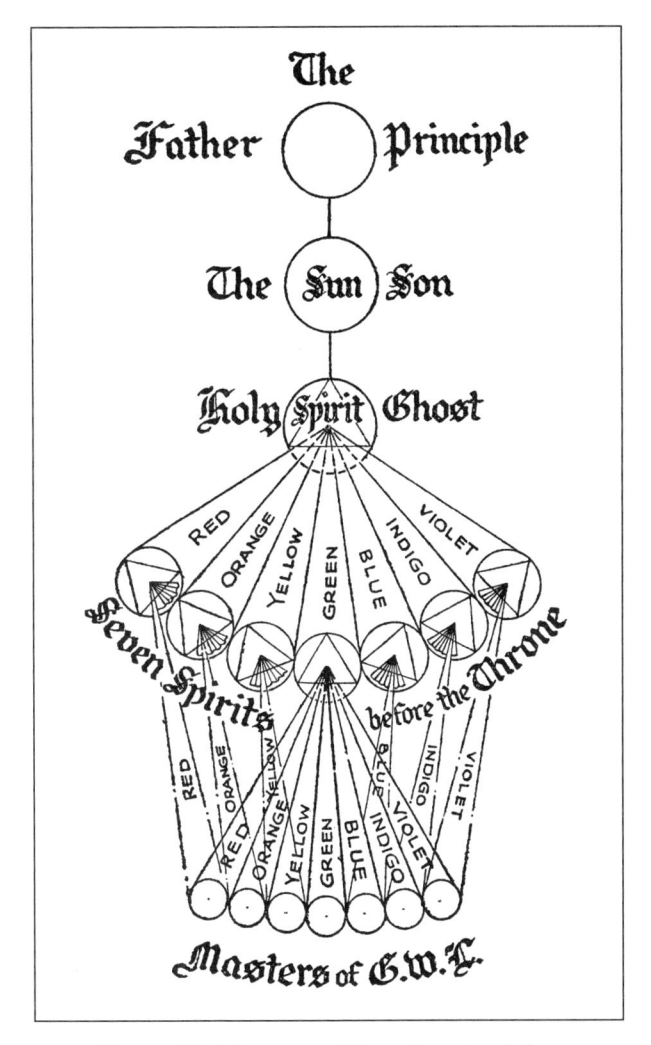

Figure 19. Masters and Rays (reprinted from
Roland T. Hunt, *Fragrant and Radiant Symphony*, 1937)[29]

the Besant/Leadbeater tradition), who govern various departments of life on earth, including power, wisdom, diplomacy, the arts, science, religious devotion, and ceremonial magic or ritual designed to work with devic consciousness. The Great White Lodge is associated with the benevolent power of so-called white magic.

Each human being is associated with one of these rays and

its color, Master, and implied life purpose. This association also expresses itself in a personality type. Through the Master, ray, and color, we attune ourselves to the Source of all being. This task requires us to align the chakras and their colors with their respective glands. Each chakra has a "centrifugal motion," and its color accelerates that motion, which "generates a magnetic force to which the gland under its control responds, thereby releasing certain chemicals necessary to the health of the bloodstream."[30]

This attunement process is enhanced by meditation on the Master, along with the use of colored lights, fragrances, musical tones, and jewels or gemstones—any of which can also help with healing physical, emotional, mental, and spiritual deficiencies (and the resulting diseases). Perhaps to suggest the all-embracing nature of the energies and forms of consciousness represented by the rays as devic beings and the Masters representing them, months, days of the week, and numbers are also said to correspond to them. It is possible (but not explicit in the *Initial Course*) that months, days of the week, and numbers provide clues about the ray to which individuals belong, based on numerological analysis of name and birthdate.[31]

Through aura analysis, it is possible to determine individuals' colors of *activity*, *rest*, and *inspiration*, thereby providing further support for the fulfillment of their life purpose and recovery from confusion and soul weariness.[32] This concept appears to be original to Whitten, who promotes the idea of an aura consultation for the determination of such colors for all students of color awareness, asserting that the gift or talent for such analysis is available only to those who have passed the "second great initiation," thus indirectly declaring what she considered to be her own spiritual status.[33] According to *The Masters and the Path*, this is the stage at which psychic abilities are mastered.[34]

The *Initial Course* was designed to help people meet the Master of their ray for spiritual guidance in the work they were to accomplish in the world. It describes a star of consciousness that represents the monad, "your own individualized spark of God. It is the real you—that which *is*."[35] This star can be carried in the solar plexus (for the first four rays) or in the forehead (for the last three). Those in the solar-plexus category will connect with the Master "in your sleep and you will bring back the experience as a beautiful dream or vision." Those in the forehead category "will simply SENSE or feel the presence the Master." Later comes "the moment when you both see and recognize him."[36]

This notion of a star of consciousness was introduced to the public in Leadbeater's *The Masters and the Path*, where he speaks of a "tiny silver star of consciousness that represents the monad."[37] According to Leadbeater, "A man may keep this star of consciousness where he will—that is to say, in any one of the seven principal centers of the body. Which of these is most natural to a man depends largely upon his type or ray." Most Westerners "nearly always keep that consciousness in the brain, in the center dependent upon the pituitary body." Others may "keep it habitually in the heart, the throat or the solar plexus."[38]

With the exception of Whitten's *Initial Course*, I have not seen references to the star of consciousness in later Theosophical literature. However, the notion resurfaced in the 1990s, in the energy healing work of Barbara Brennan, in which it is described as the *core star*. I return to this subject in the final chapter.

Color Correspondences

It is possible that Whitten's system remained unknown because no one made the effort to tabulate the apparently random lists of color correspondences in the *Initial Course* to perceive its sweep and grandeur. Ideally, the seventeen columns of correspondences I have extracted would form a single foldout spreadsheet demonstrating the move from cosmic color rays to Masters, human personality types, chakras, glands, needs, sounds, fragrances, and jewels—as if from the most spiritual to the most material elements of our universe. But publishing constraints require that I divide these columns into several tables (see pages 266–69), with some repetition

Table 14

Whitten's Major Ray Correspondences (1932)

Rays	Qualities	Colors	Masters
. . .	Cosmic urge Creation	White	Maitreya
Seventh	Inspiration Healing	Violet	Rakoczi [St. Germain]
Sixth	Intuition Devotion	Indigo	Scarus [Jesus]
Fifth	Science Invention	Blue	Hilarion
Fourth	Beauty Harmony	Green	Serapis
Third	Tact Intelligent service	Yellow	Venetian Master
Second	Wisdom Transmutation	Orange	Kuthumi
First	Will Vitality	Red	Morya

Personality Types	Chakras	Glands
. . .	. . .	. . .

Arch [crescent]
  Hypersensitive
  Idealistic
  Great artists
	Crown	Pineal

Oval
  Intolerant
  Practical
  Reformers
	Between eyes [Brow]	Pituitary

Circle
  Inertia-prone
  Adaptable
  Scientists
	Laryngeal [Throat]	Thyroid

Hexagon/square
  Greedy
  Generous
  Artists/Bankers
	Cardiac [Heart]	Memory [Mammary?]

Square
  Conservative
  Balanced
  Govt. workers
	Navel	Pancreas

Blunted triangle
  Prideful
  Understanding
  [Teachers[39]]
	Splenic	Spleen

Triangle
  Aggressive
  One-pointed
  Pioneers
	Root	Adrenals

TABLE 15
Whitten's Types and Needs (1932)

Rays	Personality Types	Physical Needs	Emotional Needs	Mental Needs	Spiritual Needs
Violet	Arch	Phosphorous	Love	Inspirational creative work	Poise/peace
Indigo	Oval	Silicon Phosphorous	Tranquility	Vision	Sense of at-one-ment
Blue	Circle	Oxygen	Stimulus	Inspiration	Unselfishness
Green	Hexagon	Nitrogen	Sympathy	Supervised systematic study	Mass or group worship
Yellow	Square	Carbon Phosphorous	Enthusiasm	Stimulation	Love
Orange	Blunted triangle	Carbon	Appreciation	Application	Peace
Red	Triangle	Hydrogen Iron	Joy	Activity	Purpose

TABLE 16
Whitten's Minor Ray Correspondences (1932)

Rays	Months	Days	Numbers	Tones	Perfumes	Jewels[40]
White	All months	...	11	Music of the spheres	White violet	Pearl
Violet	August	Monday	7	B	Violet	Amethyst Porphyry Violane
Indigo	September	Friday	3	A	Delicate oriental perfumes	Ruby
Blue	May	Thursday	1	G	Lilac Lily of the valley	Sapphire Topaz Citrine
Green	October	Saturday	8	F	Narcissus Tea rose	Jasper Agate Serpentine
Yellow	...	Wednesday	6	E	Jasmine	Emerald Jade
Orange	...	Sunday	9	D	Oriental lily	Sapphire Turquoise Sodalite
Red	January	Tuesday	5	C	Rose	Diamond Rock crystal [quartz]

for the sake of maintaining people's awareness of the basis of such correspondences in rays and colors.

Cosmic urge is a New Thought term from Ernest Holmes's *The Science of Mind* (1926), whose glossary defines it as "The desire of Spirit to express Itself." The presence of the spleen chakra in the second position indicates that Whitten was working from Leadbeater's *The Chakras*. The list of endocrine glands is based on that in Bailey's *The Soul and Its Mechanism* but revised to substitute the spleen for Bailey's sacral chakra. The substitution of memory/mammary glands for Bailey's thymus is curious.[41] Several passages in the *Initial Course* indicate that Whitten was writing primarily for a female audience.

The days of the week and musical tones are derived from a table in Blavatsky's Esoteric Instruction No. 1.[42] The perfumes appear to be a unique contribution.

The personality types appear to be derived from the tattvas of Rāma Prasād. An initial explanation lists only five types, just as there are five tattvas. Later lessons add the blunted triangle and the hexagon as "a sort of modification of the square [type], a little more pliable and rather more forward looking."[43] Here is a comparison of Prasād's tattvas (from *Śiva-Svarodaya*) and Whitten's types. (See table 17.)

Clearly, the association of the chakras with tattvas, or elements, in the Eastern system was broken in whatever process led to the creation of Whitten's types. That process may have involved an unknown intermediary who invented the system. That intermediary may have been responsible for expanding the types to seven so they would correspond with the rays, after which Whitten linked them to rays, colors, and chakras.

A few references in Whitten's *Initial Course* indicate a possible set of correspondences between personality types and crystal types: "The crystal of green is a modification of the square, almost hexagonal"; "the crystal of indigo is not fixed, varying between an oval and a hexagon, sometimes tending toward one, sometimes the other, but most often the oval."[44] Specific crystal types are not

Table 17
Tattvas, Symbols, and Colors

Chakras (Traditional)	Tattvas (Traditional)	Symbols (Prasād)	Colors (Prasād)	Chakras (Whitten)	Symbols (Whitten)	Colors (Whitten)
Fifth	Ether	Oval	All colors	Seventh	Broken arch [Crescent]	Violet
Fourth	Air	Circle	Green	Sixth	Closed arch [Oval]	Indigo
Third	Fire	Triangle	Red	Fifth	Circle	Blue
Second	Water	Crescent	White	Third	Square	Yellow
First	Earth	Square	Yellow	First	Triangle	Red

given for the other chakras/rays/colors. The notion of linking crystals and chakras does not reappear for another fifty years, with the publication Joy Gardner's *Color and Crystals: A Journey through the Chakras* (1988).

In more recent correlations of the chakras with gemstones or crystals, the abiding principle seems to be matching the colors of each. According to this principle, red gems go with the first chakra, so it is odd to find ruby associated with the sixth. Orange gems correspond to the second chakra, but Whitten's are blue. Yellow gems should be matched with the third chakra; Whitten's are green. Whitten seems to "get it right" by associating sapphire with the blue of the fifth chakra, but topaz and citrine should be matched with the third. Only amethyst in the seventh chakra lines up with current thinking on such correspondences. Diamond, too, could be matched with the seventh chakra in systems that use white instead of violet.

The issue here is that the original table in Leadbeater's *The Masters and the Path* matched up rays and jewels but not colors. The association of the seven rays with the prismatic colors in rainbow order was Whitten's unique contribution. She simply apportioned the entries in Leadbeater's table to the rays/colors/chakras in her system without revising the colors of the jewels—except in the case of sapphire, which appears twice. Leadbeater assigned it to the second ray, and Whitten assigned it to the second chakra but then added it to the blue fifth ray/chakra as a substitute for steatite.

Table 18 lays out the information available to Whitten in the period after the publication of *The Chakras* in 1927 and before the publication of her color-awareness course in letter form in 1932. It appears that she drew her ray qualities from both Leadbeater and Bailey, adding her own interpretations.

Whitten's Legacy

Bailey called her incomplete list of ray colors in *Letters on Occult Meditation* a "puzzle," thus challenging Whitten to solve it.[49] Bailey

Table 18
Rays, Chakras, and Colors (1920s–30s)

Rays/Chakras	Leadbeater's Ray Qualities (1920)[45]	Chakra Colors (1927)[46]	Bailey's Ray Qualities (1922)[47]	Ray Colors (1922)[48]	Whitten's Ray Qualities (1932)	Ray/Chakra Colors (1932)
Seventh	Ordered service Ceremony	Violet	Ceremonial magic Law	Violet	Inspiration Healing	Violet
Sixth	Devotion	Indigo	Abstract idealism Devotion	...	Intuition Devotion	Indigo
Fifth	Science Detailed knowledge	Blue	Concrete knowledge Science	Orange	Science Invention	Blue
Fourth	Beauty Harmony	Yellow	Harmony/Beauty Art/Unity	Green	Beauty Harmony	Green
Third	Adaptability Tact	Green	Activity Adaptability	Yellow	Intelligent service	Yellow
Second	Wisdom	Rose	Love Wisdom	Indigo	Wisdom Transmutation	Orange
First	Strength	Orange-red	Will Power	...	Will Vitality	Red

had stated that "complementary colors may be spoken of in occult books in terms of each other. Red may be called green and orange may be called blue,"[50] inviting Whitten to substitute blue for orange in the fifth ray and orange for indigo in the second. After that, it was a simple matter to place red and indigo in prismatic order in the blanks left by Bailey.

Alternatively, Whitten could refer to Leadbeater's *The Chakras*, swapping green and yellow so they correspond to colors given for the third and fourth rays by Bailey, and replacing rose with orange for the second ray. However, though Leadbeater referred to the colors in the chakras as rays, they are rays of vitality (prana) from the physical sun, not the "seven great streams of force of the Logos" as defined by Blavatsky, Leadbeater, and Bailey.[51] By correlating the cosmic rays of the Logos with the pranic rays of the sun, Whitten was able to link the rays, colors, and chakras. However, at this point, the connection of the chakras with Blavatsky's seven principles and their colors, as given in the chart from which Whitten drew the correspondences for colors, days of the week, and tones, was severed.[52]

Blavatsky said that "the human principles elude enumeration, because each man differs from every other. . . . Numbering is here a question of spiritual progress and the natural predominance of one principle over another." Furthermore, "the numbers and principles do not go in regular sequence, like the skins of an onion, but the student must work out for himself the number appropriate to each of his principles"—and this must be done "apart from any system of enumeration, or by association with their corresponding centers of action, colors, sounds, etc."[53] Leadbeater and Bailey had tried to honor Blavatsky's teachings on these matters, leading to much confusion, especially in Bailey's myriad versions of ray/color and chakra/color correspondences in later books. Perhaps for this reason, Whitten took the decisive step of no longer referring to the rays by number but only by color, calling them *cosmic* rays.

It should be clear from this analysis of Whitten's *Initial Course* that this simple yet obvious correlation of chakras and rainbow colors had significant hurdles to overcome in Theosophical circles in the 1920s. (See table 18.) Based on Blavatsky's writings, Bailey was in the process of evolving ever more complicated associations between rays, colors, and chakras. Without realizing it, Whitten had inserted herself into the tradition of chromotherapy initiated by Bailey's *Letters on Occult Meditation* in a way that broke decisively with the principles Bailey was developing—principles that would first become explicit in the first volume of *Esoteric Psychology* (1936). Among these principles, as noted, was the placement of the first ray, in association with red, in the seventh or highest center—in connection with the atman, the divine will; and the placement of violet in connection with the second center, because we were allegedly passing through a historic period in which the seventh ray would be actively stimulating our sexuality.

Whatever sense Bailey's principles made from the cosmic perspective, they were not usable by color therapists. There were too many inflections to remember. The seven rainbow colors provided a simple mnemonic device that any Westerner could use as a handy set of mental drawers within which to file information relevant to the purpose and proper functioning of the seven chakras.

Though Whitten was the first to list correspondences between Masters, rays, colors, and chakras, she was not the last. The I AM Activity, a movement with Theosophical roots, initiated in the 1930s by Guy Ballard (1878–1939) and his wife Edna (1886–1971), correlated Masters with colors.[54] The Bridge to Freedom, an offshoot of the I AM Activity founded by Geraldine Innocente (1915–61), added the chakras in the 1950s. The Summit Lighthouse and Church Universal and Triumphant of Mark L. Prophet (1918–73) and his wife Elizabeth Clare Prophet (1939–2009), which developed from the Bridge to Freedom, published two popular books on the chakras in the 1970s: *Studies of the Human Aura* (1971), channeled by Kuthumi (allegedly Master KH of the Theosophical tradition) and Djwal Kul (allegedly Alice Bailey's source); and *Intermediate Studies of the Human Aura* (1976), channeled by Djwal Kul.

These groups each developed a list of Masters that was different from that published by Leadbeater in *The Masters and the Path*, though with some overlap. Their coordination of colors and chakras is unique—the Bridge to Freedom and the Summit Lighthouse do not use Leadbeater's system or the rainbow system, and their respective systems differ slightly from each other (from lowest to highest, in the Bridge to Freedom: white, violet, gold and ruby, pink, blue, green, and yellow; in the Summit Lighthouse: white, violet, purple and gold, pink, blue, green, and yellow).[55] Though the Summit Lighthouse books were popular in their day, they do not seem to have influenced the development of the Western chakra system. The Bridge to Freedom system has been almost entirely forgotten.

Chapter 18
Temples of Radiance

Chromotherapy was based on the scientific correlation between color and vibrational frequency. Sound, too, was correlated to vibrational frequency. Thus the seven colors of the spectrum could be correlated to the seven notes of the diatonic scale. Just as there were sounds with frequencies above and below the threshold of human hearing, so were there colors above and below the threshold of human sight. Since the piano was divided into octaves in which the same notes repeated in ever higher ranges, it was assumed that the spectrum of light was also divided into octaves. Thus there must be octaves of light frequencies below red (infrared) and above violet (ultraviolet).

Nonphysical planes, too, came in octaves of seven subplanes. It was assumed that their ever more subtle varieties of matter corresponded to ever higher vibrational rates. It was also assumed, based on Blavatsky's teachings, that humans would develop sixth and seventh senses that would allow them to perceive astral sounds and colors.

In the mid-twentieth century, fragrances were added to the mix. It was thought that these too must be arranged in octaves and that there must be a vibrational continuum that linked smells to sounds to colors in ever rising frequencies. Though there might be gaps in human perception along this continuum, spiritual evolution would eventually fill them in with astral sense impressions—and those of even higher planes—including smells, sights, and sounds.[1]

Movements developed to employ these sense modalities in ritualistic settings, including magical orders, secret societies, and alternative churches. One example comes from an ad in a Spiritualist newsletter from 1961 for a "Temple of Radiant Reflection" sponsored by the Aquarian Cosmic Color Fellowship in Hollywood, CA: "Radiant Life Harmonics, an evening dedicated to the

Garden of the Soul, featuring a symphony of color, music, perfume, and incense, followed by a trance lecture on the Science of Color."[2] Such "temples of radiance" can be traced to the lost color teachings of Ivah Bergh Whitten.

Color Temple College (Roland Hunt)

As noted, Whitten's chief student was Roland Thomas Hunt (1900–1973). He fostered an image as a multitalented Renaissance man—anatomist, architect, artist, businessman in advertising and publicity, musician, physiologist, poet, psychologist, and spiritual healer/teacher. In his writings, he comes across as an ambitious, enthusiastic, humanitarian, idealistic, romantic visionary—and tireless self-promoter, in particular of his line of art-deco-style color healing (Spectrone) lamps. Based on the only photograph I have been able to examine and hints in his writings, Hunt seems to have been a charming, handsome, clothes-horse of a celebrity hound. He was married to artist/author Vera Stanley Alder (whom we met in an earlier chapter) for ten years from 1943 to 1953.[3]

Hunt first visited the United States in 1923.[4] By 1930, he had met Whitten. His book *The Finding of Rainbow's End, and Other Mystical Experiences in the "Mother Lode" Country in 1930* (1939), a memoir-like work of what now would be called creative nonfiction, tells the tale of geology professor Stuart White (Aaron Stuart Whitten) and his clairvoyant wife's magical discovery of a property in the California Sierras they hope to develop into a paradisiacal spiritual retreat—pending their mining of the rich vein of radium on which it rests.[5]

An earlier book, *Fragrant and Radiant Symphony* (1937), presented Hunt's spiritual synthesis of the arts of color, perfume, and sound while chronicling the development of his vision of an international movement of spiritual color workers in service of humanity, based on Whitten's teachings (AMICA), with a nucleus under his direction in England and under hers in the United States. The symbol of this movement was a pinecone, with reference to the pineal gland, which "plays such an important part in the unfolding of the etheric faculties."[6] Hunt presented elaborate, never-to-be-realized architectural plans for a futuristic "Color-Temple-College" called Lotus Lodge.

Hunt explained that, twenty-one years earlier, Whitten "was first told to leave her beautiful mansion-home and treasured possessions." The call must have come between the 1913 death of her husband and her appearance in Texas in 1920. Hunt continued: "She was instructed by the Masters to proceed to establish a color and art colony with a central club house and a half circle of individual bungalows, each in its color-note."[7] Eventually, there would be "a Yellow Temple for development of intellectual understanding, a Blue Temple for devotional purposes of a new order, and a Green Temple for the active, physical application of cosmic knowledge."[8]

Similar temples, in terms of color and purpose, are described in Besant and Leadbeater's *Man: Whence, How, and Whither* (1913), in connection with the evolution of humanity and the development of a colony in California intended to foster the development of a more spiritually advanced race whose heyday would come hundreds of years in the future.[9]

In Hunt's *The Seven Keys to Color Healing* (1940), the purposes of the AMICA movement were described as follows:

- "To increase color awareness throughout the world"
- "To employ the color wisdom individually and collectively, subjectively and objectively, in every aspect of life"
- "To take active part in world reconstruction, building sound health and harmonious environment; to improve individual and international understanding"
- "To use color's wonderful flexibility in the service of healing with spiritual awareness, psychological understanding, and the aid of physical color accessories [such as Hunt's lamps]"[10]

Progress in the movement entailed the following steps:

1. Introduction to the subject, using *What Color Means to You*
2. Class instruction or correspondence course (with individual selection of four possible subjects: color awareness, color psychology, color symbolism, or color therapy
3. Formation of independent study groups "of not more than eleven members"
4. Associate membership, with certificate, after one year of study and dedicating "at least fifteen minutes a day for one year studying color"
5. Possibility of visiting AMICA headquarters, whose address "will always remain a secret with our members, and you may not visit there until you are an associate member"[11]

Only Whitten's course on color awareness was ever made public. Hunt mentioned a second course entitled Using Color, "containing clairvoyant paintings of the chakras, charts, etc.," but it seems not to have survived.[12] The secret headquarters was probably a nonphysical or astral location, perhaps a color temple such as those described.

The Seven Keys to Color Healing brought forward portions of Whitten's course on color awareness, in particular the connection of cosmic color rays and chakras. Hunt greatly expanded Whitten's color correspondences to include metals, chemicals, and foods and specified color-based regimens and protocols for the alleviation of various physical and psychological illnesses.

As noted in my afterword to Leadbeater's *The Chakras*, Hunt's *Seven Keys* also contained a diagram showing side and front views of a human torso with the locations of the chakras marked in each, copied from plates in Leadbeater's *The Chakras*.[13] These views are laid out against a graphic representation of the seven planes. Each plane not only receives a color (with the color names running along a central vertical line labeled "The Color Aspect of the Logos and Man") but also is linked by lines to a chakra in the torso:

- **Physical**—red (root)
- **Etheric** (called "plane of chemicalization or man's disease")—orange (spleen)
- **Astral**—yellow (navel)
- **Lower Mental**—green (heart)
- **Upper Mental**—blue (throat)
- **Buddhic**—indigo (brow)
- **Nirvanic**—violet (crown)
- **Paranirvanic**—white

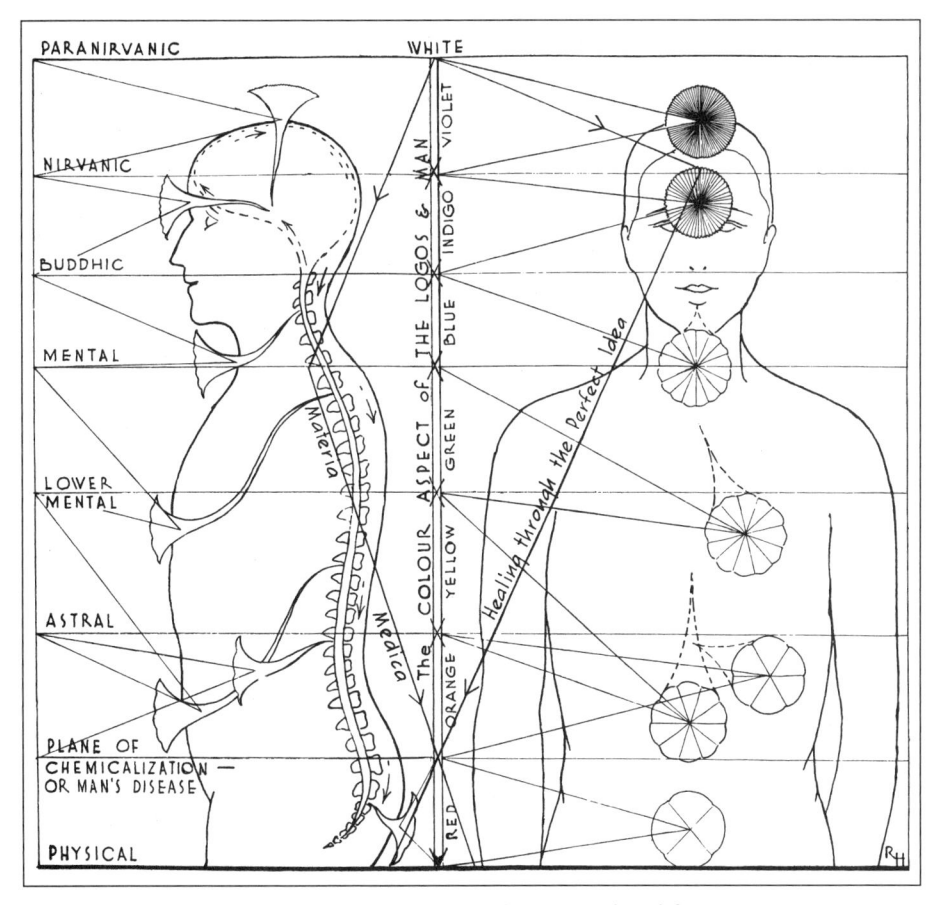

Figure 20. Chakras and Planes (reprinted from Roland T. Hunt, *The Seven Keys to Color Healing*, 1940)

Chemicalization is a Christian Science term meaning "an agitation and aggravation of old beliefs on their way to dissolution."[14] Possibly, the etheric level of being is highlighted as the plane on which disease first manifests itself before appearing in the physical body, as well as the plane on which the causes of disease may be dissolved.

This is perhaps the first graphic depiction of a connection between chakras and planes. It follows the terms Leadbeater used in a plate in *Man Visible and Invisible* (though Leadbeater treated the physical and etheric levels of being as a single plane, as he also did the lower and upper levels of the mental plane; he called the monadic plane *paranirvanic*—"beyond nirvanic"; and he added a *mahaparanirvanic* plane—"greater beyond nirvanic"—to make up seven planes in all).[15]

An outline of Hunt's diagram—without the torso, chakras, and line of color names—appeared as early as 1932, in *What Color Means to You*, suggesting that the correspondence of chakras, colors, and planes dates to the same period as the color-awareness course.[16] Though the course itself mentioned planes and subplanes in connection with the effectual range of certain colors, the graphic presentation in *Seven Keys* was clearer.

Hunt's book remained in print for the next forty years, thus keeping Whitten's association of colors and chakras current until they were eventually combined with the chakra qualities we are now familiar with in the 1970s.

After Whitten's death in 1947, Hunt and Dorothy Bailey founded the AMICA Trust in order to keep Whitten's legacy alive. The results were the publication of an expanded version of *What Color Means to You*, the pamphlet on color breathing mentioned previously, and the *Initial Course*. A year after the death of Aaron Stuart Whitten in 1958, Hunt and Bailey established the AMICA Temple of Radiance in Los Angeles and began a new a series of correspondence course lessons channeled by someone other than Whitten. Since these lessons rarely deal with chakras and colors, I do not consider them here.[17]

Cosmic Color Fellowship (S. G. J. Ouseley)

If Whitten had her international association of color workers in AMICA, her self-appointed successor, S. G. J. Ouseley (1903–57), had his "Cosmic Color Fellowship," "a worldwide organization that stands to help and serve you whatever your position or ambition is." The requirements for joining were simpler than Whitten's— nothing more than pursuing "a six-months' course in the principles of color science." Both course and membership had the purpose of "helping people to radiate new life, light, and color" by becoming "*cosmic*-minded so that they may become more sensitive to the rays flowing perpetually from the cosmic planes."[18]

Another advertisement indicated that the fellowship was founded in 1947 and existed "for the purpose of applying the principles of color and radiation in all aspects of life. It is devoted to the Science of Radiant Life. Correspondence courses in color science and chromotherapy are available."[19] A publisher's note in later editions of *The Power of the Rays* indicated that the fellowship was closed after Ouseley's death.[20]

Born Stephen Geoffrey John Ouseley, this British Theosophist and occultist was the only son of John Joseph Mulvy (sometimes Mulvey) Ouseley (1859–1930), a London-based journalist, newspaper editor, novelist, dramatist, and publisher, and his second wife. Stephen Ouseley trained to become a teacher, worked as a schoolmaster, and married twice. He seems to have lived quietly— with one notable exception.[21]

In 1931, the year after his father's death, Ouseley published a brief autobiographical memoir, *From Camaldoli to Christ: Modern Monasticism Unveiled*. His family was devoutly Catholic. The memoir resentfully described Ouseley's schooling in Catholic institutions, climaxing with a failed attempt to become a monk in the Tuscan monastery of Camaldoli, and his turning to the Church of England. The book was published by an anti-Catholic organization called Harrison Trust. Indeed, Ouseley may have been exploited by a rabidly anti-Catholic protestant priest who not only helped him publish the book but also sent him out on the lecture circuit, where he horrified audiences with tales of his sufferings in Catholic schools and the monastery. The *Tablet*, a London-based Catholic weekly, attempted to discredit the book and lectures with a series of articles that mockingly exposed various inconsistencies, exaggerations, and alleged untruths.[22] It is possible that, because of the resulting scandal, Ouseley chose to live almost invisibly and sign himself with his initials, rather than Stephen, to avoid being identified as an unreliably truthful author.

In the 1940s, following the death of his mother, Ouseley began publishing occult fiction in little magazines. He also published pieces in the *Theosophist* and the *Occult Review*, to which he was a frequent contributor.[23] Toward the end of the decade, he produced the small books he is presently known for: *A Guide to Telepathy and Psychometry* (1948), *The Science of the Aura* (1949), *Color Meditations* (1949), and *The Power of the Rays* (1951). With the exception of the first, these books were continuously in print for nearly forty years. Ouseley died prematurely in 1957, at the age of 53.

Color therapy had apparently become a hot topic in the mid-twentieth century. Ouseley's books were published by L. N. Fowler, a competitor of Hunt's British publisher, C. W. Daniel, perhaps because of Hunt's success with *The Seven Keys to Color Healing*.

Whatever Ouseley touched, he improved (by his own lights). Thus, what Whitten called color *awareness*, Ouseley called color *consciousness*. Whitten's appeal to a female audience with hints on color decoration became Ouseley's appeal to a male audience through an emphasis on abstract theory and frequent use of the term *color science*. Whitten's briefly mentioned colors of rest, activity, and inspiration, became Ouseley's categories of restful, revitalizing, and inspiring or stimulating colors, complete with lists.[24] Whitten's technique of color breathing, first described in Hunt's *Seven Keys* and elaborated in her posthumously published pamphlet, became the basis of rewrites of Hunt's book in more usable formats in *Color Meditations* and *The Power of the Rays*.[25]

On close inspection, any Ouseley material that seems genuinely new is repackaged from some earlier, unmentioned source. For example, in Theosophical literature, the seven subplanes of the physical plane are divided into solid, liquid, gaseous, and four types of ether, each more subtle than the last. Besant and Leadbeater label them with the unhelpful names of Ethers I–IV and later the only slightly more helpful names etheric, superetheric, subatomic, and atomic. In Heindel's *The Rosicrucian Cosmo-Conception*, these levels are called the chemical ether, light ether, life ether, and reflecting ether—the last containing a physical-plane reflection of the akashic records.[26] Ouseley resurrects the terms in *The Power of the Rays* but does not attribute the source.[27]

Ouseley's fundamentals are similar to Whitten's but more decisively stated:

- "The color rays are representatives of the cosmic lights—realize that they are spiritual forces perpetually flowing toward and through you."
- "The colors work through the glandular centers of the body. The principle behind color healing is the regulation of the flow of the color forces by consciously absorbing them as needed, using each ray with the specific purpose of rebuilding and revitalizing every organ of the body *through the etheric counterpart.*"
- "Regular and systematic practice will gradually transform your body, mind, and spirit. The general health will improve, and the mind will become more efficient, and the spirit-self more sensitive and developed."
- "The color method soon becomes a *subconscious* function; color being one of the fundamental elements in the universe, [it] acts on the subconscious mind which is an important source of health and vitality, whilst life in general assumes a happier outlook."[28]

Ouseley's emphasis on the etheric body and the subconscious indicates that the scope of his system was less grand than Whitten's. The purpose of Whitten's *Initial Course* was to outfit people for work on behalf of the world with knowledge about the life purpose of their ray and how to connect to the spiritual guidance of the Master of that ray. Ouseley's approach focused on health and self-improvement, as does the Western chakra system we are familiar with today.

For our purposes, Ouseley's teachings on correspondences between colors and chakras may be quickly summarized in tabular form. (See table 19 on pages 290–91.) Though he makes the same attribution of chakras to rays as did Whitten, he leaves out references to the ray names, Masters, personality types, and the minor correspondences, such as those to the days of the week and gemstones.

The functions of the cosmic color rays in Ouseley's books are more divergent from Leadbeater's and Bailey's teachings than are the functions taught by Whitten. However, Ouseley's functions look even more like a continuum of human potential rising in graded stages from material to spiritual than does Pryse's or Leadbeater's take on the chakras. Ouseley's continuum allows for a clearer alignment between elements, planes, auras, and qualities.

The column of elements is to be understood as a sevenfold manifestation of each ray/color. For example, orange has its physical/material, psychological, harmonizing/unifying, healing, inspirational/intuitive, and spiritual/higher-consciousness aspects—in addition to its usual vitalizing function. This is another way of saying that each ray contains the other rays within it. Thus there is orange-red, orange-orange, orange-yellow, orange-green, orange-blue, orange-indigo, and orange-violet. Bailey employed this nomenclature in *Letters on Occult Meditation*.[30] By following Ouseley's nomenclature, we could more easily realize the functions of the sevenfold rays by referring to orange-yellow as "the psychological aspect of vitality" or orange-indigo as "the inspirational aspect of orange."

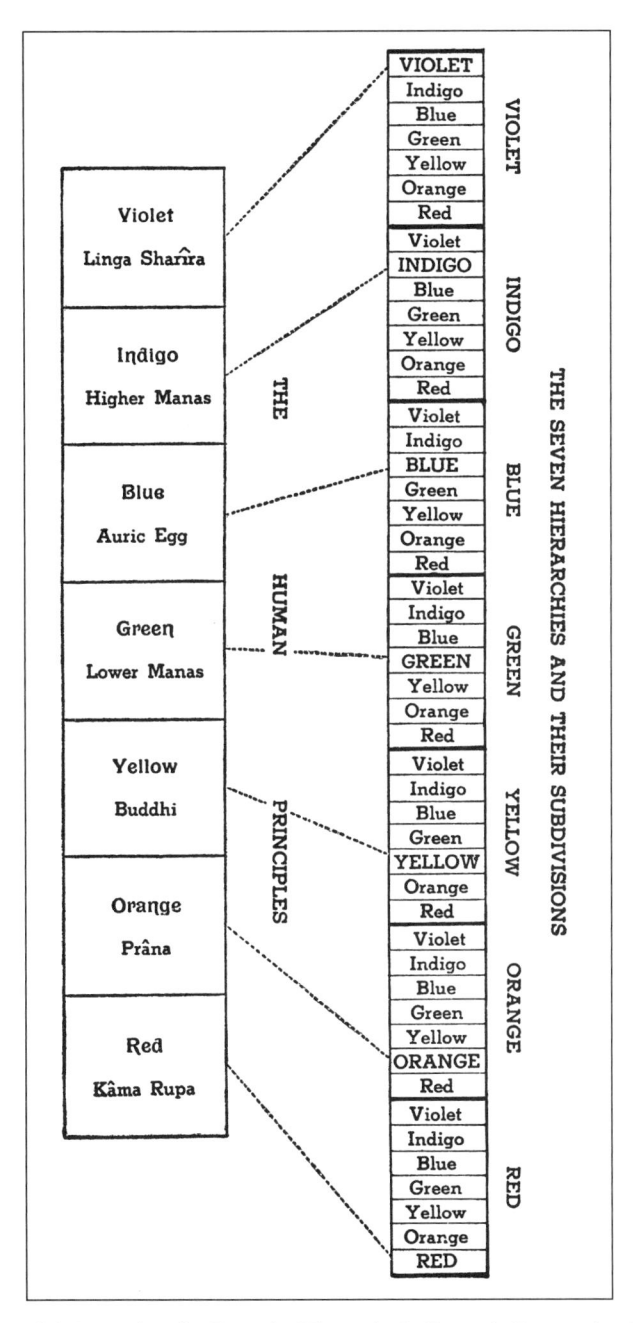

Figure 21. Mapping the Rays in Blavatsky's Esoteric Instruction No. 2
(reprinted from H. P. Blavatsky, *The Secret Doctrine*,
vol. 5: *Occultism*, 1897/1938)

The rationale for mapping the rays into one another appeared in Blavatsky's Esoteric Instruction No. 2, in the following words, accompanied by a diagram reproduced here as figure 21:

> As the seven colors of the solar spectrum correspond to the seven rays, or hierarchies, so each of these latter has again its seven divisions corresponding to the same series of colors. But in this case one color, *viz*: that which characterizes the particular hierarchy as a whole, is predominant and more intense than the others.[31]

This idea is carried forward not only in Bailey's teachings but also in Ivah Bergh Whitten's, as relayed by Roland Hunt in *Fragrant and Radiant Symphony*. Hunt reproduced Blavatsky's diagram there but eliminated the names of the principles, thus paving the way for Ouseley's radically different presentation of this correlation, as given in table 19.[32] It is important to note that Hunt's version represented a decisive break with from Blavatsky's teachings on the relationship between principles, planes, colors, and the aura.

As indicated, Blavatsky insisted that the principles should not be given an order, since their appearance in every individual represented an evolutionary stage in that person's spiritual development and would be different for everyone. Though Bailey and her followers remained true to this approach, most writers on color healing and the chakras after Whitten and Hunt portrayed the lower and higher principles, planes, layers of the aura, and chakras by arranging them to correspond to the lower and higher frequencies of light and their respective colors, from red to violet, in rainbow order. Over time, the notion of principles became submerged, as in Ouseley's books, then dropped out completely.

In table 19, the thread-self (*sūtrātman*) refers to a lesser known Theosophical concept, describing the causal body (soul) as a thread upon which an individual's lifetimes are strung like beads.[33] This is the first time the notion appears in conjunction with the chakras. It does not receive further attention in this context for another forty years. In the 1990s, it reemerges in the chakra and aura teachings of Barbara Brennan.

Another idea implied in this table of correspondences, but not fully developed until Brennan takes it up, is that aura layers and chakras may be mapped into each other. Ouseley does not go so far as to state that each layer of the aura has its own chakra system, as does Brennan. However, he indicates that the chakras are "gateways" to the aura layers and their respective planes, principles, or functions.[34]

Ouseley reversed the gland correlations of the sixth and seventh chakras. He may have been following Bailey's *Letters on Occult Meditation*, or he may have preferred the apparent logic of linking the so-called third-eye gland (pineal) with the third-eye clairvoyance of the sixth chakra. Curiously, Hunt's *Seven Keys* uses the same correlation, even though Whitten linked the pineal with the seventh chakra.[35]

The value of Ouseley's books is that they are clear, concise, and systematically presented. He was a better writer than either Whitten or Hunt—not only in organization, but also in style. He synthesized a vast amount of occult information (usually without attributing sources) into what appears to be an authoritative, perhaps innovative system. But I see Whitten as the true innovator in the color/chakra connection. Hunt was a disseminator. Ouseley was a source-amnesia-prone consolidator. If his books were not so focused on the aura and color healing, and only incidentally on the chakras, I would call them the *Wheels of Life* of 1950—but that would be unfair to Anodea Judith, who scrupulously acknowledged her sources.

Ouseley's published works never *literally* plagiarized the sources he appropriated. For example, his chapter on the Temple of Color in *Color Meditations* was derived in part from the passages on color temples in Besant and Leadbeater's *Man: Whence, How, and Whither*—but Ouseley's version was more beautifully rendered.[36]

Table 19
Ouseley's Correspondences (ca. 1950)[29]

Rays	Functions	Elements	Planes
White	. . .	. . .	Cosmic source
Violet	Spiritual power	Spiritual Higher consciousness	Divine/absolute
Indigo	Intuition	Inspirational Intuitional	Intuitional
Blue	Inspiration	Healing	Spiritual/causal
Green	Energy supply	Harmonizing Unifying	Higher mental
Yellow	Wisdom	Psychological	Lower mental
Orange	Health	Vitalizing	Astral
Red	Life	Physical Material	Physical/etheric

Principles (Blavatsky)	Aura Layers	Qualities	Chakras & Glands
...	...	...	...
Atman	Masters	Idealistic Worthy Truly great	Top of head Pituitary
Buddhi	Initiates	Wise Sincere Saintly	Mid-forehead Pineal
Buddhi-manas	Causal body Thread-self	Religious Devotional Mystical	Throat Thyroid
Manas or Antahkarana	Subjective mind Soul principle	Adaptable Compassionate Sympathetic	Cardiac plexus Heart
Kama-manas	Objective mind	Intelligent Concentrated Optimistic	Solar plexus Adrenals
Kama-prana	Emotional	Proud Vital Responsible	Spleen
Sthula-linga	Health	Sensual Commanding Domineering	Base of spine

If I had to classify Ouseley's variety of source amnesia, I would attribute it to the intentional vagueness of the author with nothing new to say who wants to impress an audience with intimations of spiritual authority, and to "justifiable" appropriation, in which claims by earlier sources of transmitting an ageless ancient wisdom appear to nullify present-day intellectual property rights.

Temple of Radiant Reflection (Mary L. Wiyninger)

History repeated itself in 1960, three years after Ouseley's death, when the Aquarian Cosmic Color Fellowship was incorporated as a nonprofit organization by Mary Lucille Wiyninger (1907–79). Note that the organization's name combined elements of Whitten's Aquarian Mystical Institute of Color Awareness and Ouseley's Cosmic Color Fellowship. Wiyninger was one of the ministers listed in the ad for the Temple of Radiant Reflection, mentioned earlier. This ad also referred to a correspondence course called "ABC's of Color Science—14 Lessons"—the same number as in Ouseley's course.[37]

I consulted a copy of Wiyninger's *Color and Cosmic Science: The ABC's of Color Science*—a single spiral-bound volume with typed, mimeographed text. I assumed this was the course of fourteen lessons mentioned in this ad and that it might contain lost correspondence school teachings by Whitten or Ouseley. It turned out to be volume 1 of 2, containing only the first seven lessons, covering the first three rays and chakras. Significant chunks of material had been lifted from Hunt's *Seven Keys* (without attribution). More startling were passages plagiarized from Whitten's *Initial Course in Color Awareness*, complete with original spelling errors. There was much new information on the endocrine glands in relation to the chakras, possibly from Ouseley. However, in the absence of examples of lost Whitten or Ouseley correspondence courses, it would be impossible to determine the degree of borrowing or influence. For both Ouseley and Wiyninger, source amnesia based on uncopyrighted, ephemeral correspondence courses may have provided the means of perpetrating a perfectly undetectable crime.

Be that as it may, Hunt's *Seven Keys to Color Healing* and Ouseley's *Color Meditations*, *Power of the Rays*, and *Science of the Aura* in the 1940s and early 1950s transmitted the association of chakras and rainbow colors to spiritual seekers of the 1960s and 1970s, so it was ready for assimilation with the chakra qualities developed within the human potential movement. The next stage in the evolution of the Western chakra system takes us to the peculiar combination of Eastern mysticism and Western psychology that prevailed at Esalen Institute of California, the birthplace of the Western chakra system as we know it.

Part 5
Scholars and Swamis and Shrinks, Oh My!
(1930s–70s)

Chapter 19
The Serpent's Brood

While Leadbeater's *The Chakras* was being disseminated in English-speaking countries throughout the world, in various Western European languages, and in India (in English), and the chromotherapists in England and America were at work on their color-based views of the chakras, inspired by Bailey's *Letters on Occult Meditation*, news of kundalini and the chakras was spreading slowly through intellectual circles in Europe. This spread was catalyzed by the 1919 publication of Woodroffe's *The Serpent Power*.

For example, in Italy, philosopher and esotericist Julius Evola (1898–1974) began publishing on tantric teachings and *The Serpent Power* in 1927 (*L'uomo come potenza; Man as power*). The book was revised and achieved its present title in 1949 (*Lo yoga della Potenza; The Yoga of Power*) and was translated into English in 1992. I found this to be a lucid philosophical and esoteric explanation of Tantra and the chakras—and no wonder, since Evola was in correspondence with Woodroffe when writing the first version.[1]

In France, philosopher and esotericist René Guénon (1886–1951) published several articles on Tantra and related subjects, including *The Serpent Power*, in the 1930s. These articles include *"Kundalini Yoga"* "Tantrism and Magic," and "The Fifth Veda"— each of which appears in a volume of Guénon's collected works, *Studies in Hinduism*. The book also provides a generous selection of Guénon's reviews of books and articles on various aspects of Hinduism, published in French and English from 1930 to 1950, demonstrating the wealth of personal, yogic, and scholarly investigations of the subject in Europe during this period. Like Crowley, Regardie, and Fortune, Guénon, an increasingly formidable voice in Western esoteric studies, also noted parallels between the kabbalistic Tree of Life and the chakras in his essay entitled *"Kundalini Yoga"* first published in 1933.[2]

However, the most important developments among the European intelligentsia for the evolution of the Western chakra system took place in Switzerland.

Jung and *The Serpent Power*

Zurich-based psychologist Carl Gustav Jung (1875–1961) also began to discuss kundalini yoga and *The Serpent Power* in public forums in the 1930s. Around the time of the First World War, Jung began drawing mandalas to monitor his psychological development.[3] He saw them as symbols of psychological wholeness that emerged from deep within us, often containing archetypal elements drawn from a vast storehouse of shared cultural imagery that he called the collective unconscious. Drawing a series of mandalas could represent "the restoration of inner peace to the self,"[4] superimposing "'a pattern of order'" onto "'psychic chaos.'"[5] Mandalas not only imply "a unity that embraces the whole of creative life"[6] but also may reveal important clues about the process of self-discovery and healing in patients undergoing analysis.

Jung's mandalas are part of the famous *The Red Book*, first published in 2009—an illustrated private diary of Jung's inner experiences during his psychological crisis, including dreams and visions. Some images from the *The Red Book* include serpents, perhaps indicating a symbolic link between kundalini and the psycho-spiritual process Jung was undergoing, which he termed *individuation*.[7]

Perhaps as a result of his interest in mandalas, Jung owned a copy of the 1919 edition of *The Serpent Power*.[8] His discovery of the book shed light on a problem patient—a European born in Java and brought up in India—whose physical and psychiatric symptoms puzzled him. The notions of kundalini and the levels of consciousness associated with the chakras provided a way for Jung to work with imagery in his patient's dreams and mandalas, resulting in the abatement of her symptoms.[9]

On October 11, 1930, Jung presented his findings on this

patient in a lecture entitled "Indian Parallels," in which he explored the possible relevance of Eastern notions of the kundalini and the chakras to Western psychology.[10] The next year, he invited a University of Tübingen Indologist, Jakob Wilhelm Hauer (1881–1962), to lecture on related subjects in Zurich ("Overview of Yoga," June 13, 1931). A later assessment of Hauer by a Jewish colleague as "most unreliable as a scholar and as a character as well" seems well founded.[11] Not only did Hauer attempt to establish a new religion based on a combination of Aryanism, Christianity, and the *Bhagavad Gītā*, he also joined the Nazi party in 1937, hoping this new religion would become the official religion of the Third Reich. After the defeat of Germany, he was interned for several years.[12]

Several days later, an Indologist from the University of Heidelberg, Heinrich Zimmer (1890–1943), lectured in Zurich at Jung's invitation ("Aspects of Yoga"; June 18, 1931). Zimmer played an important part in the development of the Western chakra system—as an influence on mythologist Joseph Campbell. To fill out the year, Jung offered a second lecture entitled "Indian Parallels" (October 7, 1931).[13]

The following year, Jung invited Hauer to return to Zurich and present a weeklong seminar on the chakras in German and English ("On Yoga—in Particular, the Meaning of the Chakras," October 3–8, 1932).[14] Another German Indologist, Frederic Spiegelberg (1897–1994), attended the seminar.[15] Spiegelberg also played an important part in the development of the Western chakra system—as an influence on Michael Murphy, founder of Esalen Institute in Big Sur, California.

Following Hauer's seminar, Jung offered four further lectures on kundalini (October 12, 19, and 26 and November 2, 1932), the first three in English and the last in German.[16] English transcripts and German lectures and translations were published privately. The English versions became somewhat more accessible the mid-1970s, through publication in abridged form in the journal *Spring: Journal of Archetypal Psychology and Jungian Thought*.[17] I mention these details to indicate that Jung's insights on the chakras and kundalini in his 1932 lectures were largely restricted to his associates, which included Zimmer, Spiegelberg, and later Campbell. Hence they did not have a direct or immediate public impact on the evolution of the Western chakra system.

As noted, in the Eastern chakra system, tantric practitioners seek to reduce and dissolve the diversity of the manifested universe until only its source remains. Western versions tend to place the chakras in an evolutionary context. Thus the individual—or society at large—progresses from something lesser to something greater, the subhuman to the superhuman. So it is with Jung's discussion of the chakras:

> The chakra system manifests itself in culture, and culture can therefore be divided into various levels such as that of the belly, heart, and head centers. Therefore we can experience and demonstrate the various centers as they appear in the life of the individual, or in the evolution of humanity.[18]

Adding to Jung's statement, we can develop a list of five principles that underlie most versions of the Western chakra system:

- The chakras illustrate progressive stages in a process of personal and social evolution.
- Their locations in the body have symbolic significance.
- These symbols are to be interpreted on the basis of Western cultural associations (e.g., digestion in the belly, feelings in the heart, thinking in the head).
- The evolutionary stages represented by the chakras may be interpreted psychologically (instead of, or in addition to, their implications for spiritual growth).
- The notion of tattvas is equivalent to the notion of elements in Western esotericism, especially alchemy (though the tattvas are usually thought of as constituent forces that evolve

the elements; whereas in alchemy the elements are usually thought of as foundational types of matter, and fire is the fourth element instead of air.[19]

Let us keep these principles in mind as we examine Jung's comments on the chakras. Since these comments are scattered throughout his lectures on the subject, I draw them together here, proceeding chakra by chakra up the spine. Jung's free associations on the functions of the chakras provide what could be called the matrix within which the psychological component of the Western chakra system formed.

For the sake of convenience in this chapter and those that follow, I adopt a uniform set of English names for the chakras, regardless of what they are called in the texts under discussion. This practice will facilitate comparison as components of the Western chakra system—especially the chakra qualities—begin to coalesce. Numbers in parentheses refer to pages in Jung's *The Psychology of Kundalini Yoga*; Jung used the Sanskrit names.

1. **Root**—the "self is asleep" (14); "a place where mankind is a victim of impulses, instincts, unconsciousness" (15); "personal bodily existence on this earth" (23); "our rational point of view of this world as the definite world" (26); "unconscious, latent, dormant" (76)
2. **Genital**—"the unconscious" (15); "the level where psychic life may be said to begin," including "the first rules of bodily decency" [toilet training] and "the beginning of moral education" (63); "error and desire" (76)
3. **Navel**—"the center of emotions" (34); "passions, wishes, illusions" (35); "disputes, anger" (63); "a center in which substances are digested, transformed" (44); "pairs of opposites" (76)
4. **Heart**—"at the diaphragm you cross the threshold from the visible tangible things to the almost invisible intan-

gible things" (44); we "discover the self" and "individuation begins" (39); "the region of what is called feeling and mind" (44); "recognition of values and ideas" (45); the level "our civilization has reached" (46); "the prospective spirit is born; it starts becoming conscious" (77)[20]
5. **Throat**—"beyond the empirical world" (42); a "world of abstract ideas and values" (47); "the seat of speech," leaving behind "error and the pairs of opposites," "renunciation of the world of images, a becoming-conscious of eternal things" (77)
6. **Brow**—"the remote future of mankind, or of ourselves" (56); the "*unio mystica* [mystical union] with the power of God"; an "experience of the self [subject] that is apparently different from the object, God" (57)
7. **Crown**—"a philosophical concept with no substance to us whatever; it is beyond any possible experience"; "no object, no God, nothing but brahman [the Absolute]" (57)

As the evolution of the Western system progresses through the remainder of the twentieth century, we shall see further incarnations of the five principles I have derived from Jung's work, as well as various resonances with this list of chakra associations.

The Chakras at Mid-Century

As influential as *The Serpent Power* proved to be among European intellectuals such as Evola, Guénon, and Jung, a French translation appeared only in 1959, followed by translations in German (1961), Italian (1968), and Spanish (1979). Subsequent English editions after the first appeared in India—but even there, a gap of nearly twenty years occurred between the third edition, of 1931, and the fourth, of 1950. The book would not become widely known in America until the Dover paperback edition was published in 1974.

After the interruption caused by World War II, European scholars resumed study and publication of works on yoga. French-

Rumanian scholar of comparative religion Mircea Eliade published an essay on the origins of the mystical practice of yoga as early as 1936; but his monumental classic, *Yoga: Immortality and Freedom*, with its section on the chakras as described in *The Serpent Power*, came out nearly twenty years later (French, 1954; English, 1958).

French Indologist and musicologist Alain Daniélou (1907–94) moved to India in 1932 and lived there for nearly forty years. He studied under various spiritual teachers and Indian musicians and wrote a chapter based on *The Serpent Power* for *Yoga: The Method of Re-Integration* (French, 1949; English, 1955), a complete exposition of the eight limbs of yoga with translations from apposite scriptures.

In India, Sivananda Saraswati had been codifying the principles of his kundalini yoga since the 1930s. The result was his classic *Kundalini Yoga* (1935). Meanwhile, since 1927, Sri Aurobindo Ghose (1872–1950) had been writing letters on his own developing yoga practice, which he called Integral Yoga—including information on the chakras. At mid-century, Aurobindo's teachings were reaching an ever wider audience, eventually having a seminal impact on the formation of the Western chakra system.

In America, Indian native Devā Rām Sukul (1895–1965)—who founded the Hindu Yoga Society in Chicago in the 1920s, which later became the Yoga Institute of America in California, and who numbered actress Mae West among his followers—published *Yoga and Self-Culture* (1947).[21] The book contained an explanation of the Eastern chakra system, useful tables of its components, such as mantras and deities, and colored illustrations of the chakra mandalas based on *The Serpent Power*. However, this was not the first time these images had appeared on American soil. British-American psychic investigator Hereward Carrington (1880–1958) published sepia versions of the chakra mandalas from the original colored illustrations for *The Serpent Power* in *Higher Psychical Development: The Yoga Philosophy* (1920).[22] Sukul's innovation was to add insets with anatomical renderings of the nerve plexuses associated with the chakras.

Meanwhile, clairvoyant investigation of the chakras continued in England with the publication of *The Science of Seership* (1929) by Theosophical clairvoyant Geoffrey Hodson (1886–1983), which contained a culminating chapter on the subject, and especially under the auspices of the Theosophical Research Center, founded in 1934.[23] The center's primary investigator was clairvoyant Phoebe Daphne Payne (1891–1974; married name, Bendit), who published a semiautobiographical account of her research in *Man's Latent Powers* (1938). The book carries forward the identification of psychic abilities with the etheric- and astral-body chakras in Leadbeater and Powell, combining this schema (including the spleen chakra) with personal observations of how the chakras appear in sickness and in health, and with respect to the development of psychic sensibilities.

As noted, Bailey introduced the concepts of blocked and balanced chakras. Payne graphically described the closing of chakras as a result of physical or emotional trauma and their opening in response to energy healing treatments—a first in the history of Western literature on the chakras and the basis for energy healing practices developed decades later.

In conjunction with her husband, Jungian psychiatrist and Theosophist Laurence J. Bendit (1898–1974), Phoebe Payne also produced *The Psychic Sense* (1943), a comprehensive theory of the development of clairvoyance through the conscious and intelligent use of the third through seventh chakras—again using the model developed by Leadbeater and Powell (illustrated in figure 12 in the present book). The Bendits' research culminated in a monograph on health and psychic development in conjunction with the growth of the etheric body from conception to adulthood in *Man Incarnate: A Study of the Vital Etheric Field* (1957; published since 1977 as *The Etheric Body of Man: The Bridge of Consciousness*).

Joseph Campbell and Sri Ramakrishna

After the war, the German Indologists interested in kundalini yoga either had gone into exile in the United States (Zimmer, Spiegelberg) or were effectively silenced by the tribulations of life in post-Nazi Germany (Hauer). With the emigration of Zimmer and Spiegelberg, tributaries of scholarly and esoteric thought on the chakras, kundalini, and Tantra were about to merge with a flood of teachings and teachers from India in the 1960s and 1970s to produce the Western chakra system.

The American mythologist Joseph Campbell (1904–87) played an important role in this confluence. Himself a professor at Sarah Lawrence College in Yonkers, New York, Campbell attended lectures by Heinrich Zimmer at Columbia University in 1942. Zimmer had moved to New Rochelle, New York, after having been stripped of his job at the University of Heidelberg by the Nazis in 1938 and lived and taught in England for several years. Campbell was born and lived for much of his adult life in New Rochelle. The two men became close friends.[24]

When Zimmer died in 1943 at the age of fifty-two, Campbell took on the task of editing and publishing his papers. In 1951, Zimmer's *Philosophies of India* was published, edited by Campbell.[25] According to religious studies scholar Jeffrey Kripal, Campbell "more or less wrote the Tantric summary and summation of Heinrich Zimmer's influential *Philosophies of India*." This contact with the teachings of Tantra was "formative" for Campbell.[26]

Equally formative was Campbell's encounter with an Eastern teacher living in New York, Swami Nikhilananda (1895–1973).[27] The swami had founded the Ramakrishna-Vivekananda Center there in 1933. He was himself a member of that lineage, having been initiated by Sri Sarada Devi (1853–1920), wife and disciple of Sri Ramakrishna, as had been Vivekananda. We have seen the impact Vivekananda had on the development of interest in yoga in the United States following his appearance at the World Parliament of Religions in 1893 and publication of his seminal *Raja Yoga* in 1896.

Sri Ramakrishna (1836–86) was an eclectic Bengali saint who had absorbed a variety of Hindu, Christian, and Muslim teachings. He became a priest of the goddess Kali in 1856 and lived for years on the grounds of a temple dedicated to her. He was initiated into Tantra from 1861 to 1863 by a female ascetic, Bhairavi Brahmani.

A disciple of Ramakrishna, Mahendranath Gupta, began to record Ramakrishna's teachings in Bengali in 1882 and continued to do so until the latter's death four years later, assembling them into five volumes, published from 1902 to 1932. Swami Nikhilananda undertook the translation of these volumes into English and asked Campbell to edit the results, published in a single volume, *The Gospel of Sri Ramakrishna* (1942)—destined to become a spiritual classic.[28] The book sports an enthusiastic blurb from Zimmer.

Kripal claims that "something of these two texts"—*Philosophies of India* and *The Gospel of Sri Ramakrishna*—could be said to "carry through Campbell's entire corpus as a constant guiding inspiration."[29]

In 1953, Campbell met Jung in Switzerland (and would return there for the Jungian Eranos Conferences in 1957 and 1959). In 1954 and 1955, he traveled in India with Swami Nikhilananda, visiting the Theosophical Society's international headquarters in Adyar, near Madras (now Chennai), where he met Daniélou, at that time director of the Adyar Library and Research Center.[30]

After his return to the United States, Campbell began lecturing at the Cooper Union for the Advancement of Science and Art in New York City in 1958. That year he gave what appears to be his first public lecture describing the workings of kundalini and the chakras. Backing up Kripal's noting of the importance of Tantra in Campbell's work, I have discovered references to kundalini and the chakras in the following writings by Campbell. This is not an exhaustive list. The bracketed initials stand for the titles of these publications, to be used in my presentation of the Ramakrishna/Campbell list of chakra qualities:

1971—*Myths to Live By* ("The Inspiration of Oriental Art," a chapter based on the 1958 Cooper Union lecture) [*MLB*]

1974—*The Mythic Image* (a lavishly illustrated explanation of the Eastern chakra system in a section entitled "The Lotus Ladder" [*TMI*]

1975—an article in *Psychology Today* (December issue) entitled "Kundalini Yoga: Seven Levels of Consciousness" [*PT*]

1988—*The Inner Reaches of Outer Space: Metaphor as Myth and as Religion* (three chapters: "Metaphors of Psychological Transformation"; "Threshold Figures"; "The Metaphorical Journey"

1990—*Transformations of Myth through Time* (two chapters on kundalini yoga)

2003—*Myths of Light: Eastern Metaphors of the Eternal* (includes "Raja Yoga: The Serpent of the Cakras," based on a lecture of October 17, 1966) [*MOL*]

Campbell's approach to the chakras was to use and translate their Sanskrit names and describe them in terms of *The Serpent Power* as lotuses, listing the number of their petals and their colors. However, he carefully collated the few passages in *The Gospel of Sri Ramakrishna* in which the saint described his experience of kundalini and the chakras into a list of states of consciousness associated with each. It is important to note that Ramakrishna's conversations were recorded during the period that Blavatsky was living in India. They were published in Bengali before the appearance of *The Serpent Power*. Therefore, these utterances of a tantric initiate must have had for Campbell an anthropological authenticity that he could not have accorded to those of any later teacher, who might have been influenced by the Theosophical Society's interpretations of Hindu mysticism or Woodroffe's scholarly, though experiential, European bias.

Ramakrishna's teachings on kundalini and the chakras were neither systematic nor exhaustive. Thus it is equally important to note that the list of chakra qualities that Campbell touted in his lectures was derivative and interpretive: Campbell made inferences and filled in the blanks. For this reason, I refer to a Ramakrishna/ Campbell chakra system. This system played a key role in the development of the Western system by supplying the qualities currently associated with the first three chakras.

The following list is a correlation of some of Ramakrishna's teachings on the chakras. Numbers in parentheses refer to pages in *The Gospel of Sri Ramakrishna*, which uses the Sanskrit names.

1. **Root**: The key word for what the aspirant must transcend is presumably "worldliness" (169).
2. **Genital**: The key word is presumably "women," i.e., sexuality; Ramakrishna was speaking to an all-male audience (169).
3. **Navel**: The key word is presumably "gold," i.e., greed, possessiveness (169).[31]
4. **Heart**: The aspirant has a "first glimpse of spiritual consciousness" (151); the mind "sees the individual soul as a flame" (245); "the mind of the aspirant is withdrawn from the three lower centers. He feels the awakening of Divine Consciousness and sees the Light" (499).
5. **Throat**: "The mind becomes free from all ignorance and illusion" (151); "the devotee longs to talk and hear only about God" (499).
6. **Brow**: "The aspirant sees the form of God" though "with a slight barrier between the devotee and God" (500); "it is like a barrier of glass in a lantern, which keeps one from touching the light" (245).
7. **Crown**: "The mind merges in Brahman. The individual soul and the Supreme Soul become one. The aspirant goes into samadhi. His consciousness of the body disappears. He loses the knowledge of the outer world. He does not see the manifold any more. His reasoning comes to a stop" (245).

This is the matrix from which Campbell drew his account of the chakras. Compare the following collation of Campbell's views, modeled on his presentation in the lecture from 1958 published in *Myths to Live By* (108–14). I have added clarifying elements from other presentations, using initials to refer to works listed previously. Campbell used the Sanskrit names of the chakras.

1. **Root**—"spiritual torpor," "just hanging on" (*MLB*, 108); behavioristic psychology (*PT*, 78); "uninspired materialism, governed by 'hard facts'" (*TMI*, 341); "holding on to a life that is no life at all because there is no joy in it, no vitality in it, but just grim, dogged existence" (*MOL*, 29). [Note the resonance between "spiritual torpor" and Jung's remark on the self being asleep.]
2. **Genitals**—"everything means sex," Freudian psychology (*MLB*, 109); pleasure (*MOL*, 30) [Note the resonance with Jung's association with desire.]
3. **Navel**—"will to power," Adlerian psychology (*MLB*, 109); "violence" (*TMI*, 350); "consuming everything, being master of everything, eating everything, turning it into your own substance," "drive to succeed," conquest and defeat, whether military, financial, or erotic" (*MOL*, 30–31) [Note the resonance with Jung's association with digestion; Adlerian psychology was originated by Alfred Adler (1870–1937) and deals with the development of individuality through probing issues of self-esteem (such as the inferiority complex), will and power.]
4. **Heart**—"specifically human, as distinct from sublimated animal, aims and drives become envisioned and awakened," art, religion, philosophy (*MLB*, 109); "transcendence of the self and ordinary human emotions—so that love, for instance, becomes compassion, detached and impersonal," Jungian psychology (*PT*, 78); "powers of art and the spirit" (*MOL*, 31) [Note the resonance with Jung's remark about birth of the spirit.]
5. **Throat**—"purification," "removing all interpositions of the world between oneself and the vision of God" (*MLB*,

113); "spiritual effort, asceticism, and the beginning of spiritual fulfillment," where the purpose of purification is "to subdue the senses" (*PT*, 78); "ascetic, monkish disciples," "purgation," "religious zeal," "conquering one's outward-going tendencies, turning all inward" (*MOL*, 35) [Note the resonance with Jung's remark about renunciation.]

6. **Brow**—"the mystic inward eye opens, and the mystic inward ear," experience of "the whole sight and sound of the Lord . . . whose radiance resounds," "the soul beholds its perfect object, God," bliss (*MLB*, 113); "'conditioned rapture'" [*savikalpa-samādhi*] whose purpose is "to behold the ultimate image of God . . . the beatific vision" (*PT*, 78); *saguṇa-brahman*, the "qualified absolute," where ecstasy still includes perception of I and Thou (*TMI*, 380–81); "'third eye,'" "inner sight," "ultimate vision of the Lord of the World, that human form of the divine that transcends the human" (*MOL*, 35) [Note the resonance with Jung's remark about God as object.]

7. **Crown**—"the absolute, nondual state beyond all categories, visions, sentiments, and feelings," "the soul and its god, the inward eye and its object, are extinguished. There is now neither an object nor a subject, nor anything to be known or named" (*MLB*, 113–14); "'unconditional rapture' [*nirvikalpa-samādhi*] or pure bliss" (*PT*, 78); *nirguṇa-brahman*, the "unqualified absolute" (*TMI*, 381); "beyond duality," "all phenomenology is transcended" (*MOL*, 37–38) [Note the resonance with Jung's remark about "no God, no object, only brahman."]

Campbell often linked the root chakra with the dragons of Western folklore and their penchant for hoarding gold and keeping girls in caves, thus creating a bridge to kundalini as the serpent power and Ramakrishna's comments on women and gold.[32] The qualities of worldliness, women, and gold associated with the first three chakras in the Ramakrishna/Campbell system were carried over into the Western chakra system as *survival*, *sex*, and *power*. The others remained true to the Eastern notion of the chakras' representing ever-more-expansive states of consciousness but were supplanted.

Ramakrishna's chakra system was experiential and he was a validator, despite the incompleteness of his descriptions. Campbell's chakra system was interpretive; he was a consolidator of information from Ramakrishna and Jung. The latter's system, providing a wealth of possible Western meanings for the symbolism of the chakras as described in *Ṣaṭ-Cakra-Nirūpaṇa*, was formative, and Jung was an innovator.

Chapter 20
Kundalini Hot Springs– Esalen Institute

It may come as a surprise both to contemporary yoga practitioners and New Age esotericists that the Western chakra system as we know it today—a particular list of chakra qualities combined with the seven colors of the rainbow in prismatic order—originated in the peculiar mix of Eastern mysticism, behavioral psychology, and multiple bodywork modalities that came together at Esalen Institute in Big Sur, California, in the 1960s and 1970s. The institution developed from seminars organized by founders Michael Murphy (b. 1930) and Richard (Dick) Price (1930–85) on land owned by Murphy's family in 1962. Two years later, it received its name, Esalen Institute, derived from a local Native American tribe, the Essalen (by then extinct). There were natural hot springs on the property and cliff-top views of the Pacific.[1] One 1970s resident described Esalen as

> an outrageous, avant-garde center for the exploration of "those trends in education, religion, philosophy, and the physical and behavioral sciences which emphasize the potentialities and values of human existence." The institute draws some of its colorful dynamics from its location amidst the violently peaceful cliffs and woods of the Big Sur coastline, south of Carmel.[2]

Esalen was the birthplace of the human potential movement, a fixture of 1960s counterculture, and precursor to the New Age movement of the 1980s and beyond. According to Kripal, the foremost chronicler of Esalen's colorful personalities and history, the phrase *human potential* was coined in 1965 by Michael Murphy and *Look* magazine editor George Leonard as a riff on Aldous Huxley's "human potentialities." Huxley's *The Perennial Philosophy* (1945) was an early "foundational" influence on Esalen.³

Kripal indicates that Dick Price was inspired by "Sinhalese Theravada Buddhism, Japanese Zen, and Chinese Taoism."⁴ Price appears not to have played a role in the development of the Western chakra system. Murphy's role, based on his interest in Indian mysticism and yoga, was pivotal.

Michael Murphy and Sri Aurobindo

In 1950, Murphy attended what for him was a life-changing seminar on comparative religion taught by German-American Indologist Frederic Spiegelberg at Stanford University. We met Spiegelberg in the previous chapter, in connection with Jung's kundalini yoga seminars in the 1930s. After losing his professorship at Dresden University in 1937, when the Nazis were purging academia of Jewish faculty and staff, Spiegelberg fled to the United States and joined the Stanford faculty in 1941. Just before his encounter with Murphy, Spiegelberg spent two weeks at the Sri Aurobindo Ashram in Pondicherry, India, in 1949.⁵

Sri Aurobindo, a poet, philosopher, mystic, and yogi who had started off as a revolutionary working for the freedom of the Indian people from British rule, originated a system for the development of ever-more-expansive states of consciousness in an evolutionary progression achievable through meditation. These states were called higher mind, illumined mind, intuitive mind, overmind, and supermind. Aurobindo named his system Integral Yoga, noting that "it takes up the essence and many processes of the old yogas—its newness is in its aim, standpoint and the totality of its method."⁶

The aim of Integral Yoga was "to establish the Divine Consciousness and the Divine Power in men's hearts and the earthly life, not for a personal salvation only, but a divine life here." The possibility of such a synthesis of the earthly and the divine "seemed to me as nearly as possible the integral truth about them and I have therefore spoken of the pursuit of it as the integral yoga."⁷

Having met Sri Aurobindo not long before the latter's death, Spiegelberg passed his enthusiasm for Integral Yoga on to Murphy, who read Aurobindo's treatise on the subject, *The Life Divine*, which became a lifelong inspiration. According to Kripal, Murphy "made a vow both to himself and to the divine by Lake Lagunitas on January 15, 1951, to dedicate the rest of his life to this Aurobindian vision."[8] In 1956–57, several years after Aurobindo's death, Murphy spent sixteen months at the Pondicherry ashram.[9]

In the meantime, in 1951, Spiegelberg had invited a student of Aurobindo, Haridas Chaudhuri (1913–75), to come to the United States as a faculty member of Spiegelberg's just-founded American Academy of Asian Studies in San Francisco. Chaudhuri founded the Cultural Integration Fellowship (CIF) shortly after his arrival in the States. In 1956, when Spiegelberg's organization closed, CIF took over its mission and eventually became the California Institute for Integral Studies. (Price had been at Stanford at the same time as Murphy, though they had not met; they encountered each other for the first time at CIF in 1960.) Chaudhuri, who wrote several books on Aurobindo, was invited to lead a seminar at Esalen on Integral Yoga in 1964.[10]

Aurobindo's teachings on the chakras are scattered throughout a series of letters to his students written from 1927 to 1950. Three small selections of letters on yoga were published in the 1930s, a four-volume set from 1947 to 1951 (*Letters of Sri Aurobindo*), a two-volume set in 1958 (*On Yoga*), and a three-volume set in 1970 (*Letters on Yoga*).[11] Thus these teachings were continuously available in the decades preceding the founding of Esalen.

Here is Aurobindo's continuum of human potential:[12]

- **Physical**—first chakra (root): "commanding the physical consciousness and the inconscient [i.e., sub- or unconscious]"; having to do with nerves and sensations[13]
- **Vital**—astral consciousness,[14] divided into four parts:[15]
    1. **Lower vital** (physical vital)—second chakra (genital): "commanding the little greeds, lusts, desires,

the small sense movements"; drives, such as "food desire, sexual desire, small likings, dislikings, vanity, quarrels, love of praise, anger at blame, little wishes"

2. **Middle vital**—third chakra (navel): passions, such as "ambition, pride, fear, love of fame, attractions and repulsions"; "commanding the larger life-forces and the passions and larger desire-movements"
3. **Central/emotional vital**—fourth chakra (heart): "commanding the higher emotional being"; emotions such as "love, joy, sorrow, hatred"
4. **Higher/mental vital** (also called vital mind)—fifth chakra (throat): "commanding expression and all externalization of the mind movements and mental forces" (as in speech[16]); thought or verbal expression of "emotions, desires, passions, sensations"

- **Thinking mind**—sixth chakra (brow): "commanding thought, will, vision"; also the third eye
- **Higher mind**—seventh chakra (crown—above the head): "commanding the higher thinking mind and the illumined mind and reaching upwards to the intuition and overmind"
- **Illumined mind**—also centered in the seventh chakra
- **Intuitive mind**—beyond, but transmitted through, the seventh chakra
- **Overmind**—"a sort of delegation from the supermind (this is a metaphor only) which supports the present evolutionary universe in which we live here in Matter";[17] beyond, but transmitted through, the seventh chakra
- **Supermind**—"self-determining Truth of the Divine Consciousness,"[18] "in which there can be no place for the principle of division and ignorance"; "a full light and knowledge superior to all mental substance or mental movement";[19] correlated with *satya-loka* (world, or plane, of truth), "the highest of the scale connected with this universe"[20]
- **Supreme**—*saccidānanda* (existence/consciousness/bliss);

"not a world, it is supracosmic";[21] equivalent to "Divine Consciousness"[22]

Aurobindo provided a list of colors and numbers of petals associated with the lotuses/chakras. The numbers of petals are traditional. However, the colors seem eccentric, unrelated to earlier systems, from Tantra to Leadbeater. They played no role in the development of the Western chakra system. Yet the continuum of human potential implied by Aurobindo's teachings became a central metaphor for much that occurred at Esalen and in the larger human potential movement. This metaphor was also the matrix that birthed the Western chakra system as we know it.

Thus, for Esalen, Aurobindo's vision of the chakra system was formative, and he himself was an innovator—despite the fact that within the larger context of Aurobindo's Integral Yoga, the chakra system played a relatively minor role. Meditators were to transcend the states of consciousness represented by the chakras to achieve the intuitive mind, supermind, and overmind, expansions of consciousness that went beyond the higher and illumined mind of the seventh chakra.

Esalen and Energy

Another central metaphor at Esalen was the notion of *energy* (frequently capitalized)—a difficult to define word that has become ubiquitous in New Age discourse. In science classes, we learn about physical energy and how it is stored (potential energy) and released (kinetic energy). We understand that energy is absorbed by some chemical reactions, as when atoms bond with molecules, and is released in others, when such bonds dissolve. We see energy released in fire and understand that the release of energy through nuclear fission can be used to produce electrical power or atomic bombs. But things get fuzzy when we try to understand subtle energies and their effects, such as kundalini, the chakras, auras, and so on.

In New Age contexts, the word *energy* is often accepted as foundational and intentionally left vague and unexplained or surrounded by pseudoscientific diagrams and speculation linking it with quantum physics. I was much surprised when I looked up the word in my *American Heritage College Dictionary*, 4th edition, and discovered the following definition, which seems to suit all purposes—even New Age ones: "The capacity for work or vigorous activity; exertion of vigor or power; vitality or intensity of expression." In other words, energy is not a thing but a condition or state of a physical or nonphysical thing, system, or agent, whether described as organic or inorganic, or as with or without consciousness.

Because Esalen was attempting to target and trigger the development of human *potential* (derived from the Latin word for *powerful*), it focused on the release of personal and group energy to express increased vitality and achieve greater fulfillment in life—physical, sexual, emotional, social, and spiritual. As Kripal indicates, Esalen "believed in the reality and power of Energy as a mystical and erotic force."[23] As in Indian Tantra, the exploration of this force could be pursued along mystical or erotic lines. The former led to right-hand-path practices, hence Michael Murphy's emphasis on the "'right-hand' metaphysics of meditation and Sri Aurobindo's writings." Kripal identifies Aurobindo as "a right-handed Tantric philosopher," though for political reasons, Aurobindo himself avoided identification of his Integral Yoga with Tantra.[24] According to Kripal, the erotic side of this mystical energy at Esalen and in American counterculture "from its sexual revolution and psychedelia to its explicit and consistent borrowing from Tantric Asia—can easily be read as a left-handed American Tantric tradition." Murphy himself saw it as such.[25]

A history of the development of Western notions of the purpose and functioning of kundalini energy from their Eastern counterparts would parallel the present account of the development of the Western chakra system. Kripal's *Esalen* provides background on the Indian context and locates the primary point of transmission of erotic and mystical interpretations of kundalini into American culture at Esalen. He does not deal with the key role of the Theosophical Society as the earliest nexus for this East/West transmission, some seventy years before the founding of Esalen. For example, Blavatsky's *Theosophical Glossary*, published in 1892 in London and New York, defined *kundalini-shakti* as follows:

> The power of life; one of the forces of nature; that power that generates a certain light in those who sit for spiritual and clairvoyant development. It is a power known only to those who practice concentration and yoga.[26]

Clearly, this was the mystical, or right-hand, interpretation of kundalini. In early Theosophical literature, the sexual interpretation was mentioned only to be disparaged—for example, in Leadbeater's *The Inner Life*, in which the premature arousal of kundalini was said to excite "the most undesirable passions," turning people into "satyrs, monsters of [sexual] depravity."[27] George Sydney Arundale (1878–1945), Besant's successor as international president of the Theosophical Society, provided a more moderate view, some twenty-five years later, in *Kundalini: An Occult Experience* (1938), in which kundalini is described as "the feminine aspect of the creative force of evolution."[28]

According to Arundale, whose views on kundalini and sexuality may have been modified by his having married an Indian woman, Rukmini Devi (1904–86), the development of kundalini may be accompanied by what contemporary New Agers call sacred sexuality:

> Sexual vitality and activity are very closely allied to kundalini, for both are supremely creative in their nature, and the development of one is bound to stir the development of the other. All sexual urge must be under complete control, at the will of the individual, and must be

in a condition of what may be called sublimation, that is to say it must be recognized as a sacrament and therefore to be used in reverence and in a spirit of dedication. Sex-differentiation in all its various implications is one of God's earliest gifts to His children—often abused and grossly used, but at last learned to be approached as the true priest approaches the altar. Only those who thus approach the divinity of sex may be safely entrusted with that later gift of kundalini, which can be handled with safety and profit by the tried and trusty alone.[29]

Meanwhile, in America, since about 1900, the nation's first native-born tantric yogi, Pierre Bernard (1875–1955), had been teaching a kundalini- and sexuality-based form of yoga that trod a thin line between promiscuous hedonism and evolutionary ascent to the divine—and repeatedly getting in trouble with moral authorities and the law. Some of these teachings originated from a Syrian-Bengali guru who met Bernard in Lincoln, Nebraska, in 1889, when Bernard (then known as Perry Baker) was seventeen. Bernard lived and studied with this guru for eighteen years, in various locations. Their teachings may have passed into the eclectic mix at Esalen through Ida Rolf (1896–1979), originator of the bodywork modality called Structural Integration, or Rolfing. Rolf was a student of Bernard in the 1920s.[30]

Another influence on Esalen's notion of a mystical and erotic evolutionary energy was Wilhelm Reich (1897–1957), a controversial Austrian-American student of Sigmund Freud (1856–1939). Reich expanded on Freud's concept of libido—the instinctual sexual drive that motivates desire, lies behind physical and emotional expressions of love, and may be sublimated in intellectual, creative, and spiritual activities—into a cosmic and universal force he called orgone. Though function of orgone is similar to that of kundalini, I have not been able to determine how, if at all, Reich may have been influenced by Indian teachings on the subject.

Reich was driven out of several European psychological associations and persecuted for his beliefs and practices by American authorities, who burned his books and jailed him. He died in prison. However, his legacy flowed into Esalen through his students Alexander Lowen and John Pierrakos, originators of Bioenergetics, a bodywork modality that involved the breaking down of body armoring against the free experience of pleasure / life-force flow / sexual energy / kundalini. Reich had identified seven zones of body armoring, an endeavor the folks at Esalen saw as a form of independent Western scientific validation of the existence of the Eastern chakra system.[31]

A further influence on Esalen's notion of mystical and erotic evolutionary energy was Indian kundalini experiencer Gopi Krishna (1903–84). Though George Arundale was an early memoirist of the personal experience of kundalini awakening, Gopi Krishna published detailed descriptive and speculative accounts of his own kundalini awakening in tandem with the development of Esalen, in books such as *Kundalini: The Evolutionary Energy in Man* (1967), whose second edition (1970) contained an introduction by Spiegelberg. Kripal notes that this book was a classic "within the California counterculture of the 1970s."[32]

The publication of books on tantric sexuality—notably Omar Garrison's *Tantra: The Yoga of Sex* (1964)—began around the time of Esalen's founding and proliferated in the 1970s in connection with the spread of teachings by contemporary tantric gurus from India, such as Bhagwan Shree Rajneesh (1931–90; now known as Osho). The result was a movement called neo-Tantra, which celebrated sexual liberation and mystical enlightenment along left-hand-path lines.

Psychotherapist Bernard Gunther, who spent thirteen years at Esalen and originated Esalen-style massage as a means of awakening and revitalizing the senses, and who became a devotee of Rajneesh, wrote books on the chakras (*Energy, Ecstasy, and Your Seven Vital Chakras*, 1978) and neo-Tantra (*Neo-Tantra: Bhagwan Shree Rajneesh on Sex, Love, Prayer, and Transcendence*, 1980).[33] A more extreme version of left-hand neo-Tantra emerged in the writings of Jonn Mumford, a disciple of tantric guru Satyananda Saraswati, and others, mentioned in chapter 4. The most overt of his books is *Sexual Occultism: The Sorcery of Love in Practice and Theory* (1975), revised as *Ecstasy through Tantra*, 1998.

Neo-Tantra, when not an excuse for the pursuit of sensual gratification, taught the harnessing of sexual energy to achieve transcendent states of consciousness and liberation from the socially conditioned self. The Western chakra system that originated at Esalen taught the harnessing of vital energy that could express itself sexually but was not limited to erotic or reproductive experience, to achieve physical, emotional, social, and spiritual satisfaction or self-realization. Sexuality was included, but enjoyed as an expression of human potential at the level of the second chakra rather than as an ultimate goal in itself. Thus it could be said that the Esalen version of the chakras represented more of a middle path than an exclusively left-hand tradition equating sexuality, bliss, and transcendence or an exclusively right-hand path of sublimating sexuality through meditative practice. The key word *energy*, with its erotico-mystical connotations, represented this middle way.

Chapter 21
Handbooks to Higher Consciousness

According to Kripal, "Psychology was one of the three central pillars of Esalen announced in early brochures, along with psychical research and drug-induced mysticism." Furthermore, when it comes to Esalen, "what looks 'New Age' turns out to be a synthesis of psychoanalysis and mystical philosophy."[1] So it is with the birth of the Western chakra system. In this and the following chapter, I chronicle some of the psychologists/mystics who midwifed this birth.

Transcendent Needs (Abraham Maslow)

The father of humanistic psychology, Abraham Maslow (1908–70) was arguably the godfather of Esalen. He arrived on the scene early, accidentally, if not synchronistically. Driving down the Pacific Coast Highway past Big Sur late at night in the summer of 1962, Maslow and his wife pulled into what they thought was a motel. It turned out to be Big Sur Hot Springs (the Esalen Institute had not yet been named)—and the whole staff was reading Maslow's recently released *Toward a Psychology of Being* (1962).[2]

A key element of Maslow's contribution to American psychology is his "hierarchy of needs," defined by his biographer Edward Hoffmann as the "inborn array of physiological and psychological needs encompassing the *basic needs* and *metaneeds*. As a lower need is fulfilled within us, a newer and higher need tends to emerge." By *metaneeds*, a Maslowian coinage, Hoffmann meant our motivation to fulfill ourselves through the pursuit of ideal objects such as "truth, beauty, and justice."[3]

Psychotherapist Mark Koltko-Rivera notes that many basic psychology textbooks cite early examples of Maslow's hierarchy of needs from 1943 and 1954 publications. This hierarchy has five levels, whereas articles published just before Maslow's death indicated that he was considering the addition of a sixth category.[4] Here is Koltko-Rivera's "rectified" version of Maslow's hierarchy of needs, based on "The Farther Reaches of Human Nature," a 1969 article in the inaugural issue of the *Journal of Transpersonal Psychology* (presented in ascending order):

1. Physiological (survival) needs
2. Safety needs
3. Belongingness and love needs
4. Esteem needs
5. Self-actualization
6. Self-transcendence[5]

In a 1979 article in the *American Theosophist*, psychotherapists Thomas B. Roberts and Robert H. Hannon compared Maslow's hierarchy of needs with the chakra system. The coauthors noted that if we divide Maslow's lowest level into survival and sexual needs, we then have seven levels and a rough correlation to the chakra system. Though it may be that any attempt to mark seven stages of a continuum of human potential from materially to spiritually motivated states of being will end up with similar subdivisions, I find this presentation remarkably aligned with Blavatsky's seven principles (added in brackets):

1. **Root**—biological needs, food, water, shelter, freedom from pain [sthula—dense body]
2. **Genital**—sex and reproduction [linga—subtle body (one meaning of *linga* is "phallus")]
3. **Solar plexus**—security via power and control [prana—life force]
4. **Heart**—love, devotion, caring for others [kama—desire]
5. **Throat**—vocal expression, verbal knowledge [manas—mind]

6. **Third eye**—psychic visualization, intuition, vision of the ultimate, inner direction and self-reference [buddhi—intuition, spiritual intelligence, or soul]
7. **Crown**—peak, or transcendent, experience, unites man with infinite [atman—highest self][6]

Roberts and Hannon's version of the chakra system so closely resembles the one we are used to seeing in recent books on the chakras that it seems probable that the Western list of chakra qualities came together prior to 1979. I do not believe that Maslow or his hierarchy of needs was directly responsible for the Western chakra qualities. However, I suspect a reciprocal influence between Maslow and the folks at Esalen. Maslow supplied them with the term *survival* for the function of the first chakra, whereas developments at Esalen in the 1960s encouraged Maslow to divide the fifth level of his original hierarchy of needs into two, adding the category of self-transcendence.

I noted a similar progression in the development of the Eastern chakra system in my chronology. The five-chakra system added a sixth chakra when the lowest split into two, and later added a seventh when the new highest chakra split into two. This is not to say that Maslow's hierarchy of needs was influenced by reading about the chakras. Hoffman indicates that Maslow began reading "books on Eastern philosophy, especially Taoism" as early as 1942[7]—a year before he published his first version of the hierarchy of needs. But in the absence of a detailed reading list from this period, it is useless to speculate.

For the development of Esalen's version of the chakras, Maslow was an innovator and his hierarchy of needs, though not yet a chakra system, was formative.

The Only Dance There Is (Ram Dass)

Another fixture at Esalen was Baba Ram Dass (Richard Alpert, b. 1931). Trained as a psychologist, Ram Dass was an early self-experimenter with the use of psychedelics to produce altered and mystical states of consciousness. He went to India in 1967, found his guru, and received his name, returning to America in 1969 and becoming a guru of the counterculture movement. Kripal notes that he was present at Esalen as early as 1964 (guiding Michael Murphy on an LSD trip) and after his trip to India in May 1969 (as a presenter).[8]

In 1970, Ram Dass gave a lecture under the auspices of the Menninger Foundation in Topeka, Kansas, in which he described the chakras; the lecture was subsequently published in two parts in the *Journal of Transpersonal Psychology* in 1970 and 1971 and in book form in 1974 as *The Only Dance There Is*. Incidentally, Anodea Judith notes in *Wheels of Life* that this was "The first book I read with the word *chakra*. The book that got me started on all this."[9] In the wave of popularity following the 1971 publication of Ram Dass's bestselling book of spiritual autobiography and instruction, *Remember, Be Here Now*, many 1970s readers likely could have made a similar claim.

Ram Dass's version of the chakras represents a clarification of the Ramakrishna/Campbell version. I do not know how or when he would have been exposed to this system. Kripal notes that Campbell first presented at Esalen Institute in 1966 and gave seminars at Esalen Center in San Francisco during its first season, in October 1967, entitled "Freud, Jung, and Kundalini Yoga" and "The Lessons of Kundalini Yoga for Western Psychology."[10] Ram Dass was probably already in India by the time of the latter. Here is Ram Dass's list of chakra qualities:

1. **Root**—survival of the individual as a separate being; security
2. **Genital**—sensual gratification and sexual desires and reproduction; linked to Freud
3. **Solar plexus**—connected with power, with mastery, with ego control; linked to Adler
4. **Heart**—"Buddha's compassion"; linked to Jung, archetypes, collective unconscious; compassion
5. **Throat**—"deeper within"; higher planes of light, energy,

or form; perceptual organization of universe identified with ideas, not gross body or personality
6. **Brow**—causal plane; cosmic perspective; wisdom, laws, realm of pure ideas
7. **Crown**—merging "back into the oceanic"; going "back into the one"; "Buddha state"[11]

Ram Dass states that when you are "climbing this ladder, at each new level there is a new way in which you receive energy or transmute energy in the universe."[12] This ladder image, as well as the mentions of Freud, Adler, and Jung, comes directly from Campbell. The qualities listed for the fifth through sixth chakras reflect the increasing expansion of consciousness implied in Ramakrishna's descriptions of the chakras but are more specific than Campbell's version. Mention of the causal plane in the above list, and of the astral plane elsewhere in this lecture, indicates that Ram Dass was familiar with Theosophical concepts.[13]

Just as Ram Dass drew from Campbell, later authors drew from Ram Dass. Though the larger public did not hear of this list until 1974, I place it chronologically in 1972, when the journal version was published. The line of transmission of Ram Dass's ideas on the chakras may have passed to other faculty and staff at Esalen through this article, through his presence on campus, or in other undocumented ways. I see Dass as a disseminator and his description of the chakras as explanatory.

Here Comes Everybody (William Schutz)

American psychologist William Schutz (1925–2002) was on the faculty at Esalen from 1967 to 1975, arriving just as his bestselling book *Joy: Expanding Human Awareness* came out. With "humorous charm," he promptly declared himself the "'first emperor of Esalen'" and established the "Flying Circus," a band of workshop leaders who promoted the group-oriented therapeutic and self-exploration practice he called "open encounter," both at Esalen and beyond. According to Kripal, "The phrase was meant to both attract attention and confess a certain dangerous playfulness, a kind of bold showmanship, perhaps even a level of trickery."[14] The trickery was ostensibly therapeutic, since the working method of open encounter was to use any available and agreed upon means to break down social and personal inhibitions against authenticity with oneself and others.

In his next book, *Here Comes Everybody: Bodymind and Encounter Culture* (1971), Schutz described the evolution of his method. First came "the T-group (*T* for training) originated by the National Training Laboratories in 1947," focused "primarily on group process." Then came "sensitivity training" in the early 1950s, with a focus on "individual dynamics." Psychologist Carl Rogers (1902–87), with whom Schutz worked in the 1950s, came to refer to such "personally oriented" groups as "encounter" groups. Schutz's own focus was what he called "open encounter," which "aims at personal growth and realization of human potential, and admits a wide range of other types of activities into the experience." Such activities might include "dramatic methods, fantasy, hypnosis, nonverbal, meditation, mysticism, massage, sensory awareness, and a wide variety of methods involving the body and energy."[15]

To achieve "openness and honesty,"[16] open encounter groups often used confrontational methods that were considered controversial. Such methods received much media attention in the late 1960s and early 1970s—including the 1969 film *Bob and Carol and Ted and Alice*, which detailed the comedic effects of two couples' attempts at "marital honesty" after one of them attended such a group.[17] However, the workshop format that has been a primary means of disseminating information about the Western chakra system for decades (and that is currently promoted at holistic learning centers such as Omega Institute in Rhinebeck, New York or at yoga retreat centers such as Kripalu Center for Yoga and Health in Lenox, Massachusetts) originated in Esalen's encounter group methods. The confrontational edge may be gone, but the experiential self-help basis of such learning remains.

Schutz went on to describe the philosophy behind his methods: "Open encounter is based on the belief that man is a unified being and functions on many levels at once: physical, emotional, intellectual, interpersonal, social, and spiritual." Not only is there "a life flow in man on all of these levels" but also, "physical blocks lead to physical illness, emotional blocks to mental illness, intellectual blocks to underachieving, social blocks to incompatibility, war, and violence, and spiritual blocks postpone a realization of the total man." For the psychologist and bodyworker, "Removal of blocks is the therapeutic task."[18]

The continuum of human potential from physical to spiritual is mirrored in Schutz's list of chakra qualities (I have interpolated words from the first citation in the previous paragraph to make the connection clear):

1. **Root**—grand potential, primitive energy [physical]
2. **Genital**—sexual energy [physical]
3. **Solar plexus**—assertiveness, anger [emotional]
4. **Heart**—affection, love [emotional]
5. **Throat**—communication, expression [intellectual, interpersonal, social]
6. **Brow**—intuition [intellectual/spiritual]
7. **Crown**—cosmic consciousness [spiritual][19]

The emphasis on energy blockages and their removal through therapeutic methods is fundamental to the "neo-Reichian" styles of bodywork practiced at Esalen, such as Lowen's Bioenergetics.[20] Though the notions of blocked and imbalanced chakras can be traced back to Bailey, their endorsement by the psychologists and bodyworkers at the forefront of the human potential movement enshrined them in the Western chakra system. These pioneers developed physical and psychological methods for identifying and removing energy blocks that went beyond Bailey's proposals in *Esoteric Healing* (whether or not they were aware of such proposals). Their acceptance of the principle of a continuum of human potential from physical to spiritual was sufficient to guarantee a fluid boundary between Western psychological and Eastern mystical applications of the chakras, regardless of whether their methods were explicitly identified with them. Lowen's Bioenergetics were not so identified; but those of his colleague John Pierrakos, originator of Core Energetics, were so identified.

Schutz admitted to being a "neophyte" with regard to "the concepts used for the spiritual levels of man" in his discussion of kundalini and the chakras.[21] But that did not prevent him from appropriating these ideas to diagnose psychological issues and recommend procedures for remedying them:

> A man in an encounter group is having difficulty establishing a love relation (fourth chakra) with a woman in the group. She reports that she feels some phoniness in his approach and feeling. What frequently results is that he has a sexual desire (second chakra) for her and is not acknowledging that this issue must be dealt with first. Or sometimes he has great hostility toward women (third chakra) that he is also not dealing with. The order of the chakras supports the idea that in order to reach the highest levels of joy and ecstasy, or even real affection, the sexual and aggressive feelings must be dealt with satisfactorily.[22]

Here I detect several ways of thinking that become endemic in Western teachings on the chakras to the present day. The chakras are not only reduced to tokens referring to Western psychological constructs but also are seen primarily in terms of behavioral motivations. Blockage of life-force flow through the chakras means we do not get what we want. Flow means we do. Thus the chakras are virtually cut off from their roots in Eastern mysticism as signifiers for states of consciousness and become psychological and meditative focal points for achieving personal happiness. This is the basis for most subsequent New Age approaches to the chakras.

To the extent that Schutz is here a spokesperson for an

approach to the chakra system originating in and promulgated by Esalen, I believe it is safe to say that the Western chakra system as we currently know it would not exist without Esalen's radical reinterpretation of its structure, purpose, and use. Critics of the Western appropriation of Eastern teachings on the chakras may lay the blame on a legion of New Age interpreters publishing books on the subject from the 1980s to the present, but the real blame—if blame there is—should perhaps be laid at the door of Esalen in the late 1960s and early 1970s.

Like Dass, Schutz was a disseminator and his description of the chakras was explanatory.

The Handbook to Higher Consciousness (Ken Keyes Jr.)

A mystic and natural (rather than trained) psychologist, Ken Keyes Jr. (1921–95) was exposed to polio at age twenty-five. He became quadriplegic and was confined to a wheelchair for the rest of his life. Nevertheless, Keyes became a wealthy real-estate mogul. In 1970, just before turning fifty, he attended a life-changing workshop at Esalen. Spiritual exploration, experiments with mescaline and communal living, a spontaneous enlightenment experience, and attempts to resolve issues of jealousy and sexual addiction led to the development of his "Living Love" method of self-help and self-realization, which he subsequently taught at Esalen. This method became the basis for his *Handbook of Higher Consciousness*, a multimillion-copy bestseller, first published as *Living Love* in 1972.

The chakras—dubbed the "seven centers of consciousness"—played an essential role in the *Handbook*. The list is modeled after that promulgated at Esalen, with one key difference in the qualities assigned to the fifth chakra.

1. **Root**—security/food/shelter
2. **Genital**—sensation/sex
3. **Solar plexus**—power/domination/wealth

4. **Heart**—love/compassion
5. **Throat**—cornucopia/well-being
6. **Brow**—conscious awareness
7. **Crown**—cosmic consciousness[23]

Students of the Eastern chakra system may recognize the function of Keyes's fifth chakra as that of the minor chakra called hrit, traditionally located between manipura (third chakra) and anahata (fourth chakra). According to Goswami, hrit contains the celestial wish-fulfilling tree of Hindu myth—hence Keyes's introduction of the word *cornucopia*. Keyes may have learned of this minor chakra from *The Serpent Power* or Leadbeater's *The Chakras*, each of which contains a brief description of hrit chakra and mentions the wish-fulfilling tree.[24] Despite its wide dissemination, Keyes's list of chakra qualities did not become the dominant one. However, the quality of abundance is sometimes associated with the fifth chakra and probably has its origin in this list.

Perhaps more important to the evolution of the Western chakra system is Keyes's focus on improving the quality of personal satisfaction in physical, emotional, mental, and spiritual life through overcoming negative aspects of the chakras, associated with addiction, and replacing ("reprogramming") them with positive aspects, associated with freedom from addiction—a psychological self-help reinterpretation of the original function of the chakra system, in Tantra, as a means of achieving spiritual liberation. This was an amplification of the personal satisfaction approach to the chakras espoused by Schutz, but in the form of a widely disseminated practical manual for achieving such satisfaction. Without drawing directly from Keyes's work, many later New Age books include lists of negative and positive chakra qualities. Thus his influence may be felt more in the transmission of principles than of terms.

Keyes was a pioneer of the self-help movement, and his *Handbook to Higher Consciousness* was one of the must-read self-help books of the 1970s. I see him as a validator and his chakra system as experiential.

Total Orgasm (Jack Lee Rosenberg)

In his own words, Jack Lee Rosenberg (1932–2015) "got to be known as 'the dentist who teaches sex.'"[25] As a practicing dentist, he discovered Esalen in 1963 and became involved in the many forms of bodywork and group and individual therapy available there. He was also a meditator and yoga practitioner and later became a psychotherapist. Rosenberg integrated what he learned at Esalen, and elsewhere, into a program of exercises for freeing up sexual energy in individuals and couples, publishing the results, *Total Orgasm*, in 1973.

Rosenberg once heard Campbell speak on the chakras,[26] and his discussion of the subject resembles that in Campbell's *Myths to Live By*, published two years earlier. But there is material unique to each list, so it is not possible to say that Rosenberg's derives solely from that book. Perhaps he was also recounting what he remembered from one of Campbell's lectures at Esalen or in San Francisco:

1. **Root**—"not moving out into the world"; "just hanging on and existing"
2. **Genital**—sex; "one's whole existence in life is centered around sex"; Freudian psychology
3. **Navel**—power; "to turn things into the self, taking in"; "to be on top, to be in control, to incorporate, to consume, to achieve power, to be a winner"; Adlerian psychology
4. **Heart**—love; transformation; union of opposites; loss of ego sense or selfness; "reaching out with love"; Jungian psychology
5. **Throat**—purification of lower chakras; inner light, inner sound; monasticism, spiritual disciplines; "moving out of the world and turning to the inner world"
6. **Brow**—third eye; "spiritual power and knowledge"; "high-

est sphere of inner authority"; "beholding the image of the world of God"

7. **Crown**—"past all pairs of opposites and one with God"[27]

Rosenberg was a disseminator and his system was explanatory.

The lists of chakra qualities provided in this chapter demonstrate the competing currents present at Esalen in the early 1970s: the Ramakrishna/Campbell system and the Aurobindo/Esalen system. In the next chapter, I demonstrate how these two lists were merged to form the list of chakra qualities we usually see today—the first three chakras from Ramakrishna/Campbell and the remaining four from Aurobindo/Esalen.

Chapter 22
The Birth of the Western Chakra System

The year 1975 represented the centenary of the founding of the Theosophical Society. Ninety-five years had elapsed since the TS unwittingly initiated the transfer of ancient tantric teachings on the chakras from Eastern yoga into Western esotericism and psychology. Only three stages remained in the long gestation period of the Western chakra system. The first involved a disciple of Sri Aurobindo and the second, the collaboration of an Indian guru living in America with two devotees who were Western-trained psychiatrists.

Yoga Psychology (Haridas Chaudhuri)

We met Sri Aurobindo's disciple Chaudhuri in chapter 20 as the founder of the Cultural Integration Fellowship in San Francisco, where Michael Murphy and Dick Price lived prior to founding Esalen. In 1975, Chaudhuri contributed and essay entitled "Yoga Psychology" to Charles Tart's anthology *Transpersonal Psychologies* (1975), including an account of Aurobindo's chakra system. Tart (b. 1937) was a frequenter of Esalen who achieved notoriety as a parapsychologist. Here is a list of key terms culled from Chaudhuri's discussion of the chakras:

1. **Root**—material world
2. **Genital**—vital, instinctual, sexual
3. **Navel or solar plexus**—power
4. **Heart**—soul/unselfish; unconditional love and higher values
5. **Throat**—communication, self-projection, and creative inspiration to others; "realizing one's own Self as a unique individual, as an intrinsically valuable spiritual being, as

an active center of creative energy"; achieving a "pure and distinctive awareness of things as they are in their uniqueness or suchness"; residence of the goddess of speech
6. **Brow**—wisdom and divine command (from higher Self); third eye; spiritual enlightenment, self-mastery, and cosmic consciousness (defined as "synoptic vision of the world as a whole"); "Being . . . as destiny or the purpose of life, freely chosen on the basis of awareness of one's true Self as related to the cosmic whole"; self-realization "as awareness of one's true Self as a creative center of the cosmic whole"
7. **Crown**—transcendental consciousness, defined as "cognition of the nontemporal depth dimension of Being"[1]

Chaudhuri was a disseminator of Aurobindo's teachings. His version of the chakras, though clearly presented, was merely explanatory. With the birth of the Western chakra system, the attributions of the first two chakras fall away, to be replaced by items from the Ramakrishna/Campbell list. Comparing this list with Aurobindo's teachings on the chakras in chapter 20, we see that power, from the Ramakrishna/Campbell list, has already replaced Aurobindo's attribution to passion. The remaining attributions are in line with the Aurobindo/Esalen lists provided in the previous chapter.

The Yogi and the Shrinks (Swami Rama)

The next-to-last gestational stage in the development of the Western chakra system occurred a year later, with the publication of a popular and influential book, *Yoga and Psychotherapy: The Evolution of Consciousness* (1976) by the Indian guru Swami Rama (1925–96) and two Western psychiatrists, Rudolph Ballentine (b. 1941) and Allan Weinstock (b. 1940; also known as Swami Ajaya, an initiate of Swami Rama, and as Dr. Allan Ajaya).

Swami Rama came to the United States in 1969 and underwent an extensive series of tests of his yogic control over supposedly involuntary mechanisms in the physical body at the Menninger

Clinic in Topeka, Kansas in 1970 and 1971. These tests made quite a splash in the worlds of yoga and psychology and were touted as providing scientific validation for the existence of yogic powers. Subsequently, Swami Rama established the Himalayan Institute in Honesdale, Pennsylvania, for spiritual education, humanitarian projects, and the promotion of holistic health. Ballentine, a pioneer of holistic medicine, directed the institute for twelve years.[2]

Here is a list of key words culled from a chapter of *Yoga and Psychotherapy* entitled "The Seven Centers of Consciousness." There is a separately titled section for each chakra and I have italicized the words used in these titles:

1. **Root**—*fear/paranoia*/survival
2. **Genital**—*sensuality/sexuality* [Freud is mentioned, indicating Campbell's influence; there is also a quotation from Keyes's *Handbook to Higher Consciousness* about addictions connected to the first and second chakras.]
3. **Solar plexus**—*domination/submission* [Adler is mentioned and first three chakras are called instinctual, indicating Campbell's influence; a footnote refers to Maslow's "motivational hierarchy"—i.e., his hierarchy of needs.]
4. **Heart**—*emotion / empathy* / compassion / selfless love (called the transition between instinctual lower and "more evolved consciousness" of higher chakras) [Original links are made to Rogerian therapy (so-called person- or client-centered psychotherapy) and that of Erich Fromm (1900–80), possibly with reference to his 1956 bestseller *The Art of Loving*.]
5. **Throat**—*nurturance / creativity* / receiving grace [Though the inclusion of grace seems eccentric, *expression* is implied through mention of devotional singing, chanting, verbalizing, painting, and dream interpretation.]
6. **Brow**—*intuitive knowledge* / third eye / introspection / inner vision / clairvoyance
7. **Crown**—*highest state of consciousness* / samadhi[3]

The Campbell influence in this list may be explained by the prior publication of *Myths to Live By*, *The Mythic Image* and the *Psychology Today* article discussed in chapter 19. The Esalen influence comes through Keyes's *Handbook to Higher Consciousness* (first, second, and fourth chakras). The resemblance between descriptions of the sixth chakra's functions by Chaudhuri and Rama is probably explained by traditional Indian associations rather than influence of the former on the latter.

Rama, Ballentine, and Ajaya were consolidators. Their version of the chakras, pooling sources listed in the previous paragraph, was interpretive.

Child of Bodymind (Ken Dychtwald)

The last gestational stage came a year later, in 1977, when the Esalen list of chakra qualities and the chromotherapists' list of rainbow colors finally came together. Ironically, the individual responsible for this culmination was, and has probably remained, unaware of his historical role in bringing about the birth of the Western chakra system.

Ken Dychtwald (b. 1950) called himself a "humanistic psychotherapist" in his first book, *Bodymind: A Synthesis of Eastern and Western Approaches to Self-Awareness, Health, and Personal Growth*, based on his experiences while living at Esalen from 1970 to 1974. He is better known these days as a specialist in the psychology, sociology, and economics of aging. Dychtwald's popular book developed from his doctoral dissertation. It was an attempt to turn the integrated physiological (body) and psychological (mind) approaches to physical, emotional, mental, and spiritual well-being into a grand theory of everything human, which he called bodymind. (As we saw in the discussion of Schutz, the word was already in use at Esalen before the publication of *Bodymind*.)

Dychtwald defined bodymind as "the evolutionary storehouse of all life's potentials."[4] His book describes various methods used at Esalen for exploring bodymind in theoretical, practical, and personal terms. He states:

My own interest in Kundalini yoga began when I first realized that the Kundalini perspective on psychosomatic structure and process is in some ways remarkably similar to some of the Western approaches, such as bioenergetics, Reichian energetics, Rolfing, and chiropractic.[5]

As noted, Esalen fostered the view that Eastern kundalini and the biophysical, erotic, and mystical energy associated with these Western forms of bodywork were mutually validating. With Bioenergetics tracing its lineage through Reich's theory of orgone energy (which Kripal indicates is a "neologism derived from 'orgasm' and 'organism'"[6]) back to Freud's concept of libido; and with Rolfing having originated in part from a transmission of Eastern tantric teachings through Pierre Bernard, the notion of spiritual East meets scientifically validating West was an inevitable discovery for anyone who spent time at Esalen.

According to Kripal, Reich saw orgone as

> a subtle cosmic energy that links the sentient and non-sentient worlds and expresses itself through the various mediums of the pulsing rhythms of simple-cell organisms, the intensely pleasurable contractions of the human orgasm, the healing charisma of Christ, and atmospheric weather patterns. Even when he is not explicitly invoked or perhaps even known about, Reich is—very much like his concept of the orgone—somehow everywhere at Esalen.[7]

To this "streaming, intensely blissful cosmic energy residing in the human body that needs to be released through various physical manipulations" in the bodywork modalities and psychological approaches promulgated at Esalen, Kripal juxtaposes "the central categories of many Asian Tantric yoga systems, including the Shakti or 'occult energy' that streams through the aspirant's body during initiation and spiritual ecstasy"—as well as kundalini, the seven chakras (linked to Reich's seven rings of body armor ascending along the spinal column), and prana as "'life-energy.'"[8] But he does not perceive that at Esalen the central metaphor uniting these Western and Eastern streams of thought on energy is Aurobindo's continuum of human potential and its associated list of chakra qualities. The Maslowian actualization of these qualities is what the meditative spiritual practices of the East *and* the physical and psychological manipulations of bodywork and open encounter of the West mutually aim for.

Dychtwald's book opens dramatically with his being examined in the nude in a workshop, before a large group of people, by John Pierrakos (1921–2001). Pierrakos is reading Dychtwald's personality from the structure of his body and posture with great detail and accuracy. Pierrakos was an important influence on Barbara Brennan, author of *Hands of Light* (1989), a bestselling book on energy healing with a strong focus on the chakras. I return to Brennan's work in the final chapter.

Dychtwald continues with accounts of Rolfing sessions, open encounter groups, and experiences with various other physical and psychological approaches to releasing human potential, such as yoga and meditation. These accounts cover a range of roles, from client or participant to witness or facilitator, from personal experiment and self-reflection to private consultations and group process. Though *Bodymind* is not, strictly speaking, a memoir, it may be one of the most revealing records of what was going on therapeutically at Esalen in the early 1970s, from daily life and practice to the theory behind it all and what it was supposed to accomplish.

The Esalen approach to the chakras described in Schutz's *Here Comes Everybody* serves as a metaphor for organizing Dychtwald's speculations on the connections between the human body and our feelings about self and others, our thoughts and beliefs, and our aspirations toward self-transcendence. Indeed, Dychtwald observes that the location of the chakras "suggests a path along which an individual might travel on his personal road to optimal bodymind health and a full realization of his human potentialities" [9]—thus ringing changes on Esalen's central metaphor of the continuum of human potential, as implied in Aurobindo's teachings on chakras and states of consciousness. Even the term *bodymind* may have originated in Aurobindo's letters on yoga:

> There is too an obscure mind of the body, of the very cells, molecules, corpuscles. . . . This body-mind is a very tangible truth; owing to its obscurity and mechanical clinging to past movements and facile oblivion and rejection of the new, we find in it one of the chief obstacles to permeation by the supermind force and the transformation of the functioning of the body. On the other hand, once effectively converted, it will be one of the most precious instruments for the stabilization of the supramental light and force in material Nature.[10]

Implicit in Dychtwald's use of this metaphor is the idea that the chakras are where body and mind meet. This notion hearkens back to Besant's and Leadbeater's teachings that the etheric-body chakras are the links between the physical body and the subtle bodies, with the astral/emotional body and the mental and causal bodies representing what Dychtwald calls mind. He lists Leadbeater's *The Chakras* in his bibliography—and Leadbeater specifically addresses the function of the etheric-body chakras as links between the physical and subtle bodies in that book.

The implication of the chakras being where the body and the mind meet is that they, as well as the human potentialities they represent, are a metaphorical map of the bodymind. I am reminded of David Gordon White's definition of tantric practice in Asia:

> An effort to gain access to and appropriate the energy or enlightened consciousness of the absolute godhead that courses through the universe [i.e., kundalini, orgone, or Esalen's "energy"], giving its creatures life and the potential for salvation [liberation from psychological and

social conditioning]. Humans in particular [hence human potential] are empowered to realize this goal through strategies of embodiment [such as bodywork]—that is, of causing that divine energy to become concentrated in one or another sort of template, grid, or mesocosm [the chakras as map of the bodymind]—prior to its internalization in or identification with the individual microcosm.[11]

In White's understanding of Tantra, the macrocosm of godhead and the microcosm of the individual require an intermediary factor that he calls mesocosm (whole in the middle). This mesocosm is a metaphorical blending of macro and micro, of universe and individual, a map of potential to be fulfilled or realized. The Eastern chakra system is one such mesocosmic map.

Translated back into the terms of Esalen's human potential movement, mind (as defined by Aurobindo as ever-expanding states of consciousness from thinking mind to supermind) is the macrocosm and the human body is the microcosm. The bodymind is the mesocosm and the chakras are its template, grid, or map. They list the levels and qualities to be achieved in order to realize our physical, emotional, psychological, and spiritual liberation from social conditioning that prevents full use and enjoyment of body *and* mind.

Dychtwald's list of the chakras in *Bodymind* refines what we saw in Schutz, with the first three chakras reflecting Ramakrishna/Campbell and chakras four through seven reflecting Aurobindo. I have highlighted the key words that get carried forward into later presentations of the Western chakra system:

1. **Root**—grand human potential, primitive energy, and basic *survival* needs
2. **Genital**—*sexual* drives and primary interpersonal relationships
3. **Solar plexus**—raw emotions, *power* drives, and social identification

4. **Heart**—feelings of affection, *love*, and self-expression
5. **Throat**—*communication*, expression, and self-identification
6. **Brow**—powers of mind and heightened self-awareness
7. **Crown**—self-realization or *enlightenment*[12]

The notion of a continuum of human potential is retained, though by now it is thoroughly psychologized, reflecting both Maslow's hierarchy of needs and an implied process of individuation in which people must disentangle themselves from the needs and drives of the first three chakras to achieve an ever more developed sense of self, involving expression, identification, awareness, and realization.[13] By "powers of mind" Dychtwald implies not only cognition (Aurobindo's thinking mind), but also intuition or psychic abilities (Aurobindo's higher mind)—as indicated by his later listing of abilities such as telepathy, precognition, and clairvoyance in connection with the sixth chakra. He even uses the familiar esoteric term *third eye* to describe this chakra. Thus the missing key words for the sixth chakra—*intuition* and *third eye*—are indeed associated with his version of the chakra system, despite their absence from this list of qualities.[14]

In researching the present book, I hypothesized that someone who was familiar with the list of chakra qualities developed at Esalen and with the chromotherapists' association of the chakras with the colors of the rainbow must have brought these qualities and colors together to birth the Western chakra system as we know it. I believe that person was Ken Dychtwald. We have seen the similarity of his list of chakra qualities to that most commonly in use today. Let us now consider how he brought the colors into association with this list.

The dust jacket of the first edition of *Bodymind*, published in June 1977, pictures a faceless human silhouette seated in meditation with the chakras represented by colored bands in the rainbow order—possibly to hint at a connection between the chakras and Reich's rings of body armor. The chakras are more specifically located in the body throughout the book in psychedelic black-and-white illustrations based on this form. The originals of these illustrations were likely in color. Oddly, the text does not mention the chakra colors. Dychtwald may have decided or been advised not to include them in order to boost the cachet of his book amongst his psychological peers. The reason for this surmise will become clear momentarily. The rainbow-colored jacket design was replaced by others in subsequent paperback editions of the book.

To promote *Bodymind*, Dychtwald contributed an article to the July/August 1977 issue of *Yoga Journal*: "Bodymind and the Evolution to Cosmic Consciousness." Here, Dychtwald stated that "each chakra corresponds to a particular color vibration with the lowest chakra projecting the color red and each ascending chakra projecting the next color of the rainbow: orange, yellow, green, blue, indigo, and violet for the seventh chakra." He then listed the chakra qualities as given above, adding the phrase "expanded mental powers" to his description of the sixth chakra.[15]

About the seventh chakra, he said that it "corresponds to the highest level of human development, the point at which all of the bodymind's tensions and conflicts have been resolved and its potentials have been tapped. Its attainment demands complete awareness of self, and mastery of all the previous chakra elements and qualities." He listed several names for this state: "enlightenment, samadhi, nirvana, God consciousness, and cosmic consciousness." These passages are quoted almost verbatim from *Bodymind*—including the following résumé of descriptions of chakra functions (I have added the chakra locations for clarity):

1. **Root**—survival
2. **Genital**—sexuality
3. **Solar plexus**—power
4. **Heart**—love
5. **Throat**—communication
6. **Brow**—self-reflection/self-awareness
7. **Crown**—wisdom / self-realization / cosmic consciousness[16]

This article appears to be the first printed instance in which the rainbow colors are linked to the Esalen chakra qualities using words similar to those encountered in most subsequent descriptions of the Western chakra system. The qualities listed for the first five chakras are often exactly reproduced in these descriptions. Those for the sixth and seventh chakras differ slightly but usually have similar connotations—such as insight for the sixth chakra and enlightenment for the seventh. By this time, the third-eye connection with the sixth chakra had been around for so long, starting with the Theosophical Society, that its presence in any list of chakra qualities was practically automatic and traditional, even at Esalen. So its absence from Dychtwald's *Yoga Journal* article hardly provides an opportunity for later innovation.

There are no books by chromotherapists in the bibliographies of *Bodymind* and the *Yoga Journal* article. However, both sources list one of the earliest manuals of neo-Tantra published in America: Omar Garrison's *Tantra: The Yoga of Sex* (1961). Garrison describes the Eastern chakra system as presented in *The Serpent Power*, with special emphasis on the occult powers associated with the development of each chakra. He adds the endocrine glands in a more sensible order than Alice Bailey's (gonads, adrenals, pancreas, thymus, thyroid, pituitary, pineal), then states that each chakra "has a characteristic dominant color" and that these colors "correspond to the seven visible rays of light that comprise the spectrum—namely, red, orange, yellow, green, blue, indigo and violet."[17]

After citing Leadbeater's *The Chakras*, Garrison proceeds to emend Leadbeater's color system. The second chakra is no longer associated with the spleen, but with the genitals. However, the function of Leadbeater's second chakra as the distributor of vitality rays throughout the body is retained. Garrison makes the third chakra yellow and the fourth green, thus imposing the rainbow order absent in Leadbeater. Yet he makes the first chakra orange (red-orange in Leadbeater) while retaining Leadbeater's original rose-red color for the second chakra—thus seeming to switch the order of red and orange in the spectrum and demonstrating what might be called the law of conservation of confusion. A further instance occurs when Garrison contradicts his earlier statements about the endocrine glands and the chakras by directing the indigo ray to the brow chakra and the *pineal* gland and the violet ray to the crown chakra and the *pituitary* gland.[18]

Dychtwald was apparently unfazed. He silently corrected both issues in his book (glands) and article (glands and colors). Thus was born the Western chakra system as we know it. Though it might be safer to say that the correlation between Esalen chakra qualities and rainbow colors was established by the mid-1970s, I like to think of June 1977 as the actual birthdate—corresponding to the publication of *Bodymind* and the period when the July/August issue of *Yoga Journal* containing his article would have hit the newsstands.[19]

As mentioned, many Internet-based writers trace the association of chakras and rainbow colors to Christopher Hills, who also published a book in 1977 that linked the chakras and the rainbow colors—using a dramatic and memorable cover image that is ubiquitous on the Web (Dychtwald's is not). However, Hills's book, *Nuclear Evolution: Discovery of the Rainbow Body*, used an alternative list of chakra qualities that had a minor influence on later writings—I have seen only a single instance outside Hills's own circle—so it cannot be said to represent the Western chakra system as we know it today. Furthermore, the acknowledgments pages of *Nuclear Evolution* are signed "July 1977," which means that *Bodymind* and the *Yoga Journal* article were published first.

In terms of the chakra qualities, Dychtwald appears to be merely a disseminator. In terms of bringing together the Esalen chakra qualities and the chromotherapists' rainbow colors, he could be perceived as a consolidator. However, if we look at the focus of *Bodymind* on personal and group experience of the chakra system as a means of organizing perceptions of inner growth and its impact on bodily and social or relational expression, then we should perhaps classify him as a validator of the Esalen vision of the chakras

Table 20
Evolution of Chakra Qualities (1970s)

Chakras	Maslow (1969)	Ram Dass (1970–71)	Schutz (1973)	Rosenberg (1973)
Crown	Self-transcendence	Buddha state	Cosmic consciousness	One with God
Brow	Self-actualization	Wisdom	Intuition	Third eye
Throat	Esteem needs	Deeper within	Expression	Purification
Heart	Belongingness & love needs	Compassion	Affection Love Communication	Love
Solar plexus	Safety needs	Power Mastery Ego control	Assertiveness Anger	Power
Genital	. . .	Sense gratification Sexual desire Reproduction	Sexual energy	Sex
Root	Physiological & survival needs	Survival Security	Grand potential Primitive energy	Just existing

Keyes (1974)	Chaudhuri (1975)	Rama (1976)	Dychtwald (1977)
Cosmic consciousness	Transcendental consciousness	Highest state Samadhi	Wisdom Self-realization Enlightenment
Conscious awareness	Wisdom Divine command Third eye Spiritual enlightenment Self-mastery Cosmic consciousness	Intuitive knowledge Third eye Introspection Inner vision Clairvoyance	Self-reflection Self-awareness
Cornucopia	Communication Self-projection Creative inspiration Speech	Nurturance Creativity Receiving grace	Communication
Love	Soul Unconditional love Higher values	Emotion Empathy Compassion Selfless love	Love
Power	Power	Dominance Submission	Power
Sensation	Vital Instinctual Sexual	Sensuality Sexuality	Sexuality
Security	Material world	Fear Paranoia Survival	Survival

as a continuum of human potential. Thus his book presents an experiential chakra system validated by acute inner and outer psychological observation rather than clairvoyance.

Table 20 demonstrates the evolution of the chakra qualities at Esalen during the nearly ten-year period between Maslow's addition of self-transcendence to his hierarchy of needs in 1969 to Dychtwald's one-word versions of the chakra qualities in 1977, including authors discussed in the two preceding chapters. I have not included the Ramakrishna/Campbell list—it is represented by the lists of Ram Dass and Jack Lee Rosenberg, which were derived from it.

Part 6
Light-Wheels Roll On
(1980s and Beyond)

Chapter 23
Way of the Dodo— Extinct Systems

The situation in the latter half of the 1970s was not unlike that of earlier phases of human evolution when several species of hominid were present on the planet, such as Neanderthals and Homo sapiens. In the 1980s, Dychtwald's version of the chakra system was gaining evolutionary ground, whereas the systems described in the present chapter gradually disappeared from most New Age presentations of the chakras and became extinct.

Under the Hood (Peter Rendel)

Theosophist and sound healer Peter Leland Rendel (1925–2003) wrote a much-cited but now-forgotten book, *Introduction to the Chakras* (1974). An important reference for at least twenty years, the book sold more than 100,000 copies and was translated into nine languages. It was mentioned by Anodea Judith in the annotated bibliography of *Wheels of Life* as "probably the best I've read on the subject!"[1]

Rendel did not list his own sources. His focus is on the elements and the tattvic tides as taught in Rāma Prasād's *Nature's Finer Forces*, which he blended with alchemy, hermeticism, the astrological zodiac, and the kabbalistic Tree of Life. Rendel also provided minimal instruction on developing the chakras through breathing techniques probably derived from Prasād. There was no information on chakra colors.

This modest booklet of sixty-five pages offered a rational, though esoteric, explanation of the structure of the chakra system that became the basis for later authors' syntheses of the Esalen qualities (all but divorced from their tantric roots and thoroughly psychologized), the chromotherapists' colors, Western esotericism, and the Theosophical principles that were originally responsible for transmitting ancient teachings on the chakras from East to West. Rendel provided a list of chakra qualities based on symbolic interpretation of the elements:

1. **Root**—earth (solidity, security, satisfaction)
2. **Sacral**—water (fluidity, ripeness, smoothness)
3. **Solar plexus**—fire (warmth, expansiveness, joviality)
4. **Heart**—air (lightness, gentleness, mobility)
5. **Throat**—ether (space, sound, change)
6. **Brow**—mind (mentation, thought, time)
7. **Crown**—spirit (bliss, union, eternal now)[2]

Though these words were not carried forward into later chakra systems, Rendel's book may be as responsible as *The Serpent Power* for later systems that link chakras and elements—because he thoroughly westernized the qualities associated with the elements. I see him as a consolidator and his system as an interpretive peek under the hood at the thought processes that produced the Western chakra system.

Energy and Ecstasy (Bernard Gunther)

Psychotherapist Bernard Gunther (Bernard Gutwillig; (1929–2013) was a student of Fritz Perls (1893–1970), the originator of gestalt therapy and an early resident teacher at Esalen. Gunther worked at Esalen from about 1964 to 1970, practicing what he called "sensory awakening" (according to Kripal, exercises intended "to awaken the senses and allow the individual to live more fully in the here and now"). Gunther takes credit for developing Esalen-style massage, which Kripal styles as "perhaps *the* central Esalen healing practice: full-body contemplative massage," historically done in proximity to the hot springs and with both therapist and client in the nude—"a largely silent and deeply sensuous ritual of the enlightenment of the body over the ocean."[3] Gunther was also a devotee of Bhagwan Shree Rajneesh in the 1970s, living for several years at his guru's ashram in Poona, India, under the name Swami Deva Amit Prem.[4]

Gunther brought out his version of the chakra system a year after Dychtwald's. *Energy, Ecstasy, and Your Seven Vital Centers* (1978) was a manual of chakra development, published well in advance of the flood to come a decade later. It contained psychedelic color illustrations of the chakras as well as instructions in "various forms of passive meditation, symbolic visualization, and subtle touch methods" designed to "increase your energy, creativity, relaxation, health, and spiritual well-being."[5] Its chart of correspondences could perhaps be considered the premier 1970s synthesis of teachings on the chakras, just as Judith's *Wheels of Life* performs that function for the 1980s. These correspondences included the following:

- **Names**—from Leadbeater's *The Chakras* (in Gunther's bibliography)
- **Functions** (sex, health, power, compassion, creativity and self-expression, paranormal powers, liberation)—from various Esalen lists[6]
- **Endocrine influences**—from Bailey's *Esoteric Psychology* (in Gunther's bibliography)
- **Colors**—from Leadbeater
- **Symbols**—from Jack Schwarz's *Voluntary Controls*, to be discussed later (not in Gunther's bibliography)
- **Sounds**—from traditional tantric teachings on the seed syllables (transliterated in a way that makes the connection less clear than in other books—e.g., *la* for *laṃ*, *ba* for *vaṃ*, *ra* for *raṃ*, and so on; *ah* given for the brow and *om* for the crown, which is nontraditional, possibly distributing the sound AUM over both chakras)
- **Elements**—from traditional tantric teachings on the tattvas
- **Senses**—from traditional tantric teachings on the tattvas
- **Planets**—from a suggestion by Rendel (Saturn is linked with the first chakra, followed by the remaining planets in order of their proximity to the sun, with Mercury associated with the fifth chakra, the Sun and Moon with the sixth chakra, and no planet for the seventh)[7]

- **Positive and negative emotions**—from an unknown source, possibly original: (1) passion vs. frustration/rage; (2) well-being vs. anxiety; (3) power/desire vs. fear/guilt/doubt; (4) joy vs. grief; (5) inspiration vs. repression; (6) ecstasy vs. obsession; (7) bliss
- **Physical and mental diseases**—from an unknown source, possibly original

The diseases are mostly associated with the areas of the body where the chakra is located. For example, hemorrhoids are linked with the root chakra, gallstones with the solar-plexus chakra, and angina with the heart chakra.[8] Listing positive and negative emotions and diseases associated with the chakras is now commonplace in New Age presentations of the chakras—but this was an early instance. Previous teachings on the chakras, especially in the Bailey, Ramakrishna/Campbell, and Keyes systems, tended to regard the three lower chakras as problematic and unsafe, indicating that their dangers could be transcended only through the development of the four higher chakras. Gunther's system is more even-handed: the lower chakras have an upside and the upper chakras have a downside.

Gunther's book also represents one of the first appearances in print of exercises designed to balance the chakras—a frequently encountered approach in later New Age books, especially as the notion of the chakras began to spread into various alternative healing modalities in the 1980s.

Energy, Ecstasy, and Your Seven Vital Chakras was popular, going through at least ten printings by 1989. Perhaps because of its basis in Leadbeater's fusing of the first two chakras and substitution of the spleen chakra for the second chakra, which creates confusion for readers familiar with the genital or sacral chakra in the second position, the book appears to have been superseded and forgotten.

Despite the apparently innovative psychedelic portrayals of the chakras in Gunther's book, I see him as a consolidator rather than an innovator. Even though he provided exercises for the development of the chakras and should perhaps be considered a validator presenting an experiential chakra system, the conceptual basis of this system, as well as much of its imagery and implementation in practice, did not originate with him. They were borrowed—in an egregious instance of source amnesia—from Jack Schwarz.

The Holy Grail (Jack Schwarz)

Dutch-American spiritual and self-help teacher Jack Schwarz (Jacob Schwarz; 1924–2000) was involved in experiments at the Menninger Foundation similar to those undergone by Swami Rama. Though not a yogi, Schwarz had the ability to regulate his own brain waves in measurable ways and to control supposedly involuntary physiological processes such as heart rate, blood pressure, circulation to limbs, perception of pain, neutralization of injected toxins, and rapid healing of wounds. The name for scientific studies of such abilities was *voluntary controls*, hence the title of his second book: *Voluntary Controls: Exercises for Creative Meditation and for Activating the Potential of the Chakras* (1978). Schwarz also had the ability to perceive auras.

Schwarz developed a program of meditative exercises involving breathing and visualization of colors and images. He built this program around Leadbeater's teachings on the chakras, including the spleen chakra in second position and the color system of red-orange, pink, green, yellow, blue, indigo, and purple. To these, Schwarz added visualizations of the symbols related to the yantras of the five elements in the Eastern chakra system. However, he rearranged their order and added two more, so each chakra had a symbol.

The practice is to activate each chakra, one at a time, through regulated breathing, while focusing on the color and symbol of the chakra. In the final stages, the symbols are assembled into an image of a chalice, the Holy Grail—in some legends, the wine cup used by Christ and his disciples at the Last Supper; in others, the receptacle into which Christ's blood flowed when his side was pierced by a

Table 21
The *Voluntary Controls* Chakra System (1978)[9]

Chakras	Glands	Colors	Functions	Traditional Yantras	Symbols
Crown	Pineal	Purple	Third eye Total integration Enlightenment	[Lotus]	Lotus
Brow	Pituitary	Indigo	Synthesizing	...	Six-pointed star
Throat	Thyroid	Blue	Creative expression Willpower Volition	Circle	Crescent
Heart	Thymus	Yellow	Transmutation Integration Purification	Six-pointed star	Cross
Solar plexus	Adrenals	Green	Life-preserving	Triangle	Circle
Spleen	Spleen Pancreas Liver	Pink	Life-regulating	Crescent	Triangle
Root	Gonads	Red-orange	Life-promoting	Square	Square

Roman spear during the crucifixion. The seeking of the Holy Grail is the subject of many tales, such as that of King Arthur and his knights, and is said to symbolize our quest for realizing the highest and best in ourselves. Schwarz's chalice has two arms on its crosslike stem, and the bowl resembles a head, open at the top to receive spiritual energy from above, with a seven-petaled lotus, representing the crown chakra, floating in the bowl. The first three chakras form the base of the chalice.

Table 21 displays Schwarz's teachings on the chakras. I include a column for the traditional Eastern system yantras to facilitate comparison with Schwarz's innovations.

Schwarz did not include a bibliography. However, readers may recognize resonances with several earlier discussions in the present book. The combination of breath control with visualizing colored symbols of the elements (tattvas) derives from Rāma Prasād, via the early developers of the Golden Dawn magical tradition. The visualization of colors in connection with the chakras while ascending the spine goes back to Blavatsky's kundalini practice, as presented in her Esoteric Instructions.

The functions are unique—I have not encountered a similar list elsewhere. I suspect this list is derived from Bailey, who associates the heart chakra with the transmutation of desire into love, the throat chakra with creative and artistic expression, and the brow chakra with synthesis. In Bailey's writings, the three lower chakras deal with life force in various ways, but I do not find the exact phrasings used by Schwarz.[10]

The notion of constructing a chalice representing the bowl of the Holy Grail resting on a cross seems like a major innovation—a claiming of the Eastern tantric chakra system by Western Christianized esotericism. However, there is an Eastern precedent. In *Foundations of Tibetan Mysticism*, Anagarika Govinda (whom we first met in chapter 2) explains the basis for meditation on the five chakras of Tibetan Buddhism, in which "the psychic Centers of the body become the five storeys [*sic*] of the sacred temple"—a chorten. Such temples are "religious monuments developed from the

Indian *stupa*, which originally served as receptacles for the relics of the Buddha and his chief disciples." The root center (which combines the first two chakras of tantric Hinduism) is the first story, represented by a "yellow square or cube." The navel center is the second story, represented by a "white disc or sphere." The heart center is the third, represented by a red triangle, cone, or pyramid. The throat center is the fourth, represented by a green, upward-turned "hemispherical body." And the "Brain or Crown Center" (which combines the brow and crown chakras of tantric Hinduism) is the fifth story, represented by a "blue flaming drop."[11]

Figure 22 illustrates the chakras of the Tibetan system and their relationship to the elements and their symbols. The chakras are numbered from 1 to 6, with an indication of which chakras from the Hindu system are paired at the root and crown. To avoid confusion, I do not use the Hindu or Tibetan names. Govinda himself uses the English names given here. In figure 23, the square, triangle, and circle should be imagined as lying on a horizontal plane as the basis for the cross.

Schwarz's book was released in April 1978. I have not been able to determine whether its publication preceded or followed that of Gunther's *Energy, Ecstasy, and Your Seven Vital Chakras*, which provided a more elaborate presentation of the same exercises, with photographs and diagrams depicting the images and actions to be visualized. The psychedelic paintings of the chakras in Gunther's book incorporate the symbols given in Schwarz's system, mixing them with elements of the traditional diagrams from *The Serpent Power*. Though Gunther does not claim to have generated the system ("The following symbolic chakra exercises are some of the most powerful this writer has ever experienced"[12]), he clearly puts his personal stamp on it—and never mentions Schwarz as the source.

If I had to choose a motivation for Gunther's source amnesia concerning Schwarz's work, I would select *original synthesis* or *"justifiable" appropriation*, or both. The system of exercises surrounding Gunther's presentation of Schwarz's work was unique to Gunther, as was his carefully thought-out table of chakra correspondences—itself an original synthesis of existing information on the chakras. In addition, Schwarz advocated the decentralizing of spiritual authority in passing on an eclectic system such as his:

> From each of the many books I have read, I have extracted the material relevant to my own needs and perspectives and dismissed the rest. Every one of them has confirmed

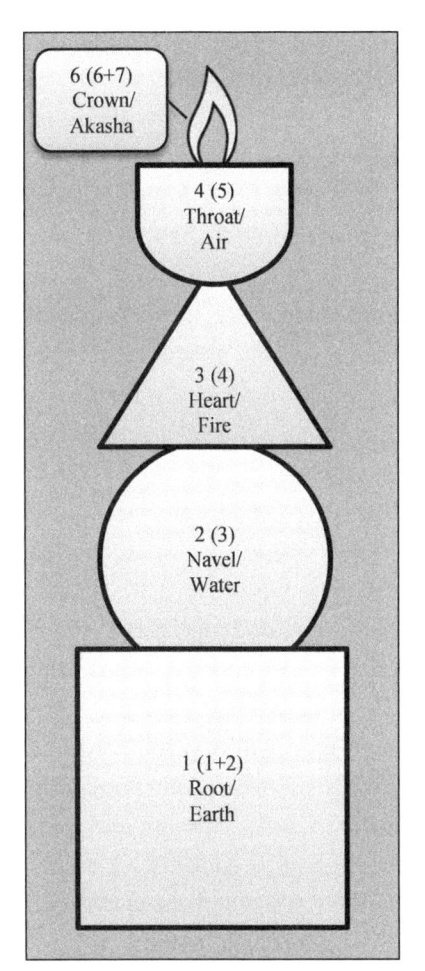

Figure 22. Tibetan Chakras as Chorten (after Anagarika Govinda, *Foundations of Tibetan Buddhism,* 1969)

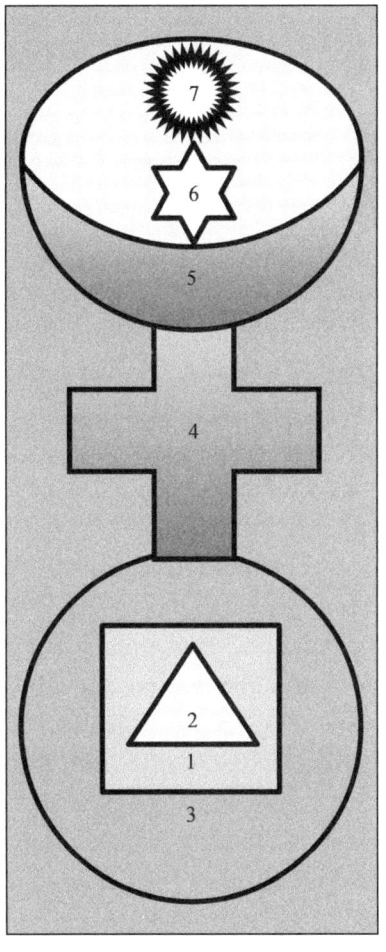

Figure 23. Western Chakras as Holy Grail (after Jack Schwarz, *Voluntary Controls,* 1978)

me, sometimes with only one sentence. This is the important thing. All my gurus have enabled me to realize that I am not the only one who is envisioning the world in a certain way. But they have also helped me to understand that the model created by all my perspectives is unique to me. That model is important to others only when it encourages them to make their own models.

What will people do with the experiences they have if they take this book seriously and practice the exercises? Will they say, "This is Jack Schwarz's method"? No. If they have followed the instructions carefully, they will be developing their own methods.[13]

These are generous words, inviting people to have their own experience, to undergo self-initiation rather than depend on the external authority of a guru or spiritual teacher. Yet these words are also an invitation for "justifiable" appropriation, as well as an apologia for Schwarz's own source amnesia and probably for that of many New Age authors. In the end, as far as Schwarz's intellectual property rights are concerned, it may not have mattered—his book, like Gunther's, went through ten or more printings and was available until at least 1992.

The focus of Schwarz's chakra system was experiential. Yet in his approach to this system, he was an innovator (of the Holy Grail connection), consolidator (of material from Leadbeater and other sources), and clairvoyant validator.

While writing this book, I picked up a wallet-sized card providing a précis of the chakra system in a New Age bookstore. Schwarz's symbols for the chakras were included, though they were assigned to the rainbow colors rather than to Leadbeater's colors, as in Schwarz's books. Friends of mine have noted these symbols on handouts provided in classes on the chakras and wondered about their origin; their source and use in Schwarz's *Voluntary Controls* chakra system have been forgotten.

Mansions of Color (Christopher Hills)

A fascinating and flamboyant combination of self-made, independently wealthy business entrepreneur and visionary economic and political philosopher, Christopher Hills (1926–97) was also a yogi, metaphysician, and clairvoyant researcher of consciousness. The quasi-hagiographic Wikipedia entry on Hills scrupulously documents his pioneering discovery, development, and worldwide sale of spirulina as a nutritional supplement; conferring with political giants such as Indian Prime Minister Jawaharlal Nehru about what to do about the Dalai Lama's exile from Tibet in 1959; spearheading a worldwide conference on science and yoga in India; and establishing New Age educational and intentional communities in the heart of London (Centre House) and near Santa Cruz, California (University of the Trees).

This was apparently an intellectual and spiritual giant of a man with a great vision and a big heart. Like Schwarz, he could control so-called involuntary physiological responses at will. He was also a master dowser/diviner who developed a theory he called Supersensonics, which attempted to reconcile the world of psychic phenomena with physical laws.

Hills originated a system for delineating personality types in *Nuclear Evolution: A Guide to Cosmic Enlightenment* (1968). He based this system on the rainbow-colored rays described in Theosophical teachings, from Blavatsky to Bailey, and those of the chromotherapists. The rays were portrayed in terms of human evolutionary stages—reflecting personality and social types—an idea explored in the first volume of Bailey's *Esoteric Psychology* (1936). Wikipedia states that "by 1960 Christopher Hills had accumulated a large metaphysical library on frequent trips to Samuel Weiser Books in New York"; so we should not be surprised at the resonances between his writings and those of earlier esotericists, even when the latter are not mentioned by him as sources.

The personality types were derived from the Lüscher color

test, developed by Swiss psychotherapist Max Lüscher (b. 1923) as a means of typing people through color preferences, which he believed were universally mapped into personality traits. The test was developed from Lüscher's doctoral dissertation, first published about 1949. It became hugely popular in the 1970s, after Lüscher published his findings and a version of the test that could be self-administered, *The Lüscher Color Test* (1969).

Hills's application of the Lüscher colors included black but eliminated brown and gray, substituting the missing rainbow colors of orange and indigo. In honor of the yogic practice he had developed since the 1960s, Hills also mapped the traditional eight limbs of yoga from the *Yoga Sūtra* of Patañjali into his system. In the 1977 edition of *Nuclear Evolution* (subtitled *The Discovery of the Rainbow Body*), Hills brought in the seven chakras as well.

Here is the matrix from which Hills's chakra system evolved. Page numbers refer to the 1968 edition of *Nuclear Evolution*; words in italics and bold refer to those chosen for his final list, which are paired with the eight limbs, on page 83:

- **Red**—mating instinct (12–13); ***sensation*** (46); touch contact (83); *yama* (ethical precepts)
- **Orange**—herd instinct (13); exploration or ***ambition*** (50); social contact (83); *niyama* (moral precepts)
- **Yellow**—love of change (16–17); ***thinking*** (52); asana (posture practice)[14]
- **Green**—possessiveness (17–20); "self-security, self-measuring, or self-confirmation and assurance" (56); "measurer of time" (60); ***vital force*** (83); pranayama (breath control)
- **Blue**—love of authority (20–22); "fixer of time," memory (60); ***mental concepts*** (83); *svādhyāya* ("study" or "contemplation"; a substitution for *pratyāhāra*, "sense withdrawal")
- **Indigo**—"intuitive sensitivity or taste" (25–26) ; ***intuition*** (63); dharana (concentration)

- **Violet**—awareness of an enduring order (29–31); *imagination* (66); dhyana (meditation)
- **Black**—will (69); *self-surrender* (83); samadhi (ecstasy)

The more developed presentation in the 1977 edition appears in table 22. Note the presence of the spleen chakra, indicating a debt to Leadbeater.

As in the previous version, Hills includes black as the will. Beyond violet, black represents the void, the Absolute. In terms of time sense, it refers to an "abstraction of the future unknown self."[17]

Despite the radically different list of chakra qualities associated with Hills's system, other characteristics of what I call the Western chakra system are present: names, connection to nerve plexuses and endocrine glands, and rainbow colors.[18] Hills's attempt to link time, space, light, consciousness, and color to the chakras and spiritual evolution of humanity, as individuals and en masse, is unique and innovative. He was aware of the Ramakrishna/Campbell list of chakra qualities, as transmitted in Ram Dass's *The Only Dance There Is*—Hills contrasts his list with that of Dass, indicating that he has shifted sexuality from second to first chakra and power from third to second chakra.[19]

In 1979, Norah Hills (1916–95), Christopher's wife at the time, published a simplified account of the *Nuclear Evolution* chakra system: *You Are a Rainbow* (1979). The book included interviews with Hills's students at the University of the Trees about what knowing their color and chakra type (as determined by Hills) meant to them. The reverence of these young community members for their guru-like teacher comes through, as well as their eagerness to develop the positive and work through the negative aspects of their type.

You Are a Rainbow inspired what appears to be the only publication by a nonstudent of Hills that carried forward elements of the *Nuclear Evolution* (1977) system: *Seven Mansions of Color* (1982; still in print) by Canadian New Age musician and meditation teacher Alex Jones. Jones supplies a basic manual of color healing based on

Table 22
Chakras according to Christopher Hills (1977)[15]

Chakra	Color	Personality Type	Consciousness	Orientation	Time Sense[16]
Crown	Violet	Imaginative	Cosmic	Divine order	Timelessness
Third eye	Indigo	Intuitive	Future	Future	Present as future
Throat	Blue	Idealistic	Conceptual	Memory	Fixer of time
Heart	Green	Acquisitive	Security	Security	Chronological time
Solar plexus	Yellow	Intellectual	Analytical	Thinking	Planning for future
Splenic	Orange	Social	Group	People	Present applied to future
Genital	Red	Sensation	Physical	Action	Immediate moment

the chakras and cites several authors and titles now familiar to us, including Woodroffe's *The Serpent Power*, Hunt's *The Seven Keys to Color Healing*, Leadbeater's *The Chakras*, and Ouseley's *The Power of the Rays* and *The Science of the Aura*.

Curiously, *Seven Mansions of Color* provides an unintentional exposé of the sources of *Nuclear Evolution*'s take on the chakras. Though Alice Bailey is not mentioned by Christopher or Norah Hills, she comes into Jones's book via Ouseley's *The Power of the Rays*. In a chart in *Seven Mansions of Color* entitled "Vibration Relationship of the Spectrum of Colors," Jones lists colors, musical notes, "Quality Intelligence" (probably "Quality/Intelligence"), and centers, drawing the qualities and types of intelligence from Ouseley and Hills, respectively. In compiling the table, Jones appears to discover mutually confirmatory resonances—thereby revealing the basis of both Hills's and Ouseley's systems in Bailey's account of the ray qualities, as linked to the rainbow colors by Hunt's teacher, Ivah Bergh Whitten.[20]

There is no sign in Jones's book of exposure to the Ramakrishna/Campbell or Aurobindo/Esalen list of chakra qualities. Thus, in its clarity and completeness, as well as its modesty, *Seven Mansions of Color* could be called an epitome of the chromotherapists' views of the chakras as they evolved in the sixty years after the publication of Bailey's *Letters on Occult Meditation*, as well as a personal synthesis of information on the chakra system using Hills's version as template.

Hills's system could be considered a British-generated contender for the title of Western chakra system. However, for lack of advocacy by later writers (with the exception of Jones), this system disappeared from view. Given the hegemony today of the system presented in Dychtwald's *Bodymind* and *Yoga Journal* article, Hills's presentation seems eccentric, despite its brilliance. Yet it may have value beyond being a merely historic, dead-end evolutionary stage of the Western chakra system.

If we were to reconsider *Nuclear Evolution* in the light of the view advocated by Besant and Leadbeater, that each subtle body has its own chakra system, then perhaps we could link Hills's system, with its emphasis on individual and social types of intelligence, to the mental body. Thus *Nuclear Evolution* could be a treatise on the existence and evolution of mental-body chakras, whereas the lifestyle-oriented descriptions of the chakra system found in present New Age books, coming out of Esalen, could be considered accounts of the etheric-body chakras. The etheric body deals with vitality and life force; the Esalen-based systems, as noted, deal directly with such energy.

Though there are several long-out-of-print books on Hills's chakra system and "theory of nuclear evolution" by his students, devotees, and colleagues at the University of the Trees, *Nuclear Evolution* is surprisingly still available from the publisher. Perhaps his system merits reconsideration in terms of a multiple-body perspective on the chakras, to be discussed in the final chapter of this book.

I would call Hills an innovating consolidator and validator of a chakra system intended to be experiential rather than merely interpretive. However, in *Nuclear Evolution* (1977), theorizing about possible applications took precedence over how-to exercises, so the book sits on the cusp of being interpretive or experiential. Clearly, Jones was merely an explanatory disseminator of this system— along with Norah Hills and others in the University of the Trees community who wrote about it.

Chapter 24
The Great Chakra Controversy

Dychtwald's pairing of the chromotherapists' rainbow colors with Esalen's chakra qualities soon began to spread into alternative healing modalities beyond those taught at Esalen. For example, in 1982, five years after the release of *Bodymind*, Maruti Seidman (b. 1948), published the following list, nearly identical to Dychtwald's, in a guide to Polarity Therapy:

1. **Root**—red; material and survival needs
2. **Genital**—orange; creativity, desires, sensuality, lust
3. **Navel**—yellow; willpower, "how we view ourselves"
4. **Heart**—green; love, compassion, self-expression
5. **Throat**—blue; speech, self-expression, communication
6. **Third eye**—indigo; intuition, perception, devotion, higher awareness
7. **Crown**—violet; cosmic consciousness, god-realization[1]

Polarity Therapy focuses on the five elements taught in Āyurveda. The writings of Dr. Randolph Stone (1890–1981; born Rudolf Bautsch), founder of Polarity Therapy, demonstrate his familiarity with the chakras associated with these elements.[2] Yet, as late as 1976, the two upper chakras were not being used by therapists trained in this system.[3] Seidman not only added these chakras to his teaching and healing methods but also provided an early published example of a technique for chakra balancing, a core practice in many forms of alternative healing.[4]

Despite its developing hegemony, Dychtwald's list was not without competitors. In 1985, the California-based freelance writer, radio show host, and book review editor of *Yoga Journal*, Dio Urmilla Neff (b. 1946), published an article whose title perfectly expressed the evolutionary status of the Western chakra system in the 1980s: "The Great Chakra Controversy."[5] Her questions and answers included the following:

- *How many chakras are there?* (anywhere between three, according to the Russian mystic Gurdjieff, and twenty-three, according to the Taoist spiritual teacher Mantak Chia)[6]
- *Where are they located?* (especially the third chakra, said to be in the area of the navel in the East and the solar plexus in the West)
- *What about the spleen chakra of the Theosophists?* (easily dismissed as the result of Victorian prudery over the genital chakra)
- *How are they perceived?* (by yogis, clairvoyants, channels, and open-minded physicians and scientists using unusual testing devices, from crystal pendulums to electrical sensors)
- *What do they look like?* (glowing vortices of energy with waves corresponding to the petals described in ancient texts—as Leadbeater perceived them, though Neff's source is Arthur Powell)
- *What does the diversity of opinions on such matters mean?* (possibly a sign of the evolutionary level of the observer or of the person or society under observation)[7]

Neff did not deal with the chakra colors. Yet, in mock despair, she noted:

> The functions commonly ascribed to the root and second chakras have often been transposed, along with the glands said to be associated with those chakras!
> Why all this mystifying disagreement? Why doesn't everyone's "chakra map" agree?[8]

Perhaps the most startling aspect of the article is that Neff supplied a sidebar listing "Functions of the Major Chakras (Traditional)." Once again the law of conservation of confusion struck: Neff provided a navel/solar-plexus chakra *and* a spleen chakra, placed the heart chakra in the position of the throat chakra, and omitted the throat chakra—while giving the usual heart chakra functions to the spleen and the throat chakra functions to the heart. I assumed this was a misprint—the spleen should have been the heart and the heart the throat—until I noticed that Neff included the transpersonal point mentioned in chapter 4 of this book in connection with the system published by Brugh Joy in *Joy's Way*. This system includes a navel and spleen chakra, passes over the heart chakra in favor of a chakra between the shoulder blades in the back of the body (not indicated by Neff), and adds the transpersonal point.

A corrected list of these "traditional" chakra qualities follows. Note the new factor—the negative emotions resulting from blockage in each chakra:

1. **Root**—physical survival, emotional and physical safety versus fear of death, fear of abandonment
2. **Genital** (simply called second here)—sexual energy; lovemaking versus jealousy, perversion
3. **Solar plexus**—social identity, confidence, personal/transpersonal power versus dominance, submission, fear
4. **Heart**—energy, compassion, connectedness to other beings versus hatred, heartlessness, sense of isolation
5. **Throat**—love [probably should be shifted to heart], self-expression, verbal communication versus blocked self-expression, inability to communicate
6. **Brow**—intuition, clairvoyance, ability to meditate versus absence of intuitive perception, inability to meditate
7. **Crown**—spiritual illumination versus unenlightened state[9]

The basis of this list of chakra qualities (after removal from association with the *Joy's Way* chakra locations) is the merging of Ramakrishna (lower three chakras) and Aurobindo (upper four chakras) that developed at Esalen ten to fifteen years earlier. Yet this list—along with the *Joy's Way* locations, published just six years earlier—is now called traditional! Neff's source amnesia is the result of either unintentional vagueness or broken transmission.

Wheels, Colors, and Crystals (Anodea Judith and Joy Gardner)

Clearly, it was time to bring order into chaos. And that is just what Anodea Judith (b. 1952) did with her 1987 *Wheels of Life*—the first formal codification of the Western chakra system, including names, locations, endocrine glands, rainbow colors, and the Esalen-originated chakra functions—and many other correspondences about which there is less agreement in writings of subsequent authors, including with foods, gemstones, incense, metals, planets, and sephiroth.[10]

The synthesizing tendency demonstrated in *Wheels of Life* was in the air. A year later, a competing book, *Color and Crystals: A Journey through the Chakras*, was published by holistic healer Joy Gardner (b. 1944).[11] Once again, we see the now familiar Western chakra system names, locations, endocrine gland associations, rainbow colors, and chakra functions—though the functions are greatly expanded to include information on balanced, excessive, and deficient energy expressed in each chakra. Again, there is a variable list of correspondences, primarily focused on gemstones and "tarot archetypes."

These books set the tone for many publications by later writers on the chakras, with *Wheels of Life* as a manual of self-development and spiritual awakening using the chakras and *Color and Crystals* as a manual of healing of self and others through balancing the chakras. Both books are experiential as well as interpretive in their assembly of preexisting information on the chakras and organization of that information in revealing new ways, so their authors may be considered as validating consolidators.

Chakra Science (Hiroshi Motoyama and Others)

The synthesizing tendency of the 1980s was strong in other countries. I have already mentioned Satyananda Saraswati's *Kundalini Tantra* (1981) as a synthesis of traditional lore on the Eastern chakra system and Theosophical ideas. The book also included a program of yoga-based exercises for developing the chakras and scientific data corroborating their existence provided by a Japanese student of Satyananda, Hiroshi Motoyama (b. 1925), who invented a device to measure electrical charges released in the areas of the physical body that correspond to the locations of the chakras and acupuncture points in the subtle body.

Motoyama produced numerous publications in the 1970s dealing with his research, which laid the foundation for subsequent books linking the South Asian nadis and chakras with Southeast Asian acupuncture meridians and points. He also published *Theories of the Chakras: Bridge to Higher Consciousness* (1981), which accompanied his scientific data with comparisons of ancient and contemporary views on the chakras, including selections from the Yoga Upanishads, *Ṣaṭ-Cakra-Nirūpaṇa*, Leadbeater's *The Chakras*, and Satyananda's teachings. Motoyama included a chakra-by-chakra account of his own kundalini awakening—a rare personal testimony by someone equally familiar with Eastern and Western chakra systems and skilled in personal observation of advanced states of consciousness and in designing scientific tests for objective validation.

Satyananda's chakra system is experiential. If we accept his status as a realized spiritual master, then his approach is that of a consolidating validator, despite the lack of personal testimony in *Kundalini Tantra*. Motoyama's purpose in writing his book was in part to disseminate Satyananda's system. Therefore, he might be classed as a disseminating validator.

Motoyama was one of several researchers during the 1960s and 1970s who were actively engaged in scientific study of the chakras.

Others included David Tansley and Valerie Hunt (both discussed later); and Shafica Karagulla (1914–86), a Turkish-American psychiatrist who worked with Dutch-American Theosophical clairvoyant Dora van Gelder Kunz (1904–99) to determine the usefulness of clairvoyant perception of the chakras as a diagnostic tool for physical and mental illness. As a young girl, Kunz had been trained by Leadbeater to develop her natural clairvoyant gifts, so it is no surprise that she used and expanded on the system he developed in *The Chakras*. Karagulla first wrote about Kunz in *Breakthrough to Creativity: Your Higher Sense Perception* (1967), in which she was called Diane and DVG. Karagulla and Kunz co-authored *The Chakras and the Human Energy Fields* (1989), one of the last serious treatments of Leadbeater's system in Western chakra literature. Kunz would be classified as a clairvoyant validator.[12]

German Developments (Klausbernd Vollmar and Others)

In Germany, the 1980s laid the foundation for a literature on the chakras and alternative healing that is rivaled only by that in the United States. After the 1927 German translation of Leadbeater's *The Chakras*, the pioneering publication, based on *The Serpent Power*, was by Werner Bohm (1896–1959): *Chakras: Lebenskräfte und Bewußtseinszentren im Menschen* (Chakras: Life-power and consciousness centers in man, 1953).[13] This book was continually in print (under various titles and in several languages, including English) for the next forty years.

The first native synthesis was apparently by Klausbernd Vollmar (b. 1946), *Fahrplan durch die Chakren* (1985; English translation, *Journey through the Chakras: Exercises for Healing and Internal Balancing*, 1987). The book provides a version of the Western chakra system that is not yet fully informed by the Ramakrishna/Aurobindo/Esalen chakra qualities. However, it uses the familiar names, locations, endocrine gland associations (derived from Bailey), and colors, combined with Eastern chakra lore such as the Sanskrit names, seed syllable mantras, and elements. It also absorbs information from Rendel's *Introduction to the Chakras,* including for the first time in tabular form, the association Rendel made between chakras and the four temperaments of medieval medicine (phlegmatic, choleric, sanguine, melancholic).[14]

There are also correspondences to astrological signs and planets; tarot cards; and Bach flower remedies, a form of homeopathic healing popular in Europe, based on herbal essences. The correlation with the twenty-two major arcana of the tarot (minus the Fool) is unique in that it associates seven cards each with the three major kundalini channels, ida, pingala, and sushumna. The book focuses both on self-redevelopment and healing. Here is the list of chakra qualities (note service in the heart—an indication of Bailey's influence):

1. **Base**—release, grounding, overcoming suffering (phlegmatic)
2. **Sacral**—surrender, release of what cannot be digested (choleric)
3. **Navel**—mastery of desire, power, ambition (sanguine)
4. **Heart**—service, overcoming distance, hatred, restlessness (melancholic)
5. **Throat**—real communication, integration, peace (awake)
6. **Third Eye**—intuition, overcoming nihilism (enlightened)
7. **Crown**—unification of the higher and lower self (Master)[15]

Vollmar was living and working at the Findhorn Community in Scotland during the writing of the book and may have pioneered his version of the chakra system in workshops in England.[16] The Findhorn Community, famous as a self-sustaining New Age center developed from the inner guidance of its followers (including information on how to grow abundant food in apparently barren local soil), had been placed on the map of American spiritual seekers by William Irwin Thompson in *Passages about Earth* (1973). Thompson was also familiar with Esalen Institute and established his own intentional community, Lindisfarne, on Long Island, as a fusion of the ideals represented by Esalen and Findhorn.[17]

Further research will likely locate the Findhorn Community as a major nexus of transmission of New Age ideas between America and Europe—moving in both directions. For example, German Reiki healer Bodo Baginski (1952–2012) spent time at Findhorn before publishing *Reiki—Universale Lebensenergie* (1985; English translation, *Reiki: Universal Life Energy*, 1988), the first book to link the chakra system with a mode of energy healing pioneered in 1922 by Mikao Usui (1865–1926), a Japanese Buddhist.[18] This was a remarkable and controversial innovation by Baginski and his coauthor and partner, Shalila Sharamon (b. 1948).[19] The transmission of Reiki teachings from Usui through his students and from Japan to the West did not include any reference to the chakras. Reiki purists deny there is such a connection. However, since the mid-1990s, many books on the chakras and Reiki have so popularized connections between the teachings and practices of each that such connections are well on their way to becoming "traditional."

Baginski and Sharamon's version of the Western chakra system includes the familiar names, locations, and endocrine gland associations (based on Bailey) but not the colors. The chakra qualities are identical to those of the Ramakrishna/Aurobindo/Esalen list, demonstrating that by 1985 this list had been transmitted to Europe.[20]

Bohm was a disseminator of the *Eastern* chakra system, explicating *The Serpent Power* in German, as Evola had done in Italian and Guénon in French. Vollmar produced an experiential system based on the consolidation of material from many sources. Hence I would describe him as a consolidating validator. Baginski and Sharamon were innovators, since Reiki and the chakras had never before been brought together. Their experiential system was formative for the many later books on this hybrid form of energy healing. Perhaps they could best be classed as innovating validators.

Bailey Revisited
(David Tansley and Zachary Lansdowne)

Another 1980s trend was the attempt to consolidate and codify Bailey's teachings on the chakras, especially for healers. This trend culminated in the publication in the United Kingdom of *The Raiment of Light: A Study of the Human Aura* by David V. Tansley (1984) and in the United States of *The Chakras and Esoteric Healing* by Zachary F. Lansdowne (1986).

David V. Tansley (1934–88) had pioneered research into the Bailey system by means of radionics, "a method of diagnosis and therapy which is primarily concerned with the utilization of subtle force fields and energies, for the purpose of investigating and combating the causes of disease[s] which ravage humanity and the other kingdoms of nature."[21] Radionics was a form of what is now called vibrational or energy medicine and sought to develop and scientifically validate means of absent healing (patient not present) or distance healing (patient miles away from practitioner). Tansley's first publication was *Radionics and the Subtle Anatomy of Man* (1972). Tansley wrote several further, highly technical books on the subject. *The Raiment of Light* provides an excellent introduction to such work for the lay reader, including information on the development of radionics.

Zachary Lansdowne (b. 1944), trained as an engineer and psychologist and at one time active in the Theosophical Society in Boston, produced what for many years was perhaps the most concise manual of chakra healing based on Bailey's teachings.[22] It digested Tansley's work and provided useful comparisons of the ways several authors on the chakras besides Bailey positioned the endocrine glands. He even drew on scientific research by a student of Christopher Hills (Victor Beasley, *Subtle-Body Healing*, 1979).

Readers familiar with the Western chakra system will find no references to colors or the Esalen chakra qualities in Lansdowne's book—only the names, locations, and gland affiliations. It seems that later authors have often mined Bailey's work for qualities to associate with the chakras, simply adding words they found relevant to the Esalen-based list of survival, sexuality, power, love, communication, illumination, and enlightenment (for example, linking *creativity* to the description of the throat chakra). Thus Lansdowne's book could be called a more refined development of an evolutionary offshoot from an earlier stage of the development of the Western system.

Tansley would be a consolidating validator, using scientific instruments rather than inner-sense experience. Lansdowne would be a consolidating disseminator.

Pranic Healing (Choa Kok Sui)

Master Choa Kok Sui (1952–2007) was born in the Philippines to a Chinese family of business people. His father was Christian (Protestant) and his mother Buddhist. He attended Roman Catholic schools, got a college degree in chemical engineering, and established his own business. From the age of twelve, he read voraciously in all areas of mysticism and the occult, developing his own clairvoyant abilities in his twenties. The system of pranic healing he pioneered was a masterly synthesis of what he read, building on Theosophical teachings on subtle bodies, planes, and chakras from Arthur Powell and Alice Bailey. He claimed to have verified Leadbeater's clairvoyant observations of the chakras through work with clairvoyants he called Mang Mike and Mang Nenet. Aspects of acupuncture and chi kung were also incorporated into pranic healing. Some aspects of the system were channeled from an inner teacher to whom Sui refers as Lord Mahaguru Mei Ling, identified with past incarnations as the god-man Rama of Hindu mythology and the legendary founder of Tibetan Buddhism, Padmasambhava.[23]

The system debuted in a book published in 1987, *The Ancient Science and Art of Pranic Healing* (first released in the United States in 1990 as *Pranic Healing*). Translated into more than thirty languages, the book initiated an international movement that continues to grow and develop after Sui's premature death.[24] The Pranic Healing chakra system includes twelve chakras, as follows:[25]

1. **Basic**—usual first chakra, located at the base of the spine
2. **Sex**—usual second chakra, located in the area of the genitals
3. *Meng mein*—Chinese for "gate of life," located at the back of the navel[26]
4. **Navel**—alternative name and location for the third chakra
5. **Solar plexus**—alternative name and location for the third chakra
6. **Spleen**—Leadbeater's third chakra
7. **Heart**—usual fourth chakra
8. **Throat**—usual fifth chakra
9. **Ajna**—Tantric name for the sixth chakra, but located in the center of the head
10. **Forehead**—usual location of the sixth (brow) chakra
11. **Crown**—usual name for the seventh chakra, located at the crown of the head
12. **Soul star**—alternative location for the seventh chakra, located above the head[27]

Thus Sui resolved the great chakra controversy by absorbing the puzzling variations in earlier systems. Now there is a sex chakra *and* a spleen chakra, thus reconciling Leadbeater, the *Ṣaṭ-Cakra-Nirūpaṇa*, and the system that emerged at Esalen. Now there is a solar-plexus chakra *and* a navel chakra, as in Brugh Joy's system, thus uniting the many Western systems that used either one or the other. The heart chakra, omitted from Joy's system, has been restored. In some Eastern writings, it was unclear whether there was a sixth chakra in the center of the head or at the brow—Sui's system has both. Similarly, it was unclear whether the seventh chakra was at the crown or above the head. Not only does Sui's system have a chakra in both locations, but also it has appropriated and renamed the transpersonal point described by Joy.

Aside from syncretism, the primary innovation here is the addition of the meng mein chakra, not present in any Eastern or Western system, ancient or modern. One wonders whether it was a minor chakra (Sui notes that it "is only 1/3 to 1/2 the size of the other major chakras"²⁸) that was added to make up the mystical number twelve. In connection with the twelfth chakra, Sui cites two verses from Revelation in which a city with twelve gates and a tree with twelve fruits are mentioned (Rev. 21:12; 22:2).²⁹

Another innovation is that the spleen, solar plexus, and heart chakras present themselves in two forms, one at the front, the other at the back of the body. The meng mein shows only at the back and the basic chakra also appears at the back, as in Leadbeater's *The Chakras*. Thus there are seven front chakras, five back chakras, one chakra in the center of the head, one at the crown, and one above the head.³⁰

As noted, the first appearance of a clairvoyantly perceived chakra opening at the back of the body occurred in Leadbeater's *The Chakras*. Two years later, another "back chakra" was noted in Geoffrey Hodson's *The Science of Seership*—identified with the spleen. (See figure 24.)

The awareness of back chakras seems to have receded into the background for the next fifty years, until Joy noted a chakra between the shoulder blades that opened toward the back of the body in 1979—instead of a heart chakra at the front of the body.³¹ Besides Sui, two other authors from the mid-1980s, John Pierrakos and Barbara Brennan (discussed in the next chapter), perceived front and back manifestations of five chakras—sexual, solar plexus, heart, throat, and brow.

Though Sui assigns colors to each chakra, they are blends of multiple colors rather than the single colors of the Western system. There is no prismatic order. Rather, the colors are based on the movements of prana, identified in terms of the six colors that make up so-called white prana (the prism colors minus indigo). Leadbeater identified and illustrated five colors of prana in *The Chakras*—orange-red, rose, green, yellow, and blue-violet. *Pranic Healing* splits the orange-red and blue-violet pranas into two pranas each and omits Leadbeater's rose-colored prana.³²

Sui's color illustrations of the chakras as clairvoyantly perceived are based on Leadbeater's, but show more detail. They could

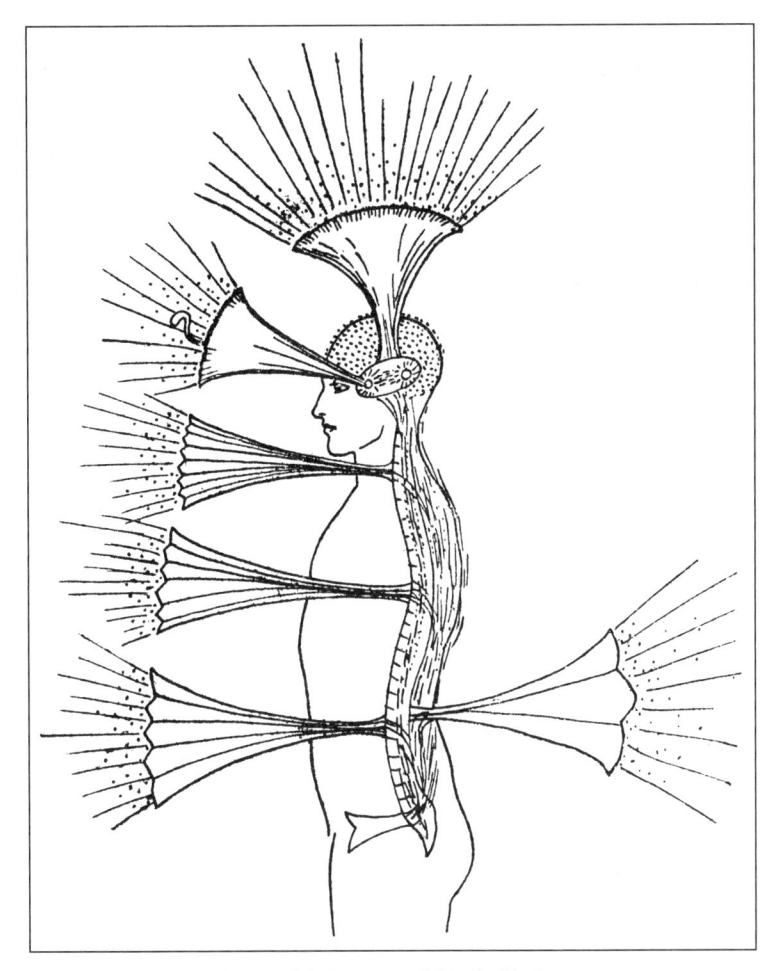

Figure 24. Front and Back Chakras
(reprinted from Geoffrey Hodson, *The Science of Seership*, 1929)

be said to be more refined or subtle—perhaps more three-dimensional (or multidimensional). Also, there are five more of them.

There are no chakra qualities in the Pranic Healing system. The chakras are considered only with respect to the health or disease of the parts of the body they are said to sustain. Thus Pranic Healing is not a system of self-development or spiritual awakening, except to the extent that it provides instruction in how to develop the clairvoyant abilities necessary to be an effective healer.

It teaches techniques of directing the flow of prana through the chakras to promote healing, providing explicit protocols of chakras, colors, meditations, and gestures for hundreds of physical and mental health problems. However, Pranic Healing is closely associated with techniques of self-development and spiritual awakening originated by Sui, which he called Arhatic Yoga. *Arhat* is a Sanskrit word for "Adept," primarily used in Buddhism.

Further description of Pranic Healing or Arhatic Yoga would go beyond the purposes of this book.[33] Suffice it to say that both systems indicate that the United States is not the only country in which innovative teachings on the chakras have been developed and exported throughout the world. If the Western chakra system described in the present book was a result of mining, reinterpreting, and synthesizing Eastern teachings on the chakras with Western esotericism, then Pranic Healing and Arhatic Yoga seem to return the favor. In Sui's work, Western teachings have been similarly plumbed, reinterpreted, and synthesized, but with reference to Eastern teachings, such as acupuncture and chi kung. Sui would be an example of an innovative, consolidating validator.

Going Within (Shirley MacLaine)

In 1984, actress Shirley MacLaine (b. 1934) published a bestselling memoir, *Out on a Limb*, detailing her exploration of reincarnation, channeling, and other spiritual and New Age approaches to life. By 1987, she was teaching workshops on the chakras and had designed a line of chakra-based jewelry, using gemstones keyed to the rainbow color system. In 1989, she released a self-help book based on the chakra workshops, *Going Within: A Guide for Inner Transformation*.[34] Here is MacLaine's lineup of the chakras:

1. **Base**—red; adrenals; grounding, survival, our "understanding of the physical dimension"
2. **Sexual**—orange; ovaries, testes; our "creative attitudes on relationships, sex, and reproduction"

3. **Solar plexus**—yellow; pancreas, spleen; "clearinghouse for emotional sensitivities and issues of personal power," "emotional integration"
4. **Heart**—green; thymus; love, "acceptance of others, and acceptance of the love within self"
5. **Throat**—blue; thyroid; "individual self-expression *without* judgment" [original emphasis]
6. **Third Eye**—indigo; pituitary; "idealism and imagination," "inner vision" and "outer expression of that inner vision"
7. **Crown**—"*violet* or sometimes *white*" [original emphasis]; pineal; "unlimited consciousness and Divine purpose" eventually reaching "the feeling of integration with God"[35]

The endocrine gland associations come from Bailey. Later in her discussion of the chakras, MacLaine also references links between the chakras and seven-year cycles of development—another notion derived from Bailey.[36]

We saw that Ella Adelia Fletcher linked white to the highest of Blavatsky's seven principles, atman; and that the Western chakra system developed from the matrix of these principles, which would link white to the seventh chakra. Nevertheless, most Western systems adopt the seven colors into which so-called white light is refracted by a prism as they were presented by Sir Isaac Newton in 1671. Newton divided the continuum of light from red to violet into seven segments to bring it into accord with the seven astrological planets, the days of the week, and so on. Later scientists determined there were only six primary and secondary colors (no indigo).[37] Thus, if all colors derive from white light, then the colors of the six lower chakras (with the sixth being violet) must blend into the white light of the seventh chakra. Yet, as rational as this set of associations seems, it remains a minority opinion within writings on the Western system.

In a sense, MacLaine's version of the chakra system resolves the great chakra controversy—it is a concise expression of all the elements of the Western chakra system with a minimum of occult

Table 23
The Western Chakra System (ca. 1990)

Numbers	Names	Locations[39]	Glands[40]	Colors	Qualities[41]
Seventh	Crown	Anterior fontanel	Pineal or pituitary	Violet/White	Enlightenment Cosmic consciousness
Sixth	Brow / Third Eye	Cavernous plexus	Pituitary or pineal	Indigo/Violet	Intuition Imagination
Fifth	Throat	Laryngeal or pharyngeal plexus	Thyroid	Blue	Communication Creativity
Fourth	Heart	Cardiac plexus	Thymus	Green	Love Compassion
Third	Solar plexus / Navel	Solar plexus	Pancreas Spleen	Yellow	Will Power
Second	Genital/ Sacral	Prostatic or vaginal plexus	Gonads Adrenals	Orange	Sexuality Sensuality
First	Root	Sacral plexus	Adrenals Gonads	Red	Survival Grounding

correspondences, designed for self-development and reversing the assignment of the pineal gland to the sixth chakra and the pituitary to the seventh in Judith's *Wheels of Life*. MacLaine's association becomes standard in later books on the chakras and Judith's choice remains contoversial. (Interestingly, Gardner assigned the pituitary and the pineal glands *both* to the sixth and the seventh chakras—a resolution of this issue that, as noted, goes back to Hodson's *The Science of Seership*.[38])

On October 4, 1990, Shirley MacLaine appeared on *The Tonight Show*, seen by millions of TV viewers in America. While being interviewed by the skeptical show host, Johnny Carson, MacLaine affixed Velcro-backed rainbow-colored circles representing the chakras to Johnny Carson's clothing and head while he complained about looking like Bozo the Clown.[42] Just as I assign the birth of the Western chakra system to June 1977, I see the date of MacLaine's TV appearance as the moment when the system went mainstream, despite—or perhaps because of—Carson's razzing and MacLaine's good-humored backchat.

MacLaine was a disseminating validator. The result of her TV appearance was an explosion of books on the chakras in English, published in the United States and translated throughout the world, as well as books written and published in other Western countries.

Tracing these developments—especially the hybridization of the Western chakra system with alternative healing modalities, such as acupuncture, massage, shamanism, and others—lies beyond the scope of this book. Though we have pursued the evolution of the Western chakra system from the times of Madame Blavatsky to those of Shirley MacLaine—the results are shown in table 23—there is one further component to discuss—an esoteric subtext that has surfaced from time to time in these pages and that possibly represents the final stage in this evolution.

Chapter 25
The Multidimensional Rainbow Body

We have seen how the names, locations with reference to nerve ganglia, associations with endocrine glands, colors, and chakra qualities were added in stages as the notion of the chakras moved from East to West. We have seen how the chakra qualities were derived from the influence of Eastern yogis Ramakrishna and Aurobindo on Western psychologists and scholars. The list of qualities that came out of Esalen was a continuum of human potential, ranging from physical and emotional to mental and spiritual. For most teachers, students, writers, readers, and users of the chakras, the psychological approach of the human potential movement would suffice as a map for self-development and healing of self and others.

But there was also an esoteric dimension, corresponding to the original Eastern approach to the chakras, not as a continuum of human potential, but as a map of discrete states of consciousness or worlds, realms, or planes. As noted, Hindu scriptures listed seven such planes, from *bhu-loka* (the earthly world or physical plane) to *satya-loka* (the enlightened or liberated plane of highest truth). The most developed form of the link between chakras and realms occurred in the Radhasoami tradition in India. This link was carried over into Theosophical traditions by Blavatsky, principally in her Esoteric Instructions, which linked principles and planes of consciousness to the aura and implied connections to the chakras without making such connections explicit.

Working from hints and clues in Blavatsky's writings after her death, Besant developed a set of terms and definitions for bodies and planes, based on the seven principles. Each body existed first as an undeveloped sheath (kosha), then as a partially developed body, able to perceive on a particular plane, and finally as a fully developed vehicle of consciousness, able to move freely on that plane.[1] Leadbeater pursued the clairvoyant investigation of the relationships between auras, bodies, and planes. However, he did not make a direct link between a particular chakra, body, and plane. He assumed that each body had a chakra system and listed the functions of the chakras, or centers, in the etheric and astral bodies. These lists are so alike that a case could be made that similar functions could be found in the chakra systems of the higher subtle bodies.[2]

Based on Bailey's *Initiation: Human and Solar*, Vera Stanley Alder linked the chakras to planes and subplanes and to major and minor initiations (expansions of consciousness). The mastery of each chakra in a particular body is a minor initiation. When these have all been mastered, a major initiation occurs, transferring the locus of learning and growth to the next-higher plane and body.[3] This framework goes a step beyond Leadbeater, implying that the chakra functions he outlined for the etheric and astral bodies are actually a roadmap for mastering those bodies center by center, subplane by subplane—and that such a roadmap duplicates itself in each higher body.

Since Alder's book came out in 1939, various correspondences between chakras, layers of the aura, bodies, and planes have emerged from time to time—though rarely. For instance, in Osho's *In Search of the Miraculous*, comprising lectures given in India in 1970 (when he was known as Bhagwan Shree Rajneesh), several lectures dealt with the connection between chakras and bodies. Further, this material was linked with information on how the bodies develop in seven-year cycles and may be correlated with evolutionary stages of human culture. The details need not detain us—they originate in Bailey, though with the names of the bodies somewhat altered. Suffice it to say that this was a case of source amnesia. The important point is that in Osho's description, each chakra was associated with one body. There was no indication that the bodies are present in layers of the aura or that the bodies each have their own chakra system.[4]

In America, the link between chakras and layers of the aura

resurfaced in the 1980s in *Opening Up to Your Psychic Self* (1982) by Petey Stevens, a founder of Heartsong Center for Expanded Perception in the San Francisco Bay area in 1976. Stevens also expanded the number of chakras to twelve.

The most advanced correlation I have seen between chakras, aura layers, bodies, and planes, occurs in the writings of Barbara Ann Brennan (b. 1939). I would argue that her correlations represent the final stage in the evolution of the Western chakra system—a codification of its esoteric dimension. However, there are problems with her nomenclature. A revision restoring the original Theosophical terms for the bodies and planes may be in order, thus bringing the development of the Western chakra system full circle, back to its roots in the East/West transfer that occurred under the auspices of the Theosophical Society in India, beginning in 1880.

Hands versus Wheels (Brennan and Bruyere)

If the psychological approach to the chakra system that developed at Esalen had its roots in Jung's kundalini yoga seminars, as transmitted by Heinrich Zimmer to Joseph Campbell and by Frederic Spiegelberg to Michael Murphy, the lineage that produced Barbara Brennan's version originated, surprisingly, with Freud. This line of transmission passed from Reich, a student of Freud, to Alexander Lowen and John Pierrakos, originators of Bioenergetics, to Brennan, who worked with Pierrakos after he split from Lowen to develop Core Energetics.

The depth of this influence may be perceived by the similarity of material discussed in Pierrakos's *Core Energetics: Developing the Capacity to Love and Heal* (first published in Germany in 1986) and Brennan's *Hands of Light* (self-published in 1987, commercially published in 1988). Both books deal with Freudian/Reichian character types (oral, masochistic, schizoid, psychopathic/aggressive, and rigid), as perceived clairvoyantly in terms of the aura and chakras.[5] Both books also posit the existence of front and back expressions of the chakras, as does Choa Kok Sui in *Pranic Heal-*

ing. Brennan's system represents the most developed formulation of this idea.[6] It is probable that Sui and Pierrakos arrived at their conclusions independently; Brennan built on Pierrakos's work.

But Brennan's book is more than a popularizing restatement of *Core Energetics*. Other currents that inform *Hands of Light* derive from Brennan's natural clairvoyance, which she first experienced as a child and later developed at the Phoenicia Pathwork Center in Phoenicia, New York, under the guidance of channel Eva Pierrakos, John's wife; and Brennan's training as a scientist (degrees in "upper atmospheric physics") and "six years at NASA's Goddard Space Flight Center" in the 1960s.[7]

A third current originated within the teachings of clairvoyant Rosalyn Bruyere (b. 1946), author of *Wheels of Light: A Study of the Chakras* (self-published, 1989; commercially published, 1994).[8] In the 1970s, Bruyere was asked to participate in a scientific study by UCLA psychologist Valerie Hunt (1916–2014). The purpose of the study was to investigate the energetic effect of Rolfing on the chakras, as perceived by a clairvoyant (Bruyere), and by scientific instruments designed to gather information on fluctuations of electrical charges in the skin in the areas where the chakras were located. Readings were taken before, during, and after the Rolfing process in the ten-session sequence specified by Rolf in her program of Structural Integration.[9]

Bruyere developed her own vision of the chakra system, which is at odds, on several counts, with the Western system as presented here. The colors are red through violet in the first six chakras, with white in the seventh (and no indigo). The pineal is in the sixth position and the pituitary in the seventh. The second chakra is associated with Peyer's patches (in the ileum of the small intestine) or the lymphatic system. The elements appear in an order at variance with all other Eastern and Western systems. To make matters more confusing, the chakras are identified in terms of planes, the names of which are also at variance with earlier teachings.[10] Table 24 compares Bruyere's system with Eastern and Theosophical ideas—not to make correlations, but to demonstrate inconsistencies.

Table 24
Chakras according to Rosalyn Bruyere (1988)

Chakras	Colors	Elements in Bruyere	Elements in Eastern System	Planes in Bruyere	Planes in Theosophy
Seventh	White	Magnetum[11]	...	Ketheric	Divine
Sixth	Violet	Radium	Mind	Celestial	Monadic
Fifth	Blue	Ether	Ether	Etheric	Nirvanic
Fourth	Green	Earth	Air	Astral	Buddhic
Third	Yellow	Air	Fire	Mental	Mental
Second	Orange	Water	Water	Emotional	Astral/emotional
First	Red	Fire	Earth	Physical	Physical/etheric

Bruyere grafted aspects of Native American mythology onto the chakra system, which explains the order of the first four elements, derived from Hopi teachings. The variations in names of the planes are more difficult to fathom—with the exception of ketheric, which is derived from Kether, the crown sephirah in Kabbalah.[12]

Bruyere made an interesting and useful contribution by linking relationships to the chakras. We connect to parents and grandparents through the root chakra (they are our roots). We connect to children and spouses through the emotional aspect of the second chakra. In the third chakra, associated with mind, we experience friends, classmates, intellectuals, and politicians. In the fourth or heart chakra, we connect to "heart-chakra teachers" such as Jesus, Yogananda, and Mother Teresa. In the fifth chakra, we encounter religious leaders and divine rulers, such as the Pope, the Dalai Lama, the Karmapa (another high Tibetan lama). In the sixth chakra, we encounter spirit teachers and spiritual friends; and in the seventh, prophets, gurus, and saints.[13]

It appears that Bruyere's version of the chakras is discontinuous. Like the Eastern system (and unlike the Western), it is not a progressive evolutionary continuum. Each chakra represents a distinct state of consciousness and the chakras are not stacked on top of one another in a progressive way. Thus the function of each chakra in Bruyere's system is determined on the basis of what could be called horizontal rather than vertical associations. Hence, in Bruyere's system, the heart chakra refers to heart-based spiritual teachings. But is the Pope, Christ's representative on earth (fifth chakra), higher and more evolved than Jesus, the son of God (fourth chakra)? Would Mother Teresa be flattered to discover that her evolutionary spiritual status was equal to that of Jesus (both accessed through the fourth chakra)?

A progressive or evolutionary (vertical) reading of the chakras would stipulate that the beings associated with the fifth chakra were more evolved than those associated with the fourth and that those associated with the fourth would be of equal development with one another. A horizontal reading does not require such progression. We reach the beings of each level by contacting them through a chakra quality that expresses the nature or our relationship to them and what we can learn from them, not who or what they are in evolutionary terms.

Bruyere is a validating innovator, in the sense that she built up her own chakra system on the basis of personal investigation and validated it later through discovering resonances with other spiritual teachings. Thus her system is both formative and (in her popular workshops) experiential. It has the same downside we saw in the formative systems of Blavatsky and Bailey—it is messy and chaotic, in need of a consolidator. Brennan played that role for Bruyere in *Hands of Light*.

I would classify Brennan as an innovative, consolidating validator. Her system was built up by validating the observations of others with her own, then consolidating these observations by means of her own intuition, resulting in an innovative synthesis. Based on personal testimony and passed on to readers and students, Brennan's system is also experiential. Furthermore, she scrupulously noted and thanked her sources. Though Brennan borrowed Bruyere's terms (and acknowledged the debt), she synthesized this information with material from other sources, such as Jack Schwarz's *Human Energy Systems* (1980; the book that followed *Voluntary Controls*).[14]

Hands of Light uses the familiar names and locations for the chakras. The chakra colors are the same as Bruyere's. It lists the endocrine gland associations from Bailey's *Esoteric Healing* (cited in the bibliography), with the pituitary in the sixth and the pineal in the seventh positions.[15] However, Brennan's list of chakra qualities diverges significantly from that of the Western system as portrayed in the present book. These qualities are in some respects closer to those of the bodies and planes described by Besant than the latter are to Bruyere's terminology.[16] I have added speculations on how Brennan's terms might correspond with Theosophical terms in brackets:[17]

1. **Base** (root)—"physical functioning and physical sensation—feeling physical pain or pleasure" [physical/etheric body and physical plane]
2. **Sacral** (genital)—"emotional life and feelings" [astral/emotional body and astral plane]
3. **Solar plexus**—"mental life," "linear thinking" [mental body and lower mental plane]
4. **Heart**—love of "not only our mates, but also humanity in general" [astral body (love of mate); buddhic body (love of humanity) and buddhic plane]
5. **Throat**—"a higher will more connected to the divine will," "power of the word," "speaking things into being, listening and taking responsibility for our actions" [atmic or nirvanic body and plane—where atmic derives from atma or atman, often referred to in Theosophical literature as an expression of divine will]
6. **Forehead** (brow)—"celestial love" that "extends beyond the human range of love and encompasses all life" [should be the monadic body and plane, though the description fits the buddhic plane]
7. **Crown**—"higher mind, knowing and integration of our spiritual and physical makeup" [should be the divine body and plane; but the description fits the causal body and higher mental plane]

This pairing of Brennan with Besant demonstrates that there are hiccups in the steady progression of evolutionary stages from one chakra, body, and plane to the next. I might expect to see the causal body in the fourth position, following the mental body, but instead it is displaced into the seventh position. Aspects of the astral and buddhic bodies and planes are duplicated on other levels. Let us examine these correlations more closely.

Auras, Bodies, and Planes

As Brennan portrays Bruyere's system of identifying the layers of the aura, the physical plane corresponds to the first three chakras and the etheric, emotional, and mental bodies. The fourth chakra corresponds to the astral plane and body, representing a bridge between the physical and spiritual planes. Then the pattern of etheric, emotional, and mental is repeated in chakras five through seven, corresponding to the spiritual plane.[18]

In Besant, the first plane is the physical, whose higher levels are called etheric. The second plane is astral/emotional, and the third plane is mental. Just as there are two bodies on the physical plane, the physical body and the etheric body, so there are two bodies on the mental plane, the mental body and the causal body. The transition between the lower and higher bodies occurs at the midpoint of the mental plane. The *personality* is associated with the physical, astral/emotional, and mental bodies, and the *individuality*, or soul, with the causal body. Beyond the causal level of the mental plane are the buddhic plane and the nirvanic plane—the highest manifested plane in our reality/learning system. These are sometimes called the spiritual planes.[19]

At first glance, there seems to be little correlation between Brennan and Besant. However, the first three chakras and bodies in Brennan correspond to the personality in Besant—the physical/etheric, astral, and mental bodies. The astral-body turning point in Brennan is similar in function to what Blavatsky called the psychic plane, a combination of the upper astral and lower mental planes, as described by Besant.[20] On the other side of the psychic plane in Blavatsky, the spiritual planes begin—just as, in Brennan, they begin on the other side of her astral plane. While the nomenclatures differ, the functions are the same.

Brennan calls the fifth layer of the aura the etheric template (physical aspect). This layer "contains all the forms that exist on the physical plane in a blueprint or template form." She makes clear that the etheric body is not to be confused with the etheric template layer of the aura.[21] In Theosophical literature, the blueprint for a *specific* physical form, including the human body, is associated with the etheric body. The level of being in which the blueprints of *all* physical forms may be found is the causal level—the upper mental plane, home of archetypes.[22]

Brennan's celestial body, associated with the sixth chakra, reflects the emotional aspect of the spiritual plane. As indicated, Brennan correlates this layer of the aura with "a love that extends beyond the human range of love and encompasses all life." In Theosophical teachings, such love is associated with the unity consciousness of the buddhic plane.

In Brennan, the ketheric template, or causal body, is identified as the "mental aspect of the spiritual plane," where we can experience oneness "with the Creator." This layer of the aura is egg-shaped and contains all the others. What Brennan calls "past life bands" play along the surface of the egg, which also "contains the life plan" for the present incarnation.[23]

In Theosophical literature, the causal body carries that name because it contains the karmic causes for each of human lifetime. In the aura, the causal level corresponds to our access to information about these causes for the present lifetime—what could be called the soul's master plan for this life. However, access to the causal level of being (the upper mental plane), also allows us to read the akashic records, which contain the history of all our previous incarnations.[24]

Blavatsky taught that we are surrounded by an auric egg, associated with what she called the seventh principle, or atman (highest self—in a sense, our creator).[25] Besant taught that the nirvanic plane, which she also called the atmic plane, refers to the self that contains the seeds for growth to be developed in the physical, astral, mental, buddhic, and nirvanic levels of being throughout the duration of our reality/learning system. Thus it could be said that the atmic level contains the master plan for our growth, not only as humans, but also in the mineral, vegetable, and animal phases through which we passed (in Theosophical teaching) before achieving the human phase in this reality/learning system. The buddhic and nirvanic levels represent our superhuman growth. To achieve the nirvanic, or atmic, level of being means to become a Master, as far as the lower planes are concerned.[26]

The ketheric template layer of the aura described by Brennan may carry information about this higher master plan. As such, it would contain the causes for all of our subhuman, human, and superhuman lifetimes, past, present, and future. Therefore, calling this level the causal body may be justified, purely in functional terms, though it may lead to confusion for those familiar with the Theosophical system of bodies and planes, in which the term represents an individual human soul.

Brennan speaks of two further layers of the aura, associated with a "cosmic plane." Little is known about them. In Besant's teachings, there are two planes beyond the nirvanic, but they are unmanifested in our reality/learning system: the monadic and divine planes.[27] For Brennan, these layers are "crystalline in nature" and "relate to who we are beyond this lifetime."[28] It might be more correct to say they relate to who we are beyond even our superhuman lifetimes. The monadic level of being could be said to contain the divine plan for *every* aspect of our evolution, from being separated from the Source at the beginning of creation to being merged with it again at the ultimate end, perhaps after our having passed through multiple reality/learning systems. In a sense, it would represent yet another—the highest—causal body.

The table on pages 396–97 summarizes this discussion, demonstrating how Brennan's system and Besant's teachings line up. I have added a column to include my own speculations on the levels of plan implied in this material, in particular the three ever-more-expansive interpretations of the term *causal body*. Brennan's system correlates planes, aura layers, bodies, and chakras; Besant's teachings correlate planes, aura layers, and bodies, but not chakras.

Multiple Bodies and Systems

Why is Brennan's system so different from others we have considered? If we accept the notion that each subtle body has its own chakra system, then it is no stretch to realize that differences in chakra systems may reflect differences in the body being described. But most teachers, students, writers, and readers assume there is only *one* chakra system and become confused when there are differences in clairvoyant observations, terminology, and descriptions. Even the formulators of such systems may not realize they may be describing part or all of the chakra system of a particular subtle body or a hybrid of more than one. Thus Brennan's placing of the causal body at the crown of her chakra system may indicate that her system maps the chakras of the causal body, as defined in Theosophical teachings—and the lower and higher bodies and planes are perceived from that perspective.

The Western chakra system described in this book is tied to the ganglia and glands of the physical body. It has to do with healing and self-development along the lines of personal happiness. In Theosophical teachings, the etheric body is our source of life force and health. The chakras in the Western system describe what we do with that life force to heal ourselves and make us happy. Thus the Esalen-derived list of chakra qualities reflects an etheric-body chakra system.

An astral-body chakra system would deal primarily with healing ourselves as emotional beings, as well as with how we direct our emotional energy toward self and others and how we deal with that energy when directed toward us. Such things are the focus of Karla McLaren's book, *Your Aura and Your Chakras: The Owner's Manual* (1997).

I have already pointed out that the social dimension of Christopher Hills's chakra system reflects the chakras of the mental body. The chakra system I developed in *Music and the Soul: A Listener's Guide to Achieving Transcendent Musical Experiences* is also a mental-body system. The first two chakras use the mind

Table 25
Brennan's and Besant's Planes

Plane (Brennan)	Aura Layer (Brennan)	Body/Chakra (Brennan)
Cosmic II	Ninth	Crystalline Little known Who we are beyond this lifetime
Cosmic I	Eighth	Crystalline Little known Who we are beyond this lifetime
Spiritual III: Mental aspect	Seventh	Ketheric template Causal body Auric egg Higher mind
Spiritual II: Emotional aspect	Sixth	Celestial Higher love Bliss
Spiritual I: Physical aspect	Fifth	Etheric template Higher will Form blueprints
Astral (physical/spiritual transition point)	Fourth	Astral Love
Physical III: Mental aspect	Third	Mental Thoughts
Physical II: Emotional aspect	Second	Emotional Feelings
Physical I: Physical aspect	First	Physical/etheric Sensations Physical blueprint

Plane/Principle (Besant)		Body/Aura Layer (Besant)	Plan (Leland)
Divine Unmanifested (Brahman)		Divine Hypothetical	. . .
Monadic Unmanifested (Paramatman)		Monadic Hypothetical	Causal III: Our experience of all reality/learning systems between being separated from and returning to Source
Nirvanic/Atmic (Atman)	I N D I V I D U A L I T Y	Nirvanic/Spiritual Blavatsky's auric egg Mastery	Causal II: Our mineral, vegetable, animal, human & superhuman experience within this reality/learning system
Buddhic (Buddhi)		Buddhic/Intuitional Unity Bliss	. . .
Upper mental (Buddhi-manas)		Causal/Soul Abstract thoughts Ideals Archetypes	Causal I: Our soul's master plan for an individual life & our entire sequence of human lifetimes on this planet Archetypal blueprints
Form/Formless transition point			
Lower mental / Upper psychic (Kama-manas)	P E R S O N A L I T Y	Mental Concrete thoughts Ideas	. . .
Astral / Lower psychic (Kama)		Astral Feelings Emotions	. . .
Upper physical (Prana-linga)		Etheric Vitality Physical blueprint	Physical blueprints
Lower physical (Sthula)		Dense physical Actions	. . .

(Aurobindo's "thinking mind"; see page 315) to influence the physical body through trance (*rhythm*) and the sensual quality of sound (*harmony*). The third and fourth chakras use the mind to influence the emotional body, through evoking angry intensity (*volume/dissonance*) or heart-opening love (*melody*). The fifth and sixth use the mind to influence the mental body itself, through laid-back or upbeat lifestyle or socializing (*tempo*), including dance music, and expressive, clever, or fantastical flights of the imagination (*form*). In a sense, all music is derived from the sixth chakra—the composers' and performers' mental-body *command* (ajna—the Sanskrit name for the sixth chakra) to bring about a reaction in a listener. The seventh chakra, associated with expanded consciousness, represents the music of the soul—and a still higher music, portraying cosmic consciousness, is associated with an eighth chakra and achieving oneness with the divine.

After the book's publication, I realized that the seventh chakra went through seven stages, each associated with a different type of spiritual music. I had enfolded the development of the causal body into the seventh chakra! Thus I learned that when writers add chakras above and beyond the crown, they may be perceiving the chakras of the *next-higher* body. It seems that our clairvoyant perceptions sometimes organize themselves in terms of multiple aura layers, bodies, and chakras forming around a central core and sometimes as full or partial chakra systems above the crown chakra, as if the next-higher body represented the next-higher floor of a building or a hazy secondary rainbow above and beyond the primary one.

In Brennan's system, the lower and higher bodies and planes were all folded into the perspective of the causal body, hence the apparent hiccups from level to level—and the eighth and ninth layers were like a secondary rainbow, reduplicating aspects of the buddhic and nirvanic planes. In *Music and the Soul*, the focal point was on the sixth chakra as an expression of the mental body. The lower bodies were ranged beneath it, two chakras per body; whereas the entire causal body was scrunched into the crown chakra and the buddhic body was represented by a single chakra, which I called the eighth, above the head. It is probable that the four chakras beyond the crown in Petey Stevens's book were also derived from higher bodies and planes.

The distortions in Brennan's system and my own remind me of concave or convex funhouse mirrors or fisheye photographic lenses. In each, the image of a normal human body is distorted, depending on the respective positions of body and mirror or body, lens, and focal point. Thus it is no wonder that etheric, astral, mental, and causal versions of the chakra system may not be recognizable when compared. Indeed, the differences between Eastern and Western systems may be derived from a similar problem of distorted perspective. If the Western system's focus on health and lifestyle reflects the etheric body, then the Eastern system's focus on liberation through self-transcendence may be another version of a causal-body system—or even a buddhic-, nirvanic-, or monadic-body system, depending on whether the goal is liberation from the personal, human, or superhuman (god-like) perspective to achieve union with atman, paramatman, or Brahman.

Multidimensional Chakras

The ideal Western chakra system would not be distorted in such ways. It would be multidimensional. The bodies and planes would be related to one another in a developmental or evolutionary continuum. Each body would have its own set of seven chakras. Each chakra would be correlated with a subplane of that body. Clairvoyants who used such a system would be able to perceive the chakras multidimensionally. They could focus their consciousness on a particular body's chakra system or on a particular chakra as it expresses itself through all the bodies.

Hands of Light suggests some basic principles of clairvoyance that could support such a system:

- "Each auric layer has its own set of seven major chakras, each located in the same place in the physical body."

- "Each of the seven chakras has seven layers, each corresponding to a layer of the auric field."
- "These chakras appear to be nested within each other like nesting glasses."
- "Each succeeding layer interpenetrates completely all the layers under it, including the physical body." (The physical body is not counted as one of the seven layers.)
- "Each chakra on each higher layer extends out farther in the auric field . . . and is slightly broader than the one below it."[29]

Two concepts from Brennan's second book, *Light Emerging*, may also be useful in the creation of an ideal Western chakra system: *hara line* and *core star*.

Brennan defines four levels of reality, each of which is the foundational support upon which the next is built. Thus the physical-body level is supported by the human-energy-field level (aura), which is supported by the hara level (having to do with life purpose and intentions), which is supported by the core-essence (or core-star) level ("the dimension of the central love of our being").[30] Perhaps the hara and core-essence levels are higher expressions of the causal body. The aura level is represented by the auric egg of the causal body, the holder of causes for the present lifetime. The hara level might by represented by the nirvanic body, as the holder of a more expansive set of causes, for *all* our lifetimes—subhuman, human, and superhuman. The core-essence level would represent the monadic body as the holder of the most expansive set of causes—those that pertain to every level of development we pass through on our journey back to oneness with the Source. (These levels are labeled Causal I, II, and III in the Plan column of table 25.)

The hara line is a personalized refinement of the hara level. It is "a laserlike line" of energy that runs down through the center of the body from an "individuation point," located "three and a half feet above the head"; through a "soul seat," located "in the upper chest area"; "down into the tan tien [source of life force, or vitality, in Asian martial and healing arts] in the lower abdomen," about "two and one-half inches below the navel"; and thence "deep into the center of the earth's core."[31] In Theosophy, the notion of sutratman, or thread soul, is similar in function. As noted, all our lifetimes are strung like beads along this thread soul. As I understand it, the thread soul emanates from the Source and extends to the core of the earth, and the chakras and bodies form along it.

The term *hara*, like *tan tien*, was borrowed from Asian martial and healing arts, where it refers to a reservoir of life force in the abdomen, as well as one of three power points along a midline of the body (hence Brennan's hara line, which simply extends the line upward and downward from these points).[32]

The core star is "the level of our inner source, or the localized divinity within us. It is from this inner source that all creativity within arises."[33] Brennan locates this core star "one and one half inches above the navel"—at the center of the body—correlating it with "the individualized divine within you."[34]

As noted, a similar concept appears in Leadbeater's *The Masters and the Path*, the "star of consciousness," which is an expression of the monad, our highest self. According to Leadbeater, this star is mobile; we may "keep this star of consciousness" wherever we wish, "in any one of the seven principle centers of the body."[35] It is not limited to the center of the body, as is Brennan's core star. Where we place it determines our entire outlook on life, our primary state of consciousness. Ivah Bergh Whitten noted that most people keep their star of consciousness in the forehead (sixth chakra) or in the solar plexus (third chakra)—the latter very close to where Brennan locates the core star. Moving the star from one center to another, as Leadbeater hints, would produce a radical shift in how we perceive the world.

The New Astral Projection

So far I have focused on the advantages of a multidimensional chakra system for clairvoyants who work with the aura. There are also advantages for out-of-body travelers or astral projectors (provided we consider the word *astral* as a general term for any subtle body—not merely the astral body—as a vehicle of consciousness to explore other planes or dimensions of being).

Here is a comparison of chakra functions provided by Leadbeater for the etheric and astral bodies, along with my extrapolation of appropriate terms that would apply to all bodies. The words in bold italics are my one-word descriptions; the italicized words within parentheses demonstrate the relationship of my terms to the Western chakra system functions. I have swapped Leadbeater's descriptions of the second and third chakras, since he originally called the navel chakra the second center in *The Inner Life* and did not move its function when he shifted it to the third center in *The Chakras*:

1. **Root**—"awakening" of the serpent power "at the astral level" [sense of being in a new subtle body, but without being able to perceive the plane on which it operates; ***embodiment*** (related to *survival*)]
2. **Genital**—sensitivity to astral "influences, though without as yet anything like the definite comprehension that comes from seeing and hearing" [sensual awareness of presence on a plane; making contact with what exists there with inner senses, as with touch; ***sensuality*** (related to pleasure aspect of *sexuality*)]
3. **Solar plexus**—conscious travel, "though with only a vague conception" of what was encountered on these "journeys" [travel within a plane; activation of a body's will-based motive power; ***motivation*** (related to *power*)]
4. **Heart**—"the power to comprehend and sympathize with the vibrations of other astral entities" so as to "instinctively

understand some of their feelings" [compassion; understanding as a means of recognizing and identifying inhabitants of a plane; *empathy* (related to *love*)]
5. **Throat**—"the power of hearing on the astral plane" [information exchange with the inhabitants of a plane; *clairaudience* (related to *communication*)]
6. **Brow**—"astral sight—the power to perceive definitely the shape and nature of astral objects, instead of vaguely sensing their presence" [ability to correlate all inner-sense impressions of a plane into a coherent whole; synthesis; *clairvoyance* (related to *third eye*)]
7. **Crown**—rounding off and completion of "the astral life" with "perfection of its faculties" [mastery of a body and plane; transcendence of the perceptual biases operating in a body and plane in preparation for learning and growth in the next-higher body and plane; *transcendence* (related to *enlightenment* or *liberation* from that body and plane)][36]

This system can explain a multitude of problems I have seen, on Internet forums, in beginners' descriptions of their astral adventures. Issues similar to these may be encountered in each higher body and plane:

- The experience of being in the astral body but not being able to feel, move, hear, or see, indicates that only the first chakra of that body is active.
- The experience of knowing you are somewhere else without being able to perceive or move indicates that the first and second chakras are active.
- Many beginning projectors can perceive and move on the astral plane, but their journeys are lonely—they encounter no astral beings. Thus the first three chakras are active, but not the fourth.
- Some projectors get frustrated when they ask questions of an astral entity (usually as mentally voiced words) and receive

no reply or a garbled reply—their fifth chakra is not sufficiently developed.
- An unstable astral environment, constantly shifting its appearance, means the sixth chakra is not working properly.
- Wanting to visit the akashic records and perpetually being rerouted or coming up against an impenetrable boundary indicates that the seventh chakra has not been mastered; a visit to the akashic records on the upper mental plane would require the causal body when neither the astral nor the mental body has been mastered.

Chakras of the Future

Taking into consideration the speculations made in this chapter about a final stage in the evolution of the Western chakra system, my ideal system of the future would entail the following:

- Free movement between the layers of the energy field and the bodies they represent
- Clear perception of the chakras in each body, separate from the others
- Multidimensional perception of each chakra along the thread soul in terms of its expression in every energy body
- Discernment of where healing or development work might be needed in any chakra in any subtle body
- Free movement of the star of consciousness between the chakras along the thread soul to experience the radically different states of consciousness represented by each chakra, body, and plane when viewed from the perspective of our highest self, the monad
- Development of sheaths into bodies, into fully functional vehicles of consciousness on each and every plane through the activation and mastery of the chakras in that vehicle and their associated subplanes

- Continual progress through the seven minor initiations associated with the chakras of each body and the seven major initiations that form the ladder of bodies and planes until we have returned at last to oneness with the Source of all being

The goal of this consummate version of the Western chakra system would be the same as that of the Eastern system: transcendence of all obstructions to realization of god-consciousness. The methods may be different—fulfilling all possibilities of human development in order to transcend them, versus reversing the process of creation through the gradual dissolution of illusions that obscure ultimate beingness, truth, reality. Yet the tantric intention to achieve liberation within the body would be the same. Perhaps only the focus would be different—an outer focus on bodies and the planes as perceived through clairvoyance and astral travel (Western) versus an inner focus on dissolving all such veils of illusion that obscure our perception of ultimate reality and oneness with the divine, through meditation (Eastern).

Besant called the path of mastering the bodies and planes that of the occultist, and the path of dissolving them as veils of illusion the path of the mystic.[37] Each is a noble and difficult work. Probably, each exists in equal measure among Eastern and Western spiritual seekers and in a multitude of equally valid methods. Even the watered-down version of the chakra system presented in so many Western books on self-help and increase of happiness through fulfillment by lifestyle, has its place—as an expression of the etheric-body stage of the ladder that ascends to oneness with Source.

Which brings me back to the Aura Cacia Aromatherapy Chakra Balancing Roll-Ons. It is conceivable that people could develop a spiritual practice employing these herbal blends of essential oils to achieve higher states of consciousness. A month of meditating on one of the chakra qualities while applying the associated roll-on would create a strong association between them, perhaps by dedicating all actions, feelings, thoughts, and spiritual aspirations to the development of that quality. Seven months of meditating in this way would allow a full traversal of the continuum of human potential implied in the Esalen chakra qualities.

Thereafter, memories associated with each month's practice—and perhaps an associated state of consciousness, or at least the feeling-tone of that period of life—could be invoked by applying the requisite roll-on. It has long been known that scents are strong encoders of memory.

Further experiments could be made in blending states of consciousness by trying every combination of two, three, four, five, or six roll-ons, ending with all seven at once. Focusing intentions on achieving certain desired outcomes—say, second-chakra sensuality, fourth chakra love and compassion, and fifth chakra communication to create an ideal loving partnership—could be strengthened by blending the appropriate roll-ons, resulting in a scent-based sympathetic magic.

What, after all, is the difference between an Eastern system seed-syllable and a chakra-balancing roll-on? States of consciousness are difficult things to grasp, to summon or dismiss at will. Why not grab onto any available handle: the colors of the rainbow, the notes of the musical scale, the sounds of a seed-syllable, or the scents of an aromatherapy roll-on? The idea is to become a complete human being, to achieve the evolutionary potential implied in the chakra qualities—what Esalen called the bodymind, and what I see as the multidimensional rainbow body.

Notes

Introduction

1. See, for example, David Gordon White, *Kiss of the Yoginī: Tantric Sex in Its South Asian Context*, xii–xv, 271–72.

Chronology

1. For the sake of consistency, I have drawn dates primarily from *The Alchemical Body: Siddha Traditions in Medieval India; Kiss of the Yoginī; Sinister Yogis; The "Yoga Sutra of Patanjali": A Biography*; and "Tantra in Practice: Mapping a Tradition," all by David Gordon White. Notes in this portion of the chronology reference specific points that may be unique to White's research or opinions. Information on Sāṃkhya comes from Gavin Flood, *An Introduction to Hinduism*, 232–34. Most biographical dates (when known) come from Wikipedia.

2. There are three further references to *nāḍī* in later Upanishads: *Kaṭha* (6.16), nearly identical to that in *Chāndogya*; *Muṇḍaka* (2.2.6); and *Praśna* (3.6.7).

3. White, *Kiss of the Yoginī*, 224–25. White traces a reference in the (later) *Bhāgavata Purāṇa* to the (earlier) *Caraka Saṃhitā*.

4. Georg Feuerstein, *Encyclopedia of Yoga and Tantra*, s.v. "Shiva."

5. Mention is also made of concentration on the breast, flanks, and organs of vision, touch, and smell (White, *Sinister Yogis*, 171–72).

6. White states that "references to the subtle body, channels (*nāḍī*), and energy centers (*cakra*) are entirely absent from this work" (*Kiss of the Yoginī*, 220). Yet *Yoga Sūtra* 3.27–28 urges meditation on the sun, moon, and polestar—which could be references to the solar and lunar channels, with the central channel as the pole around which the inner and outer universes turn; 3.30 mentions a navel chakra, traditionally the third; 3.31 mentions the throat, location of the fifth chakra; 3.33 speaks of meditation on a "light in the head" (*mūrdhan*), the location of the sixth and seventh chakras; finally, 3.35 mentions meditation on the heart, traditionally the fourth chakra. Given that the four-chakra systems that emerged in the eighth century in Buddhist Tantra focused on navel, heart, throat, and head, it seems plausible that these verses of the *Yoga Sūtra* represent at least a protochakra system.

7. *Śūraṅgama Sūtra: A New Translation, with Excerpts from the Commentary by the Venerable Master Hsüan Hua* (see bibliography, under title), 196–201.

8. Realms of the universe: earth (*bhū-loka*), atmosphere (*bhuvar-loka*), celestials (*svar-loka*, sometimes translated as "heavens"), saints (*mahar-loka*), generation (*jana-loka;* abode of progenitors), austerity (*tapar-loka;* abode of ascetics), truth (*satya-loka;* abode of Brahma). Translations from Sanjukta Gupta, "The Worship of Kali according to the *Ṭoḍala Tantra*," 480. The Sanskrit word *loka* is sometimes translated as "plane."

9. A poetic text commonly attributed to Śaṅkara, the *Saundarya-Laharī* ("Waves of beauty"; sometimes also called *Ānanda-Laharī*, "Waves of bliss"), mentions seven chakras with standard names in addition to referencing *kuṇḍalinī*. However, the authorship of this text is disputed. If it were really by Śaṅkara and his eighth- to ninth-century dates were correct, then the text would reflect the origin of the seven-chakra system and the apparent evolution of the system from four to five to six chakras over the next several centuries would be negated. If it were a later production, drawing on an already extant tradition of seven chakras with the standard names, then it would likely have emerged no earlier than the twelfth century. I make this observation only on the basis of what the chronology suggests, not on that of authoritative scholarship.

10. *Hevajra Tantra* uses alternative names for the right, left, and central channels: *lalanā* (tongue), *rasanā* (woman), and *avadhūti* (all-pervading mother) instead of *iḍā, piṅgalā*, and *suṣumṇā* (Sures Chandra Banerji, *A Companion to Tantra*, 238; translations from Keith Dowman, *Masters of Mahāmudrā: Songs and Histories of the Eighty-Four Buddhist Siddhas*, 426).

11. White, *Kiss of the Yoginī*, 227.

12. In my annotations for C. W. Leadbeater's *The Chakras: An Authoritative Edition of the Groundbreaking Classic* (xi), I placed the *Garuḍa Purāṇa* in the 900s CE, following Georg Feuerstein, *The Yoga Tradition: Its History, Literature, Philosophy, and Practice,* 298. Leadbeater cites a passage from the *Garuḍa Purāṇa* (102) that uses the six-chakra system and the familiar names of the chakras. Further research has determined that the date of the *Garuḍa Purāṇa* is problematic and portions of it may have been added in later centuries. As the present chronology indicates, the text Leadbeater quoted represents a later stage

in the formation of the Eastern chakra system and could not be from earlier than the 1100s.

13. White, *Kiss of the Yoginī*, 232.

14. For a translation of *Gorakṣa Paddhati*, see Feuerstein, *Yoga Tradition*, 400–20. The *Siddha-Siddhanta-Paddhati*, also attributed to Gorakṣanātha, elucidates a nine-chakra system, including the seven we are familiar with under their usual names (except that *sahasrāra* is called *nirvāṇa-cakra*). However, the dating of the text is problematic, so I have not included it in this chronology. White places it between the twelfth and sixteenth centuries (*Sinister Yogis*, 175).

15. *Śāradā-Tilaka Tantra* has been translated in full (see bibliography, under title); however, an abridged translation of the portion describing the chakras appears in Shayam Shundar Goswami's *Layayoga: The Definitive Guide to the Chakras and Kundalini*, 180. *Rudrayāmala* has not been translated, but an abridged translation of the portion describing the chakras appears in Goswami, 178. These texts belong to the tradition of Kashmiri Śaivism.

16. White cites the thirteenth century as a "likely" date for *Ṭoḍala Tantra* (*Alchemical Body*, 164). Sanjukta Gupta dates it in the fourteenth century ("Worship of Kali," 464). Gupta's essay includes a translation of *Ṭoḍala Tantra* (478–99).

17. White, *Kiss of the Yoginī*, 224. In Hindu Tantra, the so-called seventh (crown) chakra is not a wheel (*cakra*) but a lotus (*padma*).

18. Jeffrey Clark Ruff explains that there are two canons of Yoga Upanishads: northern, under formation from 800 to 1300 CE; and southern, including much-expanded versions of some northern texts, under formation from 1300 to 1750 ("Yoga in the *Yoga Upaniṣad*s: Disciplines of the Mystical *OṂ* Sound," 106). Twenty of the southern canon texts appear in *The Yoga-Upaniṣad-s: Translated into English on the Basis of the Commentary of Śrī Upaniṣad-Brahma-Yogin*, ed. S. Subrahmaṇya Śāstrī—my primary source in this book (hence their later placement in the chronology). Some New Age writers, especially on the Internet, assume that the name Upanishad automatically comes with an ancient pedigree and class such texts with the first Upanishads, composed some two thousand years earlier. Thus the elaborate chakra system of the Yoga Upanishads gets predated to a period when only one of its components—the nadis—was under discussion.

19. Speculative date by James Mallinson, *The Shiva Samhita: A Critical Edition and an English Translation*, x.

20. Goswami lists separate colors for each element of a chakra *maṇḍala*: petals, phonemes, the area within the *tattva* symbol, the *bīja* phoneme, the god and goddess, and the *liṅgam* (if present). See *Laya-yoga*, 276–84. Associating animals with the elements may be one of the latest developments in the evolution of the Eastern chakra system. Goswami lists only two source references to the animals: *Ṣaṭ-Cakra-Nirūpaṇa* (1577) and "*Mridanitantra*, quoted in *Amarasaṅggraha* MS." Banerji states that *Amara-Saṃgraha* dates to 1843 (*Companion to Tantra*, 121). I have not been able to trace the reference to *Mṛḍānītantra*.

21. I have not been able to determine when this link was made. As noted, the lingams in the root and heart chakras were already established in the thirteenth or fourteenth centuries, but the *Rudrayāmala* (my source for those associations) does not mention *itara-liṅga* in the sixth chakra.

Chapter 1

1. Usually, the chakras are portrayed as lotuses with varying numbers of petals—and the sixth chakra has two such petals rather than eight.

2. Bipin Behari Shom, "Physical Errors of Hinduism," *Calcutta Review*, 441. This article was published anonymously. See this chapter's note 5 for the source of the author's name.

3. In figures 1 and 2, I have reproduced diagrams from 1853 rather than the originals from the 1849 *Calcutta Review* article because the latter were rendered as three-part foldouts. The 1853, these diagrams were reengraved for a government publication called *The Sessional Papers* to fit on a single page, making them easier to reprint here.

4. Wikipedia, s.vv. "Scottish Church College," "Alexander Duff."

5. Education: editorial note in Shom, "Physical Errors of Hinduism," *Calcutta Review*, 397; name, employment, and religious affiliation from editorial note in Shom, "Physical Errors of Hinduism" in *The Sessional Papers Printed by Order of the House of Lords, or Presented by Royal Command, in the Session 1852–53*, 453; caste: Bipin Behari Shom, *Calcutta Review*, 437. Henceforward, I cite the first publication of this essay as *Calcutta Review* and the second as *Sessional Papers*.

6. It is possible that graphic representations of the chakra system were previously published in connection with explorations undertaken

by the East India Company, established in the early seventeenth century, or scholarly studies and translations from Sanskrit, beginning in the late eighteenth century. Older examples of such representations exist in museum collections throughout the world, but the engravings of Shom's maps predate reproductions of them by half a century or more. As far as I know, these maps have not been reprinted since they were first published in 1849 and 1853. However, in the absence of the originals, it is impossible to determine how much they were altered during the engraving process (witness the addition of English letters to designate the chakras for ease of reference within the text of Shom's article).

7. Shom, *Calcutta Review*, 444. I have edited Shom's account for readability, eliminating the use of upper case for technical terms, correcting unrecognizable transliterations, and rendering his use of italics for Sanskrit words more consistent.

8. Ibid., 402.

9. Feuerstein, *Encyclopedia of Yoga and Tantra*, s.vv. "mantra," "tantra."

10. Ibid., s.vv. "panca-ma-kāra," "maithunā," "vāma-mārga."

11. Shom, *Calcutta Review*, 438.

12. David Lorenzen, "Early Evidence for Tantra Religion," 33; Feuerstein, *Encyclopedia of Yoga and Tantra*, s.v. "Nātha cult."

13. Shom, *Calcutta Review*, 437.

14. Ibid.

15. Ibid., 438.

16. I have found slightly earlier references to the chakras in a scholarly work of 1843, *The Dabistān or School of Manners*, a seventeenth-century Persian text translated by David Shea (1777–1836) and Anthony Troyer (1775–1865), published in three volumes, in Paris. Three lists of the chakras are given in the second volume: one by Troyer (editor of the work) in an explanatory footnote (2:131n), the others by the original author, thought to be a Zoroastrian who traveled throughout northern India gathering information on religious customs of Hindu, Muslim, and other sects (2:131–32; 150–51). All three lists are faulty, including both correct and eccentric names and locations for the chakras. The book also refers to "*Kundeli*, 'a snake'"—one of the earliest (if not the first) references in English to kundalini (2:134).

Though the editor, Troyer, mentions that the six chakras are described "in the best treatises of the Hindu philosophers" and that "various faculties and relations with divinities and physical elements" are attributed to them, his knowledge of the system appears to be cursory (2:131n). Troyer was the secretary of the Government Sanskrit College in Benares (now Varanasi) beginning in 1835. Shea died before the translation of *Dabistān* was finished, so Troyer stepped in to complete and edit the work.

Given the unreliability of the information on the chakras in *Dabistān* and the relative inaccessibility of the translation until a one-volume, abridged edition came out in 1901, I believe that Shom's presentation in "Physical Errors of Hinduism" represents three significant firsts: (1) introduction of accurate information about the chakras in terms of names and locations; (2) presentation by a Hindu native to an English-speaking audience; and (3) publication in a generally accessible, nonscholarly public forum.

For information on *Dabistān* and Shea, see Wikipedia, s.vv. "Dabestān-e Mazāheb," "David Shea." For information on Anthony Troyer, see Gabriele Zeller and Heidrun Brückner, eds., *Otto Böhtlingk an Rudolf Roth: Briefe zum Petersburger Wörterbuch*, 369n.

17. Shom, *Calcutta Review*, 439–40. Note that the use of the word *we* in the passage quoted is problematic. The readers of the *Calcutta Review* were most likely Anglo-Indians—that is, white British citizens who lived or were born in India. Thus we are intended to understand the word *we* as *Westerners* or *Europeans*, who probably would not have included the author of the essay among their number, due to racial prejudice. Most Hindus of that time would have considered a corpse physically and spiritually unclean and would never have practiced dissection, as Shom noted (436–37).

18. Ibid., 440.

19. Rudyard Kipling, "The Ballad of East and West."

20. Sudhir Kakar, *Shamans, Mystics and Doctors: A Psychological Inquiry into India and Its Healing Traditions*, 272.

Chapter 2

1. Anagarika Govinda, *Foundations of Tibetan Mysticism according to the Esoteric Teachings of the Great Mantra "Oṃ Maṇi Padme Hūṃ,"* 93.

2. White, "Tantra in Practice: Mapping a Tradition," 9.

3. White, *Alchemical Body*, 143–44.

4. See White, *Kiss of the Yoginī*, xii–xv.

5. Kathleen Taylor, *Sir John Woodroffe, Tantra, and Bengal: "An Indian Soul in a European Body?,"* 3, 152, 202.

6. Tantric Buddhism also employs a chakra system, though it uses only five chakras—the first two chakras of the Hindu system are considered to be a single center, as are the sixth and seventh. This system has been stable since the latter part of the first millennium CE. It has had little influence on the evolution of the Western chakra system and will not be discussed further—though details of its development are included in the chronology. See Govinda, *Foundations of Tibetan Mysticism*, 129–209, for an insightful comparison of the Hindu and Buddhist chakra systems. See also figure 22 in the present book for a diagram of the Tibetan Buddhist chakra system.

7. Feuerstein, *Encyclopedia of Yoga and Tantra*, s.v. "īdā-nādī."

8. Ibid., s.v. "pingalā-nādī."

9. According to an 1894 article in the *Theosophist*, "In the ordinary person the 'serpent power' lies coiled in *mūlādhāra*, but when once aroused, it never returns there, but to the chakra above, viz., *svādhiṣṭhāna*, which is consequently the resting place of Kundalini." Thus is explained the translation of *svādhiṣṭhāna* as "her own place"—since *kuṇḍalinī-śakti* (serpent power) is considered to be female. The author's authority seems to be verse 10 of *Saundarya-Laharī* (cited as *Ānanda-Laharī*). See R. Ananta Krishna Shastry, "Some Notes on Kundalini," 279, 282.

10. *Yoga-Cūḍāmaṇi Upaniṣad*, 11.

11. See Georg Feuerstein, *Tantra: The Path of Ecstasy,* 129–30, for an explanation of *pīṭha* in terms of external and internal pilgrimage sites. The author of some notes to an 1896 *Theosophist* article entitled "The Legend of Dwārakā," which deals with the seven sacred centers of Hindu pilgrimage, links them to "the seven life-centers in man" as follows [K. Narayansami, "Notes to 'The Legend of Dwārakā,'" 218.]:

- Mūlādhāra—Dwāraka (now Dwarka)
- Svādhiṣṭhāna—Avantikā (Oujjen; now Ujjain)
- Maṇipūra—Kāñcipura (Conjeveram; now Kanchipuram)
- Anāhata—Kāśī (Benares; now Varanasi)
- Viśuddha—Māyā (Hardwar; now Haridwar)
- Ājñā—Mathurā
- Sahasrāra—Ayodhyā (Oudh; now Awadh)

12. John Woodroffe, *The Serpent Power—Being the Ṣaṭ-Cakra-Nirūpaṇa and Pādukā-Pañcaka . . . with Introduction and Commentary*, facing page 382.

13. Satyananda Saraswati, *Kundalini Tantra*, 132.

Chapter 3

1. This account of thirty-six tattvas is based on Gavin Flood, *The Tantric Body: The Secret Tradition of Hindu Religion,* 128, and refers to the tradition of Kashmiri Śaivism. The more familiar (and earlier) Sāṃkhya and Yoga systems list twenty-five tattvas, twenty of which correspond to the two sets of senses and the subtle and gross elements and are allocated to the first five chakras. See also Feuerstein, *Tantra*, 63, for a schematic diagram of the thirty-six tattvas.

2. White, *Alchemical Body*, 292–93 (absorption); *Kiss of the Yoginī*, 181 (implosion). See also *Śiva Saṃhitā* 2.78.

3. White, *Kiss of the Yoginī*, 8–14.

4. Francis King, *Tantra, The Way of Action: A Practical Guide to Its Teachings and Techniques*, 15.

5. Shom, *Calcutta Review*, 439n.

6. Feuerstein, *Encyclopedia of Yoga and Tantra*, s.v. "hatha-yoga."

7. See Mark Singleton, *Yoga Body: The Origins of Modern Postural Practice*.

8. Feuerstein, *Encyclopedia of Yoga and Tantra*, s.v. "mantra."

9. These powers (*siddhi*) include clairvoyance, precognition, levitation, astral projection, omniscience, omnipotence, and others. The subtle bodies are variously called *kośa* (sheath), *śarīra* (body), *deha* (form), *upādhi* (support; phantom), and *vahana* (carrier; vehicle). The higher realms are called *loka* and the lower realms, *tala*.

10. In Tantra, there are traditionally "six actions" (*ṣaṭ-karman*) that involve power over others in the phenomenal world: *appeasement* ("curing of diseases"), *subjugation* ("bringing a person under the practitioner's control, especially seducing a woman against her will"), *immobilization* ("stopping a person's activity"), *enmity* ("creating dissension or dislike between two persons who are attached to each other"), *eradication* ("depriving a person of his place, usually with reference to breaking an object or removing someone from a location"), *liquidation* ("taking life") (see Gudrun Bühnemann, "The Six Rites of Magic,"

448). These six actions are usually considered the domain of tantric sorcerers, followers of the left-hand path.

11. As noted, the Sanskrit term for liberation while alive is *jīvanmukta*; for liberation from rebirth after death, it is *videhamukti*.

12. See King, *Tantra*, 77–85 and 114–15 for connections between Tantra, the Golden Dawn, mantra, and Western ritual magic.

13. Satyananda Saraswati, *Kundalini Tantra*, 132.

14. Devā Rām Sukul, *Yoga and Self-Culture: A Scientific and Practical Survey of Yoga Philosophy for the Layman and the Aspirant on the Path*, 134.

15. See André Padoux, *Vāc: The Concept of the Word in Selected Hindu Tantras*, 235–304, for an in-depth discussion of the metaphysical meanings of Sanskrit vowels and consonants and their links with the thirty-six tattvas of Kashmiri Śaivism.

16. A *tanmātra* is usually described as a *faculty* or potential for perceiving sound, touch, sight, taste, or smell (see, for example, Feuerstein, *Tantra*, 65). A *jñānendriya*, representing a higher level of tattva, is an *organ* of sensation or cognition, such as hearing, touching, seeing, tasting, or smelling. Yet the distinction seems to be between *physical* senses (tanmatras) and *mental* faculties of perception (jnanendriyas). The notion of gross elements, subtle elements, and organs of sense suggests that the tanmatras somehow lie *between* external sense objects and internal sense organs, hence my use of words such as *smellables*, which are meant to suggest an intermediary phase between attributes of objects (*mahā-bhūta*, "gross elements") and their ability to be perceived by the jnanendriyas. The tanmatras are thus located at the moment when externals become internalized, while the suffix *-ables* retains the notion of potential—the potential of an object to be perceived and the potential of an individual to perceive it.

17. I have been helped in this account by Feuerstein's discussion of the thirty-six tattvas in *Tantra*, 62–66.

Chapter 4

1. W. Brugh Joy, *Joy's Way: A Map for the Transformational Journey—and Introduction to the Potentials for Healing with Body Energies*, 159. See chart of the chakras on 165–66. See also chapter 6, note 22, for further information.

2. Ibid., 196.

3. Olav Hammer, *Claiming Knowledge: Strategies of Epistemology from Theosophy to the New Age*, 180–81.

4. Ibid., 188–89.

5. Emanuel Swedenborg, *Heaven and Hell*, trans. George Dole, §106. The section numbers (§) are standardized, making it easier to consult the passages in question across various editions and translations.

6. Ibid., §104.

7. Ibid., §105.

8. Emanuel Swedenborg, *Heaven and Its Wonders, and Hell, from Things Heard and Seen*, trans. John C. Ager, §§ 97, 99.

9. Swedenborg, *Heaven and Hell*, §110.

10. Swedenborg, *Heaven and Its Wonders*, §112; the alternative translation of *uses* as "functions" or "purposes" occurs in *Heaven and Hell*, §112.

11. Swedenborg, *Heaven and Hell*, §112.

12. Examples of this belief, which applies equally to the birth process and the afterdeath process (in which the qualities acquired during the descent through the spheres must be relinquished or transcended if one is to reascend), may be found in Cicero's "Dream of Scipio," Book 6 of *De republica* (first century BCE); the hermetic text *Poimandres* (second or third century CE); and the Neoplatonic *Commentary on the "Dream of Scipio"* of Macrobius (fifth century CE).

13. See Catherine L. Albanese, *A Republic of Mind and Spirit: A Cultural History of American Metaphysical Religion*, 13–16, for an explanation of the impact of the notion of occult correspondences on nineteenth- and twentieth-century American religious and metaphysical beliefs; see 34–35 for a discussion of Agrippa and 140–42 for a discussion of Swedenborg and his influence on nineteenth-century America.

14. Henry Corbin, *The Man of Light in Iranian Sufism*, 121–31.

15. Idries Shah, *The Sufis*, 430–31. The author indicates that the *lataif* "are analogous to and often confused with the *chakra* system of the yogis" and that they are "merely concentration points" (430; original emphasis).

16. Julius Evola, *The Yoga of Power: Tantra, Shakti, and the Secret Way*, 9.

17. Satyananda Saraswati, *Kundalini Tantra*, 363–65.

Chapter 5

1. Except where otherwise noted, historical material in this chapter, up to the discussion of the first articles on Tantra in the *Theosophist*, derives from Josephine Ransom, *A Short History of the Theosophical Society*, in particular the chapter "In India: 1879–1884," 123–88.

2. Sylvia Cranston, *H.P.B: The Extraordinary Life and Influence of Helena Blavatsky*, 158.

3. These principles are the three objects of the Theosophical Society as formulated in Bombay, February 17, 1881 (Ransom, *Short History of the Theosophical Society*, 155).

4. See "Namastae! [*sic*]," the opening editorial in the first issue of the *Theosophist* in H. P. Blavatsky, *The Collected Writings of H. P. Blavatsky*, 2:84–86.

5. Biographical material on Blavatsky and Olcott and historical material on the early years of the Theosophical Society is summarized from Cranston, *H.P.B.* and from the chronologies by editor Boris de Zirkoff in *The Collected Writings of H. P. Blavatsky*, 1:liii–lxvi and 2:xxv–xxxvi. A number of Theosophical organizations trace their roots to the so-called parent society that existed prior to Blavatsky's death. Throughout this book, references to the Theosophical Society (TS) are to the organization with headquarters in Adyar, Chennai, India and its literature.

6. "The Dream of Ravan: A Mystery," pt. 4, 463; Truth Seeker, "Yoga Philosophy," 86.

7. Karl Baier, "Mesmeric Yoga and the Development of Meditation within the Theosophical Society," 155.

8. Truth Seeker, "Yoga Philosophy," 87.

9. Baier, "Mesmeric Yoga," 155.

10. Books: Listed at National Library of India website (http://www.nationallibrary.gov.in; search term: Baradkanta Majumdar). Magazine: (*Shishu*): Abhijit Battacharya, *A Guide to the Hitesranjan Sanyal Memorial Collection at Center for Studies in Social Sciences, Calcutta*, entry 114. Accessed November 25, 2015.

11. Arthur Avalon, ed., *Principles of Tantra: The Tantratattva of Shrīyukta Shiva Chandra Vidyārṇava Bhattāchāryya Mahodaya*, 539. The name given on the title page is Baradā Kānta Majumdār.

12. Baradakanta Majumdar, "Tantric Philosophy," 173.

13. Ibid.
14. Ibid.
15. Arthur Avalon, *The Serpent Power: The Secrets of Tantric and Shaktic Yoga*, 1.
16. Editorial note to Baradakanta Majumdar, "A Glimpse of Tantric Occultism," 244.
17. See, for example, H. P. Blavatsky, *Foundations of Esoteric Philosophy: From the Writings of H. P. Blavatsky*, a compilation of excerpts from *Isis Unveiled: A Master Key to the Mysteries of Ancient and Modern Science and Theology* (whose 1877 publication preceded that of Majumdar's article) and *The Secret Doctrine: The Synthesis of Science, Religion, and Philosophy* (whose 1888 publication followed it).
18. Blavatsky, *Collected Writings*, 4:164–65.
19. Singleton, *Yoga Body*, 50. Full name and birth and death dates from https://www.worldcat.org/identities/lccn-n82115364/. See Phanindranath Bose, *Life of Sris Chandra Basu*, 136–38, for further biographical information on Baman Das Basu.
20. B. B. (Baman Das Basu), "The Anatomy of the Tantras," 371n. Baman Das Basu would be familiar with these terms from Sris Chandra Basu's translation of *Śiva Saṃhitā*, published in 1887 under the title *The Esoteric Philosophy and Science of the Tantras: Shiva Sanhita* [sic]. Sris Chandra Basu (1861–1918; sometimes called Vasu; death date confirmed in Bose, *Life of Sris Chandra Basu*, 229) was the elder brother of Baman Das Basu (Bose, *Life of Sris Chandra Basu*, 28, 136).
21. The English translations of these terms come from Feuerstein, *Encyclopedia of Yoga and Tantra*, under their respective Sanskrit words.
22. *Citra* is usually designated as *citriṇī*, with a similar translation. Woodroffe notes that within the sushumna is a nadi called *vajrā* ("diamond"; not mentioned in Basu's article) and within vajra is citrini. Yet another nadi called brahma ("Absolute"; also not mentioned in Basu) is within citrini (Avalon, *Serpent Power*, 159).
23. Basu confused *brahmarandhra* (anterior fontanel, a point at the crown of the head from which the soul is said to exit at death) with *brahmadaṇḍa* (spinal column). See "Anatomy of the Tantras," 371.
24. *Triveṇī* is the location in the head where the left, right, and central channels merge. It is frequently likened to a sacred pilgrimage site in Allahabad where three rivers merge: the Gaṅgā (Ganges), the Yamunā, and the invisible Sarasvatī. See Avalon, *Serpent Power*, 111–12.

25. Kailāsa ("icy" or "crystalline") is a sacred mountain in Tibet, revered in Hinduism as well as Buddhism.

26. No female equivalent is given; perhaps the vaginal plexus.

27. Leadbeater, *Chakras*, table 2 (35).

28. Vasant G. Rele, *The Mysterious Kundalini: The Physical Basis of the "Kundali (Hatha) Yoga" according to Our Present Knowledge of Physical Anatomy*, 20–29.

29. Anodea Judith, *Wheels of Life: A User's Guide to the Chakra System* (1999), 12.

Chapter 6

1. Because of the complicated publishing history of these instructions and the multitude of formats in which they were brought out (pamphlets, books, facsimiles, and so on) as well as names by which they were called (Instructions, Papers, E. S. or E.S.T. Instructions, and so on), I have opted to call them simply Esoteric Instructions (no italics) and identify them with Arabic numerals.

2. For further information on these controversies, see Boris de Zirkoff, "*The Secret Doctrine*—Volume Three, as Published in 1897: A Survey of Its Contents and Authenticity," xxv–xliv. As the first volume of *The Secret Doctrine* was entitled *Cosmogenesis* and the second *Anthropogenesis*, the third was entitled *Occultism*.

3. The 1897 third volume of *The Secret Doctrine* was reprinted as the fifth volume of a six-volume edition of *The Secret Doctrine* issued in 1938 (called the Adyar edition). Original transcripts of notes by several participants in the Inner Group were published in Theosophical journals in the twentieth century, calling into question the authenticity of the selection, ordering, and editing of Besant's version. For a time, the fifth volume of the Adyar edition was available as a separate volume, *The Esoteric Writings of Helena Petrovna Blavatsky: A Synthesis of Science, Religion, and Philosophy*. Two editions of original transcripts were also released as *The Inner Group Teachings of H. P. Blavatsky to Her Personal Pupils (1890–91)*, by Henk J. Spierenburg. These resources are out of print. *The Collected Writings of H. P. Blavatsky*, vol. 12, contains edited versions of the first five Esoteric Instructions. A compilation by Daniel Caldwell, *The Esoteric Papers of Madame Blavatsky*, contains facsimiles of original documents pertaining to the Esoteric School,

including complete versions of six Instructions, some in multiple editions, and one transcript of Inner Group Teachings. A new edition of the Esoteric Instructions, published under this title, has been prepared recently by Michael Gomes for students of esoteric philosophy. To facilitate such study, I have cited both the *Collected Writings* edition and the Gomes *Esoteric Instructions* edition, where applicable (despite variant readings).

4. See Blavatsky, *Collected Writings*, 12:616–21 (*Esoteric Instructions*, 135–46) for the original context of these passages, which are presented in their original order.

5. Names of principles: H. P. Blavatsky, *The Key to Theosophy*, 91–92; correlated with hierarchies and aura layers: *Collected Writings*, 12:567; and with planes of existence: 12:660 (*Esoteric Instructions*, 96, 222).

6. One such set of correlations appears as a table in Esoteric Instruction No. 3 (Blavatsky, *Collected Writings*, 12:614 [*Esoteric Instructions*, foldout between 130 and 131]).

7. Blavatsky, *Collected Writings*, 12:604n (*Esoteric Instructions*, 112–13n).

8. I have not been able to trace *devakṣa*, which appears to be a coinage from *deva* (god) and *akṣi* (eye)—possibly *divya-cakṣus* (divine eye; supernatural vision). Devaksha (HPB's spelling) occurs on the Internet as an uncommon Hindi male name, translated as "having eyes like a god's."

9. Blavatsky, *Secret Doctrine*, ed. Boris de Zirkoff, *Collected Writings, 1888*, 2:289–306.

10. Ibid., 2:295.

11. "Descartes and the Pineal Gland," *Stanford Encyclopedia of Philosophy*, http://plato.stanford.edu/entries/pineal-gland/. This article cites the section of Blavatsky's *Secret Doctrine* just discussed as the origin of the third-eye/pineal connection.

12. Blavatsky, *Secret Doctrine* (de Zirkoff), , 2:298.

13. Blavatsky, *Secret Doctrine*, Adyar ed., 5:508. This note, signed "H. C.," was prepared by Herbert Coryn (1863–1927), one of Blavatsky's Inner Group students, and supposedly approved by her (ibid., 506n, 509). It has been dropped in subsequent editions of the Esoteric Instructions.

14. Feuerstein, *Encyclopedia of Yoga and Tantra*, s.vv. "shabda," "shabda-brahman."

15. Avalon, *Serpent Power*, 151–52.

16. Goswami, *Layayoga*, 276–84.

17. Mark Juergensmeyer, *Radhasoami Reality: The Logic of a Modern Faith*, 205. Information and dates concerning the Radhasoami faith and its gurus in subsequent paragraphs are from Lawrence A. Babb, *Redemptive Encounters: Three Modern Styles in the Hindu Tradition*, 20–24, 29–31.

18. Soami Ji, *Sar Bachan: The Yoga of the Sound Current*, 9–15, 20–21. Juergensmeyer notes similarities between descriptions of subtle sounds in *Sar Bachan* and by Blavatsky in *The Voice of the Silence*, 10, stating that "Nath Yoga texts" may have Blavatsky's source (Juergensmeyer, *Radhasoami Reality*, 205 and note). Indeed, these sounds are described in the section on *nāda* yoga in *Haṭha-Yoga-Pradīpikā*, 4.65–114, especially the list of subtle sounds in 4.85–86. They also appear in *Śiva Saṃhitā* 5.27.

19. Juergensmeyer, *Radhasoami Reality*, 205.

20. A. Trevor Barker, ed., *The Mahatma Letters to A. P. Sinnett from the Mahatmas M. and K.H.*, 255. K. Paul Johnson connects this letter to Saligram in *Initiates of the Theosophical Masters*, 64–65. However, he has edited the text of the letter by substituting "Salig Ram" for "Suby Ram."

21. A. P. Sinnett, *The Occult World*, 219.

22. "Babuji Maharaj observed that Mrs. Annie Besant and Colonel Alcot [sic], who was at one time the Editor of *the Pioneer* [sic], came in the august presence of Huzur Maharaj and expressed great appreciation for Sant Mat, but their companions prevailed upon them and led them astray. They remained attached to Theosophy and they never came to Satsang again" (S. D. Maheshwari, trans., *Discourses of Babuji Maharaj*, 4:51). Olcott was editor of the *Theosophist*. Besant demonstrated her familiarity with Radhasoami teachings in undated remarks published in *Talks on the Path of Occultism*, vol. 2: *The Voice of the Silence*, 126: "In India there is a school formed by a man of whom the Masters spoke highly [Saligram]." She mentioned the practice in which sounds were heard "quite clearly in the brain" and indicated that people in the north of India, where the Radhasoami movement originated, often asked her about these sounds.

23. Henry S. Olcott, *Old Diary Leaves* 5:114–18.

24. P. C. Mukherji, "The Radhaswami [sic] Society of Agra," 571. The note may have been by Olcott.

25. Brahm Shankar Mishra, *Discourses on Radhasoami Faith*, 307–9. The author refers to the chakras as "ganglia" or "nerve centers." They are located at the rectum, reproductive organ, navel, solar plexus (instead of heart), throat, and brow / pineal gland (314); the link between brow and pineal gland occurs on page 308. Brugh Joy's chakra system (*Joy's Way*) was apparently based on that of the Radhasoami faith. It also posited both a navel and a solar plexus chakra, omitted the heart chakra, and placed the thousand-petaled lotus above the head (as well as adding two chakras each in feet, knees, elbows, and hands and one between the shoulders, for a total of sixteen).

26. Leadbeater, *Chakras*, 13–14.

27. "The seat or focus of the spirit is the pineal gland" (Mishra, *Discourses*, 314).

28. For example, Blavatsky's *Voice of the Silence* mentions kundalini several times (pp. 9 and 12 and notes 24, 25, 31 on pp. 76–78), hinting that when kundalini rises from the heart to the area of the forehead it becomes possible to hear the voice of the Master and to become "a walker of the sky" (presumably an astral projector).

29. T. Subba Row, "The Idyll of the White Lotus," pt. 2, 706.

30. Wikipedia, s.v. "khagan."

31. Blavatsky, *Secret Doctrine* (de Zirkoff), 2:191n; interpolations in brackets are Blavatsky's. I have corrected the inaccurate book and hymn numbers in the *Ṛg Veda* references.

32. The earliest occurrence of the concept of koshas appears in the fourth- to third-century-BCE *Taittirīya Upaniṣad* 2.2–5.

33. It is possible that a passage in one of the Yoga Upanishads, *Maṇḍala-Brāhmaṇa* 1.2, which describes a practice of meditating on colored spaces at certain distances from the nose, as measured in fingerbreadths—four (blue), six (indigo-black), eight (red), ten (yellow), and twelve (orange red)—refers to colored layers of the aura. Some Theosophists have so interpreted this passage. See A. Marques, *The Human Aura: A Study*, 38n.

34. See, for example, Choa Kok Sui, *The Ancient Science and Art of Pranic Healing: Practical Manual on Paranormal Healing*.

Chapter 7

1. Blavatsky, *Collected Writings*, 12:620 (*Esoteric Instructions*, 142–43).
2. Blavatsky, *Collected Writings*, 12:534–35 (*Esoteric Instructions*, 36).
3. Spierenburg, *Inner Group Teachings*, 21.
4. See Blavatsky, *Collected Writings*, 12, foldout between pp. 532 and 533 (figure 5 in the present book), chart on 614, and foldout between pp. 660 and 661 (*Esoteric Instructions*, foldouts between pp. 40 and 41, 130 and 131, and 260 and 261).
5. Blavatsky, *Collected Writings*, 12:561 (*Esoteric Instructions*, 85).
6. Blavatsky, *Collected Writings*, 12:567 (*Esoteric Instructions*, 95–96).
7. Feuerstein, *Encyclopedia of Yoga and Tantra*, s.v. "nyāsa."
8. White, *Tantra in Practice*, 630.
9. Spierenburg, *Inner Group Teachings*, 10, 19; Blavatsky, *Collected Writings*, 12:516–20, 534 (*Esoteric Instructions*, 4–13, 35–36).
10. See Blavatsky, *Collected Writings*, 12:600, 604–6 (*Esoteric Instructions*, 105, 113–16) for an explanation of the rationale for esoteric blinds.
11. See Blavatsky, *Collected Writings*, 12:608–10 (*Esoteric Instructions*, 119–23) for an in-depth explanation of the auric egg or envelope.
12. The Inner Group Teachings do not make clear how to map the psychic, spiritual, and divine planes into the seven master chakras in the brain. Later meetings were devoted to demonstrating links between the seven principles experienced microcosmically in human consciousness and macrocosmically in "Kosmic consciousness" (Spierenburg, *Inner Group Teachings*, 28–40). One possible interpretation is that the seven stations along the spine represent the microcosmic, human consciousness and the seven stages in the brain represent macrocosmic, kosmic consciousness.
13. As indicated, Blavatsky's *Voice of the Silence*, 9–10, provides a list of seven sounds, representing a mystic ladder associated with raising the kundalini to the forehead chakra and perhaps beyond it, to the crown chakra: nightingale, silver cymbal, seashell, vina (Indian bowed stringed instrument), bamboo flute, trumpet, and thunder. The similar list of

sounds in *Haṭha-Yoga-Pradīpikā* 4.85–86 is associated with the fourth chakra. Radhasoami teachings associate subtle sounds with the supraterrestrial realms accessible through meditation on the sixth chakra, as in *Voice of the Silence*. See Mukherji, "Radhaswami [*sic*] Society of Agra," 710, where the sixth chakra is called *til*.

14. Spierenburg, *Inner Group Teachings*, 4. For "skull filled with akasha," see Blavatsky, *Collected Writings*, 12:698–99 (not in *Esoteric Instructions*).

15. Blavatsky instructed the Inner Group students to begin concentration "at the vertebra where the spinal cord begins," since black magic could result from concentrating in the coccygeal region, "the great line of demarcation between the animal and the man" (Spierenburg, *Inner Group Teachings*, 17). This instruction indicates that the preferred form of the practice was to begin with the linga level rather than the *sthūla* level. That would mean ending with the blue auric egg stage, which apparently corresponds to a "sacred seventh" plexus near the atlas, not known to science and not mentioned by yogis because of its sacredness (21).

16. The contents of this column are speculative. Only the order and numbering of the pituitary, the third ventricle, the pineal, and "the whole" appear in the *Inner Group Teachings*, 77—although a correlation between the cerebellum and *kāma* is also mentioned (ibid.), making it possible to add it to the series. A diagram in Esoteric Instruction No. 4 correlates the pineal gland with *buddhi* and the color yellow, and the seventh principle with "the akasha that fills the skull" and the prismatic colors / blue—a placement I have followed here (Blavatsky, *Collected Writings*, vol. 12, foldout between pp. 660 and 661 [*Esoteric Instructions*, foldout between pp. 260 and 261]).

The first three elements in the series are unknown. The original version of Esoteric Instruction No. 3 includes a diagram of the brain that was dropped in all subsequent editions but was reproduced in Caldwell's *Esoteric Papers*, 443. Twelve brain structures are identified by number. Since the diagram appears in the midst of the discussion of the chakras cited in the previous chapter, it must have something to do with the seven master chakras in the brain. Blavatsky mentions the medulla oblongata, illustrated in this diagram, as "one of the sacred centers" (*Inner Group Teachings*, 21). It makes a plausible beginning for the series of master chakras, though there is no clear indication to that effect. A second candidate from this diagram is the pons, located directly above the medulla. I have placed these speculations in brackets.

Another passage from the *Inner Group Teachings* mentions the *corpora quadrigemina* in connection with *kāma-manas* (lower mind) and places the pituitary between it and *buddhi-manas* (higher mind). The pituitary is assigned to *manas-antaḥkaraṇa*, a so-called principle linking the lower and higher mind. This state of affairs seems to apply only when the pineal gland has been activated by kundalini (25). I have included this information, too, in brackets.

Finally, the repetition of the atlas / foramen magnum from the top of column 3 at the bottom of column four suggests the continuity of the seven plexuses in the body and the seven master chakras in the brain at this important juncture—about which Blavatsky said "she herself did not use the colors above the atlas; on arriving there, as she phrased it, she 'went home'" (*Inner Group Teachings*, 17).

17. Theosophical clairvoyant Phoebe Payne correlates the corpora quadrigemina with the throat chakra and clairaudience, especially of "superphysical music," noting that this brain structure lies "immediately below the pineal gland" and has "a connection with the cochlear nerves of the ears" (*Man's Latent Powers*, 154, 152). As such, the corpora quadrigemina could perhaps be one of the master chakras, that correlated to higher *manas* and the laryngeal plexus chakra in the physical body.

18. Spierenburg, *Inner Group Teachings*, 54–55; Blavatsky, *Collected Writings*, 12, foldout between pp. 660 and 661 (*Esoteric Instructions*, foldout between pp. 260 and 261).

19. White, *Kiss of the Yoginī*, 224.

20. Satyananda Saraswati, *Kundalini Tantra*, 157.

21. Alice A. Bailey, *Esoteric Healing*, 45.

22. "Like the six superior or heavenly regions from *Sat Lok* [Blavatsky's and the *Viṣṇu Purāṇa*'s *Satyaloka* (realm of truth)] down to *Sahasdal Kamal* ["thousand-petaled lotus" at the crown], there are six lower or physical regions in *Pind* [body], which are in reality reflections of the heavenly regions" (Soami Ji, *Sar Bachan*, 13). Blavatsky: "The Lokas and Talas are reflections the one of the other" (*Inner Group Teachings*, 57; *Collected Writings*, 12:669; *Esoteric Instructions*, 256–57).

23. Such material is scattered throughout *The Secret Doctrine* and Blavatsky's journal articles in the *Collected Writings*. See Geoffrey A. Barborka, *The Divine Plane, Written in the Form of a Commentary on*

"The Secret Doctrine," 43–76 ("The Doctrine of Hierarchies") and 383–424 ("The After-Death States") for detailed exegeses of these teachings culled from both sources. Also see 158–201 ("The Septenary Law") for further information on principles, lokas, and talas.

Chapter 8

1. I have not been able to consult the 1890 first edition of *A Working Glossary*. I assume the forty-four page body of the third edition of 1892 corresponds to the original first and second editions and that the appendix was added in the third edition, expanding the work to sixty-two pages. Worldcat.org describes the first edition of 1890 as having forty-four pages.

2. Biographical information summarized from Arthur H. Nethercot, *The First Five Lives of Annie Besant*.

3. Details summarized from C. Jinarājadāsa, *Occult Investigations: A Description of the Work of Annie Besant and C. W. Leadbeater*. Jinarājadāsa has Besant and Leadbeater meeting in 1894 (8); according to Besant's biographer Arthur H. Nethercot, both Besant and Leadbeater stated that they met in 1890 (*First Five Lives of Annie Besant*, 324).

4. For the sources of information in table 5, see Annie Besant, *The Seven Principles of Man*, 113 and *Theosophy*, 25; and Kurt Leland, *Invisible Worlds: Annie Besant on Psychic and Spiritual Development*, 230–31.

5. *Atmic* is an anglicized version of *ātman* (turning a noun into an adjective), sometimes used in the 1890s as a synonym for the nirvanic plane and body (as in Besant's *The Ancient Wisdom* of 1896).

6. In *The Seven Principles of Man*, 113, Besant substitutes *prāṇa* for *linga* in relation to the etheric double, perhaps because the Sanskrit word *liṅga* refers to "subtle body" but also to "phallus." As I explained in *Invisible Worlds*, 276–79n7, the principles and bodies do not line up exactly, because a body is a compound of two or more principles. Just as the causal body is buddhi-manas, so the etheric body should be *prāṇa-liṅga*.

7. Besant, *Seven Principles of Man*, 16, 25. See also Leland, *Invisible Worlds*, 303n4 and 318n3 for more detailed information on the distinction between sense centers and sense organs and for connections

between Blavatsky's Inner Group teachings and Besant's explanations of the subject.

8. See Annie Besant, *Man and His Bodies*, 150–54, for further information on these links between bodies. Besant's descriptions of centers of sensation versus sense organs in various bodies make it seem as if there are two different systems linking the bodies. But, as I pointed out in *Invisible Worlds*, "A sense center is an operative but undeveloped chakra, providing a faculty of perception on a *lower* plane. A sense organ is a fully developed chakra, providing perception on the *same* plane" (318n3; original emphasis).

9. Besant, *Man and His Bodies*, 68–72.

10. A. E. Powell, *The Causal Body and the Ego*, 102.

11. See H. P. Blavatsky, *The Letters of H. P. Blavatsky*, vol. 1, 310–12; John Patrick Devaney, *Astral Projection or Liberation of the Double and the Work of the Early Theosophical Society*.

12. Olcott, *Old Diary Leaves*, 2:258–59.

13. Henry S. Olcott, *A Collection of Lectures on Theosophy and Archaic Religions Delivered in India and Ceylon*, 178–79. Olcott was referring to *Om: A Treatise on Vedantic Raj Yoga Philosophy*, edited by Sris Chandra Basu, published in Lahore in 1880 (reprinted in 1977 as *Vedantic Raj Yoga: Ancient Yoga of Rishies* [sic]). Presumably, plate 2 is the illustration Olcott was explaining.

14. Olcott, *Collection of Lectures*, 179.

15. Ibid.

16. My own phrasing of individual Sanskrit words as translated by I. K. Taimni in *The Science of Yoga: The Yoga-Sūtras of Patañjali in Sanskrit with Transliteration in Roman, Translation and Commentary in English*, 348.

17. Satyananda Saraswati, *Kundalini Tantra*, 143.

18. Ibid., 132–33.

19. Ibid., 131–32.

20. William Estep, *Esoteric Cosmic Yogi Science, or Works of the World Teacher*, 94–95 (eight limbs of yoga). Estep's book is a single-volume adaptation of Sabhapaty Swami's two-volume publication *Om: The Cosmic Psychological Spiritual Philosophy* (1884–90), without the original author's copious material in Sanskrit and Tamil. Estep's claim to have studied with Sabhapaty is questionable. From the time when his

book was published until his death, Estep was frequently convicted and jailed for pseudoscientific and religious fraud (http://hatch.kookscience.com/wiki/William_McKinley_Estep, accessed December 5, 2015).

21. Karl Baier, "Theosophical Orientalism and the Structures of Intercultural Transfer," 328–30.

22. Sabhapaty Swami, *Om: A Treatise on Vedantic Raj Yoga Philosophy*, 11–19 (see also the 1977 facsimile reprint, *Vedantic Raj Yoga: Ancient Yoga of Rishies*); Sanskrit names for the chakras from Estep, *Esoteric Cosmic Yogi Science*, 137–46. Thanks to Keith Cantú for help with decoding these often garbled names (email of December 11, 2015). *Bindu, nāda, kalā,* and *dvadaśānta* are attested in some traditional tantric chakra systems. See Goswami, *Layayoga*, 243–75, for scriptural references to these chakras.

23. See Estep, *Esoteric Cosmic Yogi Science*, 137–46, for descriptions of the practices involved.

24. A German translation of the 1883 edition of *Om: A Treatise on Vedantic Raj Yoga Philosophy* (retitled *The Philosophy and Science of Vedanta and Raja Yoga*), including a biographical sketch of its author, was serialized in 1908 in four issues of the Theosophical journal *Neue Lotusblüten* and published in book form in 1909. Thanks to Karl Baier, I have been able to examine a scan of a 1926 reprint, in which appears a black-and-white version of plate 2 in the present book. If that black-and-white figure also appears in the 1908 articles and 1909 book, it may be the first graphic representation of the chakra system in a German-language publication. See Sabhapatti Svami, *Die Philosophie und Wissenschaft des Vedānta und Rāja-Yoga; oder Das Eingehen in Gott*, 5.

25. C. W. Leadbeater, *Invisible Helpers*, 30–32, 130–33.

Chapter 9

1. Biographical material summarized from Wikipedia, s.v. "Rudolf Steiner."

2. Rudolf Steiner, *Autobiography: Chapters in the Course of My Life (1861–1907)*, 333n599. For this book, I draw on the seventh through eleventh installments of "Wie erlangt man Erkenntnisse der höheren Welten?," published in issues 20–24 of *Lucifer-Gnosis* (January–May 1905) and forming the basis of chapters 1 through 4 of *Initiation and*

Its Results. For simplicity's sake, these articles are cited here with the article title and page numbers only.

3. Steiner, *Initiation and Its Results*, 13–14, 42, and Steiner, "Wie erlangt man Erkenntnisse der höheren Welten?," 226, 290.

4. Steiner, *Initiation and Its Results*, 14, 36–37, 57–58.

5. Goswami lists the *vṛtti* by name in his comprehensive chart of the thirteen-chakra system in *Layayoga*, 276–84. I do not know whether Steiner was aware of the tantric tradition of assigning spiritual qualities to the lotus petals. However, the translator of Sabhapaty Swami's *Philosophy and Science of Vedanta and Raja Yoga*, Franz Hartmann (1838–1912), was living at the headquarters of the Theosophical Society in Adyar, India, when the swami was ostensibly present in nearby Madras (based on the place of publication of his major writings in Tamil and English), arriving in December 1883 (Blavatsky, *Collected Writings*, 6:xxiv) and returning to Europe in 1885 (Ibid., xlii). Hartmann and Steiner met in Vienna in 1889 (Steiner, *Autobiography*, xix, 79–80, 290nn243–44). Steiner's articles on the chakras in *Lucifer-Gnosis* preceded Hartmann's journal publication of this translation by several years. It is conceivable that Steiner's use of the notion of vrittis derived from Sabhapaty, by way of Hartmann or of colleagues they shared, such as German Theosophist Wilhelm Hübbe-Schleiden (1846–1916; ibid., xxi, 215, 324n541, 331–32n587).

6. Steiner, *Initiation and Its Results*, 13–14.

7. Ibid., 15.

8. Ibid., 16; Rudolf Steiner, "Wie erlangt man Erkenntnisse der höheren Welten?," 226; Rudolf Steiner, *How to Know Higher Worlds: A Modern Path of Initiation*, 112.

9. Steiner, *Initiation and Its Results*, 16–19; "Wie erlangt man Erkenntnisse der höheren Welten?," 227–28.

10. Steiner, "Wie erlangt man Erkenntnisse der höheren Welten?," 259. Steiner also speaks of *Seelentätigkeiten* (soul activities) in connection with these six characteristics (ibid., 257).

11. Steiner, *Initiation and Its Results*, 26–29.

12. See Annie Besant, *The Ancient Wisdom*, 328–33, for further information on these six mental attributes, which she lists as control of the mind, control of conduct, tolerance, endurance, faith, and balance.

13. Steiner, *Initiation and Its Results*, 30–35.

14. Ibid., 35; Steiner, "Wie erlangt man Erkenntnisse der höheren Welten?," 261.

15. See Leland, *Invisible Worlds*, 99–100.

16. Steiner, *Initiation and Its Results*, 57–58; Steiner, "Wie erlangt man Erkenntnisse der höheren Welten?," 323.

17. Annie Besant, *Thought Power*, 95.

18. Ibid., 76 (original emphasis).

19. Ibid., 77.

20. Steiner, *Initiation and Its Results*, 47, 50. Besant explained these qualities in *The Ancient Wisdom*, 327–33, where she listed the first as "discrimination between the real and the unreal," the second as "indifference to the unreal, the transitory," the third as given in note 12 in the present chapter, and the fourth as "desire for liberation" (333).

21. Florin Lowndes has a different interpretation. He notes that Steiner mentions a lotus with eight petals—which may be the *hṛt* chakra, the minor chakra between the navel and heart chakras. Following Steiner's linking of developmental practices to half the number of petals in each chakra, Lowndes links the attainment of the four qualifications I discuss here to the lotus with eight petals. The location of this traditional chakra is similar to that of a "preliminary" or "temporary" center in the area of the heart discussed by Steiner in *Initiation and Its Results*, 41–45, and *How to Know Higher Worlds*, 133–35. I deal with this temporary center later. See Lowndes, *Enlivening the Chakra of the Heart*, 34.

22. Radhasoami writings also tend to list the chakras from the top down. It is worth noting that Steiner's colleague in the German TS, Wilhelm Hübbe-Schleiden, spent time at the Radhasoami Satsang in Agra during his 1894–96 trip to India, as described in his *Indisches Tagebuch 1894/1896* (Indian diary), 173, 207–8—and was apparently practicing the sound-current meditation taught there (267). Radhasoami places particular emphasis on meditating on the sixth chakra (called til) to perceive higher planes, including those achieved by various degrees of saints (Mukherji, "Radhaswami [sic] Society of Agra," 709–10, 713–14 [August 1895]). Compare the previously cited passage on the sixth chakra from *Initiation and Its Results*, 57–58, in which Steiner speaks of "connection with spiritual, superhuman entities" and "currents" that "reveal the things of the higher worlds."

23. See Leland, *Invisible Worlds*, 159.

24. Steiner, *Initiation and Its Results*, 44; Steiner, "Wie erlangt man Erkenntnisse der höheren Welten?," 291. Christopher Bamford translates the phrase as "temporary center" (Steiner, *How to Know Higher Worlds*, 135).

25. Steiner, *Initiation and Its Results*, 45; Steiner, "Wie erlangt man Erkenntnisse der höheren Welten?," 291.

26. Steiner, *How to Know Higher Worlds*, 136; Steiner, "Wie erlangt man Erkenntnisse der höheren Welten?," 291. The equivalent passage in *Initiation and Its Results* renders *Häutchen* as "cuticle" (45).

27. Steiner, *Initiation and Its Results*, 42.

28. Ibid., 70–71.

29. Ibid., 71; Steiner, "Wie erlangt man Erkenntnisse der höheren Welten?," 355.

30. Steiner, *Initiation and Its Results*, 71. Note that Steiner later expunged the word *kundalini* from *Wie erlangt man Erkenntnisse der höheren Welten?* so it does not appear in later English translations.

Chapter 10

1. Blavatsky, *Collected Writings*, 3:281.

2. Olcott, *Old Diary Leaves* 3:34.

3. *The Theosophical Congress Held by the Theosophical Society at the Parliament of Religions, . . . Report of Proceedings and Documents*, 11.

4. Singleton, *Yoga Body*, 5, citing J. Gordon Melton, *New Age Encyclopedia: A Guide to the . . . New Global Movement toward Spiritual Development, Health, and Healing, Higher Consciousness, and Related Subjects*, 502 (original emphasis). The reference is to the 1890 edition. Both Singleton and Melton appear to have been unaware of Prasād's 1884 publication. Karl Baier's pioneering research into Sabhapaty Swami's writings suggests that *Om: A Treatise on Vedantic Raj Yoga Philosophy* (1880) is a better candidate for first yoga manual in English. See Karl Baier, *Meditation und Moderne: zur Genese eines Kernbereichs moderner Spiritualität in der Wechselwirkung zwischen Westeuropa, Nordamerika und Asien*, 1:363–69.

5. Rāma Prasād, *The Science of Breath and the Philosophy of the Tattwas*, 185, 248. Cited passages from this book appear with the title

Science of Breath; other references appear under the vernacular title, *Nature's Finer Forces*.

6. For a more recent complete translation with commentary, see Swami Muktibhodananda, *Swara Yoga*.

7. Prasād, *Science of Breath*: colors and shapes, 58–60 (essays); colors, 211 (verse 151); colors and shapes, 213–14 (verses 166–69). The phrase *in practice* refers to the tattva cards discussed later in this chapter in conjunction with the Golden Dawn system of magic. See King, *Tantra*, 57.

8. In 1904, Olcott refers to *Nature's Finer Forces* as the work that made Prasād known "to the whole Theosophical reading public, the world over" (*Old Diary Leaves* 3:34).

9. Biographical information from Wikipedia, s.v. "Swami Vivekananda."

10. For example, the essay "Swami Vivekananda and the Mainstreaming of the *Yoga Sutra*" in White, *"Yoga Sutra of Patanjali,"* 116–42.

11. Stefanie Syman, *The Subtle Body: The Story of Yoga in America*, 56.

12. In the revised edition of *Raja Yoga* cited in the bibliography, this drawing appears on page 51 with the following caption: "A symbolic representation of the kundalini rising through the different centers in the sushumna to the thousand-petaled lotus in the brain."

13. Swami Vivekananda, *Raja Yoga*, 34–64. Apparently, Sabhapaty Swami's *Om: A Treatise on Vedantic Raj Yoga Philosophy* was the first manual of tantric practices focused on the chakras published in English by an Indian teacher, fifteen years earlier than *Raja Yoga*. However, it was not a manual of chakra development, since its purpose was to dissolve the powers represented by the chakras in order to transcend them.

14. Blavatsky, *Collected Writings*, 12, foldout between 580 and 581, recto, plate II (*Esoteric Instructions*, foldout between 90 and 91).

15. Blavatsky, *Collected Writings*, 12, foldout between 580 and 581, verso, plate III (*Esoteric Instructions*, foldout between 94 and 95).

16. A. P. Sinnett, *The Human Aura, Transactions of the London Lodge*, no. 18.

17. Blavatsky contra Sinnett: *Collected Writings*, 12:526, 562 (*Esoteric Instructions*, 24–26; 87). Sinnett contra Blavatsky: *The Growth of the Soul: A Sequel to "Esoteric Buddhism,"* 155–58. Principles as lay-

ers of the aura: Sinnett, *Growth of the Soul*, 166–74. Blavatsky on the changing order of principles in the aura: *Collected Writings*, 12:543; 546–47 (*Esoteric Instructions*, 46, 54–55).

18. Leadbeater and the London Lodge and joint investigations of Besant and Leadbeater: Jinarājadāsa, *Occult Investigations*, 8–9.

19. See Besant, *Man and His Bodies*, 122–27.

20. A portion of this illustration, originally the frontispiece of Marques's *The Human Aura*, also appears on the front cover of the present book. Digitized versions of Marques's book do not include it, perhaps because it was a foldout.

21. This is the first publication of Fletcher's birth and death dates. Despite her brilliant career, there is no photographic or biographical information about her on the Internet related to any of the names she wrote under: E. A. Fletcher, Ella A. Fletcher, and Ella Adelia Fletcher. A notice in a Hawaiian newspaper indicated Fletcher's arrival in Honolulu in 1909 and mentioned that she was "the author of philosophic books" and was visiting her sister, Mrs. L. E. (Fannie) Thayer. See *Hawaiian Star* (Honolulu, HI), August 5, 1909. Fletcher's continuing residence in Honolulu was confirmed by data accessed on Ancestry.com, including census records and street directories; a reference to Findagrave.com with a photograph of Fletcher's grave, with birth and death dates; and other records that indicated she was born in Ohio, was raised in Galveston, Texas, and lived with her parents for an extended period in Jackson, Michigan, before beginning her editorial work in New York City (at which point she virtually disappeared from the public record, except the evidence of her publications). The 1930 US Census lists the race of her and her sister as "octoroon," meaning one of their great grandparents was black. I wonder to what degree the absence of information on Fletcher was a result of self-censorship in connection with contemporary race, gender, or even sexuality issues.

22. Unsigned review of Ella Adelia Fletcher's *The Woman Beautiful*, "New Books," *Washington Post*, March 19, 1900.

23. Wikipedia, s.v. "Williams Jennings Demorest."

24. Elizabeth Towne, "Nautilus News: A New Contributor," 1.

25. Ella Adelia Fletcher, *The Law of the Rhythmic Breath: Teaching the Generation, Conservation, and Control of Vital Force*, 191 (muladhara); 130, 337 (thousand-petaled lotus).

26. Ibid., 291–303. This list appears to be a reinterpretation of a two-part diagram in Esoteric Instruction No. 2. See Blavatsky, *Collected Writings*, 12:564 (*Esoteric Instructions*, 88–89).

27. See Flying Rolls nos. 11, 25, 26, and 30 in Francis King, *Ritual Magic of the Golden Dawn: Works by S. L. MacGregor Mathers and Others*, 75–94. A prefatory note explains the procedure, 65–69.

28. For a summary and explanation of Mathers's paper "On the Tattwas of the Eastern School," see King, *Tantra*, 77–85.

29. Back cover of Israel Regardie, *A Garden of Pomegranates: An Outline of the Qabalah*.

30. King, *Tantra*, 71.

31. Marques, *Human Aura*, foldout facing page 16. Unfortunately, this foldout has been dropped from digitized versions of the book and recent reprints. Marques linked the first three sephiroth (Kether, Chokmah, Binah) with the monad (*ātma-buddhi-manas*). The remaining seven were linked with the principles as embodied in human experience and the layers of the aura: atman (Chesed), buddhi (Geburah), higher manas (Tiphereth), lower manas (Netzach), kama (Hod), prana (Yesod), and sthula (Malkuth).

32. Aleister Crowley, *777 and Other Qabalistic Writings of Aleister Crowley, Including Gematria and Sephir Sephiroth*, vii–viii. Crowley was in India in 1902 and 1905 (http://www.lashtal.com/wiki/Aleister_Crowley_Timeline, accessed December 25, 2015). However, it has been impossible to determine whether the swami was still alive at that time. References to him peak in the 1880s and dwindle away by 1900. His death date remains unknown.

33. Ibid., 22, columns CXVII and CXVIII.

34. Blavatsky indicated that for esoteric purposes, sthula, the dense body, was not a principle but the basis of the other seven (*Collected Writings*, 12: 526 [*Esoteric Instructions*, 24])—hence the common division of manas into higher (buddhi-manas) and lower (kama-manas) to make up the full complement of seven principles.

35. Crowley revised this list a year later in "The Temple of Solomon the King," 87n. Malkuth is assigned to the first chakra, Yesod to the second, the path between Netzach and Hod to the third, Tiphereth to the fourth, the path between Chesed and Geburah to the fifth, Daath to the sixth, and Kether to the seventh. The path between the second and third

sephiroth, Chokmah and Binah, is skipped (or possibly subsumed into Daath). Thus Crowley sticks with the middle pillar of the Tree of Life.

36. First English translation: Bose, *Life of Sris Chandra Basu*, 131–32.

37. Chakra discussion: Crowley, "The Temple of Solomon the King," 86–91, http://babel.hathitrust.org/cgi/pt?id=mdp.39015088371391;view=1up;seq=98. Diagram: ibid., facing page 90.

Crowley later made notes in the margins of this diagram that identified the seven "Man of Earth" degrees in his fraternal order of ceremonial magic, Ordo Templi Orientis (OTO), with the seven chakras. In researching this book, I saw several references to a connection between the chakras and initiatory degrees in the Golden Dawn tradition. Though Crowley emerged from this tradition, the innovation appears to be his, and later Golden Dawn–based groups seem to have followed his lead. I have not seen evidence of such a correlation during the relatively brief existence of the original Hermetic Order of the Golden Dawn (1888–1901). See Baphomet XI°, "The Man of Earth Degrees and the Hindu Chakras," 193. Baphomet XI° was one of Crowley's aliases in the teen years of the twentieth century.

38. Regardie, *Garden of Pomegranates*, 93.

39. See Dione Fortune, *The Mystical Qabalah*, 71–76 for her discussion of correlations between the chakras and the sephiroth. Fortune proceeds as follows, using only the middle pillar: (1) Malkuth; (2) Yesod; (3) Tiphereth; (4) Tiphereth; (5) Daath; (6) Daath; (7) Kether.

40. I am indebted to King's *Tantra*, 38–39, for the translations of Hebrew terms for the sephiroth and for quoted remarks.

41. This mapping was suggested in a series of articles published by Fortune in 1939–40 in the journal of her organization, the Society of Inner Light, and published posthumously in book form as *The Circuit of Force: Occult Dynamics of the Etheric Vehicle* (Dion Fortune and Gareth Knight, 1998). Here, Fortune presented a well-reasoned set of correlations between the chakras and the sephiroth, including Daath, which expanded and supplanted her earlier brief mention in *The Mystical Qabalah*. She argued that the nodes where the paths connecting opposing sephiroth on the right and left pillars of the Tree of Life intersect the middle pillar represented not only certain chakras, but also the equilibration of these opposing forces (66). However, Gareth Knight

(Basil Wilby), editor of *The Circuit of Force*, suggests that if we were to use the five chakras of the Tibetan system instead of the seven of the Hindu, there is no need to go beyond the middle pillar of the Tree of Life, which has five sephiroth when Daath is included (90).

Chapter 11

1. Singleton, *Yoga Body*, 148–49 (black-and-white illustration on 149; the original is in color; see plate 8 in the present book).
2. Biographical information from Blavatsky, *Collected Writings*, 12:761–65.
3. James M. Pryse, *The Apocalypse Unsealed: Being an Interpretation of the Initiation of Ioannes, Commonly Called the Revelation of St. John, with a New Translation*, vii and subtitle (emphasis mine).
4. Ibid., 24.
5. Ibid., 15–19.
6. Ibid., 19, 41.
7. Ibid., 36–39.
8. Ibid., 46–50.
9. Ibid., 22–24.
10. Alice Bailey referenced this cross in *Esoteric Healing*, linking the two horizontal arms to the two petals of ajna chakra (149–50).
11. See Leland, *Invisible Worlds*, 276–79n7, for a detailed explanation of these terms and a discussion of the relationship between bodies and principles.
12. Pryse, *Apocalypse Unsealed*, 24. Blavatsky's *Voice of the Silence*, 12 and 77, refers to the slaying of the lunar body, identified with the personality (presumably the lower quaternary of kama-prana-linga-sthula), as well as the paralyzing of that portion of the individuality identified with the mental body (kama-manas) before the raising of the kundalini "can make of thee a god"—presumably Pryse's imperishable solar body (consciousness identified with the higher triad, atma-buddhi-manas—the monad). As David Gordon White indicates in *Alchemical Body*, one goal of yoga and other Indian spiritual traditions, including Tantra, is to produce an immortal body (1–14).
13. Spierenburg, *Inner Group Teachings*, 4.
14. Ibid., diagrams on 68, 71, and 73 and text on 14, 70, and 72. Note that Pryse is mapping the cosmos (planes) into the body in a way

that implies that the spiritual plane is linked with chakras six and seven, the psychic world with chakras four and five, the phantasmal world with chakra three, and the physical world with chakras one and two—as in figure 11 in the present book.

15. Blavatsky, *Collected Writings*, 12:695, 696 (*Esoteric Instructions*, 208, 239). (The wording is different; I follow the latter.)

16. Blavatsky, *Collected Writings*, 12:619 (*Esoteric Instructions*, 142).

17. Blavatsky, *Collected Writings*, 12: 526 (*Esoteric Instructions*, 24).

18. H. P. Blavatsky, *The Theosophical Glossary*, s.v. "antahkarana."

19. The list of principles closest to that given here appears in the transcript of the first meeting of Blavatsky's Inner Group (Spierenburg, *Inner Group Teachings*, 4).

Chapter 12

1. Biographical details summarized from Gregory Tillett, *The Elder Brother: A Biography of Charles Webster Leadbeater*, 19–40.

2. C. W. Leadbeater, *How Theosophy Came to Me*, 149–53. A less developed version of the story also appears in his *The Inner Life*, 208, and *Chakras*, 75–76.

3. Blavatsky, *Collected Writings*, 5:269.

4. Olcott, *Old Diary Leaves*, 3:394. Given that Subba Row was from Madras and Sabhapaty Swami was also located there, I wonder whether the latter was Subba Row's tantric guru.

5. Blavatsky, *Collected Writings*, 5:269.

6. Leadbeater, *How Theosophy Came to Me*, 151, 153.

7. C. W. Leadbeater, "The Aura," *Theosophist* 17:140 (December 1895). Pamphlet: *The Aura: An Enquiry into the Nature and Functions of the Luminous Mist Seen about Human and Other Bodies* (1897).

8. C. W. Leadbeater, *Man Visible and Invisible*, 71.

9. In Sarah Corbett, *Extracts from the Vahan, Including Answers by Annie Besant, A. P. Sinnett, G. R. S. Mead, C. W. Leadbeater, Bertram Keightley, Dr. A. A. Wells, and Others*, 527. This passage appears verbatim in C. W. Leadbeater, *Clairvoyance* (1899), 16–17.

10. In *Man's Latent Powers* (1938), 48–49, Theosophist and clairvoyant Phoebe Payne wrote that each chakra "acts as a vortex of energy

drawing matter of its own subtle quality into a current by its whirling action, and thus throwing a stream of force through the stalk of the vortex into the physical body. There is also a reverse action. . . ." In a later book written with her husband, Laurence J. Bendit, this reverse action is explained as follows: The inflowing energy, from chakra to center, corresponds to the organs of cognition or sensation (jnanendriyas); the outflowing energy, from center to chakra, corresponds to the organs of action (karmendriyas). Thus inflowing astral energy allows us to perceive the astral plane and outflowing astral energy allows us to act on the astral plane. See Phoebe D. Payne and Laurence J. Bendit, *The Psychic Sense*, 82–89. Much that is obscure in Besant's and Leadbeater's writings on centers and chakras is clarified by these books, published within ten years of their deaths.

11. Jinarājadāsa, *Occult Investigations*, 13, 32–34, 41–47, 66–71.

12. Annie Besant, "Thought-Forms," including color plates. See Arthur H. Nethercot, *The Last Four Lives of Annie Besant*, 58–61, for an account of the 1897 American tour, including the use of slides.

13. Biographical details summarized from Tillett, *Elder Brother*, 77–102.

14. Leadbeater, *Inner Life*, xvi.

15. Ibid., 196–98.

16. Ibid., 207.

17. Ibid., 209–10.

18. Some years later, Alice A. Bailey discussed these webs in detail in *A Treatise on White Magic* (1934), 590–93.

19. Leadbeater, *Inner Life*, 196.

20. Ibid., 199.

21. Pryse, *Apocalypse Unsealed*, viii; C. W. Leadbeater, "Force-Centers and the Serpent-Fire," 1075–94.

22. This list of colors is derived from the table in Blavatsky, *Collected Writings*, 12:614, with variant colors from the foldout between 532 and 533 (figure 5 in the present book) (*Esoteric Instructions*, foldouts between 130 and 131 and between 40 and 41).

23. C. W. Leadbeater, *The Hidden Side of Things*, 43–57.

24. Srisa Chandra Vasu, *The Siva Samhita*, 62–73.

25. See Amy Wallace and Bill Henkin, *The Psychic Healing Book: How to Develop Your Psychic Potential Safely, Simply, Effectively*, 27–30. This book has been continuously in print for more than thirty-five years.

26. *Amṛta-Nāda Upaniṣad* 34–37 lists names, locations, and colors. *Dhyāna-Bindu Upaniṣad* 94–96 lists names, locations, colors, bijas, and elements.

27. Blavatsky, *Collected Writings*, 12:699 (*Esoteric Instructions*, 199–200). (The wording is different.)

28. Leadbeater, *Chakras*, 54. James Mallinson dates the *Gheraṇḍa Saṃhitā* to ca. 1700 CE (*The Gheranda Samhita: The Original Sanskrit and an English Translation*, xiv).

Chapter 13

1. Information in this paragraph and the previous one is from Wikipedia and from Feuerstein, *Encyclopedia of Yoga and Tantra*, s.v. "Sir John Woodroffe."

2. Taylor, *Sir John Woodroffe, Tantra, and Bengal*, 148.

3. See, for example, Alice A. Bailey, *The Soul and Its Mechanism*, 94–95 (*The Serpent Power*), and *Letters on Occult Meditation*, 77–78 (*The Inner Life*).

4. Avalon, *Serpent Power*, 12.

5. Ibid., 13n.

6. White, *Kiss of the Yoginī*, 8–14.

7. See Bühnemann, "The Six Rites of Magic," 447–48.

8. Avalon, *Serpent Power*, 20–21.

9. Leadbeater, *The Hidden Life in Freemasonry*, 275; *Chakras*, 27.

10. In a presentation of publishing statistics for Quest Books on July 19, 2015, Sharron Dorr, managing editor of Quest Books, stated that the Quest edition of *The Chakras*, first published in 1972, had sold more than 200,000 copies. The book had already been in print for forty-five years by then. It has also been translated into more than a dozen languages. By 2012, when I was asked to edit a new edition, worldwide sales may have reached 600,000 copies, including those sold by Quest Books (phone conversation of August 8, 2012 with Sharron Dorr; subsequent email clarification on February 11, 2016, by Pat Griebeler of Theosophical Publishing House, Wheaton, IL).

11. Further particulars of the editing process may be gleaned from Kurt Leland, "*The Chakras*: An Editorial Report." The article includes several passages and an illustration that were dropped after the first edition. I would have included this material in the appendix of the 2013 edition if I had been aware of it.

12. Biographical information summarized from Ernest Egerton Wood, *Is This Theosophy . . .?*

13. Ibid., 297. The passage in question is as follows: "The surfaces of the streams of the primary force [i.e., vitality or prana] and the kundalini grind together at this point [in the centers along the spine], as they revolve in opposite directions and considerable pressure is caused" (Leadbeater, *Chakras*, 29).

14. Arthur Versluis notes that the true title of Gichtel's book (as translated from German into English) is *A Brief Revelation and Instruction on the Three Principles and Worlds in Man*, and that *Theosophia Practica* is a misnomer resulting from a publisher applying the title of a different work by Gichtel to this one (Arthur Versluis, *Wisdom's Children: A Christian Esoteric Tradition*, 34). Versluis has published an English translation of Gichtel's work under the title *Awakening to Divine Wisdom: Christian Initiation into Three Worlds*, including a reproduction of the original German version of plate 5.

15. Ibid., 177, 180–82. *Llewellyn's Complete Book of Chakras: Your Definitive Source of Energy Center Knowledge for Health, Happiness, and Spiritual Evolution*, by Cyndi Dale, devotes several pages (695–98) to an alchemical interpretation of the process of regeneration illustrated in Gichtel's illustrations, providing a somewhat more convincing connection between the chakras and Gichtel's planets, centers, organs, and elements.

16. Ransom, *Short History of the Theosophical Society*, 441, 452.

17. This list of colors is derived from the table in Blavatsky, *Collected Writings*, 12:614, with variant colors from the foldout between 532 and 533 (figure 5 in the present book) (*Esoteric Instructions*, foldouts between 130 and 131 and between 40 and 41).

18. Blavatsky, *Collected Writings*, 12:699 (*Esoteric Instructions*, 199–200). (The wording is different.)

19. However, there may also have been another reason, related to the teachings of Sabhapaty Swami. In *A Collection of Lectures on Theosophy and Archaic Religions*, Olcott lists the locations of the chakras in an illustration by Sabhapaty as follows: "the nasal cavity, the mouth, the root of the throat, the heart, the umbilicus, etc." (178). In a later edition, under the title *Theosophy, Religion, and Occult Science* (1885), Olcott replaced the word *etc.* with *spleen*. (152). In plate 2 in the present book, it appears that *svādhiṣṭhāna cakra* has been eliminated, but the

swami's writings indicate that it has actually been moved up to the area of the navel (Estep, *Esoteric Cosmic Yogi Science*, 138). This apparent skipping of svadhishthana and substitution of the spleen is exactly what Leadbeater presented in his description of the chakras.

20. Leadbeater, *Chakras*, 51.

21. Ibid., 48.

22. One of these diagrams (Blavatsky, *Collected Writings*, 12, foldout between 532 and 533 (figure 5 in the present book) links the colors and principles. Two others, with slightly different color correspondences, link the colors and principles with parts of the body (12:614, 630–31). See also *Esoteric Instructions*, foldouts between 40 and 41, 130 and 133, and 260 and 261.

23. Leadbeater, *Chakras*, 84.

24. Wood, *Is This Theosophy . . . ?*, 126.

25. Rishi Singh Gherwal, *Kundalini, the Mother of the Universe: The Piercing of the Six Chakras*, 146, 152. Gherwal's original given name was Rakha. Though he published under the name Gherwal, most public records use the surname Grewel. Birth and death dates from Ancestry.com.

26. Compare, for example, Sri Chinmoy, *Kundalini: The Mother Power*, a set of lectures given at New York University in 1974, pp. 6–24, with C. W. Leadbeater, *The Chakras*, 9–11. Chinmoy adopted Leadbeater's spleen chakra (absent from tantric teachings), colors, and revision of the number of petals in the sixth chakra (96 instead of 2) and seventh chakra (960 instead of 1000). For Satyananda's references to psychic abilities outlined by Leadbeater, see note 30, below.

27. See diagram in Bailey, *Esoteric Healing*, 715.

28. Jenny McFarlane, *Concerning the Spiritual: The Influence of the Theosophical Society on Australian Artists 1890-1934*, 116.

29. Rosalyn Bruyere locates the chakras "along a central axis parallel to the spinal column of the physical body" (*Wheels of Light: A Study of the Chakras*, vol. 1, 67). See also Judith, *Wheels of Life* (1999), 17.

30. For indications of Leadbeater's influence on Satyananda Saraswati, see *Kundalini Tantra,* 133–34 (ajna); 143–45 (muladhara); 154–55 (svadhishthana); 160–61 (manipura); 171–72 (anahata); 178–79 (vishuddha).

Chapter 14

1. Biographical information on Alice Bailey from Alice A. Bailey, *The Unfinished Autobiography*, supplemented by Wikipedia, s.v. "Alice Bailey."

2. Alice A. Bailey, *Initiation: Human and Solar*, 163–65.

3. Vera Stanley Alder, *The Initiation of the World*, 85–86. Information about initiation in connection with the subplanes appears in a somewhat different form in Bailey, *Initiation: Human and Solar*, 179–80.

4. Blavatsky, *Collected Writings*, 12, foldout between 660 and 661 (*Esoteric Instructions*, 260–61).

5. Alice A. Bailey, *Letters on Occult Meditation*, 212–13.

6. Ibid., 358.

7. Ibid., 359.

8. Ibid., 19.

9. Alice A. Bailey, *Esoteric Psychology* 1:142, 401–3.

10. Ibid., 1:404–6.

11. Later books by other authors sometimes identify the first chakra as sacral. Bailey calls it "the center at the base of the spine" or "base center." See, for example, Bailey, *Esoteric Healing*, 176–83, for discussions of these centers. For a list of the minor centers or chakras, see *Esoteric Healing*, 72–73.

12. Bailey, *Letters on Occult Meditation*, 71.

13. Alice A. Bailey, *The Light of the Soul: Its Science and Effect—a Paraphrase of the Yoga Sutras of Patanjali*, 309.

14. Bailey, *Soul and Its Mechanism*, 120.

15. Judith, *Wheels of Life* (1987), 20 (diagram) and 46–47 (table); (1999), 22 (diagram), 42–44 (table).

16. Bailey, *Esoteric Healing*, 142. The list did not change since it was first presented in *Light of the Soul*.

17. From Bailey, *Esoteric Psychology* 1:261. In vol. 2 of the same work a slightly different correlation of rays and centers is given: the seventh ray is moved to the first chakra, the fifth ray is moved to the second chakra, and the fourth ray is moved to the sixth chakra. The other rays remain the same (521). Bailey gives no reason for these changes. However, just as the enumeration I provide in this table pertains to the "average aspirant," so this altered version may apply to the less advanced, "average man."

18. Bailey, *Esoteric Psychology* 1:418–20, using the "esoteric colors" listed.

19. From Bailey, *Esoteric Healing* (in descending order): 145, 148–49, 153–54, 158–59, 171–72, 176, 177. This list of qualities seems to have developed gradually from book to book through a process of accretion and sifting of material on the centers. An earlier version, minus the sixth and seventh chakras, occurs in *Esoteric Psychology*, vol. 2, 523, published in 1942. Another earlier version that shares some elements of the list in this table occurs in *Esoteric Astrology* (1951), 455–56. The version from *Esoteric Healing* is the clearest and most concise of these lists, and therefore has had the most impact on the later evolution of the chakra system.

20. Bailey, *Esoteric Psychology* 1:26, 268, 261–62.

21. Ibid., 1:268–307.

22. Bailey, *Esoteric Healing*, 83, 170–72.

23. See, for example, the discussion of awakened versus unawakened chakras and over- versus under-stimulated chakras in *Esoteric Healing*, 73–88. The notion of "blocking" in the chakras is introduced on page 74 and that of improperly balanced chakras on 84. The earliest reference in the Bailey corpus to balancing chakras appears to be *A Treatise on White Magic* (1934), 595.

24. Alice A. Bailey, *Telepathy and the Etheric Vehicle*, 136.

Chapter 15

1. Herman H. Rubin, *Your Mysterious Glands: How Your Glands Control Your Mental and Physical Development and Moral Welfare*, 34, 59.

2. Ibid., facing 90.

3. Singleton, *Yoga Body*, 148.

4. Marc-Alain Descamps, author of *Histoire du Hatha-Yoga en France, passé et présent*, writes on a webpage entitled "L'histoire surprenante de l'arrivée du Hatha-Yoga en France" ("The amazing history of the arrival of hatha-yoga in France") that Cajzoran Ali was born on December 13, 1903, in Memphis, Tennessee, and died in 1975 (http://europsy.org/marc-alain/histyog.html). This information is proliferating on the Web—though both dates are nearly ten years too late, the month is wrong, and the actual location was about 750 miles away.

5. The 1900 US Census on Ancestry.com gives January 1894 and Pocahontas County. Four New York passenger lists from the 1930s, also on Ancestry.com, give either Havelock, Iowa (in Pocahontas County), or the county itself as the location, as well as the more precise date given here.

6. "Word was received here by relatives that Miss Amber Steen who has been confined in a Sioux Falls Hospital and who has underwent four operations, was taken to her home at Harrisburg [South Dakota], without any hopes of recovery. She is suffering with tuberculosis." "Havelock News," *Pocahontas (IA) Record*, December 7, 1916. Illness first announced in "County Correspondents: Havelock," *Pocahontas Record*, October 26, 1916; last mention in "Arrowettes," *Pocahontas Record*, April 26, 1917.

7. "Self-Mastery Saves Life Where Nine Operations Fail," *San Antonio Express*, August 5, 1928.

8. "Note for Leonard Walter McGilvra, 20 FEB 1897–17 NOV 1956," http://freepages.genealogy.rootsweb.ancestry.com/~fuma/ghtout/np19.htm; "Cult Leader's Nationality Puzzles New Yorkers; Claim Man a Fakir," *Norfolk (VA) Journal and Guide*, August 3, 1929. Information about Sheikh Ali's birth year also derives from this source.

9. From examining display ads in various digitized newspapers, I have documented dates, locations, and many titles for about 140 lectures by Hazrat Ismet Ali from 1926 to 1929, in Buffalo, Chicago, Cleveland, Hartford, Milwaukee, New Haven, New York City, Pittsburgh, and Syracuse, including two radio appearances in New York; I have also documented a dozen lectures by Cajzoran Ali (restricted to Buffalo and New York City) from 1927 to 1930.

10. Temple of Supreme Consciousness: William C. Hartmann, *Hartmann's Who's Who in Occult, Psychic, and Spiritual Realms in the United States and Foreign Countries*, 175.

11. "Ali's Mysticism Didn't Foretell Prison Term," *Chicago Defender*, national edition, January 18, 1930; "Prosecutor to Bring Fugitive from West Indies," *Chicago Daily Tribune*, October 25, 1930; "Law Takes Sheikh in Native Trinidad," *Decatur (IL) Review*, October 26, 1930.

12. New York passenger lists on Ancestry.com indicate that Steen returned to the United States from France on April 19, 1931 (under the name Ann Williams); May 31, 1934 (as Ann Stein Williams); April 1,

1936 (as Ann Williams); and July 3, 1939 (as Anne Amber Williams). Addresses given in connection with these records correspond to those of relatives in Chicago or Denver.

13. Wikipedia, s.v. "Otoman Zar-Adusht Ha'nish." The date of Hanish's birth is disputed, sometimes given as 1844 or 1854. The date I provide is from a 1911 US Passport application for Otto Z. Hanish, along with his place of birth (also disputed, sometimes given as Russia or Tehran)—in Stuhm, Prussia (now Sztum, Poland). Corroborative details may be found at Ancestry.com using Otto Z. Hanish as the search name and 1866 as the birth year.

14. If Steen's journey to and initiations in India were not merely astral, then it is possible that she pursued initiation at a Radhasoami Satsang, such as that at Beas. This was one of the few spiritual organizations at the time that touted leadership by a living master and offered instant initiation to Westerners. See Juergensmeyer, *Radhasoami Reality*, 203–6, for information on the attraction of Radhasoami for Westerners.

15. See Jean-Pierre Wenger, *François Brousse: l'Enlumineur des mondes; biographie*, 94–106.

16. "She made the trip to the New York fair with her friend of many years Amber Rahanii Steen, now Mrs. Ekberg, who had likewise left most of her possessions in her Paris studio" ("Princess Olga Sherinsky [*sic*] Honor Guest at Tea Given by Mrs. H. A. Ekberg," *Homestead (FL) Leader-Enterprise*, March 10, 1950). The princess did not arrive on the same boat as Steen. Ancestry.com lists her date of arrival as July 26, 1939. Steen arrived three weeks earlier.

17. "Amber Ekberg" and "Hjalmer Ekberg" in 1940 US Census on Ancestry.com.

18. "Princess Olga Sherinsky [*sic*] Honor Guest at Tea Given by Mrs. H. A. Ekberg," *Homestead (FL) Leader-Enterprise*, March 10, 1950.

19. Steen's life during the 1940s and early 1950s, including her art club activities and travels, may be tracked by means of a digitized run of the *Homestead (FL) Leader-Enterprise* from the University of Florida at http://ufdc.ufl.edu/UF00087294/allvolumes (1931–44); and *Homestead (FL) Leader* (1944–50) at http://ufdc.ufl.edu/UF00087295/00153/allvolumes.

20. Kalyanii (Dr. Kevon Arthurs), http://yogibuzz.com/kalyanii/, accessed September 6, 2015.

21. Claude Bragdon, *Yoga for You*, frontispiece and 81–85. The frontispiece appears to have been copied from a diagram in Yogi Wassan, *Secrets of the Himalaya Mountain Masters and Ladder to Cosmic Consciousness* (1927), "Opana Yama Health and Beauty Chart," unpaginated. Wassan Singh (1882–1942) was born in the Punjab, migrated to the United States in 1907, and did the yogi lecture circuit for years. His carefully copyrighted teachings and diagrams concerning the chakras are eclectic and eccentric—and bear further study with regard to origins and influence. (Biographical information from Ancestry.com, including US Naturalization Records and Wassan Family Tree.)

22. Bragdon, *Yoga for You*, xi. Bragdon's story about meeting the woman who was the source of the communications from the Brown Brother probably refers to Rahanii/Steen. Bragdon says that this woman came to New York "from a distant Southern city . . . in June 1942" (Ibid., v). Newspaper accounts indicate that Steen was in New York at that time. See "In and Around Homestead," *Homestead (FL) Leader-Enterprise*: "Leaves soon for an extended visit in New York," April 24, 1942; "visiting in New York," June 26, 1942; "spent summer in New York," October 16, 1942.

23. Various details in this paragraph from "Mrs. Olga Shirinsky, Ex-Russian Princess," Obituary, *Miami (FL) News*, February 23, 1963. The article calls Mrs. Ekberg the princess's niece.

24. "Amber Ann Ekberg" in *Florida Death Index 1877–1998*, accessed at http://www.ancestry.com.

25. David Shea and Anthony Troyer, *Dabistān* 1:404–5. See chapter 1, note 16 for background information on *Dabistān*.

26. Cajzoran Ali, *Divine Posture: Influence upon Endocrine Glands*, 99.

27. Shea and Troyer, *The Dabistān or School of Manners: The Religious Beliefs, Observances, Philosophic Opinions, and Social Customs of the Nations of the East* (1901), 250. The author of the book, by belief a Persian Parsi (Zoroastrian), may have appealed to Steen as an exemplar of her own neo-Zoroastrian beliefs.

28. Blavatsky, *Collected Writings*, 12, foldout between 532 and 533 (figure 5 in the present book) (*Esoteric Instructions*, foldout between 40 and 41).

29. Leigh Eric Schmidt, *Heaven's Bride: The Unprintable Life of Ida C. Craddock, American Mystic, Scholar, Sexologist, Martyr, and

Madwoman, 132. Pages 131–33 provide a basic orientation to Mazdaznan and its troubled founder.

Chapter 16

1. Biographical information from Association for Research and Enlightenment (ARE), *The Official Edgar Cayce Readings*, chronologies attached to report of reading 254-1 (February 13, 1911). In the ARE indexing system, the first number refers to the series of readings for an individual or group and the second to the place the reading holds in that series. The 254 series deals with Cayce's work and this was the first reading in that series.

2. Details in this paragraph from K. Paul Johnson, *Edgar Cayce in Context: The Readings: Truth and Fiction*, except the remark on spiritualism, which represents my own view.

3. ARE, *Official Edgar Cayce Readings*; the dream is described and interpreted in reading 294-127 (September 15, 1931).

4. Ibid., report attached to reading 281-17 (May 14, 1933), citing presentation of Gladys Davis (stenographer for the Cayce readings) of June 18, 1933, at the ARE's Second Annual Congress. The number 281 refers to the Glad Helpers series of readings.

5. In my afterword to Leadbeater's *Chakras*, 109–10, I indicated that Ivah Bergh Whitten was responsible for linking the rainbow colors to the chakras through a book published by her student Roland Hunt in 1940. It appears that the Cayce association predated Whitten's. I take up this issue in the next chapter of this book, providing evidence that the chakra/rainbow correlation by Whitten goes back at least to 1932.

6. ARE, *Official Edgar Cayce Readings*, report attached to reading 281-10 (August 17, 1932), in which Gladys Davis mentions the 1909 edition of Pryse's translation of the Gospel of St. John from Greek, *The Magical Message according to Ioannes*. I have confirmed with ARE archivist Claire Gardner and librarian Laura Hoff that this book and Pryse's *Apocalypse Unsealed* are both in the ARE library.

7. Johnson, *Edgar Cayce in Context*, 124.

8. The pituitary's epithet *master gland* may have been coined by Dr. Harvey Williams Cushing (1869–1939), a pioneer of neurosurgery, who published the first research on the effects of pituitary malfunction on other endocrine glands in 1912. Reflecting on this research in 1932,

Cushing stated that even then "it was strongly suspected that this centrally placed and well protected structure in all probability represented the master-gland of the endocrine series" ("The Basophil Adenomas of the Pituitary and Their Clinical Manifestation," *Bulletin of Johns Hopkins Hospital* 50:137). This epithet is now firmly embedded in Anglophone popular culture. It does not appear in Rubin's *Your Mysterious Glands* of 1925, so I suspect that the 1932 publication represents its first appearance—about four years before the development of Cayce's version of the chakra system.

The debate about whether the pituitary, as the master gland of the body, should be assigned to the crown chakra or to the third-eye chakra continued until at least the end of the century. In 1999, Naomi Ozaniec presented perhaps the cleverest resolution of the quandary by pointing out that the Sanskrit name of the sixth chakra (*ajna*) means "command"—and therefore the pituitary, as the master gland of the body, "seems well-attributed" to the sixth chakra. Furthermore, the pineal gland has been found by scientists to be sensitive to light and should therefore correspond to the spiritual light of the seventh chakra. To Ozaniec, the fact that the pituitary has two parts and the traditional iconography of the sixth chakra has two petals seemed to close the case. (Naomi Ozaniec, *The Chakras: A Beginner's Guide*, 57).

9. Andrea Diem-Lane, *The Guru in America: The Influence of Radhasoami on New American Religions*, 50, citing Kirpal Singh. Other biographical information in this chapter from the website of David Thind, http://www.bhagatsinghthind.com/about_thind.php, accessed January 31, 2016.

10. Bhagat Singh Thind, *Master Course in the Teachings of the Sikh Saviors: Sixty Free Lectures on Divine Realization.*

11. Display ads, *New York Times*, October 22, 1927, and November 5, 1927.

12. Display ads, *New York Times*, October 1, 1927.

13. "Other Services," *New York Times*, October 29, 1927.

14. It is possible that a pamphlet by Bhagat Singh Thind, entitled *Science of Breathing and Glands: All Life on Earth Is Breath; All Else on Earth is Death* and published by Thind's son David in 2004, is a reprint of the pamphlet listed in this brochure. A number of breaths for stimulating glands such as the sex glands, adrenals, spleen, solar plexus,

thyroid, pituitary, and pineal are given, but not in this order or with any mention of the chakras.

15. Bhagat Singh Thind, *Sikh Saviors* (1934). I have supplied the year based on the days of the week and dates given for individual lectures.

16. ARE, *Official Edgar Cayce Readings*, report attached to reading 255-5 (January 10, 1931), citing letter of reading recipient of March 16, 1933.

17. Ibid., program of congress attached to report for reading 254-87 (June 30, 1935); 5747-2 (June 28, 1935).

18. Ibid., 294-141 (April 23, 1932).

19. Johnson's discussion of Cayce's version of the Lord's Prayer (*Edgar Cayce in Context*, 123–24) relies on several later sources, published decades after Cayce's death. The version given here reflects the first mention in original source material (281-29).

20. Herbert B. Puryear and Mark Thurston added these lines in 1975 in *Meditation and the Mind of Man (Based on the Edgar Cayce Readings)*, 39.

21. Biographical information from Wikipedia, s.v. "Max Heindel." The first edition of Heindel's *The Rosicrucian Cosmo-Conception, or Christian Occult Science: An Elementary Treatise upon Man's Past Evolution, Present Constitution, and Future Development* is warmly dedicated to Steiner, whom Heindel met in Berlin in 1907. This dedication was dropped in subsequent editions. Some of Heindel's terminology, such as the names of the bodies (discussed in the present chapter) and the four ethers (discussed in chapter 18) are English adaptations of terms Steiner used during his teaching years within the TS.

22. Confirmed through correspondence with ARE archivist Claire Gardner, who supplied me with a photocopy of the original Glad Helpers list in March 2015.

23. Henry Reed, *Awakening Your Psychic Powers: Edgar Cayce's Wisdom for the New Age*, 169–77 (chart on 173). Reed uses the term *water chakra*, referring to the element associated with the second chakra. It is possible that this term—which also appears in Herbert B. Puryear's *Reflections on the Path (Based on the Edgar Cayce Readings)*, 108— was chosen so that the usual name, sexual or genital chakra, did not create confusion, since in the Cayce system the gonads (first chakra) and the cells of Leydig (second chakra) are both associated with the genitals.

24. Henry Reed, *Edgar Cayce on Channeling Your Higher Self*, 100–5 (diagram on 103).

25. Reed, *Awakening Your Psychic Powers*, 172.

26. Reed, *Edgar Cayce on Channeling*, 100.

27. Ibid., 101.

28. Ibid., 102–3.

29. Rubin, *Mysterious Glands*, 183 (interstitial cells); 184 (Leydig cells).

30. Ibid., 43, 57.

31. Mishra, *Discourses*, 308. The other centers, proceeding downward from the highest, "the seat or focus of the spirit," are the throat, solar plexus, navel, genital, and rectal—there is no heart center (314).

32. Mary Ellen Penny Baker, *Meditation: A Step Beyond with Edgar Cayce*, 69.

33. Herbert B. Puryear, *Reflections on the Path*, 103–14.

34. John van Auken, *Toward a Deeper Meditation: Rejuvenating the Body, Illuminating the Mind, Experiencing the Spirit*, 204.

35. Geoffrey Hodson, *The Science of Seership: A Study of the Faculty of Clairvoyance, Its Development and Use, Together with Examples of Clairvoyant Research*, 209–18 (especially 211–12, 216). See also his frontispiece. The book does not deal with other chakra/endocrine-gland correspondences.

36. Ibid., 209.

Chapter 17

1. For example, see the review of Christopher Hills's 1977 book *Nuclear Evolution: Discovery of the Rainbow Body* on the website of M. Alan Kezlev: http://www.kheper.net/topics/chakras/books.html, accessed September 9, 2015.

2. Melton, *New Age Encyclopedia*, s.v. "chromotherapy." Pleasonton's dates from Wikipedia. Theosophical associations from Blavatsky, *Collected Writings*, 1:520–21 (Pancoast), and email of Janet Kerschner, archivist at the Theosophical Society in America, October 27, 2014 (Ghadiali); further biographical information on Ghadiali from http://www.soul-guidance.com/health/colorhealing.htm, accessed January 25, 2016.

3. Bailey, *Letters on Occult Meditation*, 246–47 (original emphasis).

4. On the Mahatma letters, the origins of the Theosophical Society, and the controversial criticisms of the Society for Psychical Research, see Cranston, *H.P.B.*, 221–26 and 265–77; and Ransom, *Short History of the Theosophical Society*, 50, 209–16.

5. Perhaps the clearest presentation of these phases of evolution and the Masters in charge of the rays occurs in Ransom, *Short History of the Theosophical Society*, 42–56.

6. Blavatsky, *Collected Writings*, 12:492 (*Esoteric Instructions*, 343–44).

7. See, for example, Esoteric Instruction No. 2, Blavatsky, *Collected Writings*, 12: 542–80, especially 561–69 and figure 5 in the present book (*Esoteric Instructions*, 44–102, especially 85–99).

8. John W. Leonard, *Who's Who in New York City and State: Containing Authentic Biographies of New Yorkers Who Are Leaders and Representatives in Various Departments of Worthy Human Achievement* (1907), s.v. "Ivah de Chipenham Richardson."

9. Ivah Bergh Whitten, *What Color Means to You and the Meaning of Your Aura*, 13, mentions "notes made during twenty-eight years" of studying personal reactions to color. The book was published in 1932, hence the date of 1904 for the inception of such an interest.

10. "Church Workers," *New York Globe and Commercial Advertiser*, April 9, 1904.

11. J. Gordon Melton, *Encyclopedia of Occultism and Parapsychology*, s.v. "chromotherapy." I inadvertently neglected to cite this source in my afterword to Leadbeater's *The Chakras*.

12. H. L. Motter, ed., *The International Who's Who: Who's Who in the World* (1912), s.v. "Louis de Coppet Bergh," gives the date of June 19, 1904, for the wedding. However, the divorce from Louis Bergh's first wife did not proceed until 1906 ("Bergh Divorce Suit in Court," *New York Sun*, July 3, 1906) and a 1906 New York City Directory still lists an address for Ivah C. Richardson, accessed at Ancestry.com. The name Ivah Bergh first appears in newspaper articles in 1908.

13. "Doings of Women from Day to Day: Musings of Mollie," *Trenton (NJ) Evening Times*, March 27, 1908.

14. "Think in Curves and Be Beautiful. Angular, Scrawny Women to Be Transformed into Junos by New Method. Teacher Tells You How. Esthetic Physical Culture is Brought to Chicago by Miss Ivah Chipenham," *Chicago Tribune*, October 23, 1907; "Fair Exponent of 'Curved

Thoughts' Says Young Wives Will Follow Her," *Chicago Tribune*, October 24, 1907. The second article contains the only photograph of Whitten I have encountered.

15. Melton, *Encyclopedia of Occultism and Parapsychology*, s.v. "chromotherapy."

16. "Louis Bergh Dies of Heart Failure," *Washington Post*, January 28, 1913.

17. Cranston, *H.P.B*, 320–21.

18. Melton, *Encyclopedia of Occultism and Parapsychology*, s.v. "chromotherapy."

19. Personal email from Janet Kerschner, archivist of the Theosophical Society in America, February 22, 2013.

20. Janet Kerschner, email of February 23, 2013. Also Ancestry.com, which holds records of Aaron Whitten's earlier marriages.

21. Eva Kathryn Harris, "Society, Women's Interests, Club News," *Amarillo (TX) Globe*, May 18, 1924.

22. 1930 US Census on Ancestry.com.

23. http://www.roerich.org/roerich-biography.php, accessed June 20, 2015. It seems doubtful that the organization was ever called Amica Master Institute of Color Awareness, as given by Melton—despite my speculation in the afterword to *The Chakras* that *Amica* was a pun on the Latin word for friendship.

24. Melton, *Encyclopedia of Occultism and Parapsychology*, s.v. "chromotherapy."

25. Ibid.

26. Ivah Bergh Whitten, *The Initial Course in Color Awareness*, 1.

27. Leadbeater, *Chakras*, 109–111.

28. I examined a copy of Whitten's *Initial Course* held by the Stanford University library. The post office box number given therein for AMICA is the same as that given out before Whitten's death in 1947. This address was changed in 1959, when Roland Hunt founded the AMICA Temple of Radiance (discussed in the next chapter). Thus the book must have been published during the interval between these events.

29. Figure 19 is based on a less elaborate illustration in Whitten's *Initial Course*, 8. Roland Hunt, the illustrator, acknowledges his source in Bailey's *Initiation: Human and Solar* (Roland T. Hunt, *Fragrant and Radiant Symphony: An Enquiry into the Wondrous Correlation of the*

Healing Virtues of Color, Sound, and Perfume. . . ., 68). However, the true source is a diagram in Bailey's *Treatise on Cosmic Fire*, 344.

30. Whitten, *Initial Course*, 12–13.

31. Roland T. Hunt's *The Eighth Key to Color: Self-Analysis and Clarification through Color* employed such numerological analysis, but only of people's names (18–27).

32. Whitten, *Initial Course*, 29.

33. Ibid.

34. C. W. Leadbeater, *The Masters and the Path*, 189 (2002)

35. Whitten, *Initial Course*, 10.

36. Ibid., 37 (original emphasis).

37. Leadbeater, *Masters and the Path*, 157 (1925; not present in 2002 ed.).

38. Ibid., 173 (2002).

39. Whitten neglected to include a role for this ray. Based on contemporaneous teachings on the seven rays, I suggest the role of teacher as a possibility. Blunted triangle: trapezoid made from cutting off the point of an equilateral triangle.

40. Leadbeater, *Science of the Sacraments*, 90–91. Ordered service: "ceremonial which invokes angelic help" (91). List also cited in Leadbeater, *Masters and the Path*, 241 (2002).

41. Whitten, *Initial Course*, 30. Note that Rubin's diagram of the endocrine system (figure 14 in the present book) includes the "milk gland (in female)" at the level of the heart, thus making plausible a link between the heart chakra and the mammary glands. I have not seen other writers on the chakras make this connection.

42. Blavatsky, *Collected Writings*, 12, foldout between 532 and 533 (figure 5 in the present book) (*Esoteric Instructions*, foldout between 40 and 41).

43. Whitten, *Initial Course*, 31.

44. Ibid., 32; 39–40.

45. Leadbeater, *Science of the Sacraments*, 90–91. Ordered service: "ceremonial which invokes angelic help" (91). List also cited in Leadbeater, *Masters and the Path*, 241 (2002).

46. Leadbeater, *Chakras*, 48–52.

47. From Bailey, *Initiation: Human and Solar*, 224; also cited in *Letters on Occult Meditation*, 358–59.

48. Bailey, *Letters on Occult Meditation*, 213.

49. Ibid., 214.

50. Ibid., 207.

51. Ibid., 358–59.

52. Blavatsky, *Collected Writings*, 12: foldout between 532 and 533 (figure 5 in the present book) (*Esoteric Instructions*, foldout between 40 and 41).

53. Blavatsky, *Collected Writings*, 12:543, 546–47 (*Esoteric Instructions*, 46, 54).

54. James R. Lewis, *The Encyclopedia of Cults, Sects, and New Religions*, s.vv. "The I AM Religious Activity," "Ascended Master Teaching Foundation" (Bridge to Freedom), and "Church Universal and Triumphant."

55. Bridge to Freedom colors from http://www.iamfree.co.za/chakra%20centres%20in%20the%20body.htm, accessed June 20, 2015, based on A. D. K. Luk (Alice Schutz), *Law of Life*, 2:406ff. Summit Lighthouse colors from Elizabeth Clare Prophet, *Intermediate Studies of the Human Aura*, plates 2–8 (between 78 and 79). Alice Schutz acted as secretary for the Ballards and Innocente.

Chapter 18

1. See Hunt, *Fragrant and Radiant Symphony*, 17–64, for his version of the scientific and metaphysical rationale for these ideas. The notion of octaves of sound and color in relation to the sixth and seventh senses (including lists of frequency ranges) originates in a note by Herbert Coryn in Besant's edition of the third volume of *The Secret Doctrine* (1897). See chapter 6, note 13 of the present book for particulars.

2. Classified ad, *Chimes*, vol. 20, no. 12 (December 1961), 32, http://www.ehbritten.org/docs/chimes_december_1961.pdf, accessed November 15, 2015.

3. Information in these paragraphs assembled from the following sources: Roland T. Hunt, *Complete Color Prescription for Rebuilding Our Bodies and Cities*, 8, and back matter; *Lighting-Therapy and Color Harmony*, including descriptions and pictures of Hunt's lamps, plus his photograph with the perfumer Prince Georges V. Matchabelli (facing page 59); and Wikipedia, s.v. "Vera Stanley Alder."

4. New York Passenger Lists, June 4, 1923, Ancestry.com.

5. Roland T. Hunt, *The Finding of Rainbow's End, and Other Mystical Experiences in the "Mother Lode" Country during 1930*, 35–45.

6. Roland T. Hunt, *Fragrant and Radiant Symphony*, 105.

7. Ibid., 189n.

8. Ibid., 188.

9. Annie Besant and C. W. Leadbeater, *Man: Whence, How, and Whither*, 375–411.

10. Hunt, *The Seven Keys to Color Healing: A Complete Outline to the Practice of Color Healing*, 127.

11. Ibid., 210–11.

12. Hunt, *Fragrant and Radiant Symphony*, 123.

13. Leadbeater, *Chakras* (2013 edition), plate 8 and figure 2.5. See plates 6 and 7 in the present book.

14. Albanese, *Republic of Mind and Spirit*, 432.

15. Leadbeater, *Man Visible*, "The Planes of Nature," plate 2, following page 22.

16. Whitten, *What Color Means to You*, 16.

17. See the two volumes of *"I Will Arise!"* (1972) attributed to Paola Hugh.

18. S. G. J. Ouseley, *A Guide to Telepathy and Psychometry: The Laws of Thought Projection and the Scientific and Practical Aspects of Psychometry*, 89. Ouseley's birth and death dates have not previously been researched and published. They were determined on the basis of records on Ancestry.com.

19. Ibid., 87.

20. S. G. J. Ouseley, *The Power of the Rays: The Science of Color-Healing*, 4.

21. Biographical information on Ouseley and his father gathered from various records on Ancestry.com.

22. The story unfolded in the following anonymously published articles: "'Ex-Monk' Stephen Ouseley: His 'Four Years' Captivity,'" *Tablet*, August 8, 1931; "'For Honest Protestants': The Harrison Trust," *Tablet*, August 15, 1931; "L'Affaire Limbrick-Ouseley," *Tablet*, September 19, 1931; "Limbrick-Ouseley," *Tablet* (London), October 24, 1931; "A Lie or a Spy," *Tablet*, November 14, 1931; "An 'Ex-Monk's' Letter," *Tablet*, January 2, 1932; "Stephen Ouseley: A Final Exposure," *Tablet*, February 27, 1932.

23. We know that Ouseley was a Theosophist from his one appearance in the *Theosophist*, which includes the words "English Section" in association with his name in the byline. S. G. J. Ouseley, "The Garden of Enchantment," 70–71.

24. S. G. J. Ouseley, *Color Meditations, with Guide to Color Healing: A Course of Instructions and Exercises in Developing Color Consciousness*, 50–51.

25. Ouseley, *Power of the Rays*, 55–56, 60–62.

26. Heindel, *Rosicrucian Cosmo-Conception*, 35–38. See Leland, *Invisible Worlds*, 310–11n3, for information on Besant's use of the term *ether*.

27. Ouseley, *Power of the Rays*, 40–41.

28. Ibid., 90–91 (original emphasis).

29. In this table, the functions, auras, and qualities derive from S. G. J. Ouseley, *The Science of the Aura: An Introduction to the Study of the Human Aura*, 17–23; the elements, planes, chakras, and glands derive from Ouseley, *Power of the Rays*, 23–30, 45, 54–57. I have added the principles to clarify the connection between planes and auras, the names of which appear to be at variance with the Besant/Leadbeater system.

Ouseley spreads seven principles over five planes, as did Besant. Thus, what he calls the divine, or absolute, plane is related to the principle of atman and would correspond to Besant's atmic, or nirvanic, plane, the highest manifested plane in our reality/learning system. In Besant, the causal body is associated with the upper mental plane. Ouseley locates it between the upper mental plane and the buddhic plane—on the cusp, as it were.

As noted, Blavatsky sometimes spoke of the *antaḥkaraṇa* ("inner instrument") as a bridge between lower mind and higher mind. Alice Bailey picked up on this notion and produced a considerable amount of channeled material on the development of the antahkarana (e.g., in *Esoteric Healing*). Thus it appears that Ouseley carved out a space between the lower and higher mental plane for the antahkarana, which he called the soul principle.

30. See Bailey, *Letters on Occult Meditation*, 204–16, in which indigo is used as the base color.

31. Blavatsky, *Collected Writings*, 12:567 and diagram on 568 (figure 21 in the present book) (*Esoteric Instructions*, 95 and 97 [diagram]).

32. Hunt, *Fragrant and Radiant Symphony*, 66.

33. Blavatsky, *Theosophical Glossary*, s.v. "sutratman."
34. Ouseley, *Power of the Rays*, 56.
35. Hunt, *Seven Keys*, 92, 106.
36. Ouseley, *Color Meditations*, 56–61; Besant and Leadbeater, *Man: Whence, How, and Whither*, 379–86. Besant and Leadbeater describe four color temples: crimson, blue, yellow, and green. Ouseley describes but one, with four divisions, situating it on the astral plane. I suspect that Ouseley's color temple may have described the "headquarters" whose address would be given out only to associate members of Bergh and Hunt's AMICA.
37. Classified ad, *Chimes*, vol. 20, issue 12 (December 1961), 32. Birth and death dates from records on Ancestry.com; organizational data from http://california.14thstory.com/aquarian-cosmic-colour-fellowship.html, accessed November 14, 2015.

Chapter 19

1. Evola, *Yoga of Power*, xiii–xiv.
2. René Guénon, *Studies in Hinduism*, 26–28. Guénon believed the correlation between the Tree of Life and the chakras "has never before been made anywhere" (26). As we have seen, he was anticipated by Crowley (1909) and Regardie (1932). Interestingly, Guénon suggests a reversal of the positions of Yesod (Foundation) and Malkuth (Kingdom), since the function of muladhara chakra is foundational (the name means "root-support") and that of svadhishthana is the "proper abode" (or kingdom) of kundalini-shakti (28). Otherwise, his version anticipates that of Anodea Judith (*Wheels of Life* [1987], 46–47) and Caroline Myss (*Anatomy of the Spirit* [1997]) by more than fifty years (see left side of figure 8 in the present book).
3. Ronald Hayman, *A Life of Jung*, 212.
4. Ibid.
5. Ibid. (Jung quoted).
6. Ibid.
7. See C. G. Jung, *The Red Book—Liber Novus*, 54, 71, 109, 111, 129, and 135, for examples of kundalini-like serpent imagery in Jung's hand-painted illustrations of dreams and visions during his psychological crisis.

8. C. G. Jung, *The Psychology of Kundalini Yoga: Notes of the Seminar Given in 1932 by C. G. Jung*, xxvi (note).

9. Ibid., 104–6.

10. Lecture titles and dates in this paragraph from Jung, *Psychology of Kundalini Yoga*, xxiv–xxv.

11. Ibid., xxii (Heinrich Zimmer quoted).

12. Biographical information from Wikipedia, s.v. "Jakob Wilhelm Hauer."

13. Lecture dates in this paragraph from Jung, *Psychology of Kundalini Yoga*, xxxiii–xxxv.

14. Ibid., xxxviii.

15. Ibid., xiv.

16. Ibid., xi.

17. Ibid.

18. Ibid., 63.

19. In his lectures on kundalini yoga, Jung frequently speculated on the connection between the elements and physiological or psychological states—thus the fire of the navel chakra is associated with the kitchen, alchemy, and digestion (ibid., 43–44) and the ether of the throat chakra with the unknowns of space beyond the thin air of the stratosphere (47).

20. Alice Bailey also made a distinction between the chakras below and above the diaphragm, but for her, the first three were awake in "average humanity," while the fourth and sixth were asleep and the fifth was just beginning to stir (*Soul and Its Mechanism*, 119–20).

21. Lewis, *Encyclopedia of Cults, Sects, and New Religions*, s.v. "Hindu Yoga Society." Birth year from Ancestry.com.

22. Hereward Carrington, *Higher Psychical Development (Yoga Philosophy): An Outline of the Secret Hindu Teachings*, between 146 and 147.

23. Theosophical Research Center founding date: E. L. Gardner, "The Theosophical Research Center (England)," 3.

24. Stephen Larsen and Robyn Larsen, *A Fire in the Mind: The Life of Joseph Campbell*, 319.

25. Ibid., 325–26.

26. Jeffrey Kripal, *Esalen: America and the Religion of No Religion*, 189.

27. Wikipedia, s.vv. "Swami Nikhilananda," "Sri Ramakrishna," "Mahendranath Gupta."

28. Larsen, *Fire in the Mind*, 283.

29. Kripal, *Esalen*, 190.

30. Larsen, *Fire in the Mind*, 362–91, 433.

31. I use the word *presumably* because Ramakrishna does not make a direct link between these key words and the associated chakras or planes of consciousness. Campbell seems to accept the following passage as indicative of the correct associations of chakras and qualities: "Where does the mind of a man ordinarily dwell? In the first three planes [i.e., chakras]. These are at the organs of evacuation and generation, and at the navel. Then the mind is immersed only in worldliness, attached to 'women and gold'" (Swami Nikhilananda, *The Gospel of Sri Ramakrishna*, 169).

32. See, for example, Joseph Campbell, *Myths of Light: Eastern Metaphors of the Eternal*, 29.

Chapter 20

1. Information in this paragraph from Kripal, *Esalen*, 27–31, 75, 99, 105 (page numbers given in ascending order rather than the order of facts cited).

2. Ken Dychtwald, *Bodymind: A Synthesis of Eastern and Western Ways to Self-Awareness, Health, and Personal Growth*, 11. Dychtwald notes that the passage in quotation marks comes from the Esalen catalog for Spring 1976 (*Bodymind*, 264).

3. Kripal, *Esalen*, 28, 86–87, 202.

4. Ibid., 75.

5. Ibid., 48, 55, 57.

6. Sri Aurobindo, *Letters on Yoga*, 1:99.

7. Ibid., 1:122.

8. Kripal, *Esalen*, 58.

9. Ibid., 47, 57, 60–62.

10. Ibid., 59, 82, 105.

11. Bibliographic information from "Publisher's Note" in Sri Aurobindo, *Letters on Yoga I: Foundations of the Integral Yoga*, *The Complete Works of Sri Aurobindo*, vol. 28 (front matter unpainted). This 2012 edition completely reorganizes the material in the 2004 reprint of the 1970 edition cited in the present book. A downloadable PDF of the 2012 edition is available at http://www.sriaurobindoashram.org/ashram/

sriauro/writings.php. The detailed table of contents should allow users of this edition to find further information on terms given in my résumé of Aurobindo's teachings on chakras and states of consciousness.

12. Except where otherwise noted, information on the chakras' functions from Aurobindo, *Letters on Yoga*, 1:364–66.

13. Aurobindo, *Letters on Yoga* 1:344.

14. Ibid., 1:76. The identification of vital and astral consciousness implies that, in Theosophical terms, the first chakra refers to the physical body, the second through fifth chakras to the astral body, the sixth chakra to the mental body, and the seventh chakra (including higher mind and illumined mind) to the causal body. Intuitive mind would relate to the buddhic body, and overmind to atman and the atmic/nirvanic body. Supermind would be *paramātman* (supreme self) and the monadic body; the supreme would be Brahman and the divine body.

15. Ibid., 1:334.

16. Ibid.

17. Ibid., 1:243.

18. Ibid., 1:239.

19. Ibid., 1:257.

20. Ibid., 1:252.

21. Ibid.

22. Ibid.

23. Kripal, *Esalen*, 195.

24. Ibid., 21, 63, 237.

25. Ibid., 21, 237.

26. Blavatsky, *Theosophical Glossary*, s.v. "kundalini-sakti."

27. Leadbeater, *The Inner Life*, 205.

28. George S. Arundale, *Kundalini: An Occult Experience*, 4.

29. Ibid., 21–22.

30. Robert Love, *The Great Oom: The Mysterious Origins of America's First Yogi*, 12–14, 29–66, 286–87.

31. Kripal, *Esalen*, 231–35; Dychtwald, *Bodymind*, 9–11, 99–102.

32. Kripal, *Esalen*, 264.

33. Bernard Gunther, *Energy, Ecstasy, and Your Seven Vital Chakras*, back cover (first edition only).

Chapter 21

1. Kripal, *Esalen*, 142, 143. In the second quotation, Kripal is comparing Esalen and *The Course in Miracles* (1975), which was encouraged, channeled, and edited by psychologists.

2. Edward Hoffman, *The Right to Be Human: A Biography of Abraham Maslow*, 272.

3. Ibid., 338, 339.

4. Mark E. Koltko-Rivera, "Rediscovering the Later Version of Maslow's Hierarchy of Needs: Self-Transcendence and Opportunities for Theory, Research, and Unification," 302.

5. Ibid., 303. Despite the similarity of title (and Kripal's statement to the contrary), this article does not appear in Maslow's posthumous book, *The Farther Reaches of Human Nature* (1971). Kripal indicates that a lecture of the same title was given in San Francisco on February 6, 1966, in connection with a nascent Esalen Center to be opened there in September 1967 (*Esalen*, 186–87).

6. Thomas B. Roberts and Ralph H. Hannon, "A Holistic Meeting of Transpersonal Psychology and Theosophy: Chakras, Needs, and Moral Development," 369, figure 3.

7. Hoffman, *Right to Be Human*, 92–93.

8. Kripal, *Esalen*, 126–27. Other biographical details from Wikipedia.

9. Judith, *Wheels of Life* (1999), 424.

10. Kripal, *Esalen*, 189–90.

11. Ram Dass, *The Only Dance There Is: Talks Given at the Menninger Foundation, Topeka, Kansas, 1970, and at Spring Grove, Maryland, 1972*, 28–32, 82–86.

12. Ibid., 83–84.

13. Ibid., 158 (mentioning astral planes and Leadbeater).

14. Kripal, *Esalen*, 166–68.

15. William C. Schutz, *Here Comes Everybody: Bodymind and Encounter Culture*, xiv. Biographical details from Wikipedia, s.v. "William Schutz."

16. Schutz. *Here Comes Everybody*, xv.

17. Ibid., 39 (discussion of the movie).

18. Ibid., xvii.

19. Ibid., 64.

20. W. Edward Mann, *Orgone, Reich, and Eros: Wilhelm Reich's Theory of Life Energy*, 60.

21. Schutz, *Here Comes Everybody*, 64.

22. Ibid., 65.

23. Ken Keyes Jr., *Handbook to Higher Consciousness: The Science of Happiness*, 48–82. The list is drawn from the chart on 48–49. Biographical material from Wikipedia, s.v. "Ken Keyes, Jr."

24. See Goswami, *Layayoga*, 212–17 and 278, for further information on hrit chakra. See also Avalon, *Serpent Power*, 382–33, and Leadbeater, *Chakras*, 98–99. Plate 10 in Goswami provides a visual image of hrit chakra with the wish-fulfilling tree.

25. Jack Lee Rosenberg, *Total Orgasm*, 212.

26. Ibid., 201.

27. Ibid., 201–5.

Chapter 22

1. Haridas Chaudhuri, "Yoga Psychology," 267–68.

2. Wikipedia, s.v. "Swami Rama"; Ballentine: http://www.thisisawar.com/AuthorsRudolph.htm, accessed November 14, 2015.

3. Swami Rama, Rudolph Ballentine, and Swami Ajaya, *Yoga and Psychotherapy: The Evolution of Consciousness*, 226–72.

4. Dychtwald, *Bodymind*, 262.

5. Dychtwald's juxtaposition of kundalini and chiropractic was probably based on the chiropractic principle that blockages (subluxations) of vital force flowing through the nerves of the spine are responsible for physical disabilities and disease (Wikipedia, s.v. "chiropractic").

6. Kripal, *Esalen*, 234.

7. Ibid., 231.

8. Ibid., 235.

9. Dychtwald, *Bodymind*, 88.

10. Aurobindo, *Letters on Yoga*, 1:340.

11. White, *Tantra in Practice*, 8–9.

12. Dychtwald, *Bodymind*, 86.

13. This movement from self-expression to self-identification, self-awareness, and self-realization may be Dychtwald's original synthesis of earlier psychological notions of the chakra qualities based on his read-

ing of a reprinted spiritual classic that gained a strong readership in the 1960s and 1970s, *Cosmic Consciousness: A Study in the Evolution of the Human Mind* (1901) by nineteenth-century Canadian physician Richard Maurice Bucke (1837–1902). See Dychtwald, *Bodymind*, 256–60.

14. Dychtwald, *Bodymind*, 236–39.

15. Ken Dychtwald, "Bodymind and the Evolution to Cosmic Consciousness," 23.

16. Ibid., 23–24; Dychtwald, *Bodymind*, 256, 258.

17. Omar Garrison, *Tantra: The Yoga of Sex*, 31–38 (chakra discussion); 56 (colors).

18. Ibid., 59–60 (red/orange and green/yellow swaps); 59 (pituitary/pineal swap—compare 37–38).

19. In a telephone interview of November 22, 2015, Ken Dychtwald informed me that he had hoped *Bodymind* would inject something personally and socially transformative into the culture. However, that *something* was not the chakra system per se, which he had used primarily as a means of providing structure to the book. He explained that the psychedelic illustrations of the chakras were by artist Jad King, but the cover had been produced by the publisher, in-house, by an unknown illustrator (who appears to have been aware of the correspondence between chakras and rainbow colors). Dychtwald said there was an additional influence on his linking of the chakras with the rainbow colors that I could not have been aware of: the music of New Age composer Steven Halpern (b. 1947), a personal friend. Halpern's album *Spectrum Suite* (1975; now called *Chakra Suite*) had been released while *Bodymind* was being written. Its seven movements were based on the chakras, the colors of the rainbow, and the seven tones of the diatonic scale. Halpern was the first to use the notion of the chakras as the basis for musical compositions—now a staple of sound-healing therapies and the genre of New Age music.

Chapter 23

1. Judith, *Wheels of Life* (1987), 504. Rendel birth date from obituary in *Insight* 45:29–31 (Summer 2004).

2. Peter Rendel, *Introduction to the Chakras*, 16 (diagram), 27–30, 33–38.

3. Kripal, *Esalen*, 244, 246 (original emphasis).

4. Gunther birth date from Ancestry.com (under "Bernard Gutwillig"); death date from Doug De Stephano (email of August 25, 2016); biographical information from Gunther, *Energy, Ecstasy*, back cover (first edition only).

5. Ibid. (all editions).

6. The third through seventh chakra qualities are identical with those of other lists coming out of Esalen, if we see "paranormal powers" in the brow chakra as an alternative for "third eye." The difference in the first two chakras may be explained by Gunther's using Leadbeater's system as a template. In that system, the base and sexual chakras are combined into one and the spleen chakra, in the second position, has been assigned the function of health because the spleen regulates the body's immune system.

7. Rendel, *Introduction to the Chakras*, 63: "It seems that in relating the planets to the chakras one should observe some logical sequence such as their distance from the earth or relative speeds of movements." Gunther chose the former.

8. One less-than-obvious link is kidney disease with the brow chakra. I suspect that Gunther was referring to the medical fact that pituitary malfunctions are sometimes associated with kidney disease—and Gunther linked the pituitary with the brow chakra.

9. See Jack Schwarz, *Voluntary Controls: Exercises for Creative Meditation and for Activating the Potential of the Chakras*, 90–95.

10. Bailey, *Esoteric Healing*, 144–83.

11. Govinda, *Foundations of Tibetan Mysticism*, 181–86. Compare the cover illustration of the chakra chalice for Schwarz's *Voluntary Controls* with the body-temple illustration in Govinda (184) to see how the latter inspired the former (also figures 22 and 23 in the present book).

12. Gunther, *Energy, Ecstasy*, 47.

13. Schwarz, *Voluntary Controls*, 19.

14. Thinking and *āsana* may seem like an odd pairing. If it needs justification, I would suggest that in Patañjali's time, *posture* primarily referred to posture in meditation and that achieving a still posture resulted in a stilled mind.

15. Based on charts on pages 36 and 43 of Christopher Hills, *Nuclear Evolution* (1977).

16. The source page numbers for these qualities in Christopher Hills, *Nuclear Evolution* (1977), are as follows (from top to bottom): 356, 339, 327, 312, 292, 277, 257.

17. Ibid., 383, 385.

18. Ibid., diagrams on 56 and 58, the latter based on figure 2.5 from Leadbeater's *The Chakras* (2013), which shows the locations of the chakras in a side view of the human torso (plate 7 in the present book), but with the rainbow colors added.

19. Christopher Hills, *Nuclear Evolution* (1977), 53.

20. Alex Jones, *The Seven Mansions of Color*, 76.

Chapter 24

1. Maruti Seidman, *Like a Hollow Flute: A Guide to Polarity Therapy*, 31–32 (note the absence of endocrine glands). Seidman reissued the book as *A Guide to Polarity Therapy* in 1986, 1991, and 2000. Birth date from Ancestry.com (under Martin S. Seidman).

2. Stone's familiarity with the chakras may have derived from his having become a lifelong member of the Radhasoami faith during a visit to India in 1945. Biographical data from Juergensmeyer, *Radhasoami Reality*, 203n, and http://energyschool.com/about-dr-randolph-stone/dr-randolph-stone-chronology/ (accessed February 14, 2016).

3. "The sixth and seventh chakras are the spiritual centers of the body. We do not work with these directly in Polarity" (Sharon and Jefferson Campbell, eds., *Notes on Energy Balancing at the Polarity Health Institute*, 13).

4. Seidman, *Like a Hollow Flute*, 33–34. See also Seidman's book-length treatment of the subject, *Balancing the Chakras* (2000).

5. Neff birth date from Ancestry.com.

6. The reference to Thai-born Chinese Taoist master Mantak Chia (b. 1944) is probably to *Awaken Healing Energy through the Tao: The Taoist Secret of Circulating Internal Power* (1983), which includes a list of twenty-four "energy centers" (174–81), among them the seven chakras, identified primarily with acupuncture points and secondarily with the familiar Sanskrit names, the rainbow colors, and the endocrine glands. Neff's citing of twenty-three such centers appears to be an error.

I have seen several references to teachings of the Russian mystic George Ivanovich Gurdjieff (1866, 1872, or 1877–1949; the birth date is disputed) and the chakras, but few attempts to justify or explain the connection. A useful exposition appears in Jean Vaysse, *Toward Awakening: An Approach to the Teaching Left by Gurdjieff* (French, 1973; English,

1979). In a clearly written chapter on "centers and functions" (67–109), seven centers are described, not three. Though the word *chakra* does not appear, it would be easy to arrange the names of Gurdjieff's centers in an order that easily parallels that of the continuum of human potential evoked in the Esalen chakra qualities: (1) instinctive; (2) sexual; (3) moving; (4) emotional; (5) higher emotional; (6) intellectual; and (7) higher intellectual.

7. Dio Urmilla Neff, "The Great Chakra Controversy," 42–45, 50, 52–53.

8. Ibid., 50.

9. Ibid., 44.

10. Judith birth date from Wikipedia, s.v. "Anodea Judith."

11. Gardner birth date from https://en.wikipedia.org/wiki/User:JoyGardner, accessed June 22, 2015.

12. Karagulla birth date from Melton, *Encyclopedia of Occultism and Parapsychology*, s.v. "Shafica Karagulla"; death date from Ancestry.com. Kunz birth and death dates from Wikipedia, s.v. "Dora Kunz." Further biographical information on Kunz from Shafica Karagulla and Dora van Gelder Kunz, *The Chakras and the Human Energy Fields*, 3–4.

13. Bohm dates from id.loc.gov/authorities/names/n86137157.html, accessed November 14, 2015.

14. Rendel, *Introduction to the Chakras*, 32.

15. Klausbernd Vollmar, *Journey through the Chakras: Exercises for Healing and Internal Balancing*, 56–59 (chart).

16. Ibid., 1; also Wikipedia, s.v. "Klausbernd Vollmar"; http://www.kbvollmar.de/sonstige/biografie.html, accessed June 22, 2015.

17. William Irwin Thompson, *Passages about Earth: An Exploration of the New Planetary Culture*, 150–83 (Findhorn); 187–91 (Lindisfarne). There is also a discussion of the chakras in the essay "Of Physics and Tantra Yoga" (84–118), a mélange of interviews with physicist Werner Heisenberg and kundalini-experiencer Gopi Krishna, along with explanations of Sri Aurobindo's teachings, tantric sexuality, and occultism (including the chakras' link to Revelation)—a veritable 1970s time capsule.

18. Birth and death dates for Bodo J. Baginski from obituary at https://bantryblog.wordpress.com/2012/06/17/bodo-baginski-save-bantry-bay-committee-member-will-be-sadly-missed/, accessed June

22, 2015. Time spent at Findhorn documented in Bodo J. Baginski and Shalila Sharamon, *Reiki: Universal Life Energy: A Holistic Method of Treatment for . . . Mind, Body and Soul*, 12.

19. Sharamon birth date from http://www.reiki-land.de/rezensionen/buecher/bodo-baginski-shalia-sharamon-reiki-universale-lebensenergie.html, accessed June 22, 2015.

20. Baginski and Sharamon, *Reiki*, 75–76.

21. David V. Tansley, *Radionics and the Subtle Anatomy of Man*, back matter. Biographical data from http://www.sourcewatch.org/index.php/David_V._Tansley, accessed June 22, 2015.

22. Lansdowne birth date from Ancestry.com. Biographical information from Lansdowne, *The Chakras and Esoteric Healing*, back matter, and http://www.sevenray.org/lansdowne.html, accessed June 22, 2015. A more recent book on the subject is Alan Hopking, *Esoteric Healing: A Practical Guide Based on the Teachings of the Tibetan in the Works of Alice A. Bailey* (2005).

23. Information in this paragraph from Choa Kok Sui, *The Origin of Modern Pranic Healing and Arhatic Yoga*, 5, 8, 9, 15, 17, 108, 201–9. Death date from http://en.wikipedia.org/wiki/User:Sg_ph/Master_Choa_Kok_Sui, accessed May 8, 2015.

24. Sui, *Origin of Modern Pranic Healing*, 120.

25. Choa Kok Sui, *The Chakras and Their Functions: Compiled from the Books of Master Choa Kok Sui*, 30 (diagram).

26. Ibid., 60. *Ming men* [sic] (door of life) also appears in Mantak Chia's list of energy centers, identified with svadhishthana chakra (Chia, *Awaken Healing Energy through the Tao*, 175). Chia's book preceded Sui's *The Ancient Science and Art of Pranic Healing* by two years.

27. Sui, *Chakras and Their Functions*, 155.

28. Ibid., 59.

29. Ibid., 156.

30. Sui, *Pranic Healing*, 94–95 (diagrams). The twelfth chakra does not appear here—its existence was revealed in a later book.

31. Joy, *Joy's Way*, 165–66 (chart).

32. Choa Kok Sui, *Pranic Healing*, 172–77.

33. See Sui, *Origin of Modern Pranic Healing*, for outlines of both systems.

34. Biographical information from Wikipedia, s.v. "Shirley MacLaine."

35. Shirley MacLaine, *Going Within: A Guide for Inner Transformation*, 79–82.

36. Ibid., 83–84.

37. Wikipedia, s.v. "visible spectrum."

38. Joy Gardner, *Color and Crystals: A Journey through the Chakras*, 109, 117.

39. These locations rarely appear by name in New Age books on the chakras, such as Judith's *Wheels of Life*. However, the locations themselves have remained unchanged since they were first identified in 1888 by Baman Das Basu.

40. The glands listed first in the entries for the first three chakras correspond to Bailey's teachings and are the most common attributions, though Judith assigns the adrenals to both the first and third chakras (Judith, *Wheels of Life* [1987], 46). The glands listed second represent minority opinions, usually based on proximity of the glands in question to the physiological locations of these chakras.

41. Chakra qualities from Judith, *Wheels of Life* (1987), 46–47, with the exception of those for the seventh chakra, which derive from Esalen lists and are more common than Judith's qualities for this chakra ("understanding/knowing/bliss"). Judith has desire in the second chakra, which is a common attribution (though it sometimes appears in connection with the third chakra, as in Bailey); I have replaced it with sensuality, again from the Esalen lists. The fifth chakra is often linked to self-expression, which could be considered a combination of communication and creativity.

42. A YouTube clip of this portion of MacLaine's appearance on the *Tonight Show* can be found at https://www.youtube.com/watch?v=lQm3WlUFBZ0, accessed June 22, 2015.

Chapter 25

1. Leland, *Invisible Worlds*, 322–23n5.

2. Leadbeater, *Chakras*, 64 (astral chakras), 68–69 (etheric chakras).

3. Alder, *Initiation of the World*, 86.

4. Osho's list of the bodies is as follows: (1) physical; (2) etheric; (3) astral; (4) mental; (5) spiritual—referred to atman; (6) cosmic—referred to Brahman; and (7) nirvanic—referred to śūnya, the void (Osho, *In Search of the Miraculous*, 386–400, 442). See also the following talks

for further discussion of these subjects: "The Path of Kundalini: Authenticity and Freedom" (385–424; includes names and descriptions, plus seven-year cycles of development and connection to human cultural evolution); "The Mysteries of the Seven Bodies and Seven Chakras" (425–67); "The Occult Mysteries of Religion" (469–513); "Kundalini: The Discipline of Transcendence" (545–79); and "The Esoteric Dimensions of Tantra" (582–617). In other contexts, Osho briefly mentions Aurobindo (236, 496–97), as well as Blavatsky, Besant, Leadbeater, and Arundale—though not Bailey (654).

5. John C. Pierrakos, *Core Energetics: Developing the Capacity to Love and Heal*, 93–101; Barbara Ann Brennan, *Hands of Light: A Guide to Healing through the Human Energy Field, a New Paradigm. . . .*, 109–28.

6. Pierrakos identifies four "feeling centers," "located in the front of the body" and corresponding to the throat (fifth chakra), heart (fourth), solar plexus (third), and pubis (presumably the first). Three "will centers," located "in the back of the body," correspond to the "small of the back" (presumably the second chakra, but possibly the back side of the fused first and second chakras characteristic of Tibetan Tantra); "between the shoulder blades," but with subsidiary funnels extending to areas of the back opposite the solar plexus and throat chakras (apparently representing the back side of the throat, heart, and solar plexus chakras); and one at the occipital bone (apparently the back side of the brow chakra, but linked also to the crown chakra). The crown center "incorporates and exceeds the operations of all the anterior and posterior entries" (*Core Energetics*, 79 and figure 9). Brennan maintains the concept of feeling and will centers, but carries Pierrakos's system to its logical conclusion: "Each major chakra on the front of the body is paired with its counterpart on the back of the body, and together they are considered to be the front and rear aspect of one chakra" (*Hands of Light*, 44–45).

7. Brennan, *Hands of Light*, xvi–xvii, 5.

8. Bruyere birth date from www.astro.com/astro-databank/Bruyere,_Rosalyn, accessed June 22, 2015.

9. An edited version of Hunt's study is included in Bruyere's *Wheels of Light* as an appendix, 247–58.

10. Bruyere, *Wheels of Light*, 42–43.

11. Bruyere indicates that magnetum is "unknown to modern sci-

ence," but is mentioned in hermetic and alchemical literature (*Wheels of Light*, 39n).

12. Bruyere and other authors who link the chakras with Native American beliefs may have been inspired by the writings of Frank Waters (1902–95), who identified five-chakra-like centers in Hopi teachings (*Book of the Hopi,* 12–13 and note) and correlated legends of seven "womb caverns" or "ancestral villages" in the mythologies of several Mexican and Southwestern US tribes, including the Hopi, to "the seven psychophysical centers within man himself" (*Pumpkin Seed Point*, 136–39).

Bruyere's chakra names likely originated in kabbalistic teachings. She states that each chakra "has a physical, an emotional, a creative, and a celestial component" (*Wheels of Light*, 34). Also, the first three chakras and planes are identified with "three-dimensional reality" (41). It is possible that Bruyere's system owes something to a diagram in Blavatsky's *The Secret Doctrine* (de Zirkoff), 1:200. What Blavatsky calls the "physical material world" (the kabbalistic Assiah) corresponds to Bruyere's first three planes, three-dimensional reality, and the *physical* component of each chakra. What Blavatsky calls the "substantial or formative world" (Yetzirah) corresponds to Bruyere's astral plane and the *emotional* component of each chakra (later Theosophical teachings often correlate the astral plane with emotion). What Blavatsky calls the "intellectual or creative world" (Briah) corresponds to Bruyere's etheric plane and the *creative* component of each chakra. What Blavatsky calls the "archetypal world" (Atziluth) corresponds to Bruyere's celestial plane and *celestial* level of each chakra. In Kabbalah, this level represents "emanation" and "closeness to God" and is considered a realm of light. Indeed, Bruyere correlates the celestial plane with a "realm of light" (*Wheels of Light*, 44). Finally, what Blavatsky calls the "divine and formless world of spirit" corresponds to Bruyere's ketheric plane: "our place of mergence with God, the Oneness, the All" (*Wheels of Light*, 44). The four worlds of Kabbalah are traditionally mapped into the Tree of Life, hence Bruyere's highest plane is called ketheric, after the first and highest *sephirah*.

13. Bruyere, *Wheels of Light*, 43.
14. Brennan, *Hands of Light*, 42.
15. Ibid., 48 (figure).
16. Ibid., 43–44. In her second book, *Light Emerging: The Process*

of Personal Healing, Brennan dropped Bruyere's terms. However, as the discussion and diagrams on pp. 20–28 of *Light Emerging* indicate, she was still working with Bruyere's template—the terms and descriptions are different, but the energetic functions are the same.

17. Brennan, *Hands of Light*, 43.
18. Ibid., 47.
19. For example, see Besant, *Seven Principles of Man*, 112.
20. See Leland, *Invisible Worlds*, 289–92n8.
21. Brennan, *Hands of Light*, 47, 49, 52.
22. Etheric body as template for physical body: A. E. Powell, *The Etheric Double: The Health Aura*, 67–69; causal level as home of archetypes: Powell, *Causal Body and the Ego*, 135–36.
23. Brennan, *Hands of Light*, 47, 53, 54.
24. Leland, *Invisible Worlds*, 241 (karmic causes), 357n32 (akashic records).
25. Blavatsky, *Collected Writings*, 12:526 (*Esoteric Instructions*, 24–25).
26. Leland, *Invisible Worlds*, 357n32 (auric egg), 229–32 (monad and atmic and buddhic planes); see Besant, *The Ancient Wisdom*, 179–96, for an in-depth discussion of the atmic and buddhic planes. For mineral, vegetable, animal, human, and superhuman growth, see Besant and Leadbeater, *Man: Whence, How, and Whither*, 1–18.
27. Leland, *Invisible Worlds*, 245. Bruyere describes eighth and ninth chakras, having to do with atman and Brahman, respectively (*Wheels of Light*, 34). It appears that Brennan's eighth and ninth layers of the aura correspond to Bruyere's eighth and ninth chakras. If so, then Bruyere's Brahman would correspond to Besant's divine plane and Bruyere's atman would correspond to Besant's monadic plane—thus bolstering my identification of Brennan's higher planes with Besant's.
28. Brennan, *Hands of Light*, 230.
29. Ibid., *Hands of Light*, 43, 45, 48.
30. Brennan's four levels of reality probably derive from Bruyere's four levels of the chakras: physical, emotional, creative, and celestial—which themselves are derived from the four levels of creation in kabbalistic teachings, as indicated in note 12 in the present chapter.
31. Barbara Ann Brennan, *Light Emerging*, 289–90.
32. Wikipedia, s.v. "hara (tanden)."
33. Brennan, *Light Emerging*, 12.

34. Ibid., 306.

35. Leadbeater, *Masters and the Path*, 173 (2002).

36. Leadbeater, *Chakras*, 64. In 1910, a British Theosophist named Arthur H. Ward, a contributor to Theosophical journals since the late 1890s (and thus, despite Internet rumors to the contrary, not the same as Arthur Henry Ward [1883–1959], who wrote under the name Sax Rohmer) published *The Seven Rays of Development*, whose endpapers displayed a diagram of correspondences between the principles, bodies, planes, and rays. The resulting continuum of human potential is similar to the one I outline here—though I discovered Ward's book after having already evolved this list. Here is a summary of his diagram (I have omitted his references to the rays and added Blavatsky's names for the seven principles):

1. **Vitality** (prana)—what I call embodiment; physical plane and body
2. **Sensation** (linga)—what I call sensuality; etheric double or desire nature (kama-linga), corresponding to the upper mental plane
3. **Impulse** (kama)—what I call motivation; astral plane and body
4. **Emotion** (kama-manas)—what I call empathy; plane not listed by Ward (possibly what Blavatsky called the lower psychic plane, corresponding to the upper astral plane)
5. **Thought** (manas)—what I call clairaudience (telepathy or though transference); mental plane and body (the upper psychic plane, corresponding to the lower mental plane)
6. **Imagination** (buddhi-manas)—what I call clairvoyance; causal body or reincarnating ego and the upper mental plane
7. **Cosmic consciousness** (atman)—what I call transcendence; spiritual (atmic or nirvanic) plane and body

Note how closely Ward's terms parallel those of the standard New Age list of chakra qualities that emerged almost eighty years later:

1. Survival
2. Sexuality
3. Power
4. Love
5. Communication

6. Third eye
7. Enlightenment or cosmic consciousness

These parallels demonstrate what may be the ultimate secret of the Western chakra system: If you create a seven-stage continuum of human evolutionary potential whose poles are matter and spirit (as they are understood in Western thought), the intermediary stages are likely to pass from physical to emotional to mental to spiritual. Names for these stages may differ from one version to another, but each stage will cover roughly the same territory. Though Blavatsky's seven principles may have been the first such continuum of human potential, it has long gone unrecognized as the basis of the Western chakra system—perhaps because of the Sanskrit terms she used for each stage. As long as later writers on the chakras stuck with the notion of seven stages from matter to spirit, every iteration of the Western chakra system was simply a variation on the matrix Blavatsky established.

37. Leland, *Invisible Worlds*, 268.

Bibliography

Albanese, Catherine L. *A Republic of Mind and Spirit: A Cultural History of American Metaphysical Religion*. New Haven, CT: Yale University Press, 2007.

Alder, Vera Stanley. *The Initiation of the World*. 1939. Reprint, York Beach, ME: Weiser, 2000.

Ali, Cajzoran [Ann Amber Steen]. *Divine Posture: Influence upon Endocrine Glands*. New York: printed by author, 1928.

Arundale, George S. *Kundalini: An Occult Experience*. Madras, India: Theosophical Publishing House, 1938.

Association for Research and Enlightenment [ARE]. *The Official Edgar Cayce Readings*. DVD-ROM. Virginia Beach, VA: ARE Press, 2007.

Aurobindo, Sri. *Letters on Yoga*. 3 vols. 3rd ed. Pondicherry, India: Sri Aurobindo Ashram, 1970.

———. *Letters on Yoga I: Foundations of the Integral Yoga*. Vol. 28 of *The Complete Works of Sri Aurobindo*. Pondicherry, India: Sri Aurobindo Ashram, 2012. http://www.sriaurobindoashram.org/ashram/sriauro/writings.php.

Avalon, Arthur [Sir John Woodroffe], ed. *Principles of Tantra: The Tantratattva of Shrīyukta Shiva Chandra Vidyārṇava Bhattāchāryya Mahodaya*. 2 vols. 1913. 2nd ed. in 1 vol. Ganesh, Madras, India, 1952.

———. *The Serpent Power: The Secrets of Tantric and Shaktic Yoga*. 1919. 7th ed. 1964. Reprint, New York: Dover, 1974.

Babb, Lawrence A. *Redemptive Encounters: Three Modern Styles in the Hindu Tradition*. 1986. Reprint, Prospect Heights, IL: Waveland, 2000.

Babbitt, Edwin D. *The Principles of Light and Color, Including among Other Things: The Harmonic Laws of the Universe; the Etherio-Atomic Philosophy of Force; Chromo Chemistry; Chromo Therapeutics; and the General Philosophy of the Fine Forces; Together with Numerous Discoveries and Practical Applications*. New York: published by author, 1878. http://catalog.hathitrust.org/Record/100242678.

Baginski, Bodo J., and Shalila Sharamon. *Reiki: Universal Life Energy: A Holistic Method of Treatment for the Professional Practice,*

Absentee Healing, and Self-Treatment of Mind, Body and Soul. Translated by Christopher Baker and Judith Harrison. Mendocino, CA: Life Rhythm, 1988.

Baier, Karl. *Meditation und Moderne: zur Genese eines Kernbereichs moderner Spiritualität in der Wechselwirkung zwischen Westeuropa, Nordamerika und Asien.* 2 vols. Würzburg, Germany: Königsberg & Neumann, 2009.

———. "Mesmeric Yoga and the Development of Meditation within the Theosophical Society." *Theosophical History* 16 (July/October 2012): 151–61.

———. "Theosophical Orientalism and the Structures of Intercultural Transfer: Annotations on the Appropriation of the Cakras in Early Theosophy." In Julie Chajes and Boaz Huss, eds., *Theosophical Appropriations: Esotericism, Kabbalah, and the Transformation of Traditions*, 309–54. Beer Sheva, Israel: Ben Gurion University of the Negev Press, 2016.

Bailey, Alice A. *Esoteric Astrology.* 1951. Reprint, New York: Lucis, 2008.

———. *Esoteric Healing.* 1953. Reprint, New York: Lucis, 2009.

———. *Esoteric Psychology.* 1936–42. 2 vols. Reprint, New York: Lucis, 2002–4.

———. *Initiation: Human and Solar.* 1922. Reprint, New York: Lucis, 1992.

———. *Letters on Occult Meditation.* 1922. Reprint, New York: Lucis, 2002.

———. *The Light of the Soul: Its Science and Effect—a Paraphrase of the Yoga Sutras of Patanjali.* 1927. Reprint, New York: Lucis, 2013.

———. *The Soul and Its Mechanism.* 1930. Reprint, New York: Lucis, 2002.

———. *Telepathy and the Etheric Vehicle.* 1950. Reprint, New York: Lucis, 2008.

———. *A Treatise on Cosmic Fire.* 1925. Reprint, New York: Lucis, 2012.

———. *A Treatise on White Magic.* 1934. Reprint, New York: Lucis, 2013.

———. *The Unfinished Autobiography.* 1951. Reprint, New York: Lucis, 2008.

Baker, Mary Ellen Penny. *Meditation: A Step Beyond with Edgar Cayce.* Garden City, NY: Doubleday, 1973.

Banerji, Sures Chandra. *A Companion to Tantra.* 1999. Reprint, New Delhi, India: Abhinav, 2007.

Baphomet XI° [Aleister Crowley]. "The Man of Earth Degrees and the Hindu Chakras." In Aleister Crowley, *The Equinox: The Review of Scientific Illuminism; the Official Organ of the O.T.O.,* vol. 3, no. 10 (March 1986), 193–94. York Beach, ME: Red Wheel/Weiser, 1990.

Barborka, Geoffrey A. *The Divine Plane, Written in the Form of a Commentary on "The Secret Doctrine."* 1961. Rev. ed. 1964. Reprint, Adyar, Chennai, India: Theosophical Publishing House, 2002.

Barker, A. Trevor, ed. *The Mahatma Letters to A. P. Sinnett from the Mahatmas M. and K.H.* 1923. Reprint, Pasadena, CA: Theosophical University Press, 1992.

Basu, Sris Chandra. *The Esoteric Science and Philosophy of the Tantras: Shiva Sanhita.* 1887. 2nd ed. Calcutta: Heeralal Dhole, 1893.

Battacharya, Abhijit. *A Guide to the Hitesranjan Sanyal Memorial Collection at Center for Studies in Social Sciences, Calcutta.* Calcutta: Center for Studies in Social Sciences, 1998. http://www.iisg.nl/csssc/guide.pdf.

B. B. [Baman Das Basu]. "The Anatomy of the Tantras." *Theosophist,* 9 (March 1888): 370–373. http://www.iapsop.com/archive/materials/theosophist/theosophist_v9_n102_march_1888.pdf.

Beasley, Victor. *Subtle-Body Healing.* Boulder Creek, CA: University of the Trees Press, 1979.

Bendit, Laurence J. and Phoebe D. Bendit. *The Etheric Body of Man: The Bridge of Consciousness.* Wheaton, IL: Quest Books, 1977.

———. *Man Incarnate: A Study of the Vital Etheric Field.* London: Theosophical Publishing House, 1957.

Besant, Annie. *The Ancient Wisdom.* 1896. Reprint, Adyar, Chennai, India: Theosophical Publishing House, 2001.

———. *Man and His Bodies.* 1896. 2nd ed. Reprint, Adyar, Chennai, India, 2008.

———. *The Seven Principles of Man.* 1892. Rev. ed. Reprint, Adyar, Chennai, India: Theosophical Publishing House, 2010.

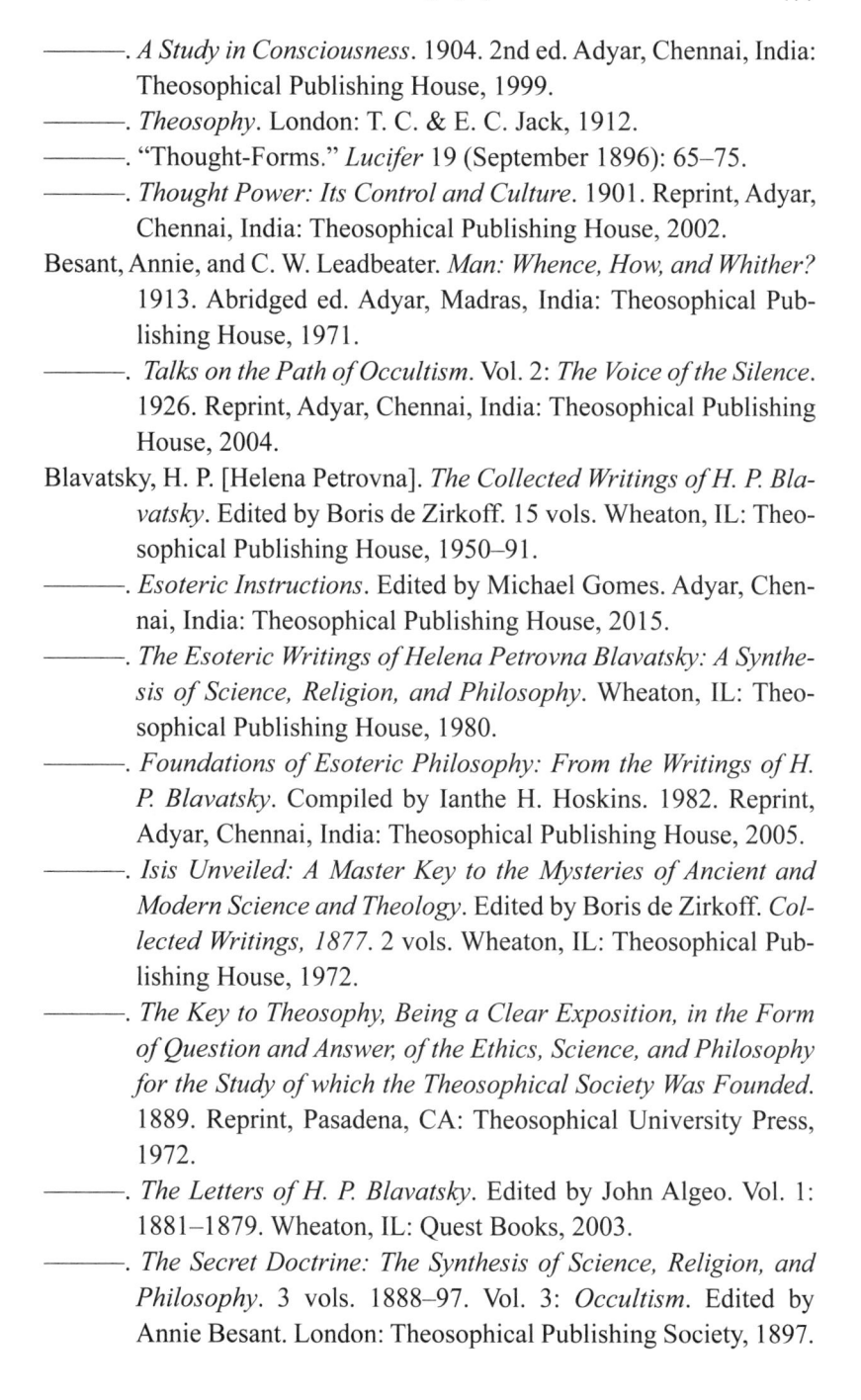

———. *A Study in Consciousness*. 1904. 2nd ed. Adyar, Chennai, India: Theosophical Publishing House, 1999.

———. *Theosophy*. London: T. C. & E. C. Jack, 1912.

———. "Thought-Forms." *Lucifer* 19 (September 1896): 65–75.

———. *Thought Power: Its Control and Culture*. 1901. Reprint, Adyar, Chennai, India: Theosophical Publishing House, 2002.

Besant, Annie, and C. W. Leadbeater. *Man: Whence, How, and Whither?* 1913. Abridged ed. Adyar, Madras, India: Theosophical Publishing House, 1971.

———. *Talks on the Path of Occultism*. Vol. 2: *The Voice of the Silence*. 1926. Reprint, Adyar, Chennai, India: Theosophical Publishing House, 2004.

Blavatsky, H. P. [Helena Petrovna]. *The Collected Writings of H. P. Blavatsky*. Edited by Boris de Zirkoff. 15 vols. Wheaton, IL: Theosophical Publishing House, 1950–91.

———. *Esoteric Instructions*. Edited by Michael Gomes. Adyar, Chennai, India: Theosophical Publishing House, 2015.

———. *The Esoteric Writings of Helena Petrovna Blavatsky: A Synthesis of Science, Religion, and Philosophy*. Wheaton, IL: Theosophical Publishing House, 1980.

———. *Foundations of Esoteric Philosophy: From the Writings of H. P. Blavatsky*. Compiled by Ianthe H. Hoskins. 1982. Reprint, Adyar, Chennai, India: Theosophical Publishing House, 2005.

———. *Isis Unveiled: A Master Key to the Mysteries of Ancient and Modern Science and Theology*. Edited by Boris de Zirkoff. *Collected Writings, 1877*. 2 vols. Wheaton, IL: Theosophical Publishing House, 1972.

———. *The Key to Theosophy, Being a Clear Exposition, in the Form of Question and Answer, of the Ethics, Science, and Philosophy for the Study of which the Theosophical Society Was Founded*. 1889. Reprint, Pasadena, CA: Theosophical University Press, 1972.

———. *The Letters of H. P. Blavatsky*. Edited by John Algeo. Vol. 1: 1881–1879. Wheaton, IL: Quest Books, 2003.

———. *The Secret Doctrine: The Synthesis of Science, Religion, and Philosophy*. 3 vols. 1888–97. Vol. 3: *Occultism*. Edited by Annie Besant. London: Theosophical Publishing Society, 1897.

———. *The Secret Doctrine: The Synthesis of Science, Religion, and Philosophy.* 1888–97. 4th ed. in 6 vols. Adyar, Madras, India: Theosophical Publishing House, 1938. [5th American ed. Wheaton, IL: Theosophical Press, 1947.]

———. *The Secret Doctrine: The Synthesis of Science, Religion, and Philosophy.* Edited by Boris de Zirkoff. *Collected Writings, 1888.* 3 vols. Adyar, Madras, India: Theosophical Publishing House, 1977.

———. *The Theosophical Glossary.* 1892. Reprint, Los Angeles: The Theosophy Company, 1973.

———. *The Voice of the Silence, Being Extracts from the Book of the Golden Precepts (First Series).* 1889. Reprint, Wheaton, IL: Quest Books, 1992. [No further volumes issued.]

Bohm, Werner. *Chakras: Lebenskräfte und Bewußtseinszentren im Menschen.* Munich, Germany: O. W. Barth, 1953.

Bose, Phanindranath. *Life of Sris Chandra Basu.* N.p.: R. Chatterjee, 1932.

Bragdon, Claude. *Yoga for You.* 1943. Reprint, New York: Knopf, 1945.

Brennan, Barbara Ann. *Hands of Light: A Guide to Healing through the Human Energy Field, a New Paradigm for the Human Being in Health, Relationship, and Disease.* New York: Bantam, 1988.

———. *Light Emerging: The Process of Personal Healing.* New York: Bantam, 1993.

Brousse, François. *Isis-Uranie ou l'Initiation majeure.* Perpignan, France: Labau, 1976.

Bruyere, Rosalyn. *Wheels of Light: A Study of the Chakras.* Vol. 1. Sierra Madre, CA: Bon Productions, 1989. [No further volumes issued.]

Bucke, Richard Maurice. *Cosmic Consciousness: A Study in the Evolution of the Human Mind.* 1901. Reprint, New York: Dutton, 1973.

Bühnemann, Gudrun. "The Six Rites of Magic." In David Gordon White, ed., *Tantra in Practice*, 447–62. Princeton, NJ: Princeton University Press, 2000.

Caldwell, Daniel. *The Esoteric Papers of Madame Blavatsky.* Whitefish, MT: Kessinger, 2004.

Campbell, Joseph. *The Inner Reaches of Outer Space: Metaphor as Myth and as Religion.* New York: Harper and Row, 1988.

———. "Kundalini Yoga: Seven Levels of Consciousness." *Psychology Today*, vol. 9, no. 7 (December 1975): 76–78.

———. *The Mythic Image*. Bollingen Series C. Princeton, NJ: Princeton University Press, 1974.

———. *Myths of Light: Eastern Metaphors of the Eternal*. Edited by David Kudler. Joseph Campbell Foundation. Novato, CA: New World Library, 2003.

———. *Myths to Live By*. 1972. Reprint, New York: Arkana, 1993.

———. *Transformations of Myth through Time*. New York: Harper and Row, 1990.

Campbell, Sharon, and Jefferson Campbell, eds. *Notes on Energy Balancing at the Polarity Health Institute*. Fall River Mills, CA: Polarity Health Institute, 1976.

Carrington, Hereward. *Higher Psychical Development (Yoga Philosophy): An Outline of the Secret Hindu Teachings*. New York: Dodd, Mead, 1920. https://ia600302.us.archive.org/32/items/higherpsychicald00carr/higherpsychicald00carr.pdf.

Cayce, Hugh Lynn. *Venture Inward*. New York: Harper & Row, 1964.

Chaudhuri, Haridas. "Yoga Psychology." In Charles Tart, ed., *Transpersonal Psychologies*, 231–80. New York: Harper and Row, 1975.

Chia, Mantak. *Awaken Healing Energy through the Tao: The Taoist Secret of Circulating Internal Power*. 1981. 2nd ed. New York: Aurora, 1983.

Corbett, Sarah. *Extracts from the Vahan, Including Answers by Annie Besant, A. P. Sinnett, G. R. S. Mead, C. W. Leadbeater, Bertram Keightley, Dr. A. A. Wells, and Others*. London: Theosophical Publishing Society, 1904. http://catalog.hathitrust.org/Record/007124954.

Corbin, Henry. *The Man of Light in Iranian Sufism*. Translated by Nancy Pearson. 1978. 2nd ed. New Lebanon, NY: Omega Publications, 1994.

Cranston, Sylvia [Anita Atkins]. *H.P.B: The Extraordinary Life and Influence of Helena Blavatsky*. New York: Putnam, 1993.

Crowley, Aleister. *The Equinox: The Review of Scientific Illuminism; The Official Organ of the O.T.O.*, vol. 3, no. 10 (March 1986). York Beach, ME: Red Wheel/Weiser, 1990.

———. *777 and Other Qabalistic Writings by Aleister Crowley, Including Gematria and Sepher Sephiroth*. Edited by Israel Regardie. 1973. Reprint, York Beach, ME: Weiser, 1986.

———. "The Temple of Solomon the King." Pt. 4. *Equinox: The Official Organ of the A∴A∴: The Review of Scientific Illuminism* 1, no. 4 (September 1910): 41–196. Reprint, New York: Weiser, 1972.

Cushing, Harvey. "The Basophil Adenomas of the Pituitary and Their Clinical Manifestation." *Bulletin of Johns Hopkins Hospital* 50 (1932): 137–95. Reprinted in *Obesity Research* 2 (September 1994): 486–508. http://onlinelibrary.wiley.com/doi/10.1002/j.1550-8528.1994.tb00097.x/pdf.

Dale, Cyndi. *Llewellyn's Complete Book of Chakras: Your Definitive Source of Energy Center Knowledge for Health, Happiness, and Spiritual Evolution*. Woodbury, MN: Llewellyn, 2016.

Daniélou, Alain. *Yoga: The Method of Re-Integration*. New York: University Books, 1955.

Devaney, John Patrick. *Astral Projection or Liberation of the Double and the Work of the Early Theosophical Society*. Theosophical History Occasional Papers, no. 6. Fullerton, CA: Theosophical History, 1997.

Diem-Lane, Andrea. *The Guru in America: The Influence of Radhasoami on New Religions*. 1995. Reprint, Walnut, CA: MSAC [Mt. San Antonio College] Philosophy Group, 2008.

Dowman, Keith. *Masters of Mahāmudrā: Songs and Histories of the Eighty-Four Buddhist Siddhas*. Albany, NY: State University of New York Press, 1985.

"The Dream of Ravan: A Mystery." Pt. 4. *Dublin University Magazine*, 43 (April 1854): 456–75. http://babel.hathitrust.org/cgi/pt?id=nyp.33433081646634;view=1up;seq=9.

Dychtwald, Ken, "Bodymind and the Evolution to Cosmic Consciousness." *Yoga Journal* 15 (July/August 1977): 22–26. https://books.google.com/books?id=cesDAAAAMBAJ&lpg=PP1&lr&rview=1&pg=PA22#v=onepage&q&f=false.

———. *Bodymind: A Synthesis of Eastern and Western Ways to Self-Awareness, Health, and Personal Growth*. New York: Pantheon, 1977.

Eliade, Mircea. *Yoga: Immortality and Freedom*. Translated by Willard Trask. 1958. Reprint, Princeton, NJ: Princeton University Press, 2009.

Estep, William. *Esoteric Cosmic Yogi Science, or Works of the World Teacher*. 2 vols. 1929. Reprint in 1 vol. Whitefish, MT: Kessinger, 2010.

Evola, Julius. *The Yoga of Power: Tantra, Shakti, and the Secret Way*. Translated by Guido Stucco. Rochester, VT: Inner Traditions, 1992.

Feuerstein, Georg. *Encyclopedia of Yoga and Tantra*. 1979. 2nd ed. Revised and enlarged. Boston: Shambhala, 2011.

———. *Tantra: The Path of Ecstasy*. Boston: Shambhala, 1998.

———. *The Yoga Tradition: Its History, Literature, Philosophy, and Practice*. 1998. Reprint, Prescott, AZ: Hohm Press, 2001.

Fletcher, Ella Adelia. *The Law of the Rhythmic Breath: Teaching the Generation, Conservation, and Control of Vital Force*. New York: Fenno, 1908. http://catalog.hathitrust.org/Record/007679679.

———. *The Woman Beautiful: A Practical Treatise on the Development and Preservation of Woman's Health and Beauty, and the Principles of Taste in Dress*. New York: W. M. Young, 1899. http://catalog.hathitrust.org/Record/012288981.

Flood, Gavin. *An Introduction to Hinduism*. Cambridge, United Kingdom: Cambridge University Press, 1996.

———. *The Tantric Body: The Secret Tradition of Hindu Religion*. London: Tauris, 2006.

Fortune, Dion [Violet Mary Firth]. *The Mystical Qabalah*. 1935. Rev. ed. San Francisco: Weiser, 2000.

Fortune, Dion, and Gareth Knight [Basil Wilby]. *The Circuit of Force: Occult Dynamics of the Etheric Vehicle*. Loughborough, Leicestershire, UK: Thoth Publications, 1998.

Gardner, E. L. "The Theosophical Research Center (England)." In *Group Work*, 2–4. London: Theosophical Research Center, 1947.

Gardner, Joy. *Color and Crystals: A Journey through the Chakras*. Freedom, CA: Crossing Press, 1988.

Garrison, Omar. *Tantra: The Yoga of Sex*. 1964. Reprint, New York: Julian Press, 1971.

Garver, Will L. *The Brother of the Third Degree*. Boston: Arena, 1894. http://catalog.hathitrust.org/Record/100552566.

Gherwal, Rishi Singh. *Kundalini, the Mother of the Universe: The Piercing of the Six Chakras*. Santa Barbara, CA: printed by author, 1930.

Gichtel, Johann Georg. *Awakening to Divine Wisdom: Christian Initiation into Three Worlds.* Translated by Arthur Versluis. St. Paul, MN: New Grail, 2004.

———. *Theosophia practica, traduite pour la première fois en français.* Paris: Chamuel, 1897.

Goswami, Shayam Shundar. *Layayoga: The Definitive Guide to the Chakras and Kundalini*. 1980. Reprint, Rochester, VT: Inner Traditions, 1999.

Govinda, Anagarika [Ernst Lothar Hoffmann]. *Foundations of Tibetan Mysticism according to the Esoteric Teachings of the Great Mantra "Oṃ Maṇi Padme Hūṃ."* 1969. Reprint, Boston: Weiser, 2001.

Guénon, René. *Studies in Hinduism*. Translated by Henry D. Fohr. 2001. Reprint, Hillsdale, NY: Sophia Perennis, 2004.

Gunther, Bernard. *Energy, Ecstasy, and Your Seven Vital Chakras*. Los Angeles: Guild of Tutors Press, 1978.

———. *Neo-Tantra: Bhagwan Shree Rajneesh on Sex, Love, Prayer, and Transcendence*. New York: Harper and Row, 1980.

Gupta, Sanjukta. "The Worship of Kali According to the *Ṭoḍala Tantra*." In David Gordon White, ed., *Tantra in Practice*, 463–88. Princeton, NJ: Princeton University Press, 2000.

Hammer, Olav. *Claiming Knowledge: Strategies of Epistemology from Theosophy to the New Age*. 2001. Reprint, Leiden, Netherlands: Brill, 2004.

Hanish, Otoman Zar-Adusht [Otto Hanisch]. *Health and Breath Culture according to Mazdaznan Philosophy (Sun-Worship)*. Chicago: Sun-Worshiper Press, 1902. ftp://ftp.mazdeen.com/21-Breath.pdf [repaginated text with original titles and figures].

Harper, Katherine Anne, and Robert L. Brown, eds. *The Roots of Tantra*. Albany, NY: State University of New York Press, 2002.

Hartmann, William C. *Hartmann's Who's Who in Occult, Psychic, and Spiritual Realms in the United States and Foreign Countries*. Jamaica, NY: Occult Press, 1925. http://www.ehbritten.org/docs/1925_hartmann_whos_who_in_occult_psychic_and_spiritual_realms_r.pdf.

Hayman, Ronald. *A Life of Jung.* New York: Norton, 2001.

Heindel, Max. *The Rosicrucian Cosmo-Conception, or Christian Occult Science: An Elementary Treatise upon Man's Past Evolution, Present Constitution, and Future Development.* Seattle, WA: Rosicrucian Fellowship, 1909. http://catalog.hathitrust.org/Record/100133409.

Hesse, Hermann. *The Journey to the East.* Translated by Hilda Rosner. New York: Farrar, Straus & Giroux, 1956.

Hills, Christopher. *Nuclear Evolution: A Guide to Cosmic Enlightenment.* London: Centre Community Publications, 1968.

———. *Nuclear Evolution: Discovery of the Rainbow Body.* Boulder Creek, CA: University of the Trees Press, 1977. [2nd edition of the above.]

Hills, Norah, ed. *You Are a Rainbow: Original Insights into the Work of Christopher Hills by Researchers Practicing His Theory of Nuclear Evolution.* Boulder Creek, CA: University of the Trees Press, 1979.

Hodson, Geoffrey. *The Science of Seership: A Study of the Faculty of Clairvoyance, Its Development and Use, Together with Examples of Clairvoyant Research.* London: Ryder, 1929.

Hoffmann, Edward. *The Right to Be Human: A Biography of Abraham Maslow.* Los Angeles: Tarcher, 1988.

Holmes, Ernest. *The Science of Mind: A Complete Course of Lessons in the Science of Mind and Spirit.* New York, NY: McBride, 1926.

Hopking, Alan. *Esoteric Healing: A Practical Guide Based on the Teachings of the Tibetan in the Works of Alice A. Bailey.* Nevada City, CA: Blue Dolphin, 2005.

Hübbe-Schleiden, Wilhelm. *Indisches Tagebuch 1894/1896.* Edited by Norbert Klatt. Göttingen: published by author, 2009. http://d-nb.info/993376584/34.

Hugh, Paola. *"I Will Arise!": The Light of Clarification.* Tacoma, WA: Fleur de Lys Foundation, 1972.

———. *"I Will Arise!": Procedures Toward Transmutation and Translation.* Tacoma, WA: Fleur de Lys Foundation, 1972.

Hunt, Roland T. *Complete Color Prescription for Rebuilding Our Bodies and Cities.* 1941. 3rd ed. Los Angeles: Paramount Press, 1962.

———. *The Eighth Key to Color: Self-Analysis and Clarification through Color*. 1965. 2nd ed. London: Fowler, 1970.

———. *The Finding of Rainbow's End, and Other Mystical Experiences in the "Mother Lode" Country during 1930*. London: Daniel, 1939.

———. *Fragrant and Radiant Symphony: An Enquiry into the Wondrous Correlation of the Healing Virtues of Color, Sound, and Perfume and a Consideration of Their Influence and Purpose*. London: Daniel, 1937.

———. *Lighting-Therapy and Color Harmony*. London: Daniel, 1941.

———. *The Seven Keys to Color Healing: A Complete Outline to the Practice of Color Healing*. London: Daniel, 1940.

Huxley, Aldous. *The Perennial Philosophy*. 1945. Reprint, New York: Harper, 2009.

Jinarājadāsa, C. *Occult Investigations: A Description of the Work of Annie Besant and C. W. Leadbeater*. Adyar, Madras, India: Theosophical Publishing House, 1938.

Johari, Harish. *Chakras: Energy Centers of Transformation*. Rochester, VT: Destiny Books, 1987.

Johnson, K. Paul. *Edgar Cayce in Context: The Readings: Truth and Fiction*. Albany: State University of New York Press, 1998.

———. *Initiates of the Theosophical Masters*. Albany: State University of New York Press, 1995.

Jones, Alex. *The Seven Mansions of Color*. Marina del Rey, CA: DeVorss, 1982.

Joy, W. Brugh. *Joy's Way: A Map for the Transformational Journey—and Introduction to the Potentials for Healing with Body Energies*. Los Angeles: Tarcher, 1979.

Judge, William Q. "Faces of Friends." *Path* 9:90–91 (June 1894). https://books.google.com/books?id=l0QUAAAAYAAJ.

Judith, Anodea. *Wheels of Life: A User's Guide to the Chakra System*. 1987. 2nd ed. St. Paul, MN: Llewellyn, 1999.

Juergensmeyer, Mark. *Radhasoami Reality: The Logic of a Modern Faith*. Princeton, NJ: Princeton University Press, 1991.

Jung, C. G. *The Psychology of Kundalini Yoga: Notes of the Seminar Given in 1932 by C. G. Jung*. Edited by Sonu Shamdasani. Bollingen Series XCIX. Princeton, NJ: Princeton University Press, 1996.

———. *The Red Book—Liber Novus*. Edited by Sonu Shamdasani. New York, Norton: 2009.

Kakar, Sudhir. *Shamans, Mystics and Doctors: A Psychological Inquiry into India and Its Healing Traditions*. 1982. Reprint, Chicago: Chicago University Press, 1991.

Karagulla, Shafica. *Breakthrough to Creativity: Your Higher Sense Perception*. Santa Monica, CA: DeVorss, 1967.

Karagulla, Shafica and Dora van Gelder Kunz. *The Chakras and the Human Energy Fields*. Wheaton, IL: Quest, 1989.

Keyes, Ken Jr. *Handbook to Higher Consciousness: The Science of Happiness*. 1972. 5th ed. Reprint, St. Mary, KY: Living Love Publications, 1978.

King, Francis. *Ritual Magic of the Golden Dawn: Works by S. L. MacGregor Mathers and Others*. 1987. Reprint, Rochester, VT: Destiny, 1997.

———. *Tantra, the Way of Action: A Practical Guide to Its Teachings and Techniques*. 1986. Reprint, Rochester, VT: Destiny, 1990.

Koltko-Rivera, Mark E. "Rediscovering the Later Version of Maslow's Hierarchy of Needs: Self-Transcendence and Opportunities for Theory, Research, and Unification." *Review of General Psychology*, 10 (December 2006): 302–17. http://academic.udayton.edu/jackbauer/Readings%20595/Koltko-Rivera%2006%20trans%20self-act%20copy.pdf.

Kripal, Jeffrey J. *Esalen: America and the Religion of No Religion*. Chicago: University of Chicago Press, 2007.

Krishna, Gopi. *Kundalini: The Evolutionary Energy in Man*. 1967. 2nd rev. ed. Berkeley, CA: Shambhala, 1970.

Lansdowne, Zachary F. *The Chakras and Esoteric Healing*. York Beach, ME: Weiser, 1986.

Larsen, Stephen, and Robin Larsen. *A Fire in the Mind: The Life of Joseph Campbell*. New York: Doubleday, 1991.

Leadbeater, C. W. [Charles Webster]. "The Aura." *Theosophist* 17 (December 1895): 134–43. http://babel.hathitrust.org/cgi/pt?id=nyp.33433087382234;view=1up;seq=140.

———. *The Aura: An Enquiry into the Nature and Functions of the Luminous Mist Seen about Human and Other Bodies*. London: Theosophical Publishing Society, 1897.

———. *The Chakras: A Monograph.* Chicago, IL: Theosophical Press, 1927.

———. *The Chakras: An Authoritative Edition of the Groundbreaking Classic.* Annotations and afterword by Kurt Leland. Wheaton, IL: Quest Books, 2013.

———. *Clairvoyance.* 1899. Reprint, Adyar, Madras, India: Theosophical Publishing House, 1968.

———. "Force-Centers and the Serpent-Fire." *Theosophist* 31(May 1910): 1075–94.

———. *The Hidden Life in Freemasonry.* Adyar, Madras, India: Theosophical Publishing House, 1926.

———. *The Hidden Side of Things.* 1913. 3rd ed. Adyar, Chennai, India: Theosophical Publishing House, 1999.

———. *How Theosophy Came to Me.* 1930. Reprint, Adyar, Chennai, India: Theosophical Publishing House, 2001.

———. *The Inner Life.* 2 vols. 1910–11. 2nd abridged ed. in 1 vol. Reprint, Wheaton, IL: Quest Books, 1996.

———. *Invisible Helpers.* 1896. Rev. and enl. ed. 1928. Reprint, Adyar, Madras, India: Theosophical Publishing House, 1986.

———. *Man Visible and Invisible.* 1902. 2nd abridged ed. Wheaton, IL: Quest Books, 2000.

———. *The Masters and the Path.* 1925. 2nd abridged ed. Reprint, Adyar, Chennai, India, 2002.

———. *The Science of the Sacraments.* 1920. 2nd ed. Reprint, Adyar, Madras, India: Theosophical Publishing House, 1991.

Leland, Kurt. "*The Chakras*: An Editorial Report." *Theosophical History* 16 (October 2014): 141–67.

———. *Invisible Worlds: Annie Besant on Psychic and Spiritual Development.* Wheaton, IL: Quest Books, 2013.

———. *Music and the Soul: A Listener's Guide to Achieving Transcendent Musical Experiences.* Charlottesville, VA: Hampton Roads, 2004.

Leonard, John, ed. *Who's Who in New York City and State: Containing Authentic Biographies of New Yorkers Who Are Leaders and Representatives in Various Departments of Worthy Human Achievement.* 3rd ed. New York: Hammersly, 1907. http://babel.hathitrust.org/cgi/pt?id=mdp.39015025876510;view=1up;seq=7.

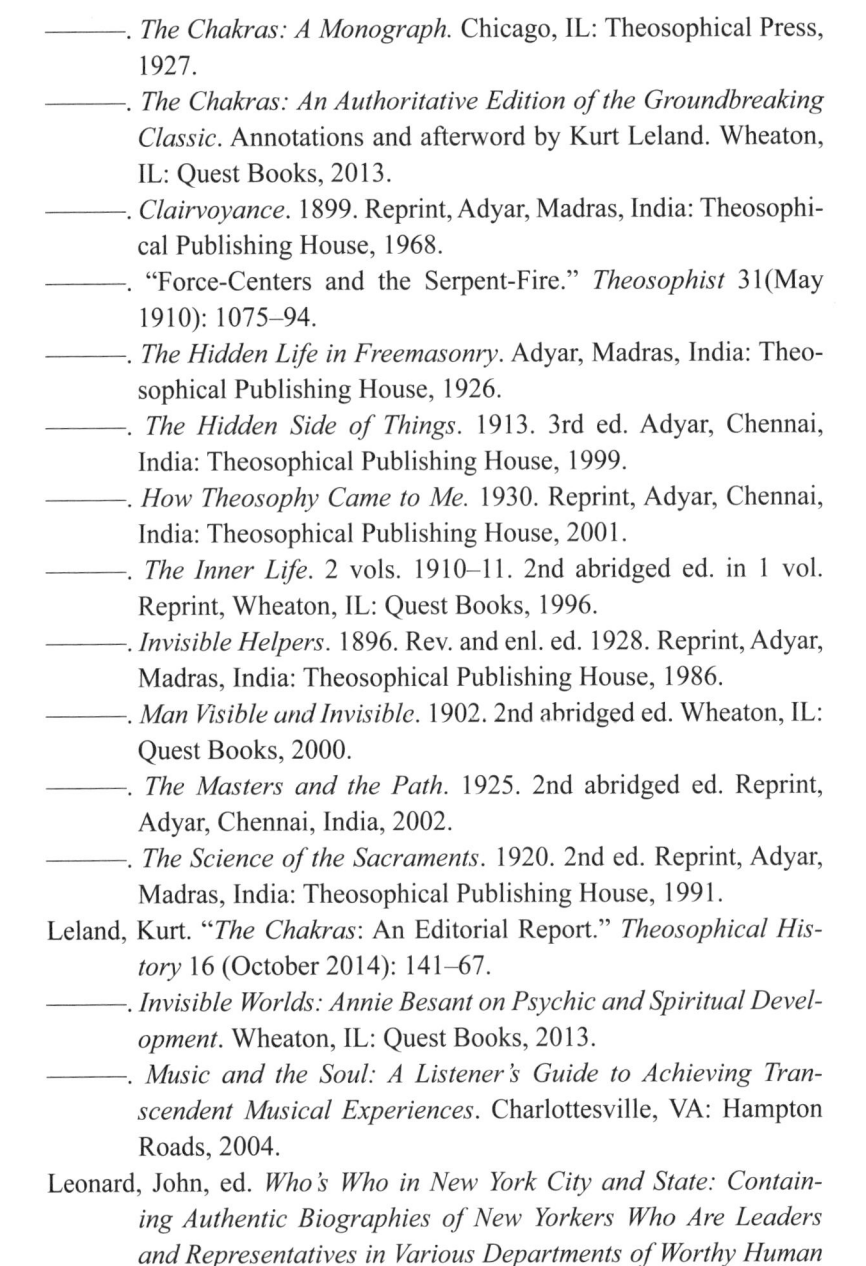

Lewis, James R. *The Encyclopedia of Cults, Sects, and New Religions.* 2nd ed. Amherst, NY: Prometheus, 2002.

Lorenzen, David. "Early Evidence for Tantra Religion." In Katherine Anne Harper and Robert L. Brown, *The Roots of Tantra*, 25–36. Albany, NY: State University of New York Press, 2002.

Love, Robert. *The Great Oom: The Mysterious Origins of America's First Yogi.* New York: Penguin, 2011.

Lowndes, Florin. *Enlivening the Chakra of the Heart: The Fundamental Spiritual Exercises of Rudolf Steiner.* 1998. 2nd ed. London: Rudolf Steiner Press, 2000.

Luk, A. D. K. [Alice Schutz]. *Law of Life.* 2 vols. Pueblo, CO: printed by author, 1959–60.

Lüscher, Max. *The Lüscher Color Test.* New York: Random House, 1969.

McFarlane, Jenny. *Concerning the Spiritual: The Influence of the Theosophical Society on Australian Artists 1890-1934.* Melbourne, Australia: Australian Scholarly Publishing, 2012.

MacLaine, Shirley. *Going Within: A Guide for Inner Transformation.* New York: Bantam, 1989.

McLaren, Karla. *Your Aura and Your Chakras: The Owner's Manual.* San Francisco: Weiser, 1998.

Maheshwari, S. D., trans. *Discourses of Babuji Maharaj.* 5 vols. Agra, India: Radhasoami Satsang Agra, 1975–78.

Majumdar, Baradakanta. "A Glimpse of Tantric Occultism." *Theosophist* 1 (July 1880): 244–45; 2 (October 1880): 3–4. http://www.iapsop.com/archive/materials/theosophist/theosophist_v1_n10_july_1880.pdf.

———. "Tantric Philosophy." *Theosophist* 1 (April 1880): 173–74. http://babel.hathitrust.org/cgi/pt?id=nyp.33433087382234;view=1up;seq=224.

Mallinson, James. *The Gheranda Samhita: The Original Sanskrit and an English Translation.* Woodstock, NY: YogaVidya.com, 2004.

———. *The Shiva Samhita: A Critical Edition and an English Translation.* Woodstock, NY: YogaVidya.com, 2007.

Mann, W. Edward. *Orgone, Reich, and Eros: Wilhelm Reich's Theory of Life Energy.* New York: Simon and Schuster, 1973.

Marques, A. [Auguste]. *The Human Aura: A Study.* San Francisco, CA: Office of *Mercury*, 1896.

Melton, J. Gordon, ed. *Encyclopedia of Occultism and Parapsychology.* 1978. 5th ed. 2 vols. Detroit, MI: Gale, 2001.

———. *Melton's Encyclopedia of American Religions.* 1978. 8th ed. Detroit, MI: Gale, Cengage Learning, 2009.

———. *New Age Encyclopedia: A Guide to the Beliefs, Concepts, Terms, People, and Organizations that Make Up the New Global Movement toward Spiritual Development, Health, and Healing, Higher Consciousness, and Related Subjects.* Detroit, MI: Gale, 1990.

Mishra, Brahm Shankar. *Discourses on Radhasoami Faith.* Benares, India: Radhasoami Satsang Benares, 1909. http://catalog.hathitrust.org/Record/002711864.

Motoyama, Hiroshi. *Theories of the Chakras: Bridge to Higher Consciousness.* Wheaton, IL: Quest Books, 1981.

Motter, H. L., ed. *The International Who's Who: Who's Who in the World.* New York: International Who's Who, 1912. babel.hathitrust.org/cgi/pt?id=wu.89097340061;view=1up;seq=7.

Mukherji, P. C. "The Radhaswami Society of Agra." Pts. 1 and 2. *Theosophist* 16 (1985): 571–76 (June), 708–14 (August).

Mumford, Jonn. *A Chakra and Kundalini Workbook: Psycho-spiritual Techniques for Health, Rejuvenation, Psychic Powers, and Spiritual Realization.* St. Paul, MN: Llewellyn, 1994.

———. *Ecstasy through Tantra.* 1998. Reprint, St. Paul, MN: Llewellyn, 2002.

———. *Psychosomatic Yoga: A Guide to Eastern Path Techniques.* 1962. Reprint, New York: Weiser, 1974.

———. *Sexual Occultism: The Sorcery of Love in Practice and Theory.* St. Paul, MN: Llewellyn, 1975.

Myss, Caroline. *Anatomy of the Spirit: The Seven Stages of Power and Healing.* New York: Three Rivers Press, 1997.

Narayansami, K. "Notes to 'The Legend of Dwārakā.'" *Theosophist* 17 (January 1896): 218–20. http://babel.hathitrust.org/cgi/pt?id=nyp.33433087382234;view=1up;seq=224.

Neff, Dio Urmilla, "The Great Chakra Controversy." *Yoga Journal* 65 (November/December 1985): 42–45, 50, 52–53. https://books.google.com/books?id=nusDAAAAMBAJ&lpg=PP1&ots=q-eFudifxg&dq=%22great%20chakra%20controversy%22%20

yoga%20journal&pg=PA42#v=onepage&q=%22great%20 chakra%20controversy%22%20yoga%20journal&f=false.

Nethercot, Arthur H. *The First Five Lives of Annie Besant*. Chicago: University of Chicago Press, 1960.

———. *The Last Four Lives of Annie Besant*. Chicago: University of Chicago Press, 1963.

Olcott, Henry S. *A Collection of Lectures on Theosophy and Archaic Religions Delivered in India and Ceylon*. Madras: A. Theyaga Rajier, 1883. http://catalog.hathitrust.org/Record/100331586.

———. *Old Diary Leaves*. 6 vols. 1895–1935. Reprint, Adyar, Madras, India: Theosophical Publishing House, 1974–75.

———. *Theosophy, Religion, and Occult Science*. London: Redway, 1885.

Osho [Bhagwan Shree Rajneesh]. *In Search of the Miraculous*. 1970. Reprint, Pune, Maharashtra, India: Osho Media, 2012.

Ouseley, S. G. J. [Stephen Geoffrey John]. *Color Meditations, with Guide to Color Healing: A Course of Instructions and Exercises in Developing Color Consciousness*. 1949. Reprint, London: Fowler, 1974.

———. *From Camaldoli to Christ: Modern Monasticism Unveiled*. London: Harrison Trust, 1931.

———. "The Garden of Enchantment." *Theosophist* 67 (November 1945): 70–71.

———. *A Guide to Telepathy and Psychometry: The Laws of Thought Projection and the Scientific and Practical Aspects of Psychometry*. London: Fowler, 1948.

———. *The Power of the Rays: The Science of Color-Healing*. 1951. Reprint, Romford, Essex, England: Fowler, 1976.

———. *The Science of the Aura: An Introduction to the Study of the Human Aura*. 1949. Reprint, London: Fowler, 1975.

Ozaniec, Naomi. *The Chakras: A Beginner's Guide*. 1999. Reprint, London: Hodder & Stoughton, 2002.

Padoux, André. *Vāc: The Concept of the Word in Selected Hindu Tantras*. Translated by Jacques Gontier. Albany: State University of New York Press, 1990.

Payne, Phoebe. *Man's Latent Powers*. London: Faber & Faber, 1938.

Payne, Phoebe D., and Laurence J. Bendit. *The Psychic Sense*. London: Faber & Faber, 1943.

Pierrakos, John C. *Core Energetics: Developing the Capacity to Love and Heal*. Mendocino, CA: LifeRhythm, 1989.
Powell, A. E. [Arthur Edward]. *The Causal Body and the Ego*. 1928. Reprint, Adyar, Chennai, India: Theosophical Publishing House, 2003.
———. *The Etheric Double: The Health Aura*. 1925. Reprint, Wheaton, IL: Quest Books, 1996.
Prasād, Rāma. *Occult Science: The Science of Breath*. Lahore, India: R. C. Bary, 1884.
———. *The Science of Breath and the Philosophy of the Tattwas: Translated from the Sanskrit with Fifteen Introductory and Explanatory Essays on Nature's Finer Forces*. 1890. 2nd rev. ed. London: Theosophical Publishing Society, 1894. http://catalog.hathitrust.org/Record/001379840.
Prophet, Elizabeth Clare. *Intermediate Studies of the Human Aura*. 1976. Reprint, Los Angeles: Summit University Press, 1980.
Prophet, Mark L. *Studies of the Human Aura*. 1971. Reprint, Los Angeles: Summit University Press, 1980.
Pryse, James M. *The Apocalypse Unsealed: Being an Interpretation of the Initiation of Ioannes, Commonly Called the Revelation of St. John, with a New Translation*. London: John M. Watkins, 1910. http://catalog.hathitrust.org/Record/100433198.
———. *The Magical Message according to Ioannes; Commonly Called the Gospel according to John; a Verbatim Translation from the Greek Done in Modern English with Introductory Essays and Notes*. New York: Theosophical Publishing Company, 1909. http://catalog.hathitrust.org/Record/100771181.
———. *The Restored New Testament, the Hellenic Fragments, Freed from the Pseudo-Jewish Interpolations, Harmonized, and Done into English Verse and Prose with Introductory Analyses, and Commentaries, Giving an Interpretation according to Ancient Philosophy and Psychology and a New Literal Translation of the Synoptic Gospels, with Introduction and Commentaries*. New York: John M. Pryse, 1914. http://catalog.hathitrust.org/Record/008419140.
Puryear, Herbert B., *Reflections on the Path (Based on the Edgar Cayce Readings)*. Virginia Beach, VA: ARE Press, 1979.

Puryear, Herbert B. and Mark Thurston. *Meditation and the Mind of Man (Based on the Edgar Cayce Readings)*. Virginia Beach, VA: ARE Press, 1975. Also 2nd edition, 1978.

Radha, Swami Sivananda. *Kundalini Yoga for the West*. Spokane, WA: Timeless Books, 1978.

Ram Dass. *The Only Dance There Is: Talks Given at the Menninger Foundation, Topeka, Kansas, 1970, and at Spring Grove, Maryland, 1972*. Garden City, NY: Doubleday, 1974.

———. *Remember: Be Here Now*. San Cristobal, NM: Lama Foundation, 1971.

Ransom, Josephine. *A Short History of the Theosophical Society*. 1938. Reprint, Adyar, Madras, India: Theosophical Publishing House, 1989.

Reed, Henry. *Awakening Your Psychic Powers: Edgar Cayce's Wisdom for the New Age*. San Francisco: Harper & Row, 1988.

———. *Edgar Cayce on Channeling Your Higher Self*. New York: Warner, 1989.

Regardie, Israel. *A Garden of Pomegranates: An Outline of the Qabalah*. 1932. 2nd ed. Revised and enlarged. 1970. Reprint, St. Paul, MN: Llewellyn, 1994.

Rele, Vasant G. *The Mysterious Kundalini: The Physical Basis of the "Kundali (Hatha) Yoga" according to Our Present Knowledge of Physical Anatomy*. 1927. 3rd ed. Revised and enlarged. Bombay, India: Taraporevala, 1931.

Rendel, Peter. *Introduction to the Chakras*. New York: Weiser, 1974.

Roberts, Thomas B. and Ralph H. Hannon. "A Holistic Meeting of Transpersonal Psychology and Theosophy: Chakras, Needs, and Moral Development." *American Theosophist* 67 (December 1979): 365–73.

Rosenberg, Jack Lee. *Total Orgasm*. New York: Random House, 1973.

Rubin, Herman H. *Your Mysterious Glands: How Your Glands Control Your Mental and Physical Development and Moral Welfare*. New York: Hand's Publishing, 1925. http://catalog.hathitrust.org/Record/009074014.

Ruff, Jeffrey Clark. "Yoga in the *Yoga Upaniṣad*s: Disciplines of the Mystical *OṀ* Sound." In David Gordon White, ed., *Yoga in Practice*, 97–116. Princeton, NJ: Princeton University Press, 2012.

Sabhapaty Swami. *Om: A Treatise on Vedantic Raj Yoga Philosophy.* Edited by Siris Chandra Basu. Lahore, India: Civil and Military Gazette Press, 1880.

———. *Om: The Cosmic Psychological Spiritual Philosophy of Communion with and Absorption in the Holy and Divine Infinite Spirit.* 2 vols. Madras, India: Hindu Press, 1884–90.

———. *The Philosophy and Science of Vedanta and Raja Yoga.* 1883. Reprint, Bombay, Chaitanya Prabha Mandali, 1950.

———. *Vedantic Raj Yoga: Ancient Yoga of Rishies.* 1880. Reprint, New Delhi: Pankaj Publications, 1977.

Sabhapatti Svami. "Aus der Philosophie und Wissenschaft des Vedānta und Rāja-Yoga, von Mahātmā Jñāna Guru Yogī Sabhapatti Svāmī. Translated by Franz Hartmann. Pts. 1–3. *Neue Lotusblüten* 1 (1908): 271–82 (July/August), 319–53 (September/October), 377–403 (November/December).

———. "Aus dem Leben des Mahātmā Jñāna Guru Yogī Sabhapatti Svāmī." Translated by Franz Hartmann. *Neue Lotusblüten* 1 (July/August 1908): 259–70.

———. *Die Philosophie und Wissenschaft des Vedānta und Rāja-Yoga; oder Das Eingehen in Gott.* 1909. Translated by Franz Hartmann. Reprint, Leipzig, Germany: Theosophisches Verlagshaus, 1926.

Śāradā-Tilaka Tantram: Translation by a Board of Scholars. 1988. Reprint, Delhi, India: Sri Satguru Publications, 2002.

Saraswati, Satyananda. *Kundalini Tantra.* 1984. Reprint, Munger, Bihar, India: Yoga Publications Trust, 1996.

Saraswati, Sivananda. *Kundalini Yoga.* Madras, India: P. K. Vinayagam, 1935.

Śāstrī, S. Subrahmaṇya, ed. *The Yoga-Upaniṣad-s: Translated into English on the Basis of the Commentary of Śrī Upaniṣad-Brahma-Yogin.* Adyar, Madras, India: Adyar Library, 1938. https://ia800304.us.archive.org/5/items/TheYogaUpanishads/TheYogaUpanisadsSanskritEngish1938.pdf.

Schmidt, Leigh Eric. *Heaven's Bride: The Unprintable Life of Ida C. Craddock, American Mystic, Scholar, Sexologist, Martyr, and Madwoman.* New York: Basic Books, 2010.

Schutz, William C. *Here Comes Everybody: Bodymind and Encounter Culture.* New York: Harper & Row, 1973.

Schwarz, Jack. *Human Energy Systems: A Way of Good Health, Using Our Auric Fields—Including Special Eye Exercises, a Tarot System and Guide to Medicinal Herbs.* New York: Dutton, 1980.

———. *Voluntary Controls: Exercises for Creative Meditation and for Activating the Potential of the Chakras.* New York: Dutton, 1978.

Seidman, Maruti. *Balancing the Chakras.* Berkeley, CA: North Atlantic Books, 2000.

———. *Like a Hollow Flute: A Guide to Polarity Therapy.* Santa Cruz, CA: Elan, 1982.

Shah, Idries. *The Sufis.* 1964. Reprint, New York: Random House, 1971.

Shastry, R. Ananta Krishna. "Some Notes on Kundalini." *Theosophist* 15 (February 1894): 276–83.

Shea, David and Anthony Troyer, trans. *The Dabistān or School of Manners.* 3 vols. Paris: Oriental Translation Fund of Great Britain and Ireland, 1843. http://catalog.hathitrust.org/Record/009734009.

———. *The Dabistān or School of Manners: The Religious Beliefs, Observances, Philosophic Opinions, and Social Customs of the Nations of the East.* Abridged ed. in 1 vol. New York: M. Walter Dunne, 1901. http://catalog.hathitrust.org/Record/100605970.

Shom, Bipin Behari. "Physical Errors of Hinduism." *Calcutta Review* 11 (April–June 1849): 397–444. http://books.google.com/books?id=SdWgAAAAMAAJ&pg=PA397#v=onepage&q&f=false.

———. "Physical Errors of Hinduism." *The Sessional Papers Printed by Order of the House of Lords, or Presented by Royal Command, in the Session 1852–53.* Vol. 29: *Reports from Select Committees of the House of Lords, and Evidence (continued): Government of Indian Territories.* London: N.P., 1853. http://books.google.com/books?id=TRlcAAAAQAAJ&pg=PA453#v=onepage&q&f=false.

Singleton, Mark. *Yoga Body: The Origins of Modern Posture Practice.* New York: Oxford University Press, 2010.

Sinnett, A. P. [Alfred Percy]. *Esoteric Buddhism.* 1883. 5th ed., annotated and enlarged. London: Chapman and Hall, 1885. http://catalog.hathitrust.org/Record/100335309.

———. *The Growth of the Soul: A Sequel to "Esoteric Buddhism."*

London: Theosophical Publishing Society, 1896. http://catalog.hathitrust.org/Record/001405886.

———. *The Human Aura. Transactions of the London Lodge of the Theosophical Society*, no. 18 (July, 1893).

———. *The Occult World*. 1881. American ed. from 4th English ed. Boston: Houghton Mifflin, 1885. http://catalog.hathitrust.org/Record/100434847.

Soami Ji. *Sar Bachan: The Yoga of the Sound Current*. 1934. 8th ed. Beas, India: Radha Soami Satsang Beas, 1987.

Spierenburg, Henk J. *The Inner Group Teachings of H. P. Blavatsky to Her Personal Pupils (1890–91)*. 2nd ed. San Diego, CA: Point Loma Publications, 1995.

Sri Chinmoy. *Kundalini: The Mother Power*. Jamaica, New York: Agni Press, 1974.

Steiner, Rudolf. *Autobiography: Chapters in the Course of My Life*. Translated by Rita Stebbing. Notes and Chronology by Paul M. Allen. Great Barrington, MA: Anthroposophical Press, 2006.

———. *How to Know Higher Worlds: A Modern Path of Initiation*. Translated by Christopher Bamford. 1994. Reprint, Great Barrington, MA: Anthroposophic Press, 2014.

———. *Initiation and Its Results: A Sequel to "The Way of Initiation."* Translated by Clifford Bax. First Americanized edition. New York: Macoy, 1909.

———. *The Way of Initiation; or How to Attain Knowledge of Higher Worlds*. Translated by Max Gysi. London: Theosophical Publishing Society, 1908.

———. "Wie erlangt man Erkenntnisse der höheren Welten?: Über einige Wirkungen der Einweihung." Pts. 1–5. *Lucifer-Gnosis*, 20 (January 1905): 225–30; 21 (February 1905): 257–62; 22 (March 1905): 289–93; 23 (April 1905): 321–25; 24 (May 1905): 353–57.

Stevens, Petey. *Opening Up to Your Psychic Self*. 1982. 2nd ed. Berkeley, CA: Nevertheless Press, 1983.

Subba Row, T. "The Idyll of the White Lotus." Pt. 2. *Theosophist* 7 (August 1886): 705–8.

Sui, Choa Kok. *The Ancient Science and Art of Pranic Healing: Practical Manual on Paranormal Healing*. Quezon City, Philippines: Institute for Inner Studies, 1987.

———. *The Chakras and Their Functions: Compiled from the Books of Master Choa Kok Sui*. Makati City, Philippines: Institute for Inner Studies, 2009.

———. *The Origin of Modern Pranic Healing and Arhatic Yoga*. Makati City, Philippines: Institute for Inner Studies, 2006.

———. *Pranic Healing*. 1987. Reprint, York Beach, ME: Weiser, 1990.

———. *Universal and Kabbalistic Meditation on the Lord's Prayer*. Makati City, Philippines: Institute for Inner Studies, 2001.

Sukul, Devā Rām. *Yoga and Self-Culture: A Scientific and Practical Survey of Yoga Philosophy for the Layman and the Aspirant on the Path*. New York: Yoga Institute of America, 1947.

Śūraṅgama Sūtra: A New Translation, with Excerpts from the Commentary by the Venerable Master Hsüan Hua. Ukiah, CA: Buddhist Text Translation Society, 2009.

Swami Muktabhodananda. *Swara Yoga*. Bihar, India: Bihar School of Yoga, 1999.

Swami Nikhilananda. *The Gospel of Sri Ramakrishna*. 1942. Reprint, New York: Ramakrishna-Vivekananda Center, 1992.

Swami Rama, Rudolph Ballentine, and Swami Alaya [Allan Weinstock]. *Yoga and Psychotherapy: The Evolution of Consciousness*. Glenview, IL: Himalayan Institute, 1976.

Swami Vivekananda. *Raja-Yoga*. 1896. Rev. ed. 1956. Reprint, New York: Ramakrishna-Vivekananda Center, 1982.

———. *Yoga Philosophy: Lectures Delivered in New York, Winter of 1895–96, on Rāja Yoga, or Conquering the Internal Nature*. London: Longmans, Green, 1896. http://catalog.hathitrust.org/Record/007913435.

Swedenborg, Emanuel. *Heaven and Hell*. 1758, Translated by George Dole. West Chester, PA: Swedenborg Foundation, 2000.

———. *Heaven and Its Wonders and Hell, from Things Heard and Seen*. 1758. Translated by John C. Ager. New York: American Swedenborg Printing and Publishing Society, 1909. http://catalog.hathitrust.org/Record/100028377.

Syman, Stefanie. *The Subtle Body: The Story of Yoga in America*. New York: Farrar, Straus and Giroux, 2010.

Taimni, I. K. *The Science of Yoga: The Yoga-Sūtra-s of Patañjali in Sanskrit with Transliteration in Roman, Translation and Commentary in English. 1961. Reprint, Adyar, Chennai, India: Theosophical Publishing House, 2010.

Tansley, David G. *Radionics and the Subtle Anatomy of Man*. Saffron Waldon, Essex, England: C. W. Daniel, 1972.

———. *The Raiment of Light: A Study of the Human Aura*. London: Routledge & Kegan Paul, 1984.

Taylor, Dana. *The Lord's Prayer, the Seven Chakras, the Twelve Life Paths*. N.p.: Attunement Press, 2009.

Taylor, Kathleen. *Sir John Woodroffe, Tantra, and Bengal: "An Indian Soul in a European Body?"* 2001. Reprint, London: RoutledgeCurzon, 2006.

The Theosophical Congress Held by the Theosophical Society at the Parliament of Religions, World's Fair of 1893, at Chicago, Ill., September 15, 16, 17: Report of Proceedings and Documents. New York: American Section Headquarters, 1893. http://catalog.hathitrust.org/Record/100139189.

Thind, Bhagat Singh. *Master Course in the Teachings of the Sikh Saviors: Sixty Free Lectures on Divine Realization*. Published by author, n.d. [1927]. Digitized pamphlet. South Asian American Digital Archive [SAADA]. https://www.saadigitalarchive.org/item/20110802-278.

———. *Science of Breathing and Glands: All Life on Earth Is Breath; All Else on Earth is Death*. Malibu, CA: David Bhagat Thind, 2004.

———. *Sikh Saviors*. Published by author, n.d. [1934]. Digitized pamphlet. South Asian American Digital Archive [SAADA]. https://www.saadigitalarchive.org/item/20130829-3130.

Thompson, William Irwin. *Passages about Earth: An Exploration of the New Planetary Culture*. New York: Harper & Row, 1973.

Tillett, Gregory. *The Elder Brother: A Biography of Charles Webster Leadbeater*. London: Routledge & Kegan Paul, 1982.

Towne, Elizabeth. "Nautilus News: A New Contributor." *Nautilus* 7, no. 12 (November 1905): 1. http://babel.hathitrust.org/cgi/pt?id=uva.x030803870.

Truth Seeker. "Yoga Philosophy." *Theosophist* 1 (January 1880): 86–87. http://www.iapsop.com/archive/materials/theosophist/theosophist_v1_n4_january_1880.pdf.

Van Auken, John. *Toward a Deeper Meditation: Rejuvenating the Body, Illuminating the Mind, Experiencing the Spirit*. Virginia Beach, VA: ARE Press, 2007.

Vasu, Srisa Chandra [Sris Chandra Basu]. *The Siva Samhita*. 1914. Reprint, New Delhi, India: Munshiram Manoharlal, 2004.

Vaysse, Jean. *Toward Awakening: An Approach to the Teaching Left by Gurdjieff*. 1979. Reprint, London: Arkana, 1988.

Versluis, Arthur. *Wisdom's Children: A Christian Esoteric Tradition*. Albany: State University of New York Press, 1999.

Vollmar, Klausbernd. *Journey through the Chakras: Exercises for Healing and Internal Balancing*. Bath, UK: Gateway, 1987.

Wallace, Amy, and Bill Henkin. *The Psychic Healing Book: How to Develop Your Psychic Potential Safely, Simply, Effectively*. New York: Delacorte, 1978.

Ward, Arthur H. *The Seven Rays of Development*. London: Theosophical Publishing Society, 1910.

Waters, Frank. *Book of the Hopi*. 1963. Reprint, New York: Ballantine, 1974.

———. *Pumpkin Seed Point*. Chicago: Sage Books, 1969.

Wenger, Jean-Pierre. *François Brousse: l'Enlumineur des mondes; biographie*. Saint-Cloud, France: Danicel Productions, 2005.

White, David Gordon. *The Alchemical Body: Siddha Traditions in Medieval India*. 1996. Reprint, New Delhi, India: Munshiram Manoharlal, 2004.

———. *Kiss of the Yoginī: Tantric Sex in Its South Asian Context*. Chicago: University of Chicago Press, 2003.

———. *Sinister Yogis*. Chicago: University of Chicago Press, 2009.

———. "Tantra in Practice: Mapping a Tradition." In David Gordon White, ed., *Tantra in Practice*, 3–38. Princeton, NJ: Princeton University Press, 2000.

———. *The "Yoga Sutra of Patanjali": A Biography*. Princeton, NJ: Princeton University Press, 2014.

White, David Gordon, ed. *Tantra in Practice*. Princeton, NJ: Princeton University Press, 2000.

———. *Yoga in Practice*. Princeton, NJ: Princeton University Press, 2012.

Whitten, Ivah Bergh. *Color Breathing: The Breath of Transmutation.* 1948. Reprint, Ashingdon, Rochford, Essex, UK: C. W. Daniel, n.d.

——. *The Initial Course in Color Awareness.* 1932. Reprint, London: AMICA, n.d.

——. *What Color Means to You and the Meaning of Your Aura.* London: Roland Hunt, 1932.

Wiyninger, Mary L. *Cosmic Science and Color: The ABCs of Color Science.* 2 vols. Hollywood, CA: School of Life, n.d.

Wood, Ernest Egerton. *Is This Theosophy . . . ?* London: Rider, 1936.

Woodroffe, John. *The Serpent Power—Being the Ṣaṭ-Cakra-Nirūpaṇa and Pādukā-Pañcaka, Two Works on Laya Yoga, Translated from the Sanskrit, with Introduction and Commentary.* 1919. 13th ed. Madras, India: Ganesh, 1986.

Working Glossary for the Use of Students of Theosophical Literature, A. 1890. 3rd ed., with appendix. New York: The Path, 1892. http://catalog.hathitrust.org/Record/010518802.

Yogi Wassan [Wassan Singh]. *Secrets of the Himalaya Mountain Masters and Ladder to Cosmic Consciousness.* 1927. Mokelumne Hill, CA: Health Research, 1973.

Zeller, Gabriele and Heidrun Brückner, eds. *Otto Böhtlingk an Rudolf Roth: Briefe zum Petersburger Wörterbuch.* Wiesbaden, Germany: Harrassowitz, 2007.

Zimmer, Heinrich. *Philosophies of India.* Edited by Joseph Campbell. 1951. Bollingen Series XXVI. Reprint, Princeton, NJ: Princeton University Press, 1969.

Zirkoff, Boris de. "*The Secret Doctrine*—Volume Three, as Published in 1897: A Survey of Its Contents and Authenticity." In H. P. Blavatsky, *The Collected Writings of H. P. Blavatsky*, 14:xv–xliv. 1985. Reprint, Wheaton, IL: Theosophical Publishing House, 1995.

Index

Sanskrit terms appear first in anglicized form, followed by the IAST form, italicized, in parentheses. Titles of Sanskrit texts appear in IAST and italics. Sanskrit names of persons, places, philosophies, religions, cults appear in IAST without italics. References to figures, tables, and plates appear in boldface.

A
Adepts, 93
   auras, 107, 114, 218–19
   laws of color, 217–18
   rays, 113–14
   See also Masters, siddhas
Adler, Alfred
   and third chakra, 309, 325, 332, 336
Agrippa, Cornelius, 84, 416n13
Ajaya, Swami (Allan Weinstock), 335
akasha (*ākāśa*), 25, 50
akashic records, 285, 393, 404
Alchemical Body (White), 436n12
Alder, Vera Stanley, 216, 278
Ali, Cajzoran. *See* Steen, Amber Ann
Ali, Hazrat Ismet. *See* Williams, E. C.
AMICA Temple of Radiance, 282, 452n28
Ānanda-Laharī. *See Saundarya-Laharī*
Anatomy of the Spirit (Myss), 74, 166, 457n2
"Anatomy of the Tantras, The" (Basu), 99–101, **100**, 105, 118, 176
Ancient Science and Art of Pranic Healing, The (Sui), 376
Ancient Wisdom, The (Besant), 144, 426n5, 429n12, 471n26
antahkarana (*antaḥkaraṇa*), 180, 425n16, 456n29
Anthroposophical Society, 141
Apocalypse Unsealed, The (Pryse), 170–82, **172, 178, 179, 181, Plate 4**
Aquarian Cosmic Color Fellowship, 277–78, 292
Aquarian Master/Mystical Institute of Color Awareness (AMICA), 260, 261, 278–80, 452n23, 452n28
   See also AMICA Temple of Radiance

Arcane School, 213
Art of Loving, The (Fromm), 336
Arundale, George Sydney, 318, 320
Association for Research and Enlightenment (ARE), 237, 243
astral-body chakras, 135–36, 185–87, 188–92, **195, 204**
astral projection, 136–37, 139–40
   chakras use in, 402–4
"Aura, The" (Leadbeater), 157, 185
Aura Cacia (company), 17, 405–6
aura layers
   Blavatsky, 157, 420n5, 432–33n17
   Besant/Leadbeater, 157–58
   Brennan, 386, 392–94, **396–97**, 398, 399–400, 471n27
   Fletcher, 160–61
   Marques, 158–59, **Plate 3**
   Ouseley, 289, **290–91**
   Sinnett, 157, 432–33n17
   Yoga Upanishads, 422n33
   See also seven principles
Aurobindo, Sri. *See* Ghose, Sri Aurobindo
Avalon, Arthur. *See* Woodroffe, John
Awaken Healing Energy through the Tao (Chia), 465n6
Awakening Your Psychic Powers (Reed), 248, 449n23
Āyurveda, 25, 26, 367

B
Babbitt, Edwin Dwight, 160, 254
Babuji Maharaj. *See* Sinha, Madhav Prasad
Baginski, Bodo, 374
Baier, Karl, 95–96, 138, 431n4
Bailey, Alice Ann, 213–25, 243
balancing chakras, 224, 443n23

color, 217–18
color healing groups, 254–55
initiations/centers, 215–17
lists of chakras, 220–21, **223**
macrocosmic perspective, 214, 225
sacral center, 219
See also under endocrine glands;
  seven rays
Bailey, Dorothy Agnes, 262, 282
Baker, Mary Ellen Penny, 252
Balancing the Chakras (Seidman),
  465n4
Ballard, Guy and Edna, 275
Ballentine, Rudolph, 335
"Basophil Adenomas of the Pituitary
  and Their Clinical Manifestation,
  The" (Cushing), 447–48n8
Basu, Baman Das, 99–101, 418nn19–
  20, 418n23
  esoteric anatomy, **100**
  list of chakras, **100**
Basu, Sris Chandra, 418n20
Bendit, Laurence J., 304, 438n10
Bendit, Phoebe D., 304
  chakras as sense organs, 437–38n10
  corpora quadrigemina, 425n17
Bernard, Pierre, 319
Besant, Annie, 131–40
  astral projection, 139
  chakras as sense organs, 135–36
  clairvoyant investigations, 132,
    157–58, 160, 187–88
  meditation, 145–46
  personality vs. individuality, 133, 392
  Rhadasoami visit, 111, 421n22
  third volume of *The Secret Doctrine*,
    102–3, 419–20nn2–3
  See also under planes
Bhagavad Gītā, 26, 28, 202, 299
Bhagwan Shree Rajneesh. *See* Osho
bhutas (*bhūta*). *See* maha-bhutas
Bible
  Matt. 6:9–13, 237
  Rev. 1:11, 173, 239
  Rev. 1:12–15, 178–79
  Rev. 1:20, 173
  Rev. 5:1, 173, 239
  Rev. 5:6, 262

Rev. 8:6, 173
Rev. 14, 173
Rev. 15:6–7, 173
Rev. 21:12, 378
Rev. 22:2, 378
bija-mantras (*bīja-mantra*), 30, 52, 63,
  88, 120
Bioenergetics, 320, 328–29, 338, 386
Blavatsky, Helena Petrovna, 93–127,
  131, 183
  AUM, 117, 120, 123
  aura, 114–15, 157, 432–33n17
  auric egg, 122, 393, 400, 423n11,
    424n15
  chakras in head/brain, 109, 138
  colors, 108, 115, **192**, **204**, 258, 288
  correspondences, 114, 117–18, **119**,
    124–25
  force centers, 98–99
  hatha vs. raja yoga, 103–4
  hierarchies of spiritual beings, 104,
    118–119, 127, **287**, 288
  kundalini practice, **121**, 122–24,
    171–74, 424–25nn14–16
  Masters, 257–58, 260
  "nadis" (chakras), 118
  sixth/seventh senses, 108, 277, 454n1
  sounds, 108, 115, 117–18, 423–24n13
  Tantrists (Tantrikas), 105
  third eye (*devaksha*), 106–7, 420n8
  See also under seven principles;
    seven rays
Bob and Carol and Ted and Alice
  (film), 327
Bodymind (Dychtwald), 337–48,
  463n19
"Bodymind and the Evolution to Cosmic Consciousness" (Dychtwald),
  343–45
Bohm, Werner, 372, 374
Book of the Hopi (Waters), 470n12
Bragdon, Claude
  encounter with Rahanii/Steen, 232,
    446n22
Brahman, 50, 194, 302, 308, 310
brahmarandhra (*brahmarandhra*),
  48–49, 51, 99, 418n23

Breakthrough to Creativity (Karagulla), 372
Breathing and Glands (Thind), 243, 448–49n14
Brennan, Barbara Ann, 386–401
  core star, 265, 400–401
  eighth/ninth aura layers, 394, 471n27
  etheric template, 392–93
  four levels of reality, 400
  front/back chakras, 386–87
  hara line, 400–401
  ketheric template, 393–94
  list of chakras, 391, **396–97**
  principles of clairvoyance, 399–400
Bridge to Freedom (movement), 275
  chakra colors, 276
Brother of the Third Degree, The (Garver), 233
Brousse, François
  initiation by Ali/Steen, 232
Bruyere, Rosalyn, 387–90
  chakra locations, 441n29
  chakras / human relationships, 389–90
  eighth/ninth chakras, 471n27
  four levels of reality, 470n12
  list of chakras, **388**
  magnetum, **388**, 469–70n11
  Native American correlations, 389, 470n12
  Peyer's patches, 387
Buddhism, 25, 28
  eightfold path, 144
  Mahāyāna, 26, 257
  Mìzōng/Esoteric School, 27, 33
  Shingon, 27, 33
  Tendai, 27, 33
  Theravāda, 26
  Vajrayāna, 33, 58
  See also Tibetan Buddhism
Buddhist Tantra
  chakras, 27, 142, 205, 413n6
Bucke, Richard Maurice, 462–63n13

C
Calcutta Review (journal), 37, 412n17
Caldwell, Daniel, 419–20n3

Campbell, Joseph, 304–11
  Esalen, 325
  Jung, 306
  list of chakras, 309–10
  Nikhilananda, 305–6
  Zimmer, 305–6
Caraka Saṃhitā, 26, 407n3
Carrington, Hereward, 303
Carson, Johnny, 19, 383
Caryāgīti, 27
causal body, 112, 136, 288, 392, 398, 471n22
  Besant vs. Brennan, 393–94
  chakras, 136
  defined, 393
Cayce, Edgar, 226–27, 237–40, 249
  chakra colors, 239
  Glad Helpers, 238–40
  list of chakras, **251**
  Pryse, 239, 447n6
  Revelation, 239, 248
  Thind, 243–44, 252
  See also under endocrine glands; Lord's Prayer
Cayce, Hugh Lynn, 248, 249
chakra (*cakra*), 17, 27
  defined, 33
  early use of word in English, 39, 411–12n16
  Oxford English Dictionary, 99
  See also Eastern chakra system; Western chakra system
Chakra and Kundalini Workbook, A (Mumford), 75
Chakra Balancing Roll-Ons. *See* Aura Cacia
chakra mandalas, 29–30, 47, 51–54, 65–67, 71, **Plate 1***A*
  colors, 67, 410n20
  components, 52, **53**
  as lotuses, 50–51
  as meditation manuals, 67
  pericarp, 52
  petals, 51, **68**, 69–71
  See also bija-mantras; devatas; linga/lingam; padmas; tattvas; vahanas; yantras

chakra qualities, 18, **382**, 468n41
  Bailey, 222–24, **223**, 443n19
  Campbell, 307–10
  evolution at Esalen, 21, 312–48,
    346–47, 384
Chakras, The (Leadbeater), 19, 201–10,
  372
Chakras: A Beginner's Guide, The
  (Ozaniec), 78
Chakras and Esoteric Healing, The
  (Lansdowne), 375
*Chakras and the Human Energy Fields,
  The* (Karagulla/Kunz), 372
*Chakras: Energy Centers of Transfor-
  mation* (Johari), 75
*Chakras: Lebenskräfte und Bewußt-
  seinszentren im Menschen* (Bohm),
  372
Chaudhuri, Haridas, 314, 334–35
  list of chakras, 334–35, **346–47**
chelas. *See* disciples
Chia, Mantak, 368, 465n6, 467n26
Chohan, 257
chromotherapy, 254, 277
Church Universal and Triumphant, 275
chiropractic, 462n5
Clairvoyance (Leadbeater), 437n9
Color and Cosmic Science (Wiyn-
  inger), 292–93
Color and Crystals (Gardner), 370
Color Breathing (Whitten), 261, 282,
  284
Color Meditations (Ouseley), 284, 289,
  293, 457n36
Commentary on the "Dream of Scipio"
  (Macrobius), 416n12
continuum of human potential,
  52–53, 139, 209, 323, 465–66n6,
  472–73n36
  Aurobindo, 314–16, 339
  Esalen, 328–29, 339–40, 345–48, 384
  Leadbeater, 190–91
  Ouseley, 286
  Pryse, 180–82, 191, **Plate 4**
  See also seven principles
Core Energetics (Pierrakos), 386–87,
  469n6

Coryn, Herbert, 420n13, 454n1
Cosmic Color Fellowship, 283
Cosmic Consciousness (Bucke),
  462n13
cosmic urge, 270
Crowley, Aleister, 163–66, **164**
  Baphomet XI°, 435n37
  meditating yogi diagram, 165–66,
    165
  Ordo Templi Orientis (OTO) degrees,
    435n27
  Sabhapaty Swami, 163, 434n32
  See also under sephirah/sephiroth
Cultural Integration Fellowship (CIF),
  314
Cushing, Harvey Williams, 447–48n8

D
Dabistān, The, 233, 235, 446n27
  early lists of chakras, 411–12n16
Daniélou, Alain, 303, 306
darshanas (*darśana*), 25, 88
Dayal, Dadu, 38
Descamps, Marc-Alain, 443n4
Descartes, René
  pineal as seat of soul, 107
devas (*deva*), 104, 113, 118, 127, 257
devatas (*devāta*), 52
Devi, Rukmini, 318
Devi, Sri Sarada, 305
Dhyani-Chohans, 113, 118, 127
Dialogues on Radhasoami Faith
  (Mishra), 111, 252, 422n25,
  422n27, 450n31
disciples, 114, 255, 256
Divine Posture (Ali/Steen), **229**,
  230–36, **234**, **Plate 8**
"Dream of Ravan, The" (*Dublin Re-
  view*), 95
"Dream of Scipio, The" (Cicero),
  416n12
Duff, Alexander, 36–37
Dychtwald, Ken, 337–47
  birth of Western chakra system,
    342–45
  description of Esalen, 312
  list of chakras, 341–42, 343, **346–47**

rainbow colors, 343
reminiscences, 463n19

E
Eastern chakra system, 47–55
    as causal-body system, 399
    characteristics, 47–55
    development, 25–30, 76–77
    in Europe, 297–300, 302–3, 374
    names/locations, **48**, 49–51,
    See also chakra mandalas; granthis; pithas; Western chakra system
East India Company, 410–11n6
East/West dichotomy, 41–43
Ecstasy through Tantra (Mumford), 321
Edgar Cayce in Context (Johnson), 449n19
Edgar Cayce on Channeling Your Higher Self (Reed), 249
elements
    alchemical, 300–301
    Blavatsky, 105, 117–18
    Bruyere, **388**, 389
    Eastern, 25, 50, 65, 153, **271**, **388**
    Pryse, 175
    Rendel, 352
    Western, 56
    Tibetan, 358, **359**
    See also tattvas; yantras
Eliade, Mircea, 75, 302–3
encounter groups, 327
endocrine glands, 21, 72, 226–27, 250–52, **251**, 382
    Ali/Steen, 227–30, **229**, **234**, 235, **251**, **Plate 8**
    Bailey, 221, **223**, 227, 251
    Blavatsky, 116
    Cayce, 240
    Garrison, 344
    Judith, 468n40
    Lord's Prayer, 244, **246**
    MacLaine, 380–81
    Rubin, 227–30, **228**, 251
    Schwarz, **356**
    Thind, 242–43
    Whitten, **266–67**

    See also pineal body; pituitary body; pituitary/pineal controversy
energy
    defined, 317
    and Esalen, 316–22
Energy, Ecstasy, and Your Seven Vital Chakras (Gunther), 321, 353–55, 358
Enlivening the Chakra of the Heart (Lowndes), 430n21
Equinox (journal), 163–64, **165**
Esalen (Kripal), 317–18
Esalen Institute, 309–48
    founding, 312–13
    human potential movement, 20, 21, 312–13, 316, 317, 341
Esoteric Astrology (Bailey), 443n19
Esoteric Buddhism (Sinnett), 183
Esoteric Cosmic Yogi Science (Estep), 137–38, 427–28n20, 440–441n19
Esoteric Healing (Bailey), 79, 222–25, 436n10, 442n11
Esoteric Healing: A Practical Guide (Hopking), 467n22
Esoteric Instructions (Blavatsky), 102–3, 170–71, 419n1, 419–20n3
    No. 1, **119**, 235–36, 270
    No. 2, 157, **287**, 288, 434n26, 451n7
    No. 3, 103–16, 157, 420n6, 424–25n16
    No. 4, 124–26, 424n16
Esoteric Instructions (Blavatsky/Gomes), 420n3
Esoteric Papers of Madame Blavatsky, The (Caldwell), 419–20n3, 424–25n16
Esoteric Psychology (Bailey), 222, 275, 353, 361, 442n17, 443n19
Esoteric Science and Philosophy of the Tantras, The (Basu), 164–65
Esoteric Section/School of Theosophy (ES), 102, 170, 213, 257–58, 419–20n3
Esoteric Writings of Helena Petrovna Blavatsky, The (Blavatsky), 419n3
Estep, William McKinley, 137–38, 427–28n20

etheric body, 104, 393, 426n6, 471n22
  chakras, 135–36, **189**, 189–92, **195**, **204**, 340
  development, 148–50, 304
Etheric Double, The (Powell), 193, **195**, 208, 219
Evola, Julius, 297
  author adopts position of, 86

F
"Farther Reaches of Human Nature, The" (Maslow), 323, 461n5
Feuerstein, Georg, 37, 62, 119–20
Findhorn Community, 373–74
Finding of Rainbow's End, The (Hunt), 278
Fletcher, Ella Adelia, 159–61, 236, 381, 433n21
  colors/principles, 161
Fortune, Dione (Violet Mary Firth), 166, 435n39, 435–36n41
Foundations of Tibetan Mysticism (Govinda), 357–58, **359**, 413n6
Fragrant and Radiant Symphony (Hunt), **263**, 278–79, 288, 452–53n29, 454n1
Free Church Institution (Calcutta), 36–37
Freud, Sigmund, 319, 338, 386
  and second chakra, 309, 325–26, 332, 336
From Camaldoli to Christ (Ouseley), 283–84
Fromm, Erich
  and fourth chakra, 336

G
ganglia. *See* nerve plexuses
Garden of Pomegranates, A (Regardie), 166
Gardner, Joy, 370
Garrison, Omar, 320, 344–45
gemstones
  colors, 88, 272
  Gardner, 270–72, 370
  Leadbeater, 272, 453n40
  MacLaine, 380
  Whitten, **269**, 270–72

Ghadiali, Dinshah P., 254
Gheraṇḍa Saṃhitā, 194–96, 199–200, 202, 439n28
Gherwal, Rishi Singh, 441n25
  on Leadbeater, 207–8
Ghose, Sri Aurobindo, 303, 313–16
  bodymind, 340
  correlation with Theosophical bodies, 460n14
  Integral Yoga, 303, 313, 316
  list of chakras / states of consciousness, 314–15
  and Tantra, 317
  See also under continuum of human potential
Gichtel, Johann Georg, 202–3, 440nn14–15, **Plate 5**
Glad Helpers. *See under* Cayce, Edgar
glands. *See* endocrine glands
"Glimpse of Tantric Occultism, A" (Majumdar), 97–98
Going Within (MacLaine), 380–83
Golden Dawn, 161–62, 166
  chakras/degrees, 435n37
  Flying Rolls, 162
Gomes, Michael, 420n3
Gorakṣanātha, 28, 59–60, 79
Gorakṣa Paddhati, 28, 409n14
Gospel of Sri Ramakrishna, The (Nikhilananda), 77, 306–8 459n31
Goswami, Shyam Sundar, 109
  animals/elements, 410n20
  chakra colors, 410n20
Govinda, Anagarika (Ernst Lothar Hoffmann)
  chakras as chorten, 357–58, **359**
  definition of Tantra, 44–45
granthis (*granthi*), 27, 54, 183
"Great Chakra Controversy, The" (Neff), 367–70
Growth of the Soul, The (Sinnett), 432–33n17
Guénon, René, 297, 457n2
Guide to Telepathy and Psychometry, A (Ouseley), 284
Gunther, Bernard, 320, 352–55
  chakra correspondences, 353–54, 464n6, 464n8

See also under source amnesia
Gurdjieff, George Ivanovich
list of centers, 465–66n6

H
Halpern, Steven, 463n19
Hammer, Olav
on Christopher Hills, 82
source amnesia, 80
Handbook to Higher Consciousness, The (Keyes), 330–31, 336, 337
Hands of Light (Brennan), 339, 386–87, 390
Hanish, Otoman Zar-Adusht (Otto Hanisch), 231, 233, 445n13
Haṭha-Yoga-Pradīpikā, 29, 76, 153, 202
subtle sounds, 63–64, 421n18, 423–24n13
Hauer, Jakob Wilhelm, 299, 305
Health and Breath Culture (Hanish), 233
Heaven and Hell (Swedenborg), 82–84
Heaven's Bride (Schmidt), 446–47n29
Heindel, Max (Carl Louis von Grasshoff), 245–48
four ethers, 285
Lord's Prayer, 245, **247**
Steiner, 449n21
Here Comes Everybody (Schutz), 327–29
Hesse, Hermann, 89
Hidden Life in Freemasonry, The (Leadbeater), **200**
Hidden Side of Things, The (Leadbeater), 191, 194–96, 210
hierarchy of needs (Maslow), 322–23, 336, 348
and chakras, 323–24, 342, **346–47**
"Higher Life, The" (Besant), 145
Higher Psychical Development (Carrington), 303
Hills, Christopher, 82, 361–66
chakra colors incorrectly attributed to, 82, 345, 450n1
list of chakras, 362–63, **364**
mental-body chakra system, 365–66
Hills, Norah, 363, 366

Hinduism
foundational texts, 25, 37
realms of universe, 26, 52, 126–27, 384, 408n8
Hindu Tantra, 27, 28, 37–38, 57–58
Histoire du Hatha-Yoga en France (Descamps), 443n4
hitas (*hita*), 25
Hodson, Geoffrey, 303–4, **253**
front/back chakras, 378, **379**
See also under pituitary/pineal controversy
Holy Grail. *See under* Schwarz, Jack
How Theosophy Came to Me (Leadbeater), 183–85
How to Know Higher Worlds (Steiner), 141
hrit chakra (*hṛt-cakra*), 50, 109, 331, 430n21, 462n24
Hübbe-Schleiden, Wilhelm, 429n5
Rhadasoami visit, 430n22
Human Aura, The (Marques), 158–59, 422n33, **Plate 3**
Hunt, Roland Thomas, 82, 261, 278–82
chakras/planes, **281**
masters/rays, **263**, 452–53n29
Hunt, Valerie, 387
Huxley, Aldous, 312–13
Huzur Maharaj. *See* Saligram, Rai

I
I AM Activity (movement), 275
indriyas (*indriya*). *See* jnanendriyas; karmendriyas
Initial Course in Color Awareness, The (Whitten), 261–75, 282, 286, 292, 452nn28–29
Initiates, 255, 256–57
Initiates of the Theosophical Masters (Johnson), 421n20
initiation(s), 215–17, 256–57, 385, 405, 442n3
Initiation and Its Results (Steiner), 141–49
Initiation: Human and Solar (Bailey), 213, 215–17, 257, 385, 452–53n29
Inner Group Teachings, 102, 117, 419–20n3

Inner Group Teachings of H. P. Blavatsky, The (Spierenburg), 419n3
Inner Life, The (Leadbeater), 188–91, 201, 217, 219, 318, 402
Inner Reaches of Outer Space, The (Campbell), 307
Innocente, Geraldine, 275
In Search of the Miraculous (Osho), 385, 468–69n4
Intermediate Studies of the Human Aura (Prophet), 275
Introduction to the Chakras (Rendel), 351–52, 373, 464n7
Invisible Worlds (Leland/Besant), 139, 426–27nn6–8, 436n11. 456n26
Isis Unveiled (Blavatsky), 93–94, 160
Isis-Uranie ou l'Initiation majeure (Brousse), 232

J
Jñānadeva, 28
jnanendriyas (*jñānendriya*), 56, 124–25, 415n16, 438n10
Jñāneśvarī (Jñānadeva), 28
Johari, Harish, 75
Johnson, K. Paul, 421n20, 449n19
Jones, Alex, 363–66
Journey through the Chakras (Vollmar), 372–73
Journey to the East, The (Hesse), 89
Joy, William Brugh, 78–79
  source of teachings, 79
  Rhadasoami influence, 422n25
  transpersonal point, 79, 369, 377
Joy: Expanding Human Awareness (Schutz), 326
Joy's Way (Joy), 78–79, 369–70
Judge, William Q., 102, 170
Judith, Anodea, 21–22, 61, 370, 457n2
  Leadbeater, 101
  Ram Dass, 325
  Rendel, 351
Juergensmeyer, Mark
  Radhasoami/Blavatsky influence, 421n18
Jung, Carl Gustav, 298–302
  alchemical elements, 300–301, 458n19

chakras, 300
  and heart chakra, 325, 332
  list of chakras, 301–2
  yoga seminars, 298–300

K
Kabbalah
  levels of reality, 470n12
  See also sefirah/sephiroth; Tree of Life
Kakar, Sudhir, 42
Karagulla, Shafica, 372
karmendriyas (*karmendriya*), 56, 124–25, 438n10
Kashmiri Śaivism, 28, 56, 70–71, 409n15, 414n1, 415n15
Kaulism, 28
Keyes, Ken Jr., 330–31
  list of chakras, 330–31, **346–47**
Kipling, Rudyard, 41
Kiss of the Yoginī (White), 198–99
Knight, Gareth (Basil Wilby), 435–36n41
Koltko-Rivera, Mark, 322–23
kosha (*kośa*), 114–15, 384–85, 414n9, 422n32
Kripal, Jeffrey J.
  Aurobindo, 317
  Campbell, 305–6, 325
  energy, 317
  Esalen, 317–18, 322, 338–39, 461n1
  Gopi Krishna, 320
  Gunther, 352
  human potential, 312–13
  Maslow, 461n5
  Murphy, 314
  Reich, 338
  Rolf, 462n5
  Schutz, 326–27
Krishna, Gopi, 320
kundalini (*kuṇḍalinī*)
  Arundale, 318–19
  awakening, 28, 318–19, 320, 371
  Blavatsky, 119–124, 422n28
  Campbell, 306–7
  defined, 36
  development within Tantra, 27–28
  early appearances in English, 95, 97

Index 507

Esalen, 317–18, 338
Jung, 298, 457–58n7
Leadbeater, 185, 318
location, 49, 53, 413n9
mother of the world, 28, 95
Pryse, 171, 173–74, 179–80
Steiner, 149–50, 431n30
Vivekananda, **155**, 156
Woodroffe, 200–201
Kundalini: An Occult Experience (Arundale), 318–19
kundalini-shakti (*kuṇḍalinī-śakti*), 131, 156, 413n9, 457n2
  defined, 318
  serpent fire, 186
  serpent power, 49
Kundalini Tantra (Satyananda), 79
  as standard model for Eastern system, 75–76
  and Theosophical teachings, 75, 210, 371, 441n30
Kundalini: The Evolutionary Energy in Man (Krishna), 320
Kundalini Yoga (Sivananda), 61, 303
Kundalini Yoga for the West (Radha), 75
"Kundalini Yoga: Seven Levels of Consciousness" (Campbell), 307
Kunz, Dora van Gelder, 372

L

Lansdowne, Zachary, 375–76
latifah/lataif, 85, 169, 416n15
Law of the Rhythmic Breath (Fletcher), 159–61, 236, 243
Layayoga (Goswami), 409n15, 428n22, 429n5
Leadbeater, Charles Webster
  aura, 185
  caduceus, **200**
  chakra characteristics/functions, 185–87, 189–91
  chakra colors, **192**, 203–7, **204**, **Plates 1B, 6**
  chakra petals and moral qualities, 190
  clairvoyant investigations, 187–88
  elimination of genital chakra, 189–90, 205–6, 440–41n19

funnel effect, 209–10, **Plate 1B**
Gichtel, 202–3, **Plate 5**
influence, 208–10, 219–20, 441n26, 441n30, 464n6
list of chakras, **192, 204**
locations, 99, 208–9, **Plates 6–7**
names, 208
petals/spokes, 199–200
phallic sorcery, 198–99
psychic powers, 190–91, **192, 195, 204**, 402–3
reversing second/third chakras, 202, 206
translations, 210, 372
vitality/prana-vayus, 191–96, **195**
See also under spleen chakra
Leland, Kurt
  esoteric vs. exoteric science, 86–89
  Leland's Law, 85
  chakras in astral projection, 402–4
  levels of plan, **396–97**
  mental-body chakra system, 395–98
  personal history with chakras, 18–19
  reality/learning system, 112–13
  researcher vs. investigator, 86
Leonard, George, 312–13
Letters on Occult Meditation (Bailey), 213, 217–20
  chromotherapy, 217, 224, 275, 297, 365
  color healing groups, 254–55
  complementary colors, 218, 272–74
  seven-fold rays, 286, 456n30
Letters on Yoga (Aurobindo), 314, 459–60n11
Leydig cells, 240, 250, 449n23
Liber 777 (Crowley), 163–64, **164**
Light Emerging (Brennan), 400, 470–71n16
Light of the Soul, The (Bailey), 220–21
Like a Hollow Flute (Seidman), 465n1
linga/lingam (*liṅga/liṅgam*)
  and astral body, 137
  bana (*bāna*), 29
  itara (*itara*), 30, 410n21
  jyotir (*jyotir*), 54, 65
  multiple meanings, 53–54, 180, 323

508   RAINBOW BODY

principle, 104, 205, 426n6
svayambhu (*svayambhū*), 29
Llewellyn's Complete Book of Chakras (Dale), 440n15
Logos, 112–13, 262, 274, 280
lokas/talas. *See under* planes
Lord's Prayer, 244–50
　Cayce, 237, 244, **246**, 248
　Heindel, 245, **247**, 248
　Sui, 250
Lord's Prayer, the Seven Chakras, and the Twelve Life Paths, The (Taylor), 250
lotuses. *See* chakra mandalas; padmas
Lowen, Alexander, 320, 386
Lowndes, Florin
　eight-petaled lotus in Steiner, 430n21
Lucifer-Gnosis (journal), 142, 428–29n2, 429n5
Lüscher, Max, 361–62
Lüscher Color Test, The (Lüscher), 361–62
lyden. *See* Leydig cells

M
MacLaine, Shirley, 380–83
　list of chakras, 380–81
　on *Tonight Show*, 19, 22, 104, 383, 468n42
Magical Message according to Ioannes, The (Pryse), 447n6
magnetum, 469n11
Mahābhārata, 26
maha-bhutas (*mahā-bhūta*), 25, 56, 124–25, 415n16
Maharaj Saheb. *See* Mishra, Brahm Shankar
Mahatma Letters, 255–57, 451n4
Majumdar, Baradakanta, 96–99
　collaboration with Woodroffe, 97
　on Tantra, 96
mandalas (*maṇḍala*)
　Jung, 298
　Tibetan, 66
　See also chakra mandalas
Man and His Bodies (Besant), 132–33, 139, 158, 427n8

Man Incarnate (Bendit), 304
Man's Latent Powers (Payne), 304, 425n17, 437–38n10
mantra (*mantra*), 29, 37, 120, 156
　defined, 62–63
Man Visible and Invisible (Leadbeater), 158, 185, 188, 259, 282
Man: Whence, How, and Whither (Besant/Leadbeater), 471n26
　color temples, 279, 289, 457n36
marmani (*marmāṇi*), 25, 26
Marques, Auguste, 158–59, **Plate 3**
Maslow, Abraham, 322–24, 336, 342, **346–47**, 348
"Master Course in the Teachings of the Sikh Saviors" (Thind), 242
Masters, **266–67**, 451n5
　DK (Djwal Khul), 213, 256, 275
　KH (Kuthumi), 213, 256, 275
　M (Morya), 184, 256
　St. Germain, 256
Masters and the Path, The (Leadbeater), 257, 265, 272, 275–76, 401, 453n40
Mathers, Samuel Liddell MacGregor, 161–62, 434n28
matrika (*mātṛkā*), 66, 70
Matsyendranātha, 27, 59–60, 79
Mazdaznan (movement), 231, 233, 236, 446–47n29
McLaren, Karla
　astral-body chakra system, 395
Mead, George Robert Stowe
　editing of *Nature's Finer Forces*, 152–53
Meditation and the Mind of Man (Thurston/Puryear), **246**, 248, 449n20
Melton, J. Gordon, 431n4
Menninger Foundation, 325, 335–36, 355
mental body, 133, 146, 218, 392
　chakras, 135, 187, 365–66, 395–398
Mishra, Brahm Shankar, 111–112, 422n25, 450n31
monad
　Besant, 133
　Blavatsky, 122–23
　defined, 104, 113

Pryse, 174, 436n12
  See also star of consciousness
Motoyama, Hiroshi, 371
Mumford, Jonn, 75, 320–21
Murphy, Michael, 299, 312–14, 317, 325, 334, 386
Music and the Soul (Leland), 395–98
Myss, Caroline, 74, 166, 457n2
Mysterious Kundalini, The (Rele), 101, 177
Mystical Qabbalah, The (Fortune), 166, 435n39, 435n41
Mythic Image, The (Campbell), 306, 337
Myths of Light (Campbell), 307
Myths to Live By (Campbell), 306, 308–9, 332, 337

N

nadis (*nāḍī*), 33, **48**, 407n2, 407n6, 409n18
  brahma (*brahma*), 418n22
  as caduceus, **200**
  chronology, 25–29
  citra/citrini (*citra/citriṇī*), 418n22
  ida (*iḍā*), 47–48, 60, 131
  in *Hevajra Tantra*, 408n10
  locations, **100**
  pingala (*piṅgalā*), 47–48, 60, 131
  sushumna (*suṣumṇā*), 47–49, 52, **53**, 60, 131, 418n22
  and Tree of Life, 163
  vajra (*vajrā*), 418n22
  Vivekananda on sushumna, **155**, 156, 432n12
nadi-shuddhi (*nāḍī-śuddhi*), 50
Nālandā, 27, 28
Nāth tradition, 28, 38, 110, 421n18
Nature's Finer Forces (Prasād), 106, 151–54, 431–32n5
  influence, 158, 159, 161–62, 243, 351, 432n8
  translation of *Śiva-Svarodaya*, 152–53
Nautilus (journal), 160
Neff, Dio Urmilla, 367–70, 465n6
  list of chakras, 369
neo-Tantra, 320–21, 344

nerve plexuses, 72, 99–101, **100**, **178**, **181**, **234**, **Plate 7**
New Age
  appropriations, 23, 46–47, 330
  confusion about Upanishads, 409n18
New Thought (movement), 160, 230
Nikhilananda, Swami, 305–6
Nuclear Evolution (Hills)
  first edition (1968), 82, 361–63
  second edition (1977), 82, 345, 362, 363–66, **364**
nyasa (*nyāsa*), 29, 119–120

O

occult correspondences, 82–86, 416n13
  discovered vs. developed, 85
  lists, 73
  motivations for, 73–74
Occult World, The (Sinnett), 183
Official Edgar Cayce Readings, The (DVD-ROM), 238, 447n1
Olcott, Henry Steel, 93–94
  astral projection, 136–37
  chakras, 97–98, 136–37
  Prasād, 432n8
  Rhadasoami visit, 111, 421n22
  Subba Row, 184
Only Dance There Is, The (Ram Dass), 325–26, 363
"On the Tattwas of the Eastern School" (Mathers), 162, 434n28
Opening Up to Your Psychic Self (Stevens), 385–86
Osho (Bhagwan Shree Rajneesh), 44, 320, 385
  list of bodies, 468–69n4
Ouseley, S. G. J., 283–92, **Frontispiece**
  color consciousness, 284
  color fundamentals, 285
  color temple, 289
  four ethers, 285
  list of chakras and planes, **290–91**
  publishing scandal, 283–84
  as Theosophist, 456n23
  See also under source amnesia
Out on a Limb (MacLaine), 380
Ozaniec, Naomi, 78

P

padmas (*padma*), 39–40, 50–51, 109, 409n17
  See also chakra mandalas
Pancoast, Seth, 254
Passages about Earth (Thompson), 373, 466n17
Path of the Saints. *See* Sant Mat
Payne, Phoebe. *See* Bendit, Phoebe D.
Perennial Philosophy, The (Huxley), 312–13
Philosophies of India (Zimmer), 305, 306
"Physical Errors of Hinduism" (Shom), **34**, **35**, 37–40, 410n5, 412n16
Pierrakos, John C., 320, 329, 339
  front/back chakras, 209, 378, 386–87, 469n6
pineal body, 106–8, 124
pithas (*pīṭha*), 49, 413n11
pituitary body, 106–8, 124
  as master gland, 240, 447–48n8
pituitary/pineal controversy, **251**, **382**
  Bailey, 227, 240, 289
  Baker, 252
  Bruyere, 387
  Cayce, 240, 252
  Gardner, 383
  Hodson, 252–53, **253**
  Hunt, 289
  Judith, 221, 383
  Mishra, 252, 422n27
  Ouseley, 289
  Ozaniec, 448n8
  Puryear, 252
  Thind, 242–43
  Van Auken, 252
  Whitten, 289
planes
  Aurobindo, 460n14
  Bailey/Alder, 215–17, 385, 442n3
  Besant, 126–27, 133–34, **134**, 392–94, **396–97**
  Blavatsky, 123, 392, 423n12, 425n22, 472–73n36
  Brennan, 392–94, **396–97**, 471n27
  Bruyere, 387–89, **388**, 470n12
  Leadbeater, 282, 455n15
  lokas/talas (*loka/tala*), 52, 54, 126–28, 384, 408n8, 414n9, 425n22
  Ouseley, **290–91**, 456n29
  Pryse, 174–76, 436–37n14
  Whitten/Hunt, 280–82, **281**
planets
  Ali/Steen, **234**, 235–36
  Cayce, 240
  Gunther, 353, 464n7
  Pryse, **172**, **181**
Pleasonton, Augustus James, 254
plexuses. *See* nerve plexuses
Poimandres, 416n12
Polarity Therapy, 367, 465n3
Powell, Arthur Edward, 193, **195**
Power of the Rays, The (Ouseley), 283–85, 293, 365
prana (*prāṇa*), 25, 47, 115
  Sui, 378–80
  tides, 153–54, 158
  vitality, 180, 191–93
prana-vayus (*prāṇa-vāyu*), 105, 172, 194–96, 205, 242, **Plate 6**
pranayama (*prāṇāyāma*), 48, 60–61, 154–56
Prasād, Rāma, 151–54
  tattva symbols/colors, 153, **271**
Preliminary Memorandum (Blavatsky), 257–58
Price, Richard (Dick), 312, 313, 334
Principles of Light and Color (Babbitt), 160, 254
Principles of Tantra (Avalon), 96, 197
Probationary Path, 144, 146–47
probationers, 255, 256, 257–258
Prophet, Mark and Elizabeth Clare, 275
Pryse, James Morgan, 170–82, 436n12, **Frontispiece**
  astrological correspondences, **172**
  Blavatsky's kundalini practice, 173–74
  chakra functions, **179**, **Plate 4**
  chakra locations, 176–80, **178**
  list of chakras, **181**
  numerological correspondences, 176, 177

and Revelation, 171, 173, 175, 178–80
speirema (kundalini), 171
Theosophical Society insignia, 177–80, **Plate 4**
See also under planes; planets
Psychic Healing Book, The (Wallace and Henkin), 194, 438n25
Psychic Sense, The (Bendit), 304, 438n10
Psychosomatic Yoga (Mumford), 75
Psychology of Kundalini Yoga, The (Jung), 301–2
Pumpkin Seed Point (Waters), 470n12
Puranas
   Bhāgavata, 27, 407n3
   Garuḍa, 202, 207, 408–9n12
   Viṣṇu, 26, 126–27, 425n22
Pūrṇānanda Giri, 29–30
Puryear, Herbert B.
   water chakra, 449n23

R
Radha, Swami Sivananda, 75
Radhasoami movement, 110–11, 241–42, 423–24n13, 430n22, 445n14
   chakras, 110–112, 422n25, 450n31
Radionics and the Subtle Anatomy of Man (Tansley), 375
Raiment of Light, The (Tansley), 375
rainbow colors, **382**
   Cayce, 239, 447n5
   Dychtwald, 342–45, 463n19
   Hunt, 280–82, **281**, 293
   Leadbeater, 203–7
   Ouseley, **290–91**, 293
   Whitten, **266–67**, 272–75, **273**, 447n5
Raja Yoga (Vivekananda), 131, 154–56, **155**, 159, 160, 432nn12–13
Rajneesh, Bhagwan Shree. *See* Osho
Ram Dass (Richard Alpert), 324–26, 363
   list of chakras, 325–26, **346–47**
Red Book, The (Jung), 298, 457n7
Reed, Henry, 248
   water chakra, 449n23
Regardie, Israel, 166, 457n2

Reich, Wilhelm, 319–20, 386
   body armor / chakras, 320, 338–39
   orgone, 338
Reiki, 374
Reiki: Universal Life Energy (Baginski and Sharamon), 374
Rele, Vasant, 101, 177
Rendel, Peter Leland, 351–52
   four temperaments, 373
   list of chakras, 352
   planets/chakras, 353, 464n7
Restored New Testament, The (Pryse), 233
Rogers, Carl, 327
   and fourth chakra, 336
Rohmer, Sax, 472n36
Rolf, Ida, 319
Rolfing, 319, 338, 387
Rosenberg, Jack Lee, 332–33
   list of chakras, 332–33, **346–47**
Rosicrucian Cosmo-conception, The (Heindel), 245, **247**, 285, 449n21
Rubin, Herman Harold, 226, 227–30

S
Sabhapaty Swami, 136–39, 163, 427–28n20, 428nn22–24, 437n4
   chakra locations, 440–41n19, **Plate 2**
   first English yoga manual, 431n4, 432n13
   list of chakras, 138–39
sacred sexuality, 44, 46, 318
Śaivism, 26, 27, 28
   See also Kashmiri Śaivism
Śakti. *See under* Śiva
Śaktism, 28, 71
Saligram, Rai, 110–11, 421n20
   meeting with Besant/Olcott, 111, 421n22
Sāṃkhya, 25, 26, 56, 70, 125, 414n1
Śaṅkara, 27, 144, 146–47, 408n9
Sanskrit alphabet, 27, 29, 51, **68**, 69–71, 199
Sant Mat, 64, 110–12, 226, 241–42
Saraswati, Swami Satyananda, 65, 77–78, 208, 210, 371
   astral projection, 137

chakras as brain functions, 89
yantras for sixth/seventh chakras, 65
Saraswati, Swami Sivananda, 61, 303
Sar Bachan (Singh), 110, 421n18, 425n22
Ṣaṭ-Cakra-Nirūpaṇa (Pūrṇānanda), 29–30, 47, 76–77, 97, 371
influence, 153, 202, 207, 311, 377
Satyananda. See Saraswati, Swami Satyananda
Saundarya-Laharī, 408n9, 413n9
Schutz, Alice, 454n55
Schutz, William, 326–30
list of chakras, 328, **346–47**
open encounter, 326–28
Schwarz, Jack, 355–60
Holy Grail, 355–57, **359**
list of chakras, **356**
on sources, 359–60
Science of Breath, The (Prasād). See *Nature's Finer Forces*
Science of Mind, The (Holmes), 270
Science of Seership, The (Hodson), **253**, **379**
Science of the Aura, The (Ouseley), 284, 293, 456n29
Secret Doctrine, The (Blavatsky), 102, 107, 113–14, 132, 260
influence, 160, 177, 214, 243, 470n12
third volume, 102–3, **119**, **287**, 419nn2–3, 420n13, 454n1
Secrets of the Himalaya Mountain Masters (Wassan), 446n21
Seidman, Maruti
chakra balancing, 367, 465n4
list of chakras, 367
sephirah/sephiroth, 162–63
Crowley, 163–164, **164**, 434–35n35
Fortune, 166, 435n39, 435n41
Guenon, 457n2
Knight, 435–36n41
Marques, 163, 434n31
New Age, 166–69, **167**
Regardie, 166
Sui, 250
Serpent Power, The (Avalon), 21, 30, 97, 109

as Eastern system, 47, **48**, 51, **53**, Plate 1*A*
influence, 233, 297, 303, 307, 344, 358, 372
Jung, 298
Leadbeater, 197–201, 202, 208, 209
translations, 302
Seven Keys to Color Healing, The (Hunt), 279–82, **281**, 284, 289, 292, 293
Seven Mansions of Color (Jones), 363–65
seven principles
basis of Western chakra system, 104, 118, 125–26, 473n36
Besant, 133–34, **134**, **396–97**, 426n6
Blavatsky, 118–19, 125–26, 157, 274, 420n5, 432–33n17
Crowley, 163
Fletcher, 160–61
Heindel, 245, **247**
list, 104
Marques, 158–59, 163, 434n31
not numbered, 157, 274, 288
Ouseley, **290–91**, 456n29
physical body not included, 180, 434n34
Pryse, 180–82, **181**
Sinnett, 157, 432–33n17
Ward, 472–73n36
Whitten/Hunt, 274, 288
Seven Principles of Man, The (Besant), 132–33, 135–36, 426n6
seven rays
Bailey, 218–19, 222, **223**, **273**, 274–75, 442n17
Blavatsky, 112–14, 118–19, **287**, 288
Leadbeater, **273**
Ouseley, 285–88, **290–91**
Whitten/Hunt, 262–64, **263**, **266–67**, 272–75, **273**
Seven Rays of Development, The (Ward), 472n36
Sexual Occultism (Mumford), 75, 321
shabda-brahman (*śabda-brahman*), 50, 64, 108
Shamans, Mystics, and Healers (Kakar), 42

Sharamon, Shalila, 374
Shirinsky, Olga, 232, 445n16, 446n23
Shom, Bipin Behari, 36–40
  mysterious maps, 33–40, **34**, **35**
Short History of the Theosophical Society, A (Ransom), 451n5
siddhas (*siddha*), 28, 37, 60, 110
Siddha-Siddhanta-Paddhati, 409n14
siddhis (*siddhi*), 28, 62, 414n9
Singh, Sawan, 241–42
Singh, Seth Shiva Dayal, 110
Singh, Yogi Wassan, 446n21
Singha, Gunga Gobinda, 38–39
Singleton, Mark, 61, 99, 431n4
  on Cajzoran Ali, 170
Sinha, Madhav Prasad, 111
Sinnett, A. P., 111, 157, 432–33n17
Śiva, 26
  eye, 107
  and Pārvatī, 152
  phallus, 29, 53, 65
  and Śakti, 37–38, 46, 52, 56, 66, 69–71
Sivananda. *See* Saraswati, Swami Sivananda
Śiva Saṃhitā, 29, 164–66, 202, 207, 414n2, 418n20
  list of chakras / psychic powers, 193–94
  subtle sounds, 421n18
Śiva-Svarodaya, 152–53, 162
Soami Ji. *See* Singh, Seth Shiva Dayal
Soul and Its Mechanism, The (Bailey), 221, 226, 227, 270, 458n20
source amnesia, 20, 79–82
  Ali/Steen, 235
  defined, 80
  Gunther, 354–55, 358–60
  Ouseley, 289, 292–293
  types, 80–81
  Wiyninger, 292–93
Spectrum Suite (Halpern), 463n19
Spiegelberg, Frederic, 299–300, 304–5, 313–14, 320, 386
spleen chakra
  Bailey, 219
  Blavatsky, 126, 149, 194, 205
  Gunther, 354, 464n6
  Joy, 369
  Leadbeater, 189–90, 202–3, 205–6, 208, 440–41n19
  Neff, 368, 369
  Steiner, 149, 194
  Sui, 377
Spring (journal), 299
Sri Chinmoy, 208, 441n26
Sri Ramakrishna, 77, 305–6, 307–8
  list of chakras, 308
star of consciousness, 264–65, 401, 404
Steen, Amber Ann, 230–36, **Frontispiece**
  as Amber Ekberg, 232
  as Amber McGilvra, 230–31
  as Ann Williams, 231
  "Brown Brother," 232, 446n22
  as Cajzoran Ali, **229**, 230–231, 243, 443n4, 444n9, **Plate 8**
  list of chakras, **234**, **251**
  as Madame Zorah, 231
  Pryse, 170, 233, 236
  as Rahanii, 232
  and Revelation, 170, 226
  See also under Bragdon, Claude; Brousse, François; endocrine glands; planets; source amnesia
Steiner, Rudolf, 141–50
  chakra development, 142–48
  etheric-body development, 148–49
  list of chakras, **143**
  lotus petals/qualities, 142, 429n5
  translations, 141
Stevens, Petey, 386, 399
Stone, Randolph (Rudolf Bautsch), 367, 465n2
Structural Integration. *See* Rolfing
Studies in Hinduism (Guénon), 297, 457n2
Studies of the Human Aura (Prophet), 275
Subba Row, T., 113, 184–85, 437n4
Subtle-Body Healing (Beasley), 375
Sui, Choa Kok, 115, 196, 209, 376–80
  Arhatic Yoga, 380
  list of chakras, 377
  ming mein chakra, 377–78, 467n26
  Pranic Healing, 376–77, 379–80

Sukul, Sri Devā Rām, 303
Summit Lighthouse, 275–76
  chakra colors, 276
Śūraṅgama Sūtra, 27
sutratman (*sūtrātman*), 288–89, 401
Swami Rama, 335–37, 355
  list of chakras, 336–37, **346–47**
Swedenborg, Emanuel, 82–84, 416n13
  law of correspondences, 82–83

T
Tablet (newspaper), 284, 455–56n22
tanmatras (*tanmātra*), 56, 124–25, 415n16
Tansley, David, 372, 375–76
Tantra
  defined, 37, 44–46
  practices, 57–58, 340–41
  practitioners, 55, 57, 151, 198, 300
  right-hand vs. left-hand paths, 38, 58–60
  six actions (*ṣaṭ-karman*), 59, 198–99, 414–15n10
  sorcery, 59–60, 198–99
  spread of, 27, 44
  See also Buddhist Tantra; Hindu Tantra
Tantras
  Amara-Saṃgraha, 410n20
  Guhyasamāja, 27
  Hevajra, 27, 408n10
  Jayadrathayāmala, 28
  Kālacakra, 28
  Kaula-Jñāna-Nirṇaya, 27
  Kubjikāmata, 28
  Mṛḍānītantra, 410n20
  Netra, 27
  Rudrayāmala, 29, 409n15
  Śāradā-Tilaka, 29, 409n15
  Tantrāloka, 28
  Tantrasadbhāva, 27
  Ṭoḍala, 29, 409n16
Tantra: The Path of Ecstasy (Feuerstein), 413n11
Tantra: The Yoga of Sex (Garrison), 320, 344–45
tattvas (*tattva*), 25, 415n16
  colors, 153, **271**, 432n7
  five, 105, 270
  and Sanskrit alphabet 69–71, 415n15
  seven, 105, 125, 172
  thirty-six, 56–57, 70–71, 414n1
  tides, 158, 162, 351, **Plate 3**
  twenty-five, 56, 71, 125
  See also elements; yantras
Taylor, Dana, 250
Taylor, Kathleen, 197
Temple of Radiant Reflection, 277–78, 292
"Temple of Solomon the King, The" (Crowley), 163–64, 434–35n35
Theories of the Chakras (Motoyama), 371
Theosophia Practica (Gichtel), 202–3, 440n14
Theosophical Glossary (Blavatsky), 318
Theosophical Research Center, 304
Theosophical Society (Adyar), 417n5
  founding, 93–94, 256, 451n4
  in India, 94–95
  insignia, 177, **Plate 4**
  motto, 242
  objects, 94, 151, 417n3
  and Sant Mat, 64, 110–12, 421n22
  and Steiner, 141
Theosophist (journal), 94–101, 110–111
Thind, Bhagat Singh, 226, 241–44, 250, **251**
  and Cayce, 243–44
Thompson, William Irwin, 373–74
"Thought-Forms" (Besant), 188, 438n12
Thought-Forms (Besant/Leadbeater), 188, 259
Thought Power (Besant), 144, 145–46
thread-self. *See* sutratman
Three Works of Occult Philosophy (Agrippa), 84
Thurston, Mark, 248, 249, 449n20
Tibetan Buddhism, 66
  chakras, 357–58, **359**, 435–36n41
Total Orgasm (Rosenberg), 332–33
Toward a Psychology of Being (Maslow), 322
Toward Awakening (Vaysse), 465–66n6

Towne, Elizabeth, 160
Transformations of Myth through Time (Campbell), 307
Transpersonal Psychologies (Tart), 334
Tree of Life, 162–69, **167**, 250, 297, 351, 457n2
  See also sephirah/sephiroth
Two Women Who Posed (Facilis), 259

U

Universal and Kabbalistic Chakra Meditation (Sui), 250
Upanishads, 25
  Bṛhadāraṇyaka, 25
  Chāndogya, 25, 194, 196, 407n2
  Kaṭha, 25, 407n2
  Maitrī, 26
  Muṇḍaka, 407n2
  Praśna, 153, 202, 407n2
  Taittirīya, 422n32
  See also Yoga Upanishads
Usui, Mika, 374

V

Vahan (journal), 185
vahanas (*vahana*), 52, 66, 414n9
Van Auken, John, 252
Vaysse, Jean, 465n6
Vedānta, 25, 27
Vedas, 25, 37, 193
  Atharva, 25
  Ṛg, 113–14
Venture Inward (Cayce), 248
Versluis, Arthur
  chakras not portrayed by Gichtel, 203, 440n14
  correct title of *Theosophia Practica*, 440n14
Viveka-Cūḍāmaṇi (Śaṅkara), 144
Vivekananda, Swami, 154–56
  birth of yoga in America, 131, 154
  chakra portrayal, **155**, 156
Voice of the Silence, The (Blavatsky), 160, 176, 421n18, 422n28, 423–24n13, 436n12
Vollmar, Klausbernd, 372–74
  list of chakras, 373
Voluntary Controls (Schwarz), 353, 355, **356**, **359**, 360, 464n11
vritti (*vṛtti*), 142, 429n5

W

Ward, Arthur H., 472n36
Warner, Alfred Edward, 209
Wassan, Yogi. *See* Singh, Yogi Wassan
Waters, Frank, 470n12
Western chakra system, 72–76
  author's ideal, 404–5
  birthdate of, 21, 345
  Blavatsky's contributions, 115–16, 127
  characteristics, 72–74, **382**
  vs. Eastern chakra system, 41–42, 54, 67, 71, 74–76, 88, **Plate 1**
  esoteric dimension, 22, 384–86
  as etheric-body system, 366, 395
  in Germany, 372–74
  goes mainstream, 22, 104, 383
  locations, 99–101, **100**, **382**, 468n39
  names, 208, 219, 221, **382**, 442n11
  principles underlying, 300–301
  typology, 76–79
  unintentional collaboration, 19–20, 23, 80
  See also chakra qualities; Eastern chakra system; endocrine glands; rainbow colors; seven principles
What Color Means to You (Whitten), 261, 280, 282, 451n9
Wheels of Life (Judith), 61, 75, 79, 353
  as standard model for Western system, 75–76
Wheels of Light (Bruyere), 387
White, David Gordon
  chakras absent from *Yoga Sūtra*, 407n6
  chakras as six plus one, 29, 125
  definition of Tantra, 45
  immortal body, 436n12
  implosion of elements, 57
  tantric practice, 340–41
  tantric universe, 45–46
  yogini (*yoginī*), 58–59, 198
Whitten, Ivah Bergh, 258–61, 279, **Frontispiece**

chakra/color correspondences, 266–69, **273**
color awareness, 261–62, 284
colors of rest/activity/inspiration, 264, 284
cosmic color, 262–65
crystals, 270–72
Leadbeater influence, 259, 265, 270, 272, 280–82
mammary glands, 270, 453n41
masters/rays, **263**, **266–67**
tattvas, **271**
as Theosophist, 260–61
types/needs, **268**
Williams, E. C.
capture/trial/conviction, 231
as Hazrat Ismet Ali, 231, 243, 444n9
Wiyninger, Mary Lucille, 292–93
Woman Beautiful, The (Fletcher), 159
Wood, Ernest Egerton, 207
role in producing Leadbeater's *The Chakras*, 201–2
Woodroffe, John, 197
as Arthur Avalon, 47
chakras/caduceus correlation, 200–201
correspondence with Evola, 297
criticisms of Leadbeater, 199–200
Indian collaborators, 47
Working Glossary for Students of Theosophical Literature, A, 131, 426n1
World Parliament of Religions, 131, 154

Y

yantras (*yantra*), 29, 52, **356**
list, 65
vs. mandalas, 56–57, 65–67
See also elements; tattvas
yoga
defined, 56
eight limbs, 60, 137–38, 303, 362–63
hatha (*haṭha*), 59–62
historical development, 25–30

kundalini (*kuṇḍalinī*), 29, 61, 156, 298, 303
laya (*laya*), 64–71, 138
mantra (*mantra*), 62–63
nada (*nāda*), 63–64
shabda (*śabda*), 64
svara (*svara*), 152, 160
Yoga and Psychotherapy (Rama), 335–36
Yoga and Self-Culture (Sukul), 303
Yoga-Bāṣya (Vedavyāsa), 26
Yoga Body (Singleton), 170, 226, 431n4
Yoga: Immortality and Freedom (Eliade), 75, 303
Yoga of Power, The (Evola), 297
Yoga Sūtra (Patañjali), 26, 56, 60, 145, 153
astral projection, 137
Bailey, 220
Hills, 362
Leadbeater, 202
protochakra system, 407n6
Vivekananda, 154
Yoga: The Method of Re-Integration (Daniélou), 303
Yoga Tradition, The (Feuerstein), 408–9n12
Yoga Upanishads, 29, 76, 126–27, 194, 202, 371
Amṛta-Nāda, 439n26
Dhyāna-Bindu, 439n26
Maṇḍala-Brāhmaṇa, 422n33
Nāda-Bindu, 126
northern/southern canons, 409n18
Śāṇḍilya, 126–27
Yoga-Cūḍāmaṇi, 413n10
You Are a Rainbow (Hills), 363
Your Mysterious Glands (Rubin), 227, **228**, 448n8

Z

Zimmer, Heinrich, 299–300, 304–6, 386

About the Author

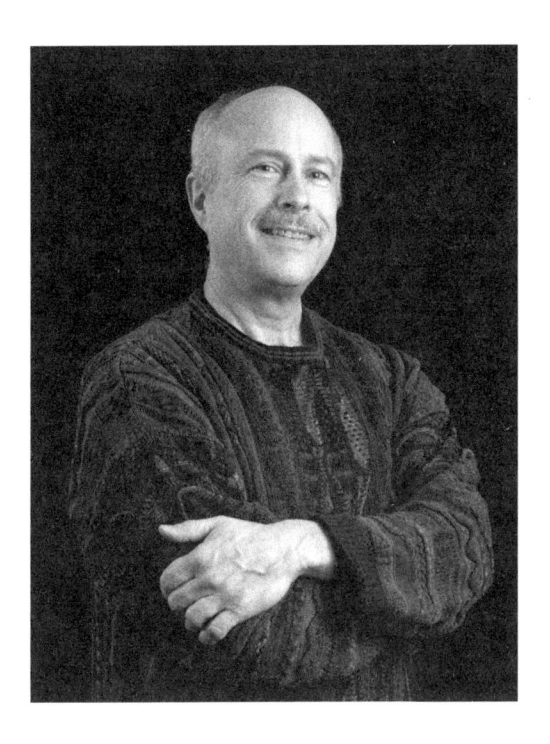

KURT LELAND has written on astral projection, near-death experiences, and the transcendent possibilities of composing, performing, and listening to music. He has edited and annotated an authoritative edition of C.W. Leadbeater's classic text *The Chakras* (1927) and a selection of Annie Besant's articles and lectures—*Invisible Worlds: Annie Besant on Psychic and Spiritual Development*. As well as being a National Lecturer for the Theosophical Society in America, he is a Boston-based classical musician and award-winning composer and maintains a consulting and teaching practice called Spiritual Orienteering.

From Ibis Press

Tantric Temples
Eros and Magic in Java

Peter Levenda

• A lavishly illustrated full-color photographic survey of the most important esoteric centers of Tantric Magic
• A scholarly presentation of Indonesian magic and its interaction with Tibetan Tantra, Hindu mysticism, and Islamic Sufism
• Provides extensive data of parallels with Western sexual magical practices

This book illustrates the history of Tantrism in Java with more than a hundred photographs of temples, statues, and iconography dedicated to the system—including the recently-excavated "white temple" of Yogyakarta—and accounts of contemporary practices in the shrines, cemeteries and secret schools of Java. Real Tantra has influenced secret societies, mystics, alchemists, Kabbalists, and magicians for hundreds if not thousands of years.

$69.00 • Hardcover • ISBN: 978-089254-169-0 • 7.5 x 10.5 • 352 pp. Profusely illustrated in full color

From Nicolas Hays

Managing the Mind
A Commonsense Guide to Patanjali's Yogasutra
Devadatta Kali

• The Yogasutra of Patanjali is described as an owner's manual for the human mind and how the mind can be used in the quest for Truth
• Presents this most important text on Yoga and meditation in clear and straightforward English
• The commentary presents a simple explanation of the realities of everyday living, the management of the mind, and the practices that lead to enlightenment

This book is a spiritual tool for the lay practitioner, while offering a path to deeper scholarship for those who choose to pursue it. It is thus an invaluable overview of yogic philosophy and language, and, at times, a controversial and innovative interpretation of this most treasure classical text. Over 2,000 years old, this treatise is as timeless today as the day it was written.

$19.95 • Paperback • ISBN: 978-0-89254-212-3 • • 6 x 9 • 192 pp.
Ebook ISBN: 978-0-89254-626-8

Ref - 84137582.

Marine Parade -
The Studio - ~~MMMW~~
~~Balmoral~~ ~~Thurs -~~
~~4 evenings~~

6 34.

Pearl Street.   26 Alistair
                   4·25 - 5pm
07804 485348   open evening.

0200'
NB 0061104

Homeless / Local Authority
          03000
              268000.

001 - -

Behind the Chicken Wire

by

Lynn Roberts

Awduresau Cymru Publishing

Copyright © Lynn Roberts 2021

Edited by Alana Davies
Cover design by AED

First published in paperback in April 2021

Lynn Roberts has asserted his right under the Copyright, Designs & Patents Act 1988 to be identified as the author of this work.

This book is a work of fiction and any resemblance to actual persons, living or dead, is purely coincidental.

All rights reserved. No part of this publication may be reproduced, stored in a retrieval system, or transmitted, in any form or by any means without the prior written permission of the publisher, nor be otherwise circulated in any form of binding or cover other than in which it is published and without a similar condition being imposed on the subsequent purchaser.

Published by © Awduresau Cymru Publishing.

18 Seaview Terrace
Swansea
SA1 6FE

It's the dawn of a new millennium in the south Wales city. The music, the cars, the fashions, the language – all are of its time. These things change, but the fight between good and evil does not.

CHAPTER ONE
December 1999

A cold bare room with a long table, twelve uncomfortable chairs and a clock. This was no place to be locked away with a band of strangers two days before Christmas eve. Outside, gusting winds threw slithers of sleet, rattling every casement window, while down on the cold grey pavements hoar-frost crawled stealthily around the city. Everyone present was listening to the constant banging and bubbling of the antiquated central heating system that was about to fail yet again. Although those concerned were still being stubborn, this latest malfunction suggested that a majority verdict couldn't be far away, as body temperatures began to drop and people were desperate to go home.

Sitting downstairs on a spare chair at the back of number one criminal court, Hook loosened his red silk tie and the top button on his faded denim shirt, as the hands of the clock in the public gallery slowly approached five minutes to five. Although there was still no news from the Jury room, he wasn't in a rush; he'd been waiting patiently for almost a year for this moment.

He generally found attending Crown Court as a witness a cleansing experience, sitting there with that godly feeling felt by infrequent Church goers whenever they sat in a pew. Yet he hated the formality of these occasions. Formal dress was for weddings, funerals and disciplinary hearings. Hook had always been a distressed-leather, jeans and T-shirt man, a legacy of his university days. Unpolished shoes screaming for attention, odd socks, and a heap of careless black hair told the world that he lived alone.

Scratching his dark stubbled throat with the rolled up list of previous convictions of both defendants, he stared idly at the attractive defence barrister sitting on the front benches just yards away. She glanced back and smiled broadly. What the hell was someone like her doing, defending two of the city's major drug dealers, he thought. Her clients were low life and scum who accepted the ruination of other people's lives, careers and families in the same casual manner they would adopt if some of the decorative bunting that surrounded their car sales empire had fallen down.

Helen Wainwright LLb, of Jarvis, Compton and Quinlan could have easily graced the catwalks of Milan or the pages of Marie Clare, he thought. She smiled again and nodded politely, causing her freshly washed blonde hair to fall down lazily over her dark eyes. With legs that an Olympian long jumper would have been proud of, counsel for the defence would have beaten Sharon Stone hands down in a lookalike competition, he thought.

Forcing a smile, he nodded back in the aloof, straight-faced manner all policemen tended to display after a two-day witness-box grilling, desperately trying to conceal the fact that, like anybody else, he didn't like being called a liar. But now that was all behind him. Today he was more than confident that the jury's verdict was going to mean a good day for the good guys.

He turned his wrist and glanced at his watch again. He knew that if the matter wasn't resolved in the next few minutes the jury would be heading for a night at a nearby hotel, and he would be putting his celebration drink on hold. He cursed under his breath but managed to manufacture a smile at the same time, as again she threw him a friendly smile.

But time hadn't diluted his annoyance. He hadn't forgotten her razor-sharp cross-examination during his evidence-in-chief only days earlier: a fiery verbal joust, with her Blue Peter smile and sarcastic suggestion that his version of events had all the credibility of a Sooty annual.

Sensing this interest in his young junior, the ruthless Hunter Jarvis QC, who headed the defence team, glanced across disdainfully, giving Hook and his blue chalk striped suit the once over. Tall, arrogant and vain, the blond haired head of chambers strutted around the judicial venues of Wales like a man who had just walked through a field of lavender on a glorious summer's day, when suddenly confronted by an open sewer. Subtle verbal fencing played no part in his cross-examinations. Jarvis tore into prosecution witnesses with all the brutality of a man trimming a hedge with a sabre. He and Hook despised each other.

But now it was almost over and all he had to do was relax and fine-tune his post-trial speech. In criminal cases, he was already four nil down in the series with Jarvis, and his end of trial gloat today needed further deliberation if he was to gain a maximum 10/10 on the smugometer.

But resorting to commiserative dialogue wasn't really in his nature. It was beginning to sound a touch childish. Perhaps just a self-satisfied smile backed up by a firm freemason handshake that had been learned from his grandfather, he thought. Yes, the old secret society squeeze with bags of firm eye contact should rattle the egotistical bastard.

Grudgingly he had to accept that Jarvis had put up an impressive defence case; the man always did, but the evidence for the prosecution had been overwhelming. If the jury hadn't been nobbled, the result was in the bag. Catching criminals was one thing, making the charges stick was something entirely different.

If ever a Crown Court trial was a foregone conclusion, the Crown versus Leonard and Michael McCann had to be it. Protracted police investigations throughout the UK and Europe clearly showed that the former South London villains, now company directors of Cars International (Wales) Limited, not only imported top of the range Mercedes and Ferrari motor cars, but also top of the range cocaine hydrochloride as well.

Although the defendants' monopolisation of the city's violent drug trade had amassed them a vast fortune, they still pursued respectability with the same ruthlessness they ran their business empire. The donation of four Vauxhall Frontera Landrovers to the force's Crime Prevention Department just prior to their arrest had been an enormous mistake and the last straw as far as Hook was concerned. He'd even been designated for the media photo call at HQ where the vehicles were officially handed over by a grinning Lennie McCann who basked in the barrage of publicity that the event attracted. Hook didn't attend. He booked sick.

High ranking senior officers including his boss, Jack Corbett, had all been lobbied and warned about the McCann's anti-social behaviour in the city, but with little success. Internal politics and an overstretched force transport budget were taking priority over the poison that was flooding out onto the city streets. Even small-time street dealers had begun to wonder if the brothers' continued liberty was somehow connected to this unholy sponsored alliance.

Banging cell doors that echoed down in the belly of the building, not only indicated the defendants were on their way back to the dock, but also that the Jury must have finally reached a verdict. Make-your-mind-up time was over.

Gradually the slumbering judiciary began to crank into action, as clerks and officials crushed cigarettes under leather soles before bursting back in through the swing doors to their positions of power. Almost like magic, four heavily built prison officers appeared up in the dock like pantomime genies, manacled to the morose 40-year-old twin brothers Lennie and Mickey McCann. Momentarily a hush descended on the courtroom.

Sweating profusely and chewing with a noisy arrogance, the defendants posed for a few seconds while their supporters, who began to fill up the public gallery, began a series of muffled cheers. When they were ready, and only when they felt it appropriate, they sat down slowly while their guards sat obediently alongside. Both brothers sported tight fitting Gorgio Armani suits, remand-wing haircuts and lashings of Tabac aftershave, in a sort of custodial makeover.

With eyes like a King Cobra and facial skin to match, the pock-marked Lennie McCann began scanning the tightly packed courtroom for one man. The one individual who had been responsible for his apple-white pallor and six-month absence from the city centre. Someone who had not only turned down the offer of a monthly brown envelope, but a man who had forced their drug operation down onto its knees.

The city's number one crime family were usually guaranteed to make it a white Christmas for all their clients, but Hook had ruined it by swarming all over them during the summer. Their criminal credibility on the streets was now under question and people in the underworld were beginning to talk. Openly. Moving from south London to Wales, where there would be easy pickings, and where they believed the Taff plod wouldn't be as attentive as their deluxe metropolitan counterparts was already proving to be a disastrous move. They hadn't bargained for Harry Hook.

Lennie twisted his steroid-developed torso around, his neck like a Komodo dragon, while his brown reptilian eyes continued to search the room.

Prior to Hook's intervention, Lennie in particular had terrorised the city with his schizophrenic violence. Bar room brawls and unpredictable behaviour fuelled by drink, drugs or whatever else was on offer made him someone to avoid. His brother Mickey was the Chief Executive of the McCann board and the brains behind the partnership. Mickey normally lit the blue touch paper while his brother was the one that exploded. When Mickey and Lennie entered a room people generally stood up. Their acquittal of a well-publicised gangland murder by Southwark Crown Court shortly before they had emigrated to Wales had given them instant respect.

Spotting Hook nearby, Mickey elbowed his brother in the chest and nodded towards the back of the court.

'Hook, you're fucking history, do you hear me?' Lennie screamed right on cue, leaping to his feet, the red marbled veins in his neck throbbing uncontrollably.

'History, that's what you are, pig.' he yelled, yanking on his cufflinks and pulling a startled guard up to his feet like a papier maché marionette.

Hook's eyes moved across to the dock as the angry cockney rant shredded the tranquillity of the packed courtroom. Only feet away, the elderly Clerk of the Court sat behind his thin trembling moustache, seemingly paralysed with shock. In something of a disorganised Mexican wave, relatives and friends of the accused seated in the public gallery, now jumped to their feet, applauding and cheering, as reinforcement officers ran from the cells below. The austere formalities of a British criminal court began to disintegrate before him.

Sitting impassively in the middle of the fracas raging around him, Hook slowly raised an eyebrow before removing some white flecks from the lapels of his jacket. Tough reputations were hard-earned in the shadowy criminal underworld, and he had no intention of relinquishing his by a look or a move. He would not appear to be embarrassed by local low life in front of a packed house. He had always played the game in the opposition faces, not in any comfort zone. He wouldn't have known how to halt, to step backwards.

Keeping the annual Crown Court guilty verdicts in double figures was a full time occupation, and sometimes the subtle bending of rules and the making of false promises were needed to handicap the pendulum that was madly swinging out of control in favour of the city's criminal superstars. Often the job took him near the edge. Sometimes he'd step over it. The high-wire had never worried him, and he certainly wasn't worried about the two-bit cockney hoodlums who screamed abuse at him just feet away. But losing their composure and rolling around the dock after such a long and tiring trial had surprised him a little. The idea of finally losing their liberty had clearly unhinged them, he thought as he checked his watch again.

After all, the brothers, in police parlance, were bang to rights, no doubt about it. Three kilos of top grade Columbian cocaine and three kilos of Turkish heroin had been discovered in a floor safe at Cars International. Two of their employees had been arrested on the French/Spanish border neat Biarritz, with five kilos of each drug hidden inside secret compartments of a Mercedes Saloon, owned by the accused.

Each worker had been given ten years by a French Court for drug smuggling, but the thought of having that sentence halved if they gave evidence for the crown in the UK made it a difficult proposition for them to refuse. With the added pledge that they could be transferred to a British prison if they made witness statements implicating the McCanns, as suggested by Hook when he visited them, had been too tempting to resist. Self-preservation versus loyalty was no contest in the world of drug trafficking.

Their witness statements at the trial provided powerful evidence, and outlined the McCanns' involvement in international drug smuggling. After taking their statements in France, he swore blind that he would urgently speak to the French authorities about reducing their sentences, and to the Home Office about a transfer to a Welsh prison.
Hook forgot.

While both defendants continued to turn the dock into Madison Square Gardens in their efforts to break free to rearrange some of Hook's twenty four facial bones, Hunter Jarvis began to smile. He was clearly enjoying every moment of this developing theatre, and Hook's public taunting at the hands of his violent clients.

Stretching his legs for a moment, Hook strolled down to the front benches, where he optimistically dropped the previous convictions papers in front of the prosecution silk Sir Hugo Evan Gladstone QC. Watching in frustration, he looked on as the portly barrister with the Falstaffian girth juggled carefully with a child's circular plastic toy. A small round game in which the object was to manoeuvre a small silver ball into a clown's huge red nose. Sir Hugo was due to retire in the new year and it showed.

'Has that distasteful exhibition of pugilism discontinued behind me?' he growled without looking up, as first the little silver ball fell in and then out of the clown's nose.

'I think they're trying to get them back into the cells to cools off. So what's the SP Sir Hugo? Five years apiece?' A frustrated Hook was in search of some reassurance.

Looking over the top of his reading glasses, and in a voice that reminded Hook of a colliery winding wheel grinding to a halt in the middle of a valley winter, he said.

'Dear heart, they'll be pissing in a tin pot for the next ten Christmases.'

Hook continued to watch with some interest until the silver ball finally came to rest in the Harlequin's nose.

'Nice one, Sir Hugo!' he said, smiling and rolling his eyes as he walked back to his seat.

The Crown Prosecution Service had already primed him that the trial judge had been impressed. He had hinted that a commendation was in the pipeline for him and his squad for apprehending the brothers, and bringing to book an international drug organisation. He smiled again, before beginning to wonder who would be next to emerge from the bottom of the pond to replace them. He knew there wouldn't be any shortage of contenders.

At first he didn't notice the scruffy attractive blonde standing near the entrance to Number One Court, clutching a tin of partially consumed Special Brew. She had a defiant look on her face, spikey gelled hair like a baby chicken, and her torn tight fitting blue jeans were in tatters. A filthy black leather jacket looked as though a chapter of heavy-drinking Hell's Angels had just pissed all over it, while a white soiled T-shirt suggested some might have missed.

He watched as she swaggered towards him, chewing and squinting through too-heavy mascara, looking for somewhere warm to sit. Within seconds of her sitting next to Hook, an ageing white-haired court usher waddled over like an Emperor penguin, croaking gently that people like her should be seated up in the public gallery.

'On your bike, numb-nuts' she snapped, sending him scurrying away in search of backup, muttering under his breath.

They didn't speak for some minutes, until Hook felt it was safe to do so.

'Your nipples are sticking out, Miss' he said, hardly moving his lips.

'That's because it's brass monkey weather on the streets' she replied, before giving an inquisitive Hunter Jarvis a sexy wink.

Inflating her chewing gum into a huge pink bubble that almost covered half her face, she waved again at the court usher who was discussing her across the room, slowly opening and closing her legs provocatively. Hook rolled his eyes.

'So what are you doing here? This isn't a Miss Wet T-shirt competition'.

'Grandad over there thinks I'm a tart, you know' she said, fiddling with her nose stud.

'For God's sake James, these are not the fucking Bafta awards,' he said.

'Christ, what time is the main bout' she said spotting a few bleeding prison guards, their hair dishevelled, standing in the dock.

Detective Trilby James' pallid complexion was bad, but she carried news that was good. Personal hygiene and an account at Armani shops had never been a prerequisite for deep undercover work, and nobody went deeper than James.

'I know you've been on pins about Operation Rotterdam,' she said. 'So I thought I'd pop in personally to update you. Keep you up to speed, Cariad.'

In an effort to keep her full-time profession a secret, he turned his back on her, while the McCanns noisily continued to question his parentage on the cell steps nearby.

'So, any developments?' he said quietly.

'One or two' she said coyly, pushing her can of lager under the seat with her foot.

'And? And?' said an exasperated Hook, still hardly moving his lips.

'We arrested six crew members and recovered 1a hundred and fifty kilos of blow, together with fifteen grand in sterling, earlier this morning.'

'Your informant?'

'Well in the clear, boss.'

A smile broke across his face, as he continued whispering out of the side of his mouth like an amateur ventriloquist at a talent contest.

'I'm going to recommend to Corbett you get a commendation from the Chief for this. Nice work, James. If you didn't resemble something from a Glaswegian rehab clinic, I'd kiss you.'

'Bed's the place for dreaming!' she replied, smiling.

'Seriously though, why don't you take some time off? You deserve it,' he whispered. 'I'll sort it out for you.'

James looked up, taken aback. Then,

'Take Christmas day and Boxing day off' he said.

She stared back and her jaw loosened, but she knew he wasn't joking. Hook set exacting standards for himself, and others were expected to follow.

It was close to six o'clock when the small door at the far end of the Court eventually opened and the Jury shuffled untidily back to their places. Hook watched them like a hawk, searching for any piece of body language that might be on show, something that could give an early indication as to their decision. Even after studying juries during his fourteen-year career, he still went through the ritual of crossing his fingers. Giving evidence in Crown Court was stressful enough, but waiting for the foreman to stand and give the thumbs-up or thumbs-down announcement was enough to start a panic attack.

Looking across at them, he knew something wasn't right. He could sense it. Some were fidgeting, while the rest just stared meekly at the floor. His eyes flashed along the front row to a couple of giggling girls and then along the back benches, but his intuition told him the black clouds were on the horizon. There wasn't a wise man or saviour in sight.

Collapsed prosecutions and surprise acquittals were not unknown to Hook, and the decaying system was getting worse by the day. In the old days it had always been fear and intimidation that influenced jurors. Nowadays it was the money. The sight of a scruffy young juror with orange hair winking at the two defendants had him dropping his head in shame.

'Oh my God James, the bastards are going to walk' he said, his voice sticking in his throat

'Let's just wait a minute' she said hopefully.

'But look at them for God's sake.'

He was right. Every single juror, including the foreman, now sat with his or her head bowed in embarrassment, avoiding glances from every corner of the room as they stared blankly at the floor.

With both elbows resting on his knees, Hook began to chew on his knuckles, like some shy kid on his first day at school. Then the anxiety in his guts began to gyrate as the 'Not Guilty' verdicts reverberated around the oak-panelled courtroom and seemed to slap him across the face.

Court etiquette dissolved in a sea of emotion, as supporters hurdled over public gallery seats, pushing over court officials like ninepins, while dubious character witnesses punched the air with juvenile shouts of 'Yes, yes!'. Both accused leapt clumsily over the brass rail of the dock into the somewhat embarrassed arms of their legal team, whom they hugged in disbelief.

He and James watched from the other side of the room as journalists raced for the telephones, while jurors joined the celebrations, backslapping the McCanns as though they had just won the Eurovision Song Contest. Hook felt as though he were having an out-of-body experience, looking down from above, watching as people began to point and glare in his direction. Helen Wainwright herself seemed a trifle stunned, and James noticed her attempts to catch Hook's eye. Both ends of Jarvis's mouth were almost touching his ears in delight, and that was too much to bear.

He was about to get to his feet when Sir Hugo and the rest of the prosecution team on their way out of the arena stopped for a moment alongside him.

'Listen, I really am terribly sorry Mr Hook. If we keep losing these battles I fear for the young in our society' growled Gladstone.

Finding it difficult to respond with any sort of facial expression, or to offer any form of handshake, Hook nodded curtly, as though he'd just lost a game of Scrabble.

Prosecution for the Crown may have felt by his demeanour that the officer in charge of the case was a bad loser. He would have been absolutely right.

'Let's get out of here, James' he said. 'People are staring at me as though I've just strangled half a dozen kittens with some piano wire.'

With footsteps echoing and rebounding off every marbled pillar, they marched hurriedly through the busy foyer towards the exit, where embarrassed faces now turned away as he approached. Not guilty verdicts always made him feel uncomfortable, almost a little responsible, as familiar heads continued to turn away. It was almost as though he had instigated some sort of trumped up charge against the brothers and suddenly he was one of the bad guys.

The loud voice that challenged them was unmistakable; it wasn't over yet, not by a long chalk. There were still a few loose ends to tie up.

'Wait, you bastard!' Lennie McCann shouted, barging through the double doors of number two court as he ran towards them, out of breath. like a rugby league loose forward on the sixth tackle.

'So who grassed us up?' he snarled, stepping into Hook's face quicker than a monkey hitting the feeder bar.

Quietly seizing her boss by the arm, James could feel the tension as his whole body began to tighten. She'd seen his eyes freeze over before and knew what would was likely to follow.

'Easy' she murmured. 'He's not worth it.'

An agitated McCann began to drop his body weight and started head-pecking, classic symptoms that the first punch was only seconds away. Moving back a touch and outside the fighting arc, Hook produced an outrageous smile.

'Hello Mr McCann. Congratulations are in order I believe. Super result for you and your brother.'

James watched as the villain's fury deflated like a party balloon.

'Listen you prick, whoever bubbled us, he's history, you comprendez?'

'You seem a touch overwrought, Leonard.'

'Don't be a smart arse, Hook. When we find out who's been grassing, I'm going to bring violence to this city you couldn't even dream of' he said, almost stabbing his finger into Hook's face.

'Grass … grass … hang on a moment now, I might be able to lay my hands on his full name and address for you by tomorrow' Hook said, pretending to search the inside pocket of his jacket. 'Okay if one of the lads phones it through, or do you want me to pin it up at the local bus station?'

Despite his calm performance, Hook was having difficulty in suppressing his anger. He turned to leave, but thick callused 'love' and 'hate' fingers dug into his shoulder, and spun him around roughly. Rule number one in Hook's book had always been that people were allowed to speak, even allowed to shout, but never allowed to touch. Already his resentment at losing the case was smouldering deep inside him like a flaming coal beneath cool ashes. The closeness of Lennie's bad breath - a legacy of his poor prison diet - swarmed over Hook's face. That was enough. Even his aunts weren't allowed that close.

Just for a second he looked across at the exit door that led out into the streets, and then into the face of the growling inbred that stood before him. He knew that the number of complaints against him for the year had reached double figures, and the hierarchy at Headquarters were watching him carefully. Leaning forward he whispered in McCann's ear,

'Now listen poppet, that big ugly broken nose of yours doesn't impress me one little bit. It simply proves that you don't duck very quickly.' Hook was quietly annoyed. He was good at annoyed. He could do annoyed. A smile broke over James lips.

'Now, I'm not into this man-to-man marking, so take your hand away from my shoulder Mr McCann, before I give you a quick demonstration of ape shit. Comprendez?' Hook had a way with words.

CHAPTER TWO

Being publicly decked in the crowded Halls of Justice by the opposition was a chance Lennie McCann just wasn't prepared to take. Skidding on his arse across the cold tiled floors of power, in front of the local paparazzi, could destroy his street cred. What's more, he could see in Hook's eyes that the detective was up for it.

In the middle of a packed foyer, McCann slowly removed his blue-pigmented fingers from the detective's broad shoulder, while his mind worked overtime for a suitably clever riposte. Something that would stop this smart-arse cop dead in his tracks.

'Fuck off' he shouted.

Heading for the main entrance, Hook had already spotted him, sitting alone on a cold hard bench alongside the cigarette machine a couple of yards away. The man, the size of a cable car, stood up slowly and barred his way. Frank Maggart, a doorman at the Blue Parrot nightclub was a formidable tough-guy, the sort of man that picked on Hell's Angels and circus strongmen. He was someone Hook knew well.

'Is this pig hassling you, Mr McCann?' he shouted across the foyer, giving Hook a stare that would have caused most men to mess their trousers.

'Frank my boy, nice to see you' said Lennie, moving straight back into Hook's face. 'But it ain't no big deal, this shit-kicker is about to leave, isn't that right?'

Hook was no shit-kicker, but perhaps it was time to leave. The opposition back-up in the black jogging bottoms, white vest and enormous denim jacket looked formidable. Standing before him, Hook tilted back his head and looked up into Maggart's face. Hook weighed up his options. His eyes barely came up to Maggart's heavily-tattooed throat. 'Cut Here' wasn't an invitation he wished to accept. In fact he wouldn't have taken on Maggart with a Kalashnikov and an armed response group.

'You heard the gentleman, piss off and take that fucking slag with you' grunted Maggart, turning even more heads in the foyer.

It was an offer both officers decided to accept. With her nerve ends beginning to jangle, James nudged his arm. She could smell the hatred.

'Let's get out of here. I'm not happy with the odds' she whispered, glancing up at the man whose huge grisly ginger head wouldn't have looked out of place in a cave mural.

'Once again, as always, it's been a pleasure to meet you, Mr Maggart' said Hook, holding out his hand politely. Maggart slapped it violently to one side.

Leaving behind prying microphones, notebooks, and over-excited newspaper men who had seen it all, Hook turned to James.

'Shoot off and get some sleep. I'll see you in the office first thing.'

Shaking his stinging red hand loosely to rid himself of the pain, he went on. 'No sense in hanging around here the way things are.'

'Fancy a coffee?' she asked brightly.

Hook shook his head.

It was snowing hard when they got outside but she didn't want to leave him. He suddenly seemed vulnerable, smaller somehow. His eyes didn't sparkle now. They looked tired and weary, darkened, stripped of their passion by a judicial system that had coughed and spluttered along for three months before cutting out. She punched his arm affectionately before bowing her head and pushing off into the freezing northerly winds that raced down from the Rhondda valleys, crushing the spiralling chimney smoke with their power. Occasionally, she glanced back, but then he was gone. She knew he needed his space, a place to be alone. She just wished it could have been her place. A small cosy Victorian riverside flat, just two miles away…

As the moon began to show between the grey December clouds, he stood outside the Crown Court, where he watched in the darkness as laughing jurors gingerly made their way down the ice-covered steps. He knew there was a lengthy celebration ahead. His money was on 'La Bodega' - a popular little wine bar in a nearby side street. Stepping back into the shadows, Hook caught sight of their delighted sponsors for the evening. The brothers McCann were trotting along behind them.

Intuition had him moving further into the doorway, as a young juror with a shaved head and some interesting self-inflicted tattoos and body piercing almost stepped on his toes, before urinating against the side of the Crown Court steps. Denim jacket, black T-shirt, torn jeans and filthy tennis shoes now seemed to be the normal attire for most jurors, he thought.

'For fuck's sake guys, hang on for me' he bellowed, zipping up his fly before racing across the street to join the others. Hook stared down at his feet as a stream of steaming urine flowed around his shoes.

Pulling up the collar on his heavy overcoat he thrust his arms into its pockets, deep and straight, until the stitching strained under his anger. He stepped over the liquid on the ground and headed off along Boulevard De Leon towards the dockside pubs two miles away. Already his efforts to put the brothers behind bars was confined to history.

Christmas fairy lights brightened the city centre, while rosy smiling faces of late night shoppers were everywhere, but Hook's eyes saw nothing. He knew full well that his boss would be back at Scrubs Lane Police Station awaiting a quick de brief on the McCann trial, but Detective Superintendent Jack Corbett would have to wait. Somehow an appointment with Jack Daniels seemed far more appropriate

'What a way to spend your bloody birthday' he muttered.

With his mind still gnawing through the prosecution evidence, he stood alone at the kerbside a mile from the courts, waiting to cross. He was about to step into the road when a squeal of tyres on the heavily gritted surface brought him smartly back to his senses. Lifting his hands, he shielded his eyes from the full headlights of the black Peugeot Cabriolet that were blinding him. Squinting desperately against the falling flakes that were stinging his eyes, he was about to jog across the road when a soft female voice called after him.

'Can I give you a lift?'

He climbed into the passenger seat, and began to stamp some circulation back into his feet, while blowing hot breath all over his gloveless hands.

Miss Wainwright smelled even nicer than she looked. The perfume was Calvin Klein, and the long black fur-collared coat she wore couldn't have been bought by Hook's monthly pay cheque. She would have looked good in a New Zealand rug he thought, as the convertible accelerated away.

Lighting up his last Gitanes, he sat back and folded his arms. Suppressing anger wasn't one of his more endearing qualities, and he sucked aggressively on a cigarette that was determined to go out. His eyes began to follow the rhythmical movement of the windscreen wipers as they did their job, pushing away the falling snow with the same ruthless ease with which she had dismissed some of his witnesses. He blew out wreaths of smoke as the car ploughed its way through the slow-moving traffic.

Accepting the lift, he knew, had been unwise. A thorough soaking followed by the onset of some flu virus from the Asian sub-continent may have been a better option, as the wordless travellers continued on through the city centre in total silence. It was almost like meeting the Sex Pistols without discussing anarchy and dope. The date may have been festive, but it was clear he was in no mood for decking anyone's hall with boughs of holly. Halted at a set of traffic lights, she finally broke the silence.

'My God Hook, you can be a pig's orphan when you want to be. You know I'm just a taxi for hire – and I don't mean my car' she said. 'It's my job to prove there's an element of doubt.'

He ignored her, carrying out an exaggerated cuticle inspection. A nine month investigation into the capital's two biggest drug dealers was down the pan, and now he had to sit and listen to the biased opinions of an overpaid, public school educated, middle class brief who didn't give a monkey's toss. He really wasn't in the mood for this patronising impromptu de-brief, but the thought that he and sobriety would soon be strangers caused him to soften for a moment.

He didn't give her a glance.

'But there was no element of doubt' he said softly. 'Fairness played no part in this equation. First, you bloody hand-picked that young ragged-arsed bunch of glue sniffers masquerading as the great British jury system.' His voice was getting louder.

'You dismissed people until you got the jury you wanted, then tried to discredit every one of my witnesses. Those people may have been nervous, but they had only come to tell the truth. You hammered one because he hadn't paid his poll tax, and another because he'd forgotten to buy a TV licence.'

'Christ, it's common knowledge they're dealing in class A drugs. The whole bloody city knows it!'

'Common knowledge never convicted anyone' she said calmly. 'Wait!'

She touched his arm as he clumsily searched for the door handle.

'It's just a game, you know that. The defence win this week, next week it's the prosecution's turn.

People have to be protected Hook, it's just the rules, it's just the bloody rules.'

'Listen' he said, sitting back now, roughly loosening his tie. 'This isn't some fucking Billy Beacon safe cycling campaign we're on about here you know...'

'Yes, yes I know, but.......'

'Yes, yes but nothing. People are injecting heroin in their feet these days so their gym teachers won't see the track marks, for Christ sake.'

'So what are we recommending here? Madame Guillotine?' she dropped her head to one side and added sarcastically, 'Community Service? Probation?'

'Funny. I like it. That's very funny, Counsel. But there's nothing funny about kids who find it easier to buy smack on the streets than bloody cider from a Londis store.'

She pulled up while the traffic ahead ground to yet another halt, and he pointed to the news headlines displayed on a placard at a news-seller's stand nearby.

'Teenager Dies in Heroin Party Overdose Tragedy'.

'So who protects them, Miss Rumpole? Tell me, who?' he was shouting now.

'Nobody, that's who, fucking nobody, because to you lot up in those bloody chambers of ignorance, the judicial system is like a nose of wax, isn't it? You twist it this way, twist it that way, just to suit your bloody selves. Because at the end of the day what's it all about? Money.'

Braking violently, Helen Wainwright skidded to a halt, forcing other motorists to swerve around her, creating reverberations of annoyance that plucked at Hook's taut nerves like a Mississippi banjo. Counsel for the defence, as one would expect from an articulate, intelligent criminal barrister, remained ice cool, calm and collected. Inside she was raging.

'Okay wise guy. Yes, the system has faults, but without it we'd be no better than the beasts of the jungle.'

Still fumbling around, he eventually found the handle that would finally remove him from this naive judicial claptrap. Throwing open the passenger door he leapt out into the real world and into the middle of traffic chaos. Still shouting he said,

'But with it, we aren't any better than them, and we moved out of the trees 25,000 years ago.'

'Well' she laughed. 'I never thought I'd see Detective Inspector Harry Hook spitting out his dummy.'

Leaning back in through the passenger door, while hanging onto his unlit Gitane between his teeth, he unzipped his battered leather briefcase and produced a small red exercise book, which he tossed into her lap.

'No, and I don't expect you ever thought you would see this either' he said. 'With my compliments Counsel. It's a record of all the telephone conversations involving your clients and some extremely dubious European gentlemen, officially recorded during our investigations. This is in complete confidence of course. Home Office red tape, you understand,' he said with heavy sarcasm. 'Unfortunately, these telephone taps are inadmissible and cannot be used in evidence, as you well know Counsel. Let's just say it's for your Christmas conscience.'

She looked puzzled. Staring at the little red book on her lap, she said,

'Is this what I think it is?'

'Lady, you'd better believe it,' he said, slamming the car door with an urgency that indicated he was halfway between annoyed and ballistic.

'That bloody shower would have found Jack the fucking Ripper not guilty' he yelled. 'And do you know what fucks me up the most? Nobody bloody cares anymore. The defence win this week, next week it's the prosecutions turn, my pimply arse.'

She watched as he moved in and out of the traffic that slowed down to allow him to cross. Reaching the opposite kerbside he paused momentarily; turning around almost as an afterthought, he shouted,

'I'm sorry about my language.'

She watched as the black curly head, now with a light covering of snow, pushed its way through the packed crowds who were watching the boisterous fairground hurdy-gurdy rides that thundered around in the middle of the Kingsway shopping parade. Looking over her shoulder and out through the rear window she stared again at the soaking wet news headline that the paper man suddenly ripped roughly from his board, abandoning it to the city's pavements.

New headlines, *'City Businessmen Sensationally Acquitted on Crown Court Drug Charges'* now took precedence over a fifteen year old's premature death.

She sat for a while listening to the high pitched juvenile screaming that came from the fairground rides, together with the loud throbbing generators that propelled them around. She knew Hook had been right. Somehow the system still had a long way to go, she thought, as she watched the scrunched-up headlines bowl along the pavement before disappearing amongst the grid-locked traffic.

Shifting in her seat she turned to look for him, but he was already gone, on the last leg of his journey towards the dockside pubs to drink with others who perhaps would understand.

Leaving behind the noise, she drove around the corner into a quiet deserted street of rundown terraced houses, in an area where there weren't too many Royal visits. She pulled over into the kerbside and stopped. Activating the central locking, she switched on an interior light. She opened the little red book somewhere near the middle, and began to read its contents, in handwriting she knew was Hook's.

Man into cars international tel no 027720/ 273846 12.20P.M.(Sounded Dutch) CALLER.. Hello Mr McCann.
MAN. Hello my son, what's the score across the water?
CALLER. Usual time date and place 50 kees of Charlie, but I have some good news.
MAN. Carry on my friend.
CALLER. Our South American friends are in full agreement and can if you so wish increase the goods to 100 kilos. But first Leonard they must have £150,000 cash up front how you say for goodwill.
MAN If the purity is kosher deal us in.
CALLER. One more thing Leonard, our Dutch Police have been nosing around, and have been making enquiries for your drugs police, is everything under control over there?
MAN. Listen, it's not a problem Henk, the drug squad over here are just pissing in the wind. We have no problems. Speak to you soon.

Helen didn't bother to read anymore but slammed the book shut. Switching off the interior light she sat for a few moments in the darkness.

'Bollocks' she muttered.

CHAPTER THREE

A pair of jaundiced eyes stared out from behind the chicken wire that enclosed the squalid toilet attendant's office, deep in the belly of the city. The dimly-lit Victorian conveniences at the far end of the Kingsway were quiet, deserted, and only the eerie sound of dripping urinals amongst the stench of stale urine and nightly stomach content could be heard. It was the sort of building you only entered if you'd already started to piss yourself.

Squinting behind tiny thick-lensed glasses that his head appeared to have outgrown, caretaker sat in his office as still as a mouse, surrounded by tins of industrial disinfectant and out of date Contact magazines. He was clearly close to retirement age. With sixty minutes of his shift remaining, his tired eyes darted back and fore between the plastic office clock and all the empty cubicles.

Large to the point of obese, his ill-fitting jet-black hairpiece, ravaged by the elements, had slipped forward again, bringing his artificial parting even closer to his left ear. The shell suit he wore had yet to grace the inside of a laundrette. He had been a paedophile long before it had become a buzzword with Social Services, the media and a variety of investigative agencies. Much of his career had been spent as a travelling pervert.

Over the years, the condemned, pungent-smelling set of toilets had become an infamous introduction bureau for a section of society who preferred to meet anonymous partners through small holes in partition walls. Somehow it seemed appropriate that the man with the biblical name should spend the greater part of his existence in a foul-smelling tiled hole, underground.

From a radio inside his office, Elvis sang *Blue Christmas*.

The sound of something being dragged down the steps caused his eyes to brighten. Turning down the volume, his dirty fingers slipped through the hexagonal mesh and he waited.

Giggling and laughing, two young boys on their way home after an evening at a city centre amusement arcade burst into the dilapidated toilets with two small mountain bikes. Dropping them noisily onto the wet concrete floor, they followed the cold breath that puffed from their mouths towards the stained urinals that suddenly towered above them. Breathing shallowly, his heartbeat slipped into top gear, as their tracksuit bottoms were slowly lowered exposing tiny pasty buttocks. Slowly he began to perspire. He had to be quick.

Whispering and chuckling, they stood shoulder to shoulder, still in their first decade of innocence, jostling each other, unaware of the wickedness that hovered only feet away behind the chicken wire. With eyes and ears alert for any parent or friend, he excitedly rummaged in the drawer of his desk for packets of sweets or chocolates. Jelly babies somehow seemed ironic as he grabbed them from his desk. Quietly, he opened the door to his office. It was always the same. The kids would be offered the sweets first, then engaged in football talk, or handed money for ice cream, anything that would secure their confidence. Sometimes he would say he knew their father or support their football team, but it was always the same. He was always 'going in their direction'. Still oblivious to his presence, the adolescents hastily dressed again before clambering up the steps towards the bright lights of the Kingsway. Mr Moses cursed under his breath. He would be going home alone tonight.

The snow was still falling, great gusts whipped up by increasingly high winds, when Billy Saduskas slipped out from a cobbled side street and into the busy Kingsway a few minutes later. The city hadn't been warm for months.

Swamped by late night shoppers and celebrating English football fans, he mingled nervously with the shaven heads and multi-coloured scarves that rampaged around the capital, totally bladdered after a notable victory.

'Welsh wanker!' someone shouted, as the mob jostled passed him.

With self-preservation uppermost in his mind, Billy moved anxiously into a shop doorway, smiled and nodded. He was too small to shout back.

He was just under five foot five in height, with thick brown hair, too long, parted in the centre but now covered by a green knitted bobble hat. Billy was in his mid-thirties, single, living alone in a nearby flat. His hobbies were playing guitar, reading and films. His occupation was selling drugs.

After watching the football fans disappear, he stepped out from the warmth of the ladies' fashion shop doorway and back onto the crowded pavement. Billy had never been a fighting man. Pulling up the stiff collar on his denim jacket as the wind bit into his neck, he hurried off towards the far end of the Kingsway. He was already five minutes late.

Arriving at the public conveniences that were encircled by rusting wrought iron spikes, he bounced down the steps. Once inside he brushed the light dusting of snow from his shoulders, pulled off his little woollen hat and held it timidly in his hands as though he had stepped into a place of religious worship. Looking about nervously, he ran some fingers through his long greasy fringe, brushing it tenderly to one side. Inside the gents it was dark and empty. The ghastly smell that rose to meet him caused him to select certain moments to inhale.

For a moment he stood at one of the cubicles pretending to urinate. Behind the chicken wire he could see that the caretaker was now dozing lightly in a striped council deckchair. Across his lap lay an ancient well-thumbed copy of Playboy magazine. Only one cubicle appeared engaged. The rest were empty.

He looked at his watch. It was ten minutes past nine but there was no sign of anyone. The squeaking sound of a rusty hinge from the end cubicle had him slowly turning around as the grey metal door opened just a few inches. With his eye still on the dozing attendant he moved promptly across the floor and slipped into the cubicle.

Pushing the door closed behind him, he said, 'Christ you are being careful tonight.'

The hand that clamped his mouth and pushed his head back against the breeze-block wall had animal strength, and took him completely by surprise. The hand that held the knife that split his skin and slid deep into his groin was even firmer. Unexpected coldness and the sudden trauma caused him to vomit through his mouth and nose. The puke squirted through the fingers that gripped his face like a steel trap.

He recognised the face that stared, deadpan, inches from him. He felt the blade roughly removed before it ripped once again into his groin, plundering his body like a hot blacksmith's iron. The tearing of flesh was excruciating and he spewed again, as lines of thin grey bile blew up out of his mouth and slowly rolled down onto his chin, dripping off the end of a week-old goatee beard. His eyes closed tightly while a thousand fragments of pain seized his whole body.

'Please don't ...'

Desperately he tried to hold onto the top of the dividing partition wall, then onto his attacker's clothing, but shock and panic had ripped away all his strength and he fell backwards. He tried to scream but the powerful fingers still gripped his face tightly, twisting his hollowed cheeks like glaziers putty before his head bounced off the side of the toilet bowl on its way to the cold wet tiled floor.

From a deep gash on the side of his head he could feel the blood start to run across his forehead and down into his eyes. Blinking furiously, his overworked heart smashed against his chest as he desperately tried to clear the blurred vision.

He didn't know if the knife was still lodged in his lower body. He could hear the sound of his own laboured breathing in the deafening crescendo of silence that had fallen on the cubicle. Above him a blurred sepia image tenderly brushed the fringe from his eyes. Even amidst surgical shock he could make out hushed sentences of sympathy. The voice was telling him things would be alright, to relax, that death was only moments away.

Out of control, his eyes began to roll in his head, and he drifted in and out of consciousness. The sound of some of his clothing being roughly torn had his eyes spinning wildly again. Seizing the top of the toilet bowl with one hand, he tried to pull himself up, but every ounce of strength had evaporated. Vainly he tried to focus again on the man at his feet, but all he could feel was the coldness of the porcelain pan that pressed tightly against his cheek, while the flow of blood was starting to seal his eyes,

'Why …?'

He thought he heard the sound of a coin being pushed into the brass slot in the cubicle next door, and the noise of someone moving around inside. The strong powerful fingers that returned to his mouth and secured his silence confirmed it.

The same hand that had stifled his cries suddenly began to cradle his head. More muffled words of concern were being whispered by the pseudo Samaritan. A banging door and the sound of feet squelching across the wet floor, fading into the night, told him that the toilet alongside was empty again.

Minutes later yet another frightening sensation began to tear through his small body,. A congealing coldness that caused a chronic shivering, as it merged with waves of fearsome panic. Somehow Billy Saduskas knew what it was. That terrifying feeling that some people must get when they know they are just about to die.

Fighting to keep his eyes alive, bone white, he shivered uncontrollably on the floor in the darkness, amidst other people's foul smelling shit and stench, while a sixth pint of blood spewed jerkily from somewhere between his legs.

Again he could sense his jeans being roughly cut, his body being flipped over onto his stomach. Eyes wide and blinking, he felt the sudden sensation of the ice-cold tiles on his belly, and something being shoved harshly into his mouth as his head was turned to one side.

Billy Saduskas stopped blinking.

It was ten minutes before ten when Sidney Moses finally awoke and pushed himself stiffly out of the torn grubby deckchair. Picking the remnants of an earlier corned beef sandwich from between unattractive cream teeth, he stretched his body towards the cracked skylight and farted. Extinguishing the one light bulb that burned in the toilet, and accompanied only by his wretched shadow, he followed the beam from his torch towards the closed door of the end cubicle. Carefully he tip-toed across the partially flooded floor that was covered with paper streamers and party hats, the aftermath of some afternoon office celebration.

He banged heavily on the door with the end of his black rubber torch, grunting a few expletives, but there was only silence. He knew it wasn't unusual for local kids to lock cubicles from the inside, before climbing up and over into the next door toilet. Sometimes they would lock all six.

'Little bastards' he muttered, picking some mucus from his nose with his fingers, while still grieving over the missed opportunity earlier.

Opening the door with his set of master keys, he began to push with both hands, but it only moved a matter of inches. Something was stopping it, something heavy on the floor. Nestling his shoulder against the door, he began to push and shove again, slowly at first but building up into a frenzy like a chronic claustrophobic trying to get out of a lift.

A few people had collapsed and died in the toilets over the years, of a heart attack or stroke, and it was of paramount importance that he got in there as quickly as possible. Altruism unfortunately played no part in this concern for others. His interest was the cash, the credit cards and the jewellery that could be pilfered before the police or paramedics arrived. The caretaker had looted dead bodies before and wasn't even averse to touching up the odd stiff, before the body bag had arrived.

Coughing and beginning to perspire, he desperately shoulder-charged the door once more as the pounds of flab trembled around his waist, the thought of the financial rewards in wallets and clothing pushing him on to even greater efforts. With Christmas just around the corner, credit cards would do just nicely, sir.

Moving an inch or two at a time, the door began to open a little until, without warning, a thick crimson stream of warm arterial blood swirled around his bright cheap trainers. Suddenly another half-gallon of red sludge squirted and spewed through the gap as a white human leg came into view.

Racing for the entrance, the blood chased him, flowing, gliding, surging towards the deathly white porcelain urinals, before disappearing with a slow grisly belch that echoed up the steps after him.

CHAPTER FOUR

Taking another deep breath that seemed to assist his balance and concentration for only seconds, a glassy-eyed Hook lunged forward again, missing the doorbell this time by inches, but he was getting closer. An almost full bottle of single malt whisky and a senior detective's co-ordination showed little respect for one another, as he repeatedly moved sideways like a Tesco shopping trolley. In the background he could hear the faint sound of police car sirens racing through the city.

Turning up four hours late for your own birthday party had to be a mistake, but he seemed to have been making them all day. Now the one person for whom he cared most in the world had also been given the treatment, and he hated himself for it.

Trying to socialize with friends after a serious crown court defeat would have been a recipe for disaster, particularly when supported by alcohol. But he knew there was no way he could have attended any celebrations before putting to bed all the demons that raged inside him. Jumping into a bottle when the system went against him was par for the course, and his pal Jack Daniels always seemed to be there when he needed to ease off the guilt pedal.

But a nice long lie-in tomorrow morning, and he would be back in their faces by the afternoon, swarming all over them like the bubonic plague. Already news of the McCann's acquittal had started to hit the streets, and dealers were already battening down the hatches and going to ground in anticipation. Most knew Mr Hook. Most would be expecting reprisals.

However, punctuality had never been one of his strongest qualities. Promptitude was confined to investigations and people who could help the cause. Those nearest were always made to suffer.

The brain knew exactly what the manoeuvre was, yet arms and eyes ravaged by alcohol failed to communicate. Lunging forward again, he stabbed out a desperate finger towards the elusive bell, finally registering a partial hit which left an imperfect palm print in blood on the clean whitewashed wall. Staring blankly at the imprint he watched as some blood trickled slowly down to the floor. Trying to recollect what he had been doing five minutes earlier was difficult enough, let alone during the previous part of the evening. He squinted at his hand again and then at the blood on the wall.

He heard the heavy security chains rattle noisily inside the small two bedroom upmarket flat, before the door opened slowly, inches at a time. Spitting on his hands, he smoothed down both sides of his unruly hair and decided to try a smile.

'What do you do for an encore, Hook? she said. 'Everyone's gone home.'

Swaying unsteadily, he turned away.

'I'm sorry. You're absolutely right. You're just a haxi for tire' he slurred, concentrating all his efforts on staying upright. Smiling weakly, he waved to her and started to walk away.

Stepping out onto the cold windy landing, Helen Wainwright grabbed him by the arm.

'You'd better come in Harry' she said.

CHAPTER FIVE

He knew instinctively, as soon as he heard it, that there was a problem. He cursed in the darkness. A detective's worst nightmare - a five am call-out after a night on the piss. His mouth felt like the back seat of a Bangkok taxi, while a little man with a toffee hammer was inside his head trying to remove a pituitary adenoma.

Sliding silently off the green shabby-chic sofa, he began to fumble in the pockets of his jacket that lay crumpled on a nearby chair. Finally after establishing exactly where he was, he quietly answered the muted tones of his mobile, while Helen slept peacefully alongside. At the other end the voice was urgent. There was no time for freshly ground coffee and croissants.

'I'm on my way' he croaked, stepping unsteadily into his neatly creased trousers at the fourth attempt

Shivering with the early effects of an awaiting hangover, he parted the venetian blinds in the lounge carefully with two fingers. Peeping out, he saw that winter had now seized the marina, a thick layer of ice surrounding the bobbing swell.

He poked a finger into the untouched birthday cake, and scooping out part of the chocolate filling, he licked it gratefully. After picking up and sipping a glass of flat Moet Chandon that made him wince, he tiptoed towards the door.

Raising her creased blonde hair from beneath a mountain of soft multi-coloured cushions and risking just one eye, Helen moaned,

'Happy birthday Hook' as the front door slammed shut behind him.

Later that morning, in a wealthy avenue of white leafless trees on the outskirts of the city, he sat alone in a khaki green Ford Transit surveillance van with its heater blasting hot air around his legs. Builders' ladders and scaffolding poles covered the roof. It was the sort of rusting van you pass in the street every day without giving it a second glance. A vehicle you would normally expect to find in the local scrap yard. Contained in the rear of the van behind blackened windows were some comfortable chairs, radios, ordinance survey maps. After years of housing overweight detectives who thrived on junk food, the inside smelt like gorilla shit and old socks, no matter what air fresheners were tried. Sometimes it smelt like gorilla shit and lavender.

He twisted his head to look out of the driver's window, catching the full force of the frosty early morning breeze that parted his hair and eliminated the need for a tumbler of Alka Seltzer.

But he was back, that was the main thing. Back out at the sharp end. Out of that stuffy Crown

Court, sitting on his arse, filling in witness expense forms, adjusting uncomfortable ties and apologising to prosecution witnesses who had been torn to shreds by the defence. He was back at what he did best: hunting down premier-league villains who sold drugs to pimple encrusted kids, who in turn sold drugs to other kids.

He sat up, watching in the wing mirror as the occupant of a detached five-bedroom mock-Tudor house closed the front door behind him, before bouncing jauntily down the driveway towards him. Nice area thought Hook to himself. The man leapt into the front passenger seat, smelling strongly of expensive cologne.

'Cheers John. Cor, it ain't 'alf cold this morning. Brass monkey weather!' said the man with the London taxi driver's accent.

Offering a hand weighed down by three heavy rings and an expensive gold Rolex, he said,

'Detective Constable Eddie Stobart. How are you?'

'Pleased to meet you' Hook said. 'Welcome to the Drug Squad.'

'Cheers John. I was just saying to my old lady, first day on the squad and I get into a bloody murder!' he said.

'Thought I'd seen enough murders up in the smoke' he continued, pulling down the sun visor mirror and checking on some recently acquired designer stubble.

'It's going to be a bit quiet down here, after the Met' Hook suggested, as he started up the van and began to move noisily towards the city.

'Well, as it 'appens, as it goes John, we've been thinking about it for ages. The old lady is Welsh and wanted to get back to her roots, and - well, ten years in and out of Clapham CID is enough to do anyone's 'ead in' he said.

'Have we met before somewhere, on a course, or some conference?' Hook said with a slight frown. 'Your face seems familiar.'

'It's possible. I'm fairly well known in the Met.'

My God thought Hook, James is going to have a field day with this pearly king, catching sight of the immaculate creases in his passenger's new denim jeans and the heavy-duty gold neck-chain that he continually toyed with.

Detective Constable 1138 Eddie Stobart ran a couple fingers through his short-cropped and heavily-gelled blond hair, his ice-blue eyes still checking his designer stubble, still occasionally checking on his furry tongue in the vanity mirror, as they headed for Scrubs Lane. He and Hook had two things in common: they were each thirty five years old and just over six foot tall.

'You know anything about this murder then, John?' said Stobart.

'Nope' said Hook, 'other than they've got a body with one of the legs hanging off.'

Leaning back leisurely with both feet propped up on the dashboard, Stobart turned casually to Hook while he began to peel the paper off a stick of chewing gum.

'You the squad driver or something, John?'

Hook smiled politely.

'Yeah, I think I am sometimes, Eddie' he said.

The grimy century-old dark stone Scrubs Lane police station loomed up in the middle of the Docklands, like a huge sore on a landscape of urban decay. From the front of the station, Stobart stared open mouthed at the grotesquely-carved stone gargoyles that screamed silently from the rooftops above and doorways below them. The deranged human and animal faces glowered back demoniacally at anyone who wished to look. It reminded Stobart of a Victorian mental hospital.

Snaking streets of terraced houses encircled the station, in an area where police sirens were as common as the Tuesday morning giro. Surrounding the station, a black spiked iron security fence served as testament to an out-of-control crime rate and a similar drugs problem, blighting a multi-cultural community into violence and generating no-go areas.

Police enquiries in the Docklands generally required a van and four uniformed officers. Hook normally took Trilby James.

'Those black stains around the ground floor, over there ...'

'That's where they tried to burn it down last month.' Hook's introduction to their place of work was helpful.

'Do people actually work here?' Stobart said, as Hook activated the security gates that led into the rear station yard.

'The boys call it Bedlam' said Hook, waving to a posse of journalists that were hanging around the front entrance as they drove in.

'What a poxy hole ‚John!' moaned Stobart.

Glum faces with alabaster complexions, half-closed eyes and bad breath dominated the noisy station canteen, where force detectives congregated in cliques, catching up on force gossip while occupying tables full of greasy fry-ups and black coffee.

The Drug Squad was already there, having seized an early corner table near the dartboard. Their mood was strangely subdued for a pre-murder breakfast briefing, but it was almost Christmas Eve and a murder investigation was just about to turn their festive arrangements into turmoil.

'Gentlemen, this is D.C. Eddie Stobart' Hook said, sitting down. 'He starts with us today.'

The former Metropolitan policeman sat down slowly at the table and joined his new colleagues, gazing with some bewilderment at his surroundings. The mess room had been pained some twenty years earlier in a depressing dark-brown and grubby-beige combo, and had all the ambience of a New Age burial chamber. The brown paint concealed many of the damp patches but the beige had failed dismally. Stobart had never been inside such an old station before.

Alongside him on a flaking wall, a poster of the much-maligned Colorado beetle and an out-of-date Drink Driving campaign poster nearly hid a few more moist patches. The canteen smelt like a Cheddar cave.

'Yes, I know what you're thinking,' said James. 'It's got character.'

Watching him closely as he shook hands with her colleagues, she was already a little suspicious of his brand new denim jacket with its upturned collar, black ZZ Top T shirt and slight hint of a facial tan.

'First day on the Drug Squad is it, cariad?' she said, grasping his outstretched hand.

'Not really. I've been on most of the squads up the smoke. SO 10, SO 13, SO 6, SO 19 and the National Crime Squad. Worn the T shirt, if you know what I mean love.'

A certain look drifted across Trilby James' face like a summer shadow, whilst a nasty fit of coughing swept across the table. After ten years as a serving police officer, she had come to despise many things. Paedophiles, rapists, and roofers who preyed on the elderly all figured high on her list. Her boss, the arrogant Jack Corbett, was another. Fat policemen with body odour hiding in office jobs; flashers, and untidy officers who left empty chip papers on her desk, they all followed closely behind. But snotty nosed, chauvinistic supercops who referred to her as 'love' were pretty high on the roll too. The boys began to look around as though someone had broken wind.

Scratching his temple, Hook bit the inside of his lip and began to rewind his watch.

'Listen Mr Commissioner,' she snapped. 'I'm Trilby James, the boys here call me James and most of my friends call me Trilby, but you can call me Sergeant if that's acceptable.'

Leaning over the table towards him DC Max Gander whispered none too quietly, 'Duw I think you've pulled, Eddie!'

It wasn't the start Stobart had hoped for, but his skin had been thickened by his service in the Met. He didn't respond to James' put-down.

'Listen guys, what's the DI in charge of this outfit like?' he said.

'He's the curly-headed guy who's just given you a lift to work, why don't you try asking him?' said James as she left the table.

Slouched on uncomfortable orange plastic chairs that tested the sacroiliac joint to the limit, detectives of all ages packed the small conference hall as the lights were softly lowered. The only absentee was the usherette with her drinks on a stick. Noisily, the video-tape began to roll into action. Hook watched the television screen carefully as the pictures unfolded before them, images that began outlining the probable route taken by the killer only hours earlier. Murder briefings would occasionally be interlaced with light-hearted black humour, which tended to mask the inner feelings of many officers subjected to the celluloid aftermath of one human being's savage behaviour towards another. On this occasion there was no banter, no humour and no quips.

After a few moments of scrambled images and the occasional sound of a passing vehicle, a chilling scene began to unravel, as the film stopped momentarily at the top of the toilet steps. Everyone watched as the camera-man zoomed into the sign on the wall. *Public Convenience.*

The video picture tremored a little, as if the operator were nervous, before descending into the empty passage below. Like everyone else, Hook followed behind the killer's eyes, as the video camera entered and panned around the urinals, sinks and toilet cubicles, prying, peeping, even intruding upon someone's fatal demise.

A grubby purple anorak and a filthy New York Yankees baseball hat, left behind by Moses, came into view, while the faint sound of Radio Three came from a cheap portable radio behind the chicken wire. The recognisable song was one of Helen's favourites. Roberta Flack's 'Killing Me Softly', a track that appeared a touch ironic considering the setting.

Most murder scenes were videoed by the force technical support unit with the body in situ, and this investigation was no different. Silently the audience listened as the slapping footsteps of the officer echoed on the soundtrack, while he moved unhurriedly across the wet floor.

Watching such films invariably motivated Hook, made him angry, as each macabre detail was branded into the mind. Death and murder with its suddenness and awful finality never really left you, and would select unexpected moments to return. In Hook's case it was generally some time after midnight.

Like many around him, he sparked up a cigarette and pecked away quickly. He wished someone could have switch off that fucking radio.

Tracking across the bloodstained floor, the camera halted for a second outside the partially open door of the end cubicle. Once again the video camera began to shake. At this point, the cameraman appeared to have difficulty in gaining access to a body that lay inside. Hook had already spotted the leg.

Then, like some of the toilets' peculiar customers, the camera suddenly swept into the adjoining cubicle, before peeking up and over the partition wall, and down into the carnage next door. Already Hook had spotted a palm print in blood on top of the white tiled wall as the camera moved slowly past.

'Poor bastard must have tried to climb out of hell' he whispered, as the body came into view.

The victim lay slain on his stomach, his hair matted in blood, his head having smashed on the concrete floor. The unrecognisable blood-splattered face was visible and appeared jammed between the porcelain toilet bowl and the cubicle wall, while his legs stretched down towards the wooden toilet door. His tiny brown piggy eyes were not closed, but stared desperately towards the now-open door. Every wall was awash with blood, concealing much of the poetic prose scribbled by the urinal's regulars.

Hook could see that the deceased's legs were crossed which indicated he'd been turned after death, or perhaps just before he had finally given up the ghost. It was too early to know if there'd been anal penetration, although nobody in the briefing would have betted against it.

Hook began to visualise the victim, thrashing about inside the small partitioned space like a gasping fish in a dried-up river.

Five partial bloodied fingerprints and a smeared palm print around the edge of the toilet bowl suggested the deceased hadn't given up easily. Brave attempts had been made to get up, shortly before blackness had removed the pain.

Two men in one toilet cubicle. Consent. They must have met by consent. If they were consenting homosexuals and knew each other, that was the end of the sports. Experience had taught him it was always easier to solve murders when people kill those they know. Killing strangers out of some evil irrational destructiveness that coincided with lunar cycles was far more complicated.

But if they weren't gay, why did they meet there of all places? Because it was fairly quiet at that time of night. And if seen or heard, their presence would have been put down to the usual sexual activity that went on there. A lot of men who went in there avoided eye contact because of its reputation. He wouldn't be identified. The lighting was poor, it was just about to close. When TV appeals for witnesses were being made, who the hell would admit to being in there?

These toilets were also at the far end of the Kingsway, well away from CCTV cameras. Once out of the Gents, there must have been a dozen quiet dark side streets where the assailant could have disappeared. Street lighting in this area, he knew, was pretty poor. There had been a big soccer match on in the city that afternoon. The capital had been buzzing.

Hook's mind was already pushing the fast forward button. They had to be consenting homosexuals, he thought. How the hell would two grown adults end up inside one cubicle otherwise? This was a murder scene with all the hallmarks of a frenetic sexual killing

One other thing he felt sure about. The bastard was big, strong and had a frightening amount of confidence to murder in a public convenience. Violent death, he knew, quickly erased any dignity the deceased deserved. Every single piece of the corpse would be washed, cut, swabbed, sawn and scraped before photographs in pretty blue ring-binders were compiled for the jury and the morbid fascination of curious CID typists.

Moments like this always affected him. With the added knowledge that after inspection, major organs were sometimes squeezed into places inside the body they hadn't been removed from, but simply stuffed like a scatter cushion. The thought had his guts performing head-springs.

Panning into the body even closer, the camera lens zoomed in and highlighted in glorious Technicolor the victim's right leg, a limb that had been stabbed and cut deeply around the groin area. His last meal of chicken tikka and rice had returned just before death, and appeared to be smeared down the front of his faded denim jacket. It seemed that the right leg of the pair of Levi jeans the victim was wearing had been cut off and was missing.

'Where's the leg off his jeans?' said Stobart leaning forward for a closer look.

'It's stuffed in his mouth' said Hook, as the lights came up.

Jack Corbett, arrogant as ever, rose from his chair and stood before them. A small thickset antediluvian Detective Superintendent with splayed feet and thick Hush Puppies. A 56-year-old who collected enemies like Hook collected fixed penalty tickets. He wore the statutory blue and white pin-striped suit with matching spotted tie and handkerchief, and a neatly blow-dried hair style that covered both ears that went out of fashion in the seventies. Deep set eyes under a bulging forehead made him someone to avoid during Halloween.

His propensity with fashion had little to do with personal pride however. There were nationwide TV appearances to be considered. Crimewatch and other news programmes. Nothing like a bit of self-publicity, with the promotion boards just around the corner. He also believed that great leadership was all about shouting

Clutching a sheaf of papers he began.

'Professor Woolfe, the Home Office Pathologist is still down at the PM, and puts death at between 9pm and 11pm last night. Now, we all know why these toilets are popular. Vice have pulled solicitors, local councillors, miners and even deep sea divers, but they still flock there.' Shuffling amongst his papers he said,

'Yes, here we are. The body has been identified as William Saduskas, a 35-year-old local man, who lived alone in a flat above a Chinese takeaway, in Steelyard Lane.'

Hook's jaw dropped as James elbowed him sharply in the ribs.

'Christ, it's your nark, little Billy!' she said.

Hook's face distorted. Moving forward to the edge of his seat, anxiety galloped around in the pit of his stomach while he glared at the victim's body.

'He's in the system with a previous for simple theft,' went on Corbett. 'Robbery doesn't seem to be the motive - £180 cash was still intact, as were all his credit cards. We've done his flat and recovered a mountain of porno videos and some of that amyl nitrate stuff the woofters use. His underpants also contained what we think may be semen stains. I think we may have a jealous boyfriend in this scenario, a lover's tiff perhaps. This is a homosexual murder, I feel very strongly about that.'

'Any witnesses been found yet, sir?' said Max Gander, better known to everyone at Scrubs Lane as Goose.

'A taxi driver remembers a couple of kids and a tall middle aged bloke in a white mac leaving the toilets at the relevant time. That's why I've asked you and some of your chums from Drugs along here this morning Goose, to see if we can establish who they are. You lot know all the low-lifes, don't you?' said Corbett sarcastically, generating some early morning laughter from his own CID team who seemed to hang on his every word.

With his mouth still open, Hook sat staring at the frozen image on the screen before him, a bloodied picture of someone he couldn't even recognise yet someone whom he'd known since his schooldays. Things started to twist dramatically in his mind. He was sure that this was no homosexual murder.

Once again this murder briefing was going to be like all the others Jack Corbett ever held. The Superintendent always talked at, talked down to officers in such a manner that people were afraid to ask questions for fear of being ridiculed in front of their colleagues. Jack Corbett scripted, produced, co-directed and starred in all his briefings.

Some years previously, Hook had been the subject of his wrath for failing to fit up a major city villain. Hook bent the rules as much as anyone and often said that the Police and Criminal Evidence Act was simply a rough guide to help out the boys. But fitting up innocent criminals who had committed no crime, no matter who they were, played no part in his investigations. The following day Corbett had transferred him to Drugs, and very rarely spoke to him again.

'Any questions so far?' shouted Corbett.

Stobart raised his hand.

'The assailant seems right wicked, but can you tell us a little more about Saduskas' injuries, sir?'

Corbett stalled for a split second before catching the eye of Chief Superintendent Larry Mulholland, the Scrubs Lane Divisional Commander, who sat alongside him. Looking around the room, the Commander turned back towards Corbett and moved his head slightly.

'Right gentlemen. This is for your ears only' ordered Corbett. 'It's not for your missus or the ladies in the canteen, it's not for your Auntie Peggy or the boys in the pub. This information doesn't go outside this room.'

A low expectant murmur began to spread around the room.

'As you already know, the right leg of the deceased's trousers was cut off and pushed into his mouth' he continued. 'He was stabbed in the groin, lacerating the femoral artery, the largest in the body. These incisional wounds were probably made with an extremely sharp knife near the top of the right thigh. This resulted in exsanguination,' said Corbett.

He loved using Professor Woolfe's medical jargon whenever possible, knowing that the majority of the conference would have little idea of its meaning. He of course pretended it was a word he was fully conversant with.

'What's exsanguination?' said Stobart blankly.

'I'm sorry' he said. 'It means the total loss of blood from the body. Saduskas would have lost as much as six pints in as many minutes. Surgical shock would take hold before the poor bastard bled to death.'

Corbett's chest was visibly puffing out. 'Questions?'

'This mutilation with the knife - was it intentional?' asked James, her hand raised. 'I mean, do we think he deliberately went for the femoral?'

'Good question. There's no doubt the assailant intended to cause serious injuries, but perhaps it was just fortuitous for him that the femoral was severed. I don't know what was going through his mind. Things will be a little clearer after the PM.'

'The assailant must have been covered in blood' James went on.

'There's little doubt that both his legs and feet would be saturated, according to the professor.'

'The toilets caretaker' she continued.

'Detective Inspector Maul has already put him through the mincer' Corbett replied. 'The man's out of the equation. We're happy he rang us as soon as he discovered the body. We'll put him through the system, but I don't believe he's our man.'

At the rear of the hall, a hand was held aloft, somewhat hesitantly, by a young CID aide from an outside division. He had probably risen at 3 a.m. that morning to travel the twenty-odd miles to the murder enquiry in the city.

'I was wondering, sir, if meals will be provided at this station, or shall we claim on expense forms for meals outside?'

His question was simple and honest, but ill timed, and Corbett slaughtered him.

'You want something to eat boy, is that it? You hungry?'

The young CID aide looked embarrassed and shook his lowered head.

'I'm investigating one of the most horrific murders this city had seen in fifty years and the best question you can come up with is whether you're eligible for a fucking free Macdonald's! If that's the best question you can come up with, I suggest you return to your station' barked Corbett.

Hook glanced over his shoulder at the young temporary detective. He couldn't have been more than twenty years old, attending his first murder investigation. Fresh faced, enthusiastic and hoping to learn from an experienced bunch of hard-nosed coppers. His bloodshot eyes showed he hadn't slept all night in anticipation. But he was young and Corbett despised youth. An ugly silence floated around the hall while Hook noticed a number of gloating puppets sitting opposite.

'I won't tell you again. Now get back to your station' repeated Corbett, approaching the young constable who sat like a stunned rabbit in the headlights of a car waiting to be knocked over. The conference watched in amazement as the constable was ordered from the hall like a naughty schoolboy, head bowed.

'The man's a pig' said James under her breath, shaking her head.

'Right has anyone got any intelligent questions?' said Corbett.

With a feeling that most bungee jumpers must get when they're halfway down, Hook took a deep breath and got to his feet.

'Well, I've known the deceased, Billy Saduskas, since he was a kid. He's been narking to me for about six years' he said. 'He was just a small time drug dealer who just seemed to disappear off the planet a couple months ago. I last saw him …'

'Where's this leading, Inspector?' said Corbett, interrupting him mid-sentence.

If you let me finish …' said Hook. He stared back defiantly. 'Billy Saduskas wasn't a homosexual. I'm one hundred per cent about that. The man was a serial womaniser. I knew his family, his kids, his ex-wife. I went to school with him. He was just a two-bit street dealer. I'd have known if he were gay. And what's more, he wasn't a bastard.' Hook sat down.

From his first day on the beat he had made it a rule that people wouldn't be allowed to bully him or push him around. He had always been courteous to others so why should he allow pompous, tubby arsed superiors to speak to him like that, he thought. The sound of chair legs scraping the wooden floorboards told you the conference was livening up.

The officer leading the investigation stayed absolutely flat-eyed. Deep inside he was over-heating. He'd always hated Hook's detective flair, his enthusiasm, his energy, his popularity, and his fucking good looks. Most of all he loathed the respect that some villains had for him. What's more he detested having to tilt his head and look up to the young head of the Drug Squad on the odd occasion they spoke.

'Porno videos, amyl nitrate, nothing stolen from the body, and I bet you a pound to a pinch of shit that your little brown hatter's got a funnel shaped arse when the professor examines him' shouted Corbett, pointing at Hook.

'Now listen, not everything in this city is connected to drugs, Mr Hook. This enquiry will be firmly directed towards the homosexual community until I direct otherwise. I want enquiries made in every gay club, bar, disco, pub, in every massage parlour. If a bloke so much as backcombs his hair I want him lifted, okay?' he said, banging the table with his podgy fist.

Rounding on Hook once more he said,

'But let me give the Drug Squad here one final word of warning. If I catch any of your men shooting off on a tangent doing their own thing, riding off into the sunset on their great white chargers trying to detect this murder on their own, they'll be back wearing a funny hat in twenty minutes.'

'And I thought we were all on the same side' whispered James out of the side of her mouth.

Most of Corbett's rhetoric was now lost on Hook, who sat with his head down, his mind stumbling around dizzily. Almost unthinkable - had one of his informants paid the ultimate penalty for informing? Was that the motive behind Billy Saduskas' death? His brain explored its recesses, searching for all the locations they had previously met. Hook knew all the dangers involved in grassing, but this informant was also a good friend, someone he'd protected from exposure like a brother.

Derelict schools, seaside bunkers and isolated forestries. Nothing was left to chance. Condemned cattle markets and back-street cinemas showing dirty French films on wet afternoons, their meeting places always changed. But the deceased was no big player in city drug trafficking. The guy was a small-time street dealer who recreationally smoked Blow. Someone who occasionally pointed him in the direction of other small acorns.

But why had he disappeared months ago? Why had he been keeping out of Hook's way? Being a grass was usually an unpopular short-term profession, with a get-out clause in the contract if things got a little hot. Back alley beatings and facial rearranging normally sent informants into early retirement, while healthcare was becoming more and more expensive. Informants could also be the most dangerous people on earth, villains or retired villains who chased easy money or the escape from prosecution or custody. Unlike Hook's narks who were mostly old friends who asked for very little.

Within half an hour the show was over, with the majority of time as usual having been spent listening to Corbett monopolising the event, commandeering every theory or motive suggested.

Sitting alone at a desk at the far end of the room, Detective Inspector Lance Maul, deputy head of the local CID and Corbett's right hand man, busily allocated officers to a variety of teams as people headed for the streets. A gormless-looking man with a face that only a mother could love, he slowly removed his old-fashioned national health reading glasses and began to scan the hall for others he could delegate.

The middle-aged Carmarthenshire lay-preacher, whose main distinguishing features were incompetence and slyness, delicately smoothed down his Oswald Moseley-styled black hair which looked as if it had been ironed into position. Chewing the arm of his spectacles, he waggled his finger in Hook's direction, and called him over. It was his first mistake of the morning.

Arriving at his desk, Hook watched him sipping tea out of his own personal yellow mug, and smiled damply at the inscription. *Sexy men drink out of yellow mugs.* The Welsh-speaking Maul was about as sexy as an out of date bag of laverbread, but, like Corbett, seemed to fancy himself as a ladies' man. James said he had eyes like a whippet and probably tucked his shirt into his underpants. She had never trusted him.

'DI Hook, DS James and DCs Gander and Stobart, I want you to liaise with Vice, and keep observations on all the public conveniences that the city has.' Maul ticked their names off his list.

'I beg your pardon, Lance?' said Hook, surprised, twisting his neck to get a look at the sheet of paper.

'You heard. Surveillance on all the toilets' he said, looking over the top of Hook's head.

'I've already told you. I've known Billy Saduskas since we were kids. His family, his background his associates, his old man. And you've got me peeping under shithouse doors. You know full well I'd be of more value on the main antecedent team, dealing with members of the family. He was a mate for Christ's sake.'

He was right of course, but Maul's decision had little to do with common sense. It was all to do with personalities. He was putting Hook in an area where he couldn't shine and impress. What's more, he knew Hook would be annoyed, but he should have realised the Drug Squad Inspector wasn't someone who was likely to pull up the handbrake and start to reverse

'Listen Maul' he said, bending over the table and beginning to hiss. 'This isn't Colonel Mustard in the fucking library with the candelabra.'

'If you've got a problem with that, boy, perhaps you had better speak to the Super over there.'

He grinned, still avoiding any sort of eye contact. Being called 'boy' caused Hook's eyes to freeze over and his Adam's apple to bounce wildly inside his neck. Maul wouldn't have been the first senior officer he'd decked.

Bending over the desk and quickly pulling her boss to one side, James intervened

'What team did you say I was on boss?'

She knew full well her Inspector could look after himself, but sometimes everybody needed a little help. This pious, self-opinionated Welsh Baptist was due for it. Some weeks earlier she had opened Maul's office desk with her nail file to take a peek at an early view of her annual staff appraisal report, but had discovered more than hymn sheets while he was in the canteen. How the hell could a man that delivered a regular Sunday morning sermon at Tabernacle Chapel come back to an office desk that had a drawer full of girlie magazines?

Stretching forward even further, she deliberately knocked his mug of scalding hot coffee off the desk, and down the front of his pin- striped trousers. Yelling, he leapt to his feet soaked by a lapful of Maxwell House, before bouncing towards the Gents like Rumpelstiltskin on amphetamines. Sniggers followed him as he raced from the hall caressing a dark stained steaming groin.

'Thanks James' muttered Hook as the four left the briefing and headed off up the corridor.

'Dim problem' she replied.

'I think that Noah's Ark fella got it all wrong' he said, as they all traipsed down the stairs together.

'Boss?' she said, looking perplexed.

'When those two slugs crawled on board, he should have tipped them back over the side' he snapped.

Turning suddenly, he placed his hand on Stobart's shoulder and stopped him in his tracks. Speaking softly, he said,

'Listen Eddie, take this the right way - but I'm not into all this 'apples and pairs' and whistle and flute' stuff. Oh, and Boss or Inspector will do. I could have a problem with 'John', you savvy?'

Later that morning, a frowning Hook slipped out of a scruffy builder's van as it pulled up on double yellow lines near the Kensington Lane public toilets and went inside, the murder of Billy Saduskas still dominating his thoughts. The lane was packed with shoppers. Unlike the Kingsway, these toilets were in a more desirable part of the city, a sort of premier league urinal where a more discerning client carried out their seedy sexual interactions. Well appointed, with the local council crest imprinted upon each cubicle door and an undamaged automatic hand drying machine. Where the more professional gentleman could cleanse his hands immediately after interfering with some total stranger. It was common knowledge that one could engage a better class of pervert at these conveniences. Cottaging was a pleasant enough way to describe the behaviour of many of its visitors, but there was nothing bucolic about what transpired there, when the day declined and shadows lengthened.

'You pointing Percy at the porcelain yet?' James whispered into her radio. The three clicks she received told her that he was set.

Human behaviour had always fascinated her and she watched with curiosity the heavily bladdered opposite gender, running, jogging or skipping past her into the toilets. She smiled as members of the prostate brigade sprinted in agony, tearing at zips and buttons, while some forgetful ageing patrons left with totally exposed under garments and zippers at half-mast. Logging every individual untidily in pencil, she noted too the young juveniles who innocently went into the place for its intended purpose..

Stopping for a moment on the opposite side of the road, between two unloading goods lorries, the middle-aged female traffic warden enthusiastically removed her large black fixed-penalty book from her pocket. It was her first confirmed kill of the day. Recognising James in the driver's seat she returned the book to her pocket with a peeved expression, staring at James as though she'd just burnt down an orphanage.

'You okay in there, boss?' James said, watching the traffic warden walk slowly away. She began to tap her radio, but there was no reply.

'Boss, you okay? You okay? Over.'

There was some urgency in her voice now, as she began to check the battery connections on her radio, but still there was silence.

A number of strange-looking individuals had gone inside during the previous forty minutes, but by her calculations there should only be two people left inside, and one of those was Hook.

'If you can hear me, give me three clicks' she said, but still her covert stayed silent.

Her hand-written log was quite clear. Hook and one other man had been in there alone for over twenty minutes. Scrambling out of the van, she ran across the busy street in front of fist-waving drivers and straight into the toilets. Bored and alone, Hook stood at one of the urinals pretending to urinate.

'Christ James, what the hell are you doing?' he muttered in a low voice. Flustered and exposed, he spun around quickly, turning his back on her.

'Your coverts on the blink. You okay, cariad?'

'Course I'm bloody okay' he said, snatching at his zip while jerking his head in the direction of the second cubicle. Peering over the top of his stall James sniggered, seeing the occupant who sat with trousers crumpled below the knee.

'Don't know what all the fuss is about boss.'

Raucous laughter had them turning on their heels as a gang of building-site workmen could be heard entering the toilets from above. Slipping into an empty cubicle, she slammed the door behind her, while Hook returned to the end stall and for some reason began to whistle *White Christmas.* He had little idea why. He didn't even like Bing Crosby. In a Police Detective training school they may have called it initiative,

That morning most of James's friends were out doing some late Christmas shopping, perhaps having lunch in Debenhams or some fancy French bistro. Some were probably putting the finishing touches to the Christmas turkey, or even the Christmas tree. But here she was, slim, attractive, twenty nine years of age, sitting in a busy city gent's khazi, listening to the forced groans and bodily functions of a dozen labourers as they noisily completed their ablutions only feet away. Somehow it didn't seem fair, she thought.

Hook too found this part of police work distasteful. It was times like this that he wished he had joined the Antiques squad, and been able to drink early morning Earl Grey out of bone china up at The Grange. Instead here he was, peeping under partition walls inside seedy piss houses which reeked of urine and Domestos. It just didn't seem civilised somehow.

It must have been a size nine, she guessed. A rather expensive classic brown Oxford brogue that first appeared underneath the adjoining wall of the next cubicle. Sitting comfortably she watched with some interest as its owner moved it further and further under the partition wall, until it began to softly touch her own badly- scuffed Reebok trainer.

The handwriting on the back of a parking ticket that followed the shoe under the wall was stylish and bold and although the ink was black, the words were clearly blue.

'I would love to touch and fondle your cock' seemed a trite forward even if she'd had one, she thought, but this was exactly the category of person the murder enquiry needed to interview. Outside, Hook still loitered patiently at his stall, having finally out-urinated every single worker. No matter how hard he tried, he still managed to look sheepish.

'They give blokes like him a hard time in prison' said a burly scaffolder as he left.

'Brown hatter' shouted the last one, giving Hook a steely stare that stopped his whistling.

James watched as the Oxford brogue was suddenly replaced by a large hairy hand that commenced to fondle her foot. Frowning in disgust, she gazed down as it began to move further and further up inside the leg of her jeans, fondling her squash socks as it went.

If she'd continued to allow this illegal massage to continue any further, she may well have been eligible for the Miss Agent Provocateur Contest 1999 she thought. Standing, she stamped firmly on the offending knuckles, producing a mouse-like scream from the adjoining cubicle.

Rushing outside to join Hook, she thumped the cubicle door.

'Open up, open up bach' she cried.

'Who ... who is it?' wailed an elderly voice.

'Michael Aspel. Now open the bloody door cariad.'

Gradually the door began to open, before an elderly gent with long white unruly hair emerged, hanging his head in shame.

'Oh my God' said James in disbelief.

'Very close sergeant, very, very close' said Hook, staring at the old man's white starched clerical collar.

With a totally unproductive morning behind them, with the exception of the ecclesiastical groper who they had formally cautioned for attempting to commit an act of gross indecency in a public place, Hook and James sat alone on a cold wintry bench opposite the little van proclaiming itself to be Dai's Mobile Tea Stall. There they watched the city centre slowly come to life. A small pile of frozen leaves being escorted by a road sweeper along the gutter flew all around their legs and into the air, as the grey clouds above pressed down on the capital. Pulling down the thick black scarf that threatened to engulf the lower half of his face, Hook launched himself into his first Gitane of the day, while James cupped her hands around a plastic cup of Dai's zebra's piss tea. She could see that his mind was all over the place.

'You still think someone knew about your relationship with Billy?'

'No, I don't think anyone knew about me and him. Anyway Billy was small time, fourth division, nowhere near the premier league.'

'Perhaps he got promoted.'

'God knows, God knows.'

'Think the McCanns are behind his murder?' she said. 'Lennie did threaten your informants after the trial, he did promise violence.'

'I hadn't seen little Billy Saduskas in months. Billy wasn't informing on them' said Hook. 'Nobody knows who first bubbled the McCanns except me. Nobody knows my nark's identity, but it certainly wasn't little Billy.'

'But what about your handler? Even you must have a handler if you're running an informant' she said. 'He must know who your nark is. What about the Informant's Register at Headquarters? His name must be in there.'

When it came to the identity of his informants, Hook trusted nobody, not even his young squad. He'd been double-crossed too many times by other detectives and by other squads over the years. His philosophy was basic and simple. He protected them ferociously and they did the same for him. The ground rules were always clearly defined before any relationship with a nark commenced. He knew only too well that people like Corbett or Maul wouldn't be averse to falsely arresting one of his close informants, with the intention of pressurising him into working for them.

'What's an Informant's Register?' he said innocently.

James just rolled her eyes.

'So what about the McCanns? Are they in the frame?' she asked.

'Corbett doesn't seem to think so' he replied. 'Me, I'm not sure.'

'So what the hell where they doing inside that cubicle?'

'If we can find that out, we're cooking on gas, but take it from me, Billy wasn't gay.'

She took a gulp of the rapidly cooling grey liquid

'What happened?' she said, pointing to his heavily bandaged hand.

'You don't want to know, Trilby' he replied. Changing the subject he said,

'So what do you make of our new man from the smoke?'

'Well, for a man who once met a second cousin of one of the Spice girls and apparently saw

Noddy Holder in Harrods, I think we may have lumbered ourselves with a bit of a Dirty Harry.'

Laughing, she got up off the bench and launched her cup of disgusting tea into a nearby litter-bin.

'Hey, it's Corbett' he said, as they watched a crowd of shoppers begin to assemble around the display window of Pay-As-U-Watch, a television shop across the road from them. Squeezing themselves to the front of the growing crowd, they listened as the Superintendent made his first television appeal to the nation,

BBC interviewer: 'Are you pursuing any particular line of enquiry at present Superintendent?'

'Yes' Corbett replied, 'extensive enquiries are being made by my officers within the gay community in the city'.

Interviewer: 'There has been some speculation this morning about links between this murder and recent major drug seizures made by the Drug Squad.'

'Pure speculation' said Corbett.

'Are you hopeful that there will be an early arrest, Superintendent?'

Posing for effect on the bottom steps outside Scrubs Lane station, a position that gave him a much-needed height advantage over his lanky female interviewer, Corbett slowly turned to the camera.

With fingers crossed behind his back in the hope that the chief constable would be watching from his office at Headquarters, Corbett said,

'Let me just say this to the people of the city. No stone will be left unturned, there will be no hiding place. This person will be caught. We will prevent him ever committing such an horrendous murder again.'

'Interesting' said Hook, as they turned away, mingling with the early morning shoppers. 'I just hope he's right.'

On the opposite side of the road the driver of a dark Mini saloon watched them carefully as they disappeared into the crowds.

CHAPTER SIX

Aberdarcy Pier stretched out into the Bristol Channel like a gigantic iron centipede, as the calm grey waters gently lapped its legs below. Wilfully the chilling December breeze tossed litter all along its back. Empty lager cans, bottles, fish and chip papers and the black corduroy trouser leg cut from a pair of trousers blew all around the pier as dawn arrived. The popular rusted section of Victorian engineering seemed deserted, abandoned by local fishermen and the retired professionals who walked its boards during the early mornings.

A small yellow-coloured council cleansing vehicle and its revolving brushes could be heard as it noisily passed the empty ticket office in its own good time, before driving straight onto the pier to carry out its weekly clean.

Clem Meredith, a council sweeper who had been responsible for the pier's condition for over twenty years, braked suddenly fifty yards from the large wooden shelter at the far end of the Pier. Even though he wasn't blessed with the best eyesight, he could see the back of the head and shoulders of a man sitting alone.

Seeing early morning anglers, joggers and stressed-out insomniacs during the winter months, when the rest of the community was asleep, was normal. Often he would stop and chat. He was a sociable man. But this morning something was different. At sixty years of age, he was even getting used to the empty discarded syringes, roach ends, home-made bongs and the condoms that he continually found in the shelter. But this early morning riser was surrounded by a large flock of seagulls that circled in and out of the shelter at will, almost concealing his body with their white feathered density. Although the man wasn't feeding them they screamed and shrieked around his head, which seemed odd.

Jumping out of his little van, he made his way along the slippery boardwalk. Approaching the shelter apprehensively, the wind from the channel began to pick up and bully the meek little workman, pushing him in all directions as he tried to stay on his feet.

Holding onto his brown suede Timberland baseball hat for grim death, he peered nervously through the shelter's broken glass side window, a decision that caused his heart to crash against his ribs.

It had to be the blood that still dripped slowly from an enormous gaping wound at the top of the right thigh and down through the stained boardwalk into the sea thirty feet below, that was attracting the birds. Shouting and hammering on the glass with his fists, he finally forced the gulls to retreat to the skies, as the remaining panes fell out and smashed loudly on the soaking boardwalk.

Meredith knew that the man was dead, by the grotesque bulging tortured eyes that mirrored his last moments before life had been taken away. Eyes of yellow and green, that stared directly at the little labourer, from a face that had slumped sideways onto an undernourished shoulder. Deciding upon his age was difficult. He looked about fifty but something pointed to a younger man who had abused chemicals. Weak paper-thin brown hair, going prematurely grey in patches, had already given up, as had his heart only an hour or so earlier. The whole body was soaked with the channel's misty spray. Rigor mortis was quietly arriving.

An unruly goatee beard and half a dozen decaying teeth could have fitted the description of anyone wandering the grounds of some mental institution, or some inner city pavement late at night. A car-boot sale overcoat, black corduroy trousers and a pair of battered Dr Marten's boots appeared to be his only worthwhile possessions. A violent discharge of vomit had defiled all three. The pier's visitor had been slaughtered like a farm animal.

Inside the victim's overcoat pocket, a mobile phone suddenly began to ring, causing Meredith to rouse from his traumatised stupor. Fidgeting nervously for the keys to his vehicle, he started to panic as the returning birds began screaming and hovering above the shelter again.

Overdosed on shock, Meredith walked back towards the pier entrance, with the sound of the mobile phone still ringing in his ears. Death to him had always been closed eyes and a feathering of rouge, underneath starched sheets in a Chapel of Rest.

Ignoring his little cleansing vehicle with the keys still in the ignition and its engine still running, he broke into an arthritic jog. Refusing to look back, his stride began to lengthen while his hat blew down into the sea. If he had, he would have seen the large white birds begin to infest the shelter again.

It was the last time he ever went onto the pier.

CHAPTER SEVEN

Detective Superintendent Jack Corbett flung open the double doors of the conference hall with an almighty crash. Bursting out into the corridor, porridge complexioned, he shouted expletive instructions to the subservient Maul who struggled to keep up. Making notes on the run was another thing he hadn't mastered.

Once again the CID head had dominated the briefing on the second murder, and insisted there was a gay connection. Sections of the gay fraternity did frequent the shelter at the end of the pier, he had said; they were quite entitled to, and the collator's office was full of information on men with previous for importuning. But many others used that shelter as well. Already Corbett was squashing all his eggs into the same basket.

The whole conference had been low key. There was no energy, no constructive input from experienced detectives. Apart from a load of shouting and possibly unfair criticism, the whole briefing had been flat and uninspired, and Corbett knew it. When Hook gave a briefing it was slightly different. He nailed your arse to the chair.

The majority of murders, Corbett knew, were domestic husband and wife jobs. A ménage a trois fuelled by corner shop vodka with the statutory bread knife were normally detected within twenty four hours; if it became a runner, forensic and DNA would bail you out. But if you were still knocking doors after three weeks, when things were starting to become stale and cold, that's when the team's enthusiasm could start to wane.

'Super! Super!' shouted Maul, catching up with him. 'The ACC's on the phone, and will you speak to the TV boys downstairs?'

His blood pressure requiring him to search his trouser pockets for his red and grey capsules, Corbett spun around angrily. With little thought given to a bunch of female station cleaners passing with buckets and mops, he shouted,

'I want every single fucking policeman back out on the street in five minutes, and I don't care if it is fucking Christmas Eve!'

'Did you know him, boss?' asked Stobart, as he and Hook also left the conference hall and made their way along the long winding corridor that smelt like an ageing grammar school classroom.

'Sorry?'

'I said, did you know this last body, Howard Harvey?'

'Oh, yeah. He was a top man at Oxford, double first in physics and chemistry. He was about your age.'

'Do you think he was a ginger beer then?'

Stopping in the corridor alongside a coffee vending machine, Hook frowned wearily, slowly transferring his gaze towards the new man, while searching his pockets for change.

'Ginger beer, queer........ get it, boss?'

'Now take this the right way, my friend' he said, pushing a few silver coins around in the palm of his hand.

'I've already mentioned I'm not into all this knees-up-mother-brown stuff with jellied ells down the Old Kent Road. Can we just stick to dialogue we'll all understand?'

'Boss.'

'Homosexual. Was he homosexual? I don't know Eddie' he said, slipping a fifty pence piece into the machine. 'I have no idea if he was homosexual.'

'Any idea what he did for a living, boss?'

'Sold drugs for the McCanns' he replied casually, nodding to a couple of CID typists who laughed and giggled as they squeezed past.

'You didn't mention any of that in the conference, boss. Won't Corbett listen to you?'

'I've got more chance of French kissing the Queen Mother, Eddie.'

'So what do you think, boss?'

'I don't think there's anything coincidental about the femoral artery being sliced again. If Corbett hasn't worked that out yet, I'm not telling him.'

'Telling him what?'

'The guy's a serial killer,' he said, kicking the side of the machine. Folding his arms he watched as it produced a cup of hot chocolate and his fifty pence piece.

The Anglo Saxon church stood silhouetted against the midnight sky, as Hook picked his way slowly through the tiny snow-covered graveyard. The Christmas Eve service had finished some hours ago, and no Midnight Mass had taken place here for many years, having surrendered that privilege to its larger sister church in the town. He made his way up the gravel footpath, passing moss-covered tombs, forgotten lopsided crosses and white marble angels that stared up at the moon.

Down in Newton Cove some two hundred feet below the deserted stone church, the wild surf crashed around the rugged west Wales coast, while the wind gently teased the small church bell. He was twenty minutes from the city, and two minutes from Christmas Day.

Stepping from the lightly falling snow into the pitch-blackness of the church porch, he tugged on the collar of his navy reefer coat and fastened it tightly, before turning to look out towards the burial ground behind him. Although many had been laid to rest some centuries ago and were separated from the living by six feet of frosted earth, he still preferred to face them. Not many things frightened him, but these late-night rendezvous at Newton Church always tested his cardiovascular system to the hilt. It was a place where people with problems occasionally met.

The deep growling voice that emerged out of the darkness could even have come from one of the crypts inside the little church.

'I see you boys busy on the telly.'

Spinning around, heart pounding, Hook said,

'Fuck! I wish you wouldn't do that! This place is beginning to unhinge me'.

'So why do we meet here?' said the man with the ponytail.

'Because people like us can only thrive in the darkness. Don't you think there's a certain honesty about meeting on sacred ground?' he said, shivering while he settled on a cold-slabbed seat next to the locked church doors.

Known amongst the criminal underworld as The Ginger Beast, Frank Maggart sprinkled small pieces of cannabis he had just heated with a silver lighter, crumbling the black Lebanese resin carefully along his home-made joint, while the flame's glow illuminated his large grisly head. Staring for a moment at a face that always reminded him of something that jumped out at you on a fairground Ghost Train, Hook said nothing. He just sat for a moment with his arms folded, enjoying the unmistakable aroma of his friend's lengthy three-skinner.

Frank Maggart and Hook had been friends since primary school. Married with half a dozen children, he no longer drank, no longer brawled in bars and had become a dedicated family man. An occasional spliff was now his only vice and Hook turned a blind eye. But the two old friends had one thing in common. They abhorred hard drugs. Maggart, who regularly helped the cause with top-class information, had never asked for, or received, a penny for doing so.

During their teenage years, they had gone off on separate paths, Hook to the University of Wales while Maggart chose the University of Life. Although their equal-status balance had dramatically changed, mainly due to The Offences Against The Person Act, 1861 and Maggart's occasional loss of liberty, their friendship had always survived.

Even when the big man had been temporarily removed from the community for provoked acts of violence, Hook had kept a special eye on his friend's family, even supporting them financially. Now it was Maggart's turn to protect his old school mate's back from the criminal underworld, a back that needed protection,

Maggart's name had never been entered in the Informant's Register at headquarters; he was too valuable a friend. Their whole conversation would end up inside Hook's head, and not on any intelligence log for all the force to see.

'Nice performance in Crown the other day,' said Hook. Smiling, Maggart tenderly laid the exotic-looking cigarette onto the edge of his lips before lighting up.

'Got anything for me?' Hook went on.

Softly twisting pieces of a rather scurvy-looking ginger beard, and looking over the top of his small round pebble-type glasses, Maggart growled again,

'Talk down at the club is that the McCanns are back at it. Surprise surprise! Fifty kees of coke are due in anytime.'

'Any idea when and where?'

'Talk it's Holland.'

'Holland,' repeated Hook, with a vacant tiredness in his eyes, his mind desperately trying to stay awake while he attempted to smother a huge yawn.

'Aye, you must know it. Small flat European country tucked in between Belgium and Germany. Does a nice line in slip-on shoes' he said.

Rubbing both hands up and down a strained and fatigued face, Hook ignored the sarcasm.

'Sorry' he said. 'I've got a few problems at the moment.'

'So I can see,' Maggart said.

There were many reasons why villains respected each other. Wealth, power, loyalty, toughness, even expensive motors. But Lennie

McCann respected Frank Maggart's legendary hardness and respect among the tough criminal under-classes. The Ginger Beast was someone to be trusted, someone to be admired. Whenever they met at The Blue Parrot Lennie disobeyed the one golden rule on the villains charter. He couldn't keep his mouth shut.

'Listen - you could have asked me all this on the 'phone earlier. Now, if you've enticed me away from my spouse in search of some tedious run-of-the-mill information, on Christmas Eve, one is likely to become irritated.'

Shivering in the icy cold porch, Hook felt like a wimp as he flapped his arms around in an effort to keep the chill at bay. Without a goose bump in sight, Maggart wore black jeans and a skimpy black T-shirt. A small white "No Fear" logo embroidered on an impressive chest seemed very appropriate. Catching sight of Maggart's pink plastic flip-flops, he shivered again.

Having rediscovered some circulation near his feet, Hook glanced at his watch.

'Just past midnight. I suppose it's Merry Christmas then'.

'Oh my God, haven't you got a home to go to?' moaned Maggart, becoming restless.

'Spit it out. What d'you want to know?'

'Billy Saduskas and Howard Harvey, what d'you think?'

'Ah, so it's murder then. When a person of sound mind and discretion unlawfully kills any reasonable creature in being, under the Queen's peace of course, with malice aforethought, either express or implied.'

Hook's eyes widened, amazed but impressed.

'Tuesday and Thursday, evening classes, A level law, my son. You should come along, brush up a little.'

'Lord Chancellor's job up for grabs or something?' said Hook, unable to stop shivering. 'Seriously Frank, what do you think?'

Inhaling slowly and enjoying every single puff of his lengthy Spliff, Maggart eventually said,

'Well BUPA must be front runners, but truthfully my money is on Lennie and Mickey. Must be in the frame somewhere. Nothing much happens in this city without them, you should know that.'

'But little Billy Saduskas - where did he fit into this scenario? They tell me he was an ounce a week street dealer,' said Hook beginning to stamp his feet again as the church bell vibrated softly overhead. 'The McCanns wouldn't be interested in small fry like him, surely?'

'Didn't you know him?' asked Maggart. 'He was in primary school roughly the same time as us.'

'Can't say I did,' Hook replied, lying like a politician.

'You've really got no idea then,' said Maggart, beginning to smirk, which had more to do with the illegal substance he was inhaling than the enjoyable banter he and Hook always shared when city low life was discussed.

'Strange that,' he muttered, beginning to adjust the rubber band on his ponytail.

'Tell me about Saduskas, before my officers find five kilos of something class A under your kids' rabbit hutch,' threatened Hook.

Maggart laughed.

'Ok. You know the McCanns own Blackline Transport down west?'

'Yes, yes I know all about their wagons.' Frank Maggart smiled again. He loved these little games with Hook.

'Ah, but if policemen got off their arses more often, forgot about those bloody computers and, like your good self, relied a little more on old fashioned foot slogging, they would have already established that the man's an HGV driver. He's been driving their lorries for months, between Holland and Spain, mainly down to Gibraltar.'

'Drugs?'

'No, no, copies of the fucking Police Gazette,' said Maggart. 'Of course it's drugs. They hide it under tons of fish bait.'

'Fish bait,' winced Hook.

'If you were Customs, would you wanna hand-check ten tons of maggots?'

'But why were he and Harvey taken out? Did they double cross someone?' said Hook. 'It's almost like a Mafia hit. These people were executed, Frank.'

'You're the sheriff Mr Hook,' said Maggart. 'You're the Sheriff.'

Standing in the car park overlooking the sea, Maggart shook his mate's hand and was about to say goodbye, when he pulled the pin on another bit of information he'd been holding back, and tossed it into Hook's frozen unsuspecting lap.

'I'm afraid one of the boys in blue is letting you down, Hooky,' he said, using Hook's nickname from school. It was a signal that he was deadly serious.

A bent cop. Rumours had been circulating for some time, but Hook had always dismissed them with the contempt he felt they deserved. Weak unsubstantiated snippets of street gossip, instigated by the drugs underworld, in efforts to slow down the progress of his highly successful team. Without exception, he had hand-picked every single member of the squad; he had come to know their families, even went to the christenings. But it was something that was always at the back of his mind, in an underworld society where squalor and opulence interbred to create villains with well-lined purses.

It was the last thing he wanted to hear, but Maggart never gave him anything unless he knew it was kosher. That was the way he worked. Operating simply on underworld chit-chat influenced by alcohol was too dangerous. If Maggart brought it up you had to take notice.

Locking into his friend's eyes, Hook paused, not blinking, waiting for a punchline that he hoped would follow, but there was no humorous repartee. He should have known better. It wasn't a subject that most people found amusing.

Visibly shaken, Hook's voice dropped to a whisper.

'Name?'

'I'm not sure. Let me work on it. All I know is that someone at Cars International drops him an envelope once a month.'

'And you think it's one of my boys?'

'Beware of false prophets in sheep's clothing Hooky. You're just establishment paupers hunting down individuals with obscene riches.'

A shadow fell across Hook's face, but he knew a thousand pounds a month in a brown envelope was a powerful aphrodisiac, and cheap at half the price for any drug syndicate who wanted to know if they were being looked at. Criminal history was full of villains who had paid good money to discover where exactly they figured on the squad's priority list. Street dealers were always grateful for a prior warning that their front door was likely to come flying off its hinges in the middle of watching Coronation Street.

Flushing out this man, he knew, was going to be difficult, but if he didn't do something quickly his team's reputation and success wouldn't be worth a cup of cold piss. All Jack Corbett needed to hear were the rumours of corruption, and the knives would be out. This wasn't something the Detective Superintendent was likely to debate. Disbanding the whole Squad, tarring the innocent and guilty alike before scattering everyone to the four corners of the force area, was something Corbett was capable of doing during his tea break.

'You know it's got to be like this,' Hook said, shaking Maggart's huge hands in the darkness.

'Don't go all sentimental on me Hooky.'

'You know what I mean Frank.'

'Friends are for life, not just for Christmas,' laughed Maggart as he leapt into the front seat of his Daihatsu Four Track.

He was about to drive off when he pulled the gear lever back into neutral and lent out of the window, his huge tattooed bicep resting impressively on the driver's door like a frozen six pound turkey.

'Be careful my boy. You're upsetting a lot of people in the city. The McCanns want you out of the ball game. Lennie was spouting off recently in that new hair salon in the Plaza arcade. He wants you taken out.'

'What's he going to do Frank, blow-dry me to death?'

Shaking his head and laughing quietly to himself, Maggart waved one last time before accelerating into the blackness with wheels spinning furiously. Hook watched for a moment as the tail-lights grew smaller before disappearing.

Christmas Eve had always been a favourite time for him, but Christmas without Helen, who had been called away to Scotland on some sort of business, depressed him. If there was corruption in the ranks, the very existence of his squad was in jeopardy. And there was a madman loose in the city. All on the anniversary of the death of his mother. Things couldn't get any worse. In the corner of the graveyard, the branches on a holly tree began to scratch the top of a nearby tomb in the wind. It had been a long day. It was time to leave.

Returning to the city, he accelerated through the white country lanes, stopping occasionally to squint at the signposts. This wasn't the night to get lost. Not more than a mile from Newton Church he passed a small dark Austin Mini parked up by a farm gate. Hook was tired and took little notice. After all, this part of the countryside was renowned for attracting courting couples.

Within seconds of him passing, the engine of the Mini started up quietly, its sidelights shining brightly.

CHAPTER EIGHT

Christmas Day brought peace and tranquillity to the deserted Docklands streets. Only the occasional domestic dispute, largely fuelled by alcohol, enticed uniform staff away from the station's television set and crates of brown ale, to repair fractured relationships amongst the community's families.

Sleeping peacefully across four chairs in the senior officers' lounge upstairs, caressing a half-empty bottle of brandy that had seduced him earlier, Goose grunted and snorted to himself. Sitting at a table in the centre of the room with his head resting on his hands and a tiny blue policeman's party helmet resting on top of his head, Hook began to stir.

Together with James, the three formed part of a skeleton staff that was manning the Murder Incident room. Each of them had drawn Corbett's short straw when the Christmas day rota had been drawn up.

Fiddling with the television remote control and flicking through the channels, a bored James said,

'Right what's it to be? Bridge over the river Kwai, The Sound of Music or The Monster from the Blue Lagoon?'

Brushing some mince-pie crumbs from his black polo-necked jumper, Hook got to his feet with a sudden burst of energy and stretched his firm but aching muscles back into action.

'How's about you and I going for that monster, Miss James?' he said reaching for his coat.

Hesitating for a moment she said,

'But what did Corbett say about the Drug Squad going off on tangents, tearing off into the sunset?'

He grinned as he slipped on his coat.

'I'll march downstairs and saddle up the white chargers. See you in a minute.'

'What about Goose?' she said.

A snore drawn up from size twelve shoes gave James her answer.

Standing on the first floor landing of a council three-storey block of flats on the edge of the city, James thumped the front door of number 5A, causing a variety of dogs to growl and snarl in concert. The property was a squalid one bedroomed flat, in an area where the occupants were either villains or policemen. Seville Villas was a block of apartments where people normally didn't open their doors. An impoverished and miserable condominium where heavy handed door-knocking normally sent residents leaving by fire escapes.

Colourful graffiti had defaced most of the walls, and 'Tony Blair is a Wancer' in post-box red, caught his eye. Funny, Hook thought. He hadn't taken Seville Villas for a staunch Tory seat. Shame about the spelling.

A TV set blared away inside, so she began to strike the door again.

'There's definitely someone in there, I can hear them,' she said.

After checking over her shoulder, she cautiously bent over and peeped through the rusting letterbox. The yellow watering eyes that met her from the other side, staring back only inches away, caused her to topple over.

'Jesus Christ' she shrieked, as Hook pulled her to her feet.

A security chain rattled loudly, and the door was partially opened. A gross, greasy-skinned man glared at them. Raising her warrant card so the occupant Sidney Moses could read it clearly, she said,

'Detective Sergeant James and Detective Inspector Hook from Scrubs Lane. We understand you're employed as an attendant at the Kingsway toilets in the city. Could we have a word please?'

The unshaven resident wore stained brown trousers, black braces and a filthy vest that had once been white. He was minus his hairpiece, and without false teeth the lower half of his face had collapsed like a cheap deckchair.

'What d'you want? I've already made my statement to you lot.'

'Yes I know, but could we have another quick word with you? Inside?' she said, wrinkling her pretty nose, which sometimes helped to break down barriers. 'Just a few loose ends to tie up, you understand, bach.' She wrinkled her nose again.

'Oh yes, I understand my dear. You bastards kept me for ages before I made that statement. No, no, you ain't coming in here without a warrant.'

She was already sampling his sewage breath, and with some relief moved back from the hardboard door that began to close.

She had almost turned full circle when a size ten light-coloured suede boot lunged forward between her legs, and kicked the door back open. In a voice that was beginning to cause a lot of curtain movement in the surrounding flats, Moses shouted,

'You pair have no right, you ain't coming in without a warrant, no way.'

Hook smiled confidently. Rummaging earnestly in the inside pocket of his jacket, he finally produced a rolled-up vehicle excise licence application form, obtained recently to tax his car. Scratching his nose with the form, Hook said,

'What was that again, Mr Moses?'

'Why didn't you say you had a warrant in the first place?' he grumbled, before turning and walking back down the hallway.

'Well, let's just say it's Christmas day, and a time of peace and goodwill to all men,' said Hook, following.

Stepping over the threshold, they followed Moses into a world of unbelievable squalor and filth, as the stench of sweat and stale dog food began to disturb their earlier turkey and pickle sandwiches. The whole floor was littered with newspaper, each containing a small heap of dog excrement, while the striped mattress on the single bed at the far corner of the room was covered in the statutory urine and spermatozoa stains. Underneath a dog barked lethargically.

James felt physically sick and when she stepped in half a kilo of dog shit behind the kitchen door, she made her excuses and left. The place was like a wallpapered cesspit, with chairs.

Hook didn't trust the two filthy seats in front of him. He remained standing as he stared into the eyes of the man who stood opposite. Someone who he believed had probably committed lots of sex offences against the young. A man with many secrets. The collators office at the station had a card on him that said he was a city toilet attendant, who possibly engaged in sexual activities with some of his customers. But Hook had always had a feeling about him, even though nobody had discovered any previous convictions. Moving under a new stone in a new city whenever there was a threat of apprehension was probably the reason. Even looking at him turned Hooks guts.

'Why you staring mate? What's your problem?' Moses said, dabbing his sweaty forehead with a dirty tea towel.

'The problem, my corpulent friend, is that I know exactly what you are, and what you represent. I know what goes on in those toilets. Quite frankly I feel like vomiting.'

'You know fuck all about me, now piss off out of my flat.'

'Just tell me what you heard that night in the toilets.'

'Nothing but what I've already told the others. I heard nothing. Now get out.'

After a short silence, Hook began to make for the door, still determined to keep the annual complaints against him under double figures. Walking along the hallway he stopped suddenly and turned. There was the slightest hint of a smirk on Moses' face.

He could see that Moses initial fear of their unannounced visit had all but evaporated, and had been replaced with a smug "you've got fucking nothing on me" look. That was another thing about Hook. He did things instinctively, particularly when people laughed at him. Moving a little closer he grabbed his hosts testicles tightly. Not crushing tight, but firm enough to cause some concern. Moses squeaked like a hamster while his eyes bulged, causing his visitor to move in even closer.

'Think of the pain you feel now,' said Hook, his face only inches away. 'Then multiply it by a hundred and you'll still have no idea of the suffering that Billy Saduskas underwent when he was butchered at your workplace.'

Tightening his grip, Hook turned his head sideways and moved his ear closer to Moses mouth.

'Now I'm sure people downstairs can already hear your distress, so are you positive you didn't hear anything that night?'

The attendant squealed again.

'Okay, okay, I heard shouting of sorts.'

Hook nodded his head and gave a partial smile.

'Course you did.'

'I thought they were having sex.'

Hook nodded and squeezed again.

'Some bloke in dark red overalls. He legged it in a hurry a bit later.'

'Name, Mr Moses?'

'I only saw the back of him, you know how dark it is in there. I didn't want to get involved. Christ, fucking let go!'

Releasing his grip, Hook moved in even closer, fixing him with a stare that had Moses gulping anxiously.

'The end cubicle. Do you think he may have come from the direction of that end cubicle, Mr Moses?'

Swallowing hard, Moses moved his head in agreement.

'Right, I'm nearly finished,' Hook said.

A short while later he joined a pale-faced James, standing out on the concrete landing after Moses had slammed his door.

'What was all that squealing about? Santa not very helpful?' she said beginning to eye him suspiciously.

'Come on, spill' she said, trying to remove the dog shit from the soles of her trainers on some nearby railings.

'On the contrary, he was extremely helpful. Some guy in dark overalls left in a hurry after some noise in a cubicle. But the guy who went into the toilets before Billy Saduskas was found, the one with the white mac, the bloke who Corbett can't trace – well, Moses remembers now, he was carrying a brief case of sorts.'

'Big deal.'

'It could be. He thinks it had the initials JH on the side.'

Feeling pleased with himself, he was moving across the windy landing when the door of another flat opened in front of him and the occupant stepped out onto some coconut matting. They hadn't seen each for over ten years. It had been a long time for both, but this man had aged a great deal more. The grey hair was wavy and would have looked distinguished in another life. He must have been in his late seventies. Primrose-yellow skin and broken red facial veins told the outside world of the influence alcohol might have had on his life. Eight-year-old charcoal grey trousers and a shabby white Pound Stretcher shirt that had once fitted, now hung lazily on his undernourished frame. Some buttons on his fly had been done up wrongly.

He looked like a man that had been down in the gutter and was still hanging around there, although something suggested that his life at some stage might have embraced success. Looking at Hook, their eyes locked and time appeared to momentarily stop. Nervously the man dropped two empty milk bottles that rolled around the floor at his feet. Unsteadily he stepped back inside and began to close the door, but Hook pushed it open and followed. James knew there was some unfinished business to be discussed.

The curtainless room was in need of decoration and smelt strongly of cats, while the furniture was cheap and forgettable. Empty bottles of gin and other addictions filled shelves and bins, while a blue foldaway Formica table in the centre of the room was cluttered with bottles of multi-coloured pills - tablets that either sent you to sleep or anxiously kept you awake. Capsules that either made you happy, or made you sad.

The silence continued, and she felt a little awkward while Hook strolled around the room, shaking bottles or reading labels. She hated it when he didn't introduce her. Literature from Alcoholics Anonymous lay torn at the bottom of a waste bin, and she wondered if it had ever been read.

The old man stood with his back to them both, in a nearby bedroom, staring through some old net curtains as he drank gin from a broken mug. Eventually Hook spoke.

'My mum died a year ago today,' he said, his voice breaking like a frozen pond.

There was little response. There seemed to be more interest in the view outside.

'Did you hear what I said?'

'It's not my problem,' slurred the old man, walking into the living room and adjusting the interference on the television.

'No, nothing ever was,' Hook said. 'I see you're still tackling life's problems head on,' he continued, picking up an empty bottle of Mogadon capsules.

'What do you know about my life, my problems?' the man snapped.

Looking over at James, he could feel nothing but returning fury and indicated towards the front door. It was time to leave. Passing the little table,

Hook dropped a couple of crumpled twenty pound notes in amongst the tablets that kept reality at bay.

Out of breath, James finally caught up with him at the end of the street. He was clearly emotional as he leant on the roof of his car.

'Christ boss, who the bloody hell was that? One of your old informants?'

Looking back down the street at the decaying flats, he said,

'No. My father.'

A short but awkward silence followed.

'Was he an alki or something?' she asked quietly.

'No, just a stressed-out GP who shared his problems with methadone.'

'Christ. An addict …' she stammered. 'I'm sorry.'

'Yeah, so was my mum,' said Hook jumping into the driving seat.

In silence, they returned to the Docklands through the empty city streets, before Hook finally decided to communicate.

'Do you mind if I ask you a personal question, James?' he said as Scrubs Lane loomed up in the distance.

Looking across at him from the passenger seat, she shook her head.

'You still got dog shit on your shoes by any chance?' he said, frowning.

Jack Corbett welcomed the full murder team back into the conference hall after the Christmas recess with all the sincerity of an American TV evangelist. Within minutes of getting to his feet, the enquiry's lack of success in turning up any significant leads was placed firmly on the gay community for their lack of co-operation. In fact, he verbally lashed just about everyone on the investigation, everyone except himself. Even his glorious smartly dressed puppets came in for some criticism for not turning up a lot more witnesses. But, surprise, surprise, the biggest criticism was levelled at Hook and his team for failing to arrest enough suspects from the public conveniences. Corbett's eye was beginning to twitch. Everyone's brief Christmas leave was over but nothing had changed, with the exception perhaps of his new black matching shirt and tie. A Christmas gift, which he was convinced made him look like Jack Nicholson.

    The Jack Reginald Corbett show was well and truly back on the road, but as far as Hook was concerned, it was racing at breakneck speed, out of control, in the wrong direction. Towards the end of yet another inauspicious briefing, he angrily thumped the table with both fists, before delivering one of his less memorable motivational one liners.

    'I want this fucker in by New Year's Eve' he said, as people began to leave.

When everyone else had gone, Hook pulled Goose to one side at the back of the hall.

'Listen Goose, pop over to my office and pick up the operational file on the McCanns and meet me ASAP outside Larry Mulholland's office.'

'Duw, I'm going to have a bollocking off the missus if I don't ask you today. She wants to know if you'll spend the New Year with us and the kids.'

Hook made a pretence of considering the offer.

'Thanks mate, but I wouldn't be much company at the moment. But cheers anyway,' he said, slapping his colleague affectionately on the arm.

Goose couldn't hide his disappointment. He protected Hook's back in the squad like an older brother, and they had become close friends. He was forty two years of age and wasn't in the best of health, but he never complained.

'You okay, you look a bit pale?'

'Just a bit of flu, boss.'

Larry Mulholland had been top banana at Scrubs Lane for three years, and in earlier times had been Hook's DI when the young Hook had shed his two-year-old silver buttons for the exciting and more comfortable graduation into plain clothes. Dignified and elegant at just under six foot five, with spiky close-cropped grey hair, the fifty seven year old gentle giant was someone highly respected by the

Dockland's community leaders. As a former SAS Commando, everyone respected him.

'Why do I have this notion that I feel I know exactly what you are about to say?' Mulholland said, as Hook knocked and entered his office.

Sitting back comfortably on a green leather sofa, Hook took a moment to admire the office, with its oak-panelled walls that hid the cracks and damp. The red Axminster with ankle-deep pile was something you would have accepted a bollocking on. With the thick green ring-binder on his lap, he began to wonder if he was doing the right thing. Operation Thunderbird, the file was called. Operation Thunderbird, the code name for the old McCann investigation. It wasn't his style to go behind his superiors' backs, even people like Jack Corbett, but the longer the team scratched fruitlessly amongst the gay population, the more chance the enquiry would fail. He wasn't looking to score points. That wouldn't have been Hook. It was confidential advice he needed, and he knew the Commander would help.

'I know I'm coming in through the back door Chief and I'm probably out of order, in fact I know I'm out of order, but if we don't.....'

Both men looked up as a double knock on the door preceded a sweeping Corbett-and-Maul entrance. Suddenly he felt a compromised, sitting there holding that huge file of papers. He knew Corbett would suss him out, and he wasn't wrong. Glowering across at Hook, Corbett threw a forensic report onto the Commander's desk.

'It's the latest from the Lab,' he said. 'It appears that two different groups of blood have been found at the scene of the Kingsway murder. Group A on the toilet floor and there was some group B around the toilet seat. The lunatic probably cut himself.'

Once again he stared suspiciously in Hook's direction and then looked down at the operational file on his lap. He could clearly see the word Thunderbird.

'Sit down a moment Jack. You may want to listen to this.'

'To what?'

'We were about to re-evaluate the possible drugs angle, anything we may have overlooked in the briefing.'

'Overlooked? Rubbish! What the hell was my last briefing for, to see who owes bloody tea money?'

Easing himself out of his high-back leather chair, Mulholland removed his reading glasses, and moved slowly towards the little gas fire at the far end of the room. Bending down, he turned the fire to full, which rewarded him with a loud bang.

Hook studied him carefully. He wasn't interested or influenced by smart clothes or current fashion trends, but he nevertheless admired the commander who stood before them. The crisp white shirt that had just come out of a Peter England box fitted him like a glove, and covered a pair of folded muscular arms Hook knew could snap a man's neck as easily as some people would break a baguette. A pressed black tie and immaculate epaulettes with a crown and silver pip had him wondering if he himself would ever make the rank of Chief Superintendent. He doubted it. He wasn't smart enough. Any buttoned up, starched collar would have driven him crazy. Thick straight creases in black serge trousers and black shiny shoes that you could see your face in completed the look, and made Corbett look like the back end of a Pantomime horse by comparison.

Placing his hands behind his back to warm them at the fire, Mulholland began to fix his Detective Superintendent with a stare that normally tightened his choke chain, reminding him quickly who was in charge of 'A' Division.

'All right, Jack. I have noted your point and I'm well aware this is your investigation, but we all have to pull together. And I mean everybody. Right?'

He spoke in the short clipped tones associated with a man used to delegating soldiers.

'To be quite frank, Chief, I don't think it is right. If you wanted to bring something up, why didn't you mention it in my conference, Hook?' said Corbett, turning to face him.

Placing his file of papers on the floor, Hook rose to his feet; there was no way he was going to have his reputation taken apart while sitting on a brand new Chesterfield.

'Who the hell do you think you are, running in here behind my back, like some bloody flash super cop?' Corbett was shouting.

Hook had waited over three years for this moment and he wasn't about to let it pass. The Oval Office may not have been the correct venue, but something had to be said. He had never been one to sit and wriggle.

This inter-departmental conflict had been festering for some time, and Larry Mulholland was more than aware of Corbett's almost tyrannical conduct towards some of his subordinates during major crime investigations. It was something they had regularly discussed. A quick decision was required though, before the bell sounded for round one.

However, in Mulholland's book, a cloudy day was no match for a sunny disposition. Cutting his young former CD aide some slack, he returned to his chair and sat back down.

'You wish to say something, Inspector?'

Hook didn't need to be asked twice. He turned towards Corbett.

'It's always the bloody same. Because it's always your conference, not everyone's. It's not a collection of other people's thoughts, ideas, feelings, gut reactions. If you don't say it, it doesn't appear to count. You treat the boys in there like bloody circus horses. Stand up, sit down, get out, keep moving. The men are simply too terrified to speak any more.'

'Inspector Hook' Mulholland said, but it was a half-hearted plea. Hook had already started and he was going to finish.

Standing closer to Corbett than a gents' tailor, Hook's semi-controlled anger threatened to explode.

'Listen, I don't give a fuck if you don't talk to me. That's you're prerogative. But for God's sake, talk to the boys in there. For what it's worth, I think you're going to need them. This isn't over yet, not by a long chalk. Make no mistake Superintendent, this reptile's going to bring you hell.'

For some time, both men glared at each other almost nose to nose. Corbett was the first to blink.

'Pull the men towards you Super, don't push them away,' said Hook, now pleading.

Corbett slumped down on the second sofa. For a moment there was an embarrassed silence. Maul had said nothing. He stared at the carpet.

In his indignation, Corbett began slapping the arm of his seat with his hand, as he continued to stare defiantly across at the Drug Squad head. His eyes appeared to be jumping about inside their sockets. By fuck he was going to make Hook pay.

'It's not a drum solo on my chesterfield I want Jack, it's ideas,' said Mulholland, adding to Corbett's discomfort.

Rubbing the palms of both hands slowly up and down a face that stretched the skin in all directions and his confidence in the same manner, Corbett sat struggling with his colossal vanity. Suddenly his reputation was under question. What if the bubble burst? he thought. He needn't have worried. It was something he'd inflated himself.

Larry Mulholland spoke again. '

'Jack, now just listen a sec. If these killings are not connected to the gays and we have a serial killer here, we really need to keep our options open. Do you remember the balls-up they made on the Yorkshire Ripper enquiry? Don't forget there was no evidence of sexual activity with either Saduskas or Harvey.'

CHAPTER NINE

After everyone had pulled their chairs around the Chief's desk, Hook began dealing everyone surveillance photographs, taken some months earlier outside Cars International, during Operation Thunderbird.

Sometimes furtive photography in black and white wasn't too professional-looking, and unphotogenic villains always seemed to stare at the pavement when a nice broad smile was required. Some of Hook's boys hadn't quite mastered the art of picture-taking by day and night, but most were good enough.

Carefully, he described the scenario relating to each, backed up by sound top-grade intelligence. Corbett watched him closely. He'd just been taken apart by the young Drug Squad upstart in front of subordinates, and that had never happened before in his entire career. Hook could see that his complexion resembled the inside of a blackberry.

'Here's a stack of the second victim, Howard Harvey. He was back and fore to the garage almost daily. We think he was probably the go-between the big city street dealers and the brothers. The boys tried but we just couldn't nail him. He was good'.

'You say he was good,' interrupted Maul, 'But my boys and I saw him regularly bumming around the city like a vagrant. He didn't have a penny to scratch his arse. Did you see the state of him down the postmortem?'

'He owned an apartment in Holland.'

'Are you sure?' Maul said.

'People didn't take much notice of him. That was intentional,' said Hook. 'As I say, he was very good. Marketing drugs was his speciality. I have no doubt he was on the McCann payroll. Don't forget the man was a qualified chemist.'

'But this is just your opinion. You have no hard evidence that he was dealing for the brothers,' said Maul.

'No I don't, although forty visits a week to the garage seems a trifle excessive if he was looking for a secondhand Renault Clio.'

Removing his glasses, Mulholland moved some facial muscles that suggested he was impressed.

'The first victim, Billy Saduskas. I recently discovered he'd been running drugs for them, between the UK and the continent,' said Hook pushing forward another photo of the HGV driver outside the garage.

'Is this backed up by anything? Have you any concrete evidence?' continued Maul, desperately trying to impress his boss, who himself was still reflecting on his earlier clash with Hook..

'Sound informant,' said Hook.

'Is he in the informants' register?' Maul asked.

'What is this Lance, some sort of divisional inquisition?'

'But you agree, both murder scenes are locations frequented by the gays,' said Maul.

'I have to,' replied Hook.

'Look, can we just push this along a bit?' interrupted Mulholland. 'Now if we believe that both victims were involved in the McCann organisation …'

Hook nodded.

'… so who are we looking at? The McCanns themselves? A rival syndicate? A double cross, bad merchandise, the beginning of some bloody turf war? Hook?'

'Well Chief, I think there's a drug connection somewhere, and if we concentrate our energies towards the brothers and their organisation, I think we'll find that connection. We know nothing moves in this city without the McCann's rubber stamping it first.'

'This isn't a personal thing between you and them,' said Maul, hanging on to Hook like a pit bull terrier. 'I mean you must have been gutted after their acquittal in Crown. Why did they sling it out in the end? Lack of evidence wasn't it?'

Disguising his annoyance was becoming difficult. But Hook breathed in slowly through clenched teeth and he smiled. Silently he counted up to five.

It was obvious that the pious Lance Maul was deliberately winding him up once more and had been doing so ever since he'd been posted to Scrubs Lane. He wasn't someone who normally dealt from the bottom of the pack, but this sycophantic charlatan was pushing him too close to the edge.

Shuffling the surveillance photographs that lay strewn over the desk, Hook slipped in a photograph that no-one had been intended to see. Intelligence-wise, the black and white picture had very little relevance; in fact Hook had kept it away from the McCann trial to protect the officer from gossip, although every surveillance photograph should have been forwarded to Hunter Jarvis and the defence.

Pushing the print slowly across the desk so Mulholland and Corbett would have a good clear sight, he said,

'One for your album, Lance. You can keep that one.'

It showed Maul shaking hands with Mickey McCann some months earlier on the forecourt of Cars International, quite legitimately purchasing a brand new Vauxhall Saloon. The picture was perfectly clear - as was the police Panda car and its uniformed driver in the background, the vehicle he had unofficially used to take him there.

Maul began to stammer as though he had just been caught rifling his daughters knicker drawer.

'If, if .... this was a secret covert operation … why wasn't my department informed of it?' he said. 'I'm a detective as well you know.'

'It's okay Lance, your secret's safe with me,' replied Hook.

'Cut it out, the pair of you' ordered Mulholland, slapping the desk with the flat of his hand.

'You going to keep the garage under obs again?' asked Corbett sharply.

'No' said Hook. 'As a result of the trial, they learnt all about our crop on the side of the mountain. There's no point.'

But he was concealing the truth, the whole truth etc. History told him that corruption came from all ranks in the service and he was determined to keep the presence of any future surveillance officers who were watching Cars International a closely guarded secret.

'Hook, I want you and your squad to resurrect the McCann enquiry and push on towards the drug angle,' said Mulholland. 'You Jack, carry on as normal. I don't want any review team finding holes in this investigation.'

'Okay Chief, we'll give it a try.' Corbett turned to Hook. 'But you will report to me first thing each morning' he snapped.

'No he won't Jack, he'll report to me,' said Mulholland.

As all three investigators began to leave the Office, Mulholland called out,

'Mr Maul, would you stay behind please?'

A look of satisfaction washed over Hook's face as he pulled the door softly behind him.

The grey threadbare industrial carpet looked as though, in an earlier life, it had lain in the departure lounge at JFK International Airport. Although the room had that strange mustiness of an old cinema, it had all the bare necessities: tables, chairs and some telephones. An L shaped, emulsion-starved office where people spent very little time. Problems were on the outside, down in the streets, not in this untidy Drug Squad office where Bob Marley posters covered mildew patches and where suspicious green plants were cultivated near windows where the light was the strongest.

Yet this meeting place was full of energy and character, where department rotas were nothing more than a rough guide. Although he tried regularly, Hook's requisition forms for furniture, carpets, or anything remotely new, never got past first base, but remained firmly at the bottom of Corbett's In tray. There had been talk for over a decade that Scrubs

Lane was having a new police station. The police authority was good at talking.

Sitting in front of a large blackboard, he was excited. The thought of being offered a second chance to take on the company directors of Drugs-R-Us began to brighten his Christmas. He'd already rehearsed his briefing, he knew it had to be good.

Hook's briefings were normally sell-out dates. Everyone was there. People on rest days, people on holidays, even one officer who had been on sick leave unexpectedly appeared. A team of dedicated investigators shoe-horned into the little space that had once been occupied by the station's traffic wardens. The wardens had since been transferred into a larger, lighter office on the ground floor.

The atmosphere in the room was tense, and similar to when firearms were drawn, during operations when people were tooled-up in the knowledge that the opposition weren't going to come quietly. Some were nervy and edgy, but everyone was concentrating as Hook got to his feet. This was no normal drugs briefing. They were being asked the supreme test for any police squad. To run down a serial killer.

His unkempt hair which looked as though it hadn't been combed since primary school, and his shabby Australian Drover's coat still half-buttoned, indicated there was little time to waste. The tiny neglected office was deathly quiet.

'Right gents' he began. James didn't complain. She was one of the boys.

'Operation Thunderbird is back in play and we've got carte blanche' he said, and those in front of him began cheering.

Flapping his arms impatiently, the cheering immediately stopped.

'That psycho is in here somewhere,' he went on, tapping the large operational file of papers on the table before him. A huge murmur of mutual agreement reverberated around the room. 'And we need to find him quick before he carries out any more unauthorised surgery. That's the good news,' he said.

'The bad news, gents, is that I need you all to forget.'

Only a few looked puzzled, while he paused. Most knew that when he referred to them as gents, the briefing was important, they knew he was going to ask them to give of their best. This wasn't a Mickey Mouse drugs bust he was about to discuss. He went on:

'I'll need you to forget rest days, annual leave, eight hour shifts. I'll need you to forget some meal breaks, and overtime payments - because my budget's gone. I'll even need you to forget New Year's Eve. I'll need your body and your soul for at least a month.'

There wasn't a sound, a cough, an uneasy nervous moan or groan; they were all with him. If any one of Corbett's men wanted to know the definition of loyalty, all they had to do was to sit in on one of Hook's briefings. Wandering around the room, he said,

'And I can't stop all the domestic strife it's going to cause, because your families, particularly at this time of year, are more important than anything. They don't deserve it and for that I apologise,' he said. 'But I need twelve ...'

It was as far as he got. Eighteen palms immediately shot towards the nicotine-stained ceiling.

'Permission to volunteer, Mr Mainwaring,' shouted Goose, making everyone laugh.

Twenty minutes later Hook had told them all they needed to know.

'It's a five o'clock start tomorrow, James. I want warrants for all the division-one heroin and cocaine dealers. Informants!' he shouted to the room, 'call a few markers in. There's a few lording about this city like the bloody Colombian cartels. And I want a new crop built somewhere near Cars International tonight. If the McCanns so much as fart, I want to be the first to know.'

'Right lads, the show's back on the road,' shouted James, as chairs and stools scraped noisily along the floor. 'Let's get our arses into gear before the bloody Government legalises it all.'

Waiting for the milk float to disappear in the distance before slipping silently out of the shadows, Eddie Stobart sprinted across the deserted wet street before hitting the front wall of the house with a sickening thud. It was 5.35am. Breathing heavily, his nervous fingers gripped the wooden handle of the seven pound sledgehammer as he raised it to shoulder height. He knew he was on trial here, and that he had to be quick and accurate. It was all to do with timing, he reminded himself. If the front door of number seven Mackintosh Lane didn't go in first time, there could be problems for everyone.

It had been a few years since he had been a sledgeman on a dawn raid, and the extra stress seemed to add twenty pounds to the unsophisticated door opener as the adrenaline began to pump. Goose, acting as second sledgeman, standing only feet away on the other side of the door, had no such worries. Relaxed and laid back, he chewed gum as he waited for Mr Commissioner to start the silent count to three. If ever a man should have been arrested for indecent composure, it was the reliable Goose. Stobart wasn't on the front line by accident; Hook wanted an early view of his new transfer. If Stobart messed up, Goose would bail him out.

As Stobart began the silent count, Goose gave him a huge reassuring wink. It had to be like this. Heroin dealers like Bubbles Kavangher tended to ignore official requests to open doors when drugs squads executed untimely search warrants.

The heavily tattooed Kavangher had been seen in a number of the surveillance photographs outside Cars International talking to Howard Harvey, and intelligence indicated that much of his merchandise might well have come from the McCanns. Out on the streets, one of the unwritten laws of drug trafficking was that nobody, but nobody, grassed on anyone else. But it was amazing what conversations went on behind closed doors in police stations, after a charge sheet had being completed by the custody sergeant, Allegiances could dissolve like sherbet if brown powder was discovered under your bed. Tongues could become extremely loose after a mug of Jack Daniels in a musty police station office, when your family's liberty was in danger. But it wasn't powder Hook was after now.

The sledge smashed against the black wooden door, missing the Yale lock by almost eight inches, causing the wood to splinter. Mature crusts of flaking paint fluttered softly away in the wind.

'Bollocks' yelled Stobart

Within two seconds, the head of the backup sledge arrived as Goose hit the lock dead centre with a force that would have rung the bell and secured a fairground coconut. Seconds later, the filthy, wretched home was occupied by big untidily-dressed men with sleep in their eyes, men who had been concealed in the rear of a nearby van. A van that continued to smell like primates shit and old socks.

Everyone was inside within eight seconds, as Mr and Mrs Kavangher were awoken from their methadone haze. Being roused at dawn by a drug squad who gently shook your shoulder was one of the draw-backs of retailing heroin in the community. The whole place gave a new meaning to the word squalor, its having run out of food, warmth, self-respect and veins.

These places never failed to affect Hook; homes where ambition, dreams and expectation were replaced by foul-smelling unflushed toilets, burnt cutlery and hypodermic syringes. Houses where everyone ran around screaming and waving their arms whenever the drug squad visited. It had rarely occurred when he had been in uniform. Perhaps the blue serge and silver buttons had a more tranquil effect, he thought.

In the corner of the room an expensive wide-screen television, video recorder and Sky unit hadn't been turned off the previous night, and the screen flickered brightly in the darkness.

'How many more times? When are you going to stop these fuckin' Mickey Mouse warrants?'

Tracey Kavangher screamed, searching for her clothing.

Switching on some lights, Hook turned his head politely while she crawled, naked, off the mattress in the far corner of the room. Small and undernourished, with dyed black hair and skin like anaglypta, she wobbled unsteadily before pulling on an old pair of Levis. In an earlier life she had been described as a stunner.

Bubbles Kavangher was a little slower in his response, as a central nervous system ravaged by morphine dreams and green-egg mornings took a little longer to kick in.

Tip toeing into a small dark depressing back bedroom upstairs, James and Goose began the search. A tiny cry and even tinier arms reached out to greet them from a grimy cot in the corner of the room. It looked like the child hadn't been out of the cot for a couple of days, which probably coincided with her last nappy change.

Gently, Goose lifted her up in his powerful arms. James searched the urine-stained cot for traces of high-grade Turkish heroin, powder that had been circulating the city for weeks. As the baby began laughing at the funny faces Goose pulled for her, Tracey Kavangher appeared in the doorway, gaunt, eyes blazing like a wounded animal, screaming and shouting.

'Kav, they've got our fucking kid! Up here, quick!'

Holding the woman away at arms' length, Goose tried unsuccessfully to reason with her, leaning back to avoid her flailing tattooed arms. In amongst all the activity the baby began to scream. Everyone screamed during drug raids.

Grabbing her as gently as a man could in the circumstances, Hook looped his forearm around her thin white neck and courteously pulled her away.

'Calm down Tracey,' he said. 'It's going to be alright.'

The thunderous noise as someone tore up the stairs suggested a different scenario. Bubbles Kavangher stood at the door with bulging watery eyes, and a nose that had been running for three years. Although thirty years old, he had the pale lean body of a fourteen year old, with a shaven head and dark brown eyes that were retreating daily behind high skeletal cheekbones.

'Put that fucking kid down, you arsehole,' he shouted.

These situations were nothing new. The squad had been here before, and had the experience to deal with most things. On occasions people did make mistakes, it was human nature, but the mistake that one of the squad had made a couple of minutes earlier, was now going to prove life threatening.

'Listen cariad, get some blankets for the child and cool down for a munute' said James, calmly approaching the demented dealer. 'This won't take long.'

It happened so quickly even Hook wasn't able to intervene. In half a second, Kavangher had grabbed James around the neck and begun choking her with his wiry forearm. Hook was about to run forward, when a hypodermic syringe was pushed under her chin.

She had never been in this position before and she felt sick with fright. Her legs felt weak as the spike occasionally pricked the skin on her throat every time she anxiously swallowed. Her right arm was hanging free, and on any other day she might have elbowed him violently in the ribs and struggled long enough for Goose or Hook to get to him, but today was somehow different. Being a heroine, she knew, could be a very short-lived profession.

Even though the enormity of the situation wasn't wasted on Hook, he stayed cool.

'Now this is getting stupid, Kav. What's the reason behind all this?' he said, coolly showing Kavangher his open palms.

'Kav? Kav? You don't know my fucking name, you arsehole. Now out, the lot of you, before she has a dose of this.'

Hook's experience and the look in Kavangher's eyes told him the man was panicking and gravely in need of medication. It was only a matter of time before the two-inch needle punctured his sergeant's neck.

Sliding his arm down the back of the baby's nappy, Goose slowly began to retrieved ten neatly folded, shit-covered newspaper spills of high purity heroin, which he threw onto the floor. The foul smelling three-day-old infant excrement had been designed to halt the progress of any drug squad nosy parker. And when people like the Kavanghers acted like this, there was generally a very good reason. They were desperately trying to divert people's attention away from the baby.

Although she still hadn't completed the first year of her life, little Indiana Kavangher was already a drug courier. Concealed smack in a used napkin was the normal way the Kavanghers perambulated brown sugar around the streets of the city.

James could see that Hook was beginning to inch his way towards them, but her eyes flashed a warning, and he reluctantly stepped back.

'I'm not leaving without her, Kav. I'm not going anywhere,' Hook said.

Screaming through saliva and stale breath which sprayed the side of James's face, the man shouted,

'You just don't understand, you bastards, do you? Nobody understands.'

Hook saw the syringe begin to move as if in slow motion.

Rushing forward Tracey Kavangher shouted as she grabbed his arm,

'Don't Kav, for fuck's sake.' She turned to the police officers. 'For God's sake, the guy's HIV. Can't you bastards see he's dying?'

Dropping the spike onto the rough floorboards, he collapsed onto his knees in tears.

Standing in the doorway beaming proudly, Stobart waved a sawn-off shotgun with a twelve inch barrel, and a photograph, he had found under the blankets of the child's pram during the search of the kitchen. The picture, in a cheap plastic frame, he handed to Hook. It was of a young man in cap and gown. Howard Harvey at Oxford.

'Okay Kav, now take your time,' said Hook squatting down beside him. Studying the photo he said, 'You know the procedure better than me. You have the right to remain silent, but I suggest you totally ignore that and say something fairly quick.'

Hook had a police caution to suit most occasions.

Snatching the photo away from Hook, Kavangher rolled over towards the wall and sat with his head bent and his knees up tight against his chest. Rocking back and fore, he clutched the frame firmly against his stomach and said,

'You think I'm behind Howard's murder, is that what you all think? For Christ sake man, the guy was my stepbrother. Okay so he was gay, that's not a crime is it? The McCanns turned him into an addict, giving him cheap smack until he was hooked, then they ran him ragged. They had him dealing for them all over the country.'

Looking at the gun, he went on, 'Yeah, I thought about shooting the brothers, they've got to be behind it somewhere. It would have made no difference to me, I'm serving one life sentence already.'

While the Kavanghers were escorted into the street outside, Tracey pulled Hook back into a small room that contained an oven, a kettle and a stolen council deckchair. He thought this must be the kitchen.

'Listen Mr Hook, can we do some business?' He thought for a while before nodding his head. Peeping around the door to make sure their conversation remained confidential, she moved a little closer. Seductively she tossed back her thinning black unwashed hair, while she fastened the fly buttons on her stained denim jeans. In spite of everything, she knew Hook was okay. He'd always tried to help in the past.

She had once been a teenager who would have turned the head on a store window dummy. Now she flashed big blue eyes that hadn't sparkled in years; vainly she attempted a smile, but her teeth had been destroyed, wasted and distorted by substances that swallowed you up with the promise of a good time, before vomiting you out on the island of Hell.

'Perhaps one day, you and I could get together, few drinks, a few laughs,' she said, rocking unsteadily on her feet.

'Perhaps one day, that would be nice' Hook said. He could be nice when he wanted to.

'Some bastard was giving Howard a hard time, and I don't think it was one of the brothers. But he was scared shitless. I know something very big was in the pipeline, and I mean big. He was here the night he was murdered, he had a call on his mobile about two in the morning and rushed off,' she whispered.

'That it, Tracey?'

'No. Search Howard's flat again,' she said. 'He had a little black book.'

CHAPTER TEN

The door must have been only inches ajar and he could hear familiar voices inside, but Hook decided he would just sneak past. Dropping his head down and to one side, like a dancing Lipizzaner stallion, he lengthened his stride and was almost past the obstacle and in the clear, when a voice burst out into the corridor.

'In here, Hook.'

Stepping into the Superintendent's office on the second floor he found both Lance Maul and Corbett in a good mood. Two half-full sherry glasses were out on the desk. Or, in Hook's mind, half empty. A chunky square glass decanter, was normally locked away in the barc trophy cabinet, stood nearby. He was fairly confident he hadn't been invited in for a drink. He acknowledged them both and smiled unconvincingly.

The decanter normally came out when the chief constable visited; it hadn't been out in a long time. Scrubs Lane was a bit like Chernobyl: people knew where it was, but nobody wanted to go there.
Handing him a small brown official-looking envelope, Corbett began to smile.

'It's the result of your promotion board, Inspector.'

Although he didn't have great expectations about the Chief Inspectors' board, which had been held the previous month, he nevertheless began to feel a tinge of excitement. His interview had gone extremely well, and Larry Mulholland himself had told him to keep his fingers crossed as there was a Chief Inspector's post coming up shortly in uniform at Scrubs Lane. Like a thrilled child opening a birthday card, he eagerly began to tear away at the envelope when out of the corner of his eye he spotted the huge grin on Maul's face.

There was a certain smugness about him, as he sipped his Harvey's Bristol Cream, with the little finger of his right hand extended grandly. Corbett too, seemed unusually amiable, a strange emotion for him at that time of the day. Hook cursed himself for being so naive. The bastards, he thought, the sanctimonious bastards. They already knew what was inside. They'd probably already steamed it open. Looking closely he noticed a minute dampness and slight curling on the envelope's flap. Celebrating, that's what they were doing. Celebrating his lack of success.

Corbett had an A-level in vindictiveness and Hook had been expecting reprisals since their altercation in the Chief Super's office the previous day. Tearing slowly until the envelope was in half, he continued until it was in equal quarters. Screwing the remains into ball, he dropped it gently into a wastepaper bin alongside Corbett's desk.

'Excuse me, Super,' he said.

The Superintendent's mood changed and Hook spotted it instantly. Corbett was post-box red and starting to show most of his false teeth.

'How do you know,' said Corbett, 'How are you so sure you bloody well failed?'

'Because you're both smiling,' Hook said with a humourless laugh.

'Listen, I want a report on my desk by tomorrow about that new designer drug, the one that's sweeping the States,' barked Corbett. 'The Chief Constable wants it for the Home Office.'

'It's called Babylon, sir,' replied Hook.

The squad was still rattling cages all over the city when Hook returned to a deserted office. Only Stobart sat alone, entering details of the heroin and sawn-off shotgun into the property stores register. Leaning over him, Hook placed his hand affectionately on Stobart's shoulder.

'Everything okay?' he asked.

'Yep! Blinding result this morning, John! I mean ... boss!'

'That's good' said Hook quietly. 'Because if you ever, ever, carry out the search of a dealer's house again in such a bloody slap-dash, unprofessional, slipshod, negligent and incompetent manner, you'll be back outside Charing Cross tube station directing tourists to the Millennium Dome.'

'Listen boss,' Stobart began, visibly shaken.

'No, no, you listen Mr Stobart. James is down at the hospital right now, having blood tests because of you. Kavangher was your man. You shouldn't have taken your bloody eyes off him for a moment. Didn't you listen to the briefing? You put James in danger. The guy's got Aids and you let him get his hands on a spike.'

The Londoner's bottom jaw dropped as guilt spread across his face like a menopausal flush He knew Trilby James had been fortunate - the syringe was new and hadn't been contaminated.

The Central Wales Drug Squad was crowded with individuals with enough idiosyncrasies to keep a trick cyclist in material for half his career. Yet welded together in a tight supervised unit, they always seemed to produce the most successful investigators. Self-motivated officers with flair and dedication, personnel with an unyielding determination to take out the scum that peddled drugs. Drinking, womanising and keeping things too close to their chests occasionally rocked the boat. Lack of professionalism, however, was something Hook wouldn't tolerate.

'You're like every guy I've ever come across from the Met. If you ain't talking about them, they ain't listening. You're working in a bullshit-free zone now, so let's start again. Clear?' he said, before turning and returning to his office.

Although he was someone not overburdened with humility, Stobart nevertheless breathed a huge sigh of relief.

'Sorted boss,' he said. 'Sorted'

Later that evening, it was the nut-brown eyes that first attracted James, the neat brown hair blended with an early speckling of grey around the temples. A soiled white T-shirt tightly drawn across a muscular chest showed off an impressive six-pack, and dirty black corduroy jeans that fitted like a glove continued to hold her interest.

At a guess, he was in James's eligible age bracket, and looked the sort of guy would always be first on the team sheet when you were selecting men for the trenches. He reminded James of one of those handsome mid-thirties men who modelled Barbour jackets in mail order catalogues, yet he had the body of a marine commando. Bronzed biceps froze James to the spot. Thrown over the back of his chair was his large brown distressed-leather coat.

She wanted to speak, but there was a slight problem. He was sitting in front of the station custody officer and just been arrested.

She and Hook had been on duty for seventeen hours and were on their way towards a few well-earned drinks, as they trotted out through the custody suite, heading for the Lamb and Flag at end of the street. Turning around in his chair, his eyes brightened as he stood up. He was slightly taller than Hook, and almost as good-looking.

Her legs felt like crabsticks as he made his way towards them. She flicked at her fringe with her fingers. She had this thing about designer stubble.

'Harry. Harry Hook!' he said, in a soft Edinburgh accent that reminded her of Sean Connery.

Hook squinted, then recognising the stranger under the harsh fluorescent lighting, he suddenly beamed.

'Good God! I don't believe it!' he said, hugging and backslapping his old acquaintance. 'It's been a long time! Eight years, isn't it? What the hell are you doing here?'

'He's here because he's been caught driving, whilst pissed on a public highway, that's why he's here,' shouted over Ivor Griffiths, one of the less sociable custody sergeants at Scrubs Lane. 'Now will you let me get on with my job Inspector?'

'Road accident, a bloke ran into the back of my hire car' the newcomer told Hook. 'I've only had three pints. Any chance of a meet later?'

'No problem. The pub at the end of the street?'

The Scotsman shook his head, looking worried, and Hook knew that something was wrong.

'See you upstairs in the Drug Squad office as soon as you've finished with the breathalyser,' he said quietly. 'Ask someone to show you up.'

Outside on the station steps, Hook said, 'I'll give the pub a miss, James. I think my mate may have a problem.'

'He's a villain isn't be?' she said. 'I can tell.'

'Well, kind of.'

'Is he married, boss?'

'Beautiful wife and two gorgeous daughters last count. Now get out of here,' he laughed.

'Shame' she said.

'Hospital tests okay this morning then?'

'Yep. I only felt a small prick' she said, struggling to keep a deadpan face.

'On your bike, James!' he said.

With the broken window-blinds in his office almost closed, and only his small desk light switched on, Hook rummaged frantically in the badly-scratched filing cabinet in the corner of the room.

A loud knock was followed by Joe Brodie, accompanied by a long dark shadow and an outstretched hand. He walked into the reunion grinning quite broadly for a man that had just been bagged.

'Sit down, Joe. I'll be with you in two secs' he said.

'You tied up in this murder, then?' said Brodie, casually surveying the many charts that surrounded them.

'Aye, I suppose you could say I've got a certain input.'

'The guy sounds like a bit of a lunatic,' Brodie said, pulling up a chair close to the desk.

'Yeah. I understand our forensic criminal psychologist has already indicated such a trait,' said Hook, beginning to smile.

'What do you make of him cutting the femoral artery? Must have been a hell of a scene of crime.'

Hook spun round.

'You're well informed. We kept that from the press' he said, staring at Brodie, searching for some sort of response.

Laughing, Brodie raised both arms above his head in submission.

'Sorry, sorry. Policemen in pubs with too much to drink. They all want to be Taggart or Morse. Everybody wants to be on Crimewatch these days.'

'The louder the voice, the lower the bloody intellect' muttered Hook, still searching for some refreshment.

Finally he found it, conveniently filed between *Complaints against the Police* and *Drinking on Duty*. A bottle of Jack Daniels, still wrapped in pretty paper, which James had given him for

Christmas. He screwed off the top and carefully poured three fingers of malt whisky into two coffee-stained plastic beakers that he'd wiped on the sleeve of his shirt.

'Sacrilege. Jack Daniels and plastic,' he said, 'I haven't got a clean mug in the place. Butler's night off.'

After both mugs had silently collided in mid-air and the seasonal compliments been exchanged, Hook sat back.

'Last I heard, you were the customs liaison officer in Jamaica. Someone told me you'd left the country because I'd come top of our surveillance course,' he said sparking up a cigarette.

'That was pure luck' Brodie laughed. 'Never beat me at arm wrestling though, did you?'

'Listen, how can I help, Joe?'

'Okay, I'll come straight to the point. I'm in deep shit. I really need some help' he said, as the grin left his face.

'Fire away.'

'Well this breathalyser. They've just charged me.'

'You still with Customs and Excise, I take it.'

'Drug Investigation Division, London.'

'We should get together, Joe,' said Hook, already a couple of moves ahead.

'Fine. But this breathalyser could prove to be a bit of a problem' he said, pushing his beaker around the desk like a kid in play school.

'The days of losing case files and blood samples are gone, Joe, you should know that by now. The days of the shredded file of evidence disappeared with black police cars. So what is it?' he said, savouring the malt whisky which he swilled around his mouth before downing it in one with a grimacing swallow.

Pulling his chair even closer to the desk and beginning to drum the top with his fingers, Joe Brodie stared tensely across the room. He knew Hook wouldn't like what was coming next. Taking a large gulp, just in case he wouldn't be allowed a second, he said,

'I'm undercover in your city.'

Hook stared at him for a moment. His features distorted angrily. Carefully he replaced his whisky on a wobbly desk, already stained by the rings of a thousand cups of coffee. Glaring back at his visitor he slowly stubbed out the partially smoked cigarette and began to raise his voice.

'You're undercover on my patch and Customs didn't have the decency to tell me?'

'I swear I had no idea you were still around here. I checked our CEDRIC computer up at the yard but none of the individuals I'm watching were targeted to anyone. It's all top secret. You know the score.'

'Oh yes, I know the score alright ,Brodie. If a Customs man told me it was snowing, I'd have to look out the fucking window, he said.

'Hang on, hang on! I knew that bastard Jack Corbett was Head of CID here, but I had no idea where you were stationed,' he said. 'You did promise you'd drop me a line after our course. Remember?'

Rubbing the lower half of his stubbled face with the palm of his hand, Hook looked across the desk at a man whose shadow now rose up along the wall behind him, and halfway across the ceiling. Tiredness, he knew, was blagging his mind of any perception or alertness. Maybe he was over reacting.

'Okay, okay,' he said, taking a deep breath before emptying down his beaker in one. 'It's just that I like know what goes on around here.'

'Absolutely. It wouldn't be you if you weren't annoyed. You haven't changed.'

Your family?'

'Terrific. Elizabeth is in her first year at Oxford and Sally is sitting her GSCEs next year. You met the wife of course,' he said, appearing grateful that everything now was back on an even keel.

'Yeah, I always used to envy you and your domesticity.'

'You married?'

Hook shook his head. Half turning in his seat, Brodie pushed the office door closed behind him.

'Look I'm down in the docks, not far from here, working for a small firm,' he said.

'A London team are bringing in cocaine. Colombian iron-ore boats. The Colombians drop it on the seabed, about two hundred kilos a time, then a couple of divers go down into the docks a fortnight later, after the ship has sailed, and recover it. I'm getting close.'

'And there's positively no local talent involved? '

'Positive, it's all down to a big London villain. They just use the docks to bring it into the U.K. It's back up in Essex in three hours.'

'So what exactly are you doing in the Docks?'

'I'm labouring for a small firm, loading and unloading the Colombian ships when they dock. The pay isn't very good, but the view is terrific,' he laughed.

'You ever come across or heard of a Lennie or Mickey McCann?' asked Hook.

'Can't say I have. What are they into?'

'Usual stuff. So - what can 1 do for you anyway?' he said, quickly changing the subject.

' Well, if my bosses find out I've been done for drink driving, I'll be pulled out of this operation and replaced. My name will be in all the papers, I'll be disqualified and my cover blown. Even my wife doesn't know exactly where 1 am. This meeting hasn't taken place - you know what I mean? You haven't met me.'

Brodie pushed out his hand and waited.

It didn't take Hook long to accept the invitation. He needed all the help he could get, but he wasn't thinking about drug trafficking. A double murder was enough to be getting on with. An undercover man skulking about the city's docklands would do very nicely, thank you sir. Someone he could pull off the substitutes' bench at short notice, and push him into the field of play. He wouldn't even have to pay him wages or overtime.

Grabbing his outstretched hand, Hook shook it vigorously.

'So, keep in touch Joe. You can either ring me here or on my mobile.'

He'd liked Brodie from the moment they had first met. A man whose hatred of drug dealers was even greater than his own. A top-flight investigator who wasn't afraid to go out on a limb. In the early days, they had worked together on joint operations, always bellowing loudly from the same hymn sheet. This guy didn't just step on traffickers' toes, he smashed them with a fucking sledgehammer. Yes, this could work out very nicely, he thought.'

Enjoying a second whisky that warmed his chest pleasantly and caused some of his fatigue to slowly ebb away, he watched Brodie in the darkness, idly trying to read all the murder information pinned or chalked around the office. He liked him all right, but that didn't mean he totally trusted him. Terrific drug agent he may have been, but he worked for Her Majesty's Customs and Excise.

'I don't see any suspects' names on the board,' Brodie said.

'That's because I keep them all in my head,' said Hook with a smile.

This was good, he thought again. Police and Customs actually working together, without either struggling to obtain pole position in the investigation. Brodie apart, he'd always had a problem with other customs officers who continually quoted some antiquated smuggling laws, which evidently gave them primacy in all prosecutions involving trafficking in the UK. All major drug importations in the docklands had previously been dealt with by local customs men. Officers who continually blustered their way into police stations and seized the reins of drug investigations that had been instigated by the police. That was until Detective Inspector Harry Hook took over the squad. Filling the plastic mugs once again, he said,

'I think we may have overlooked a small point here.'

Unruffled, the customs man raised both eyebrows, before leaning back on his chair and placing his hands behind his head.

'The drink driving. If you don't turn up in court, they'll issue an arrest warrant. They know who you are,' he said.

With an exaggerated head-shake and a convincing scowl, Brodie disagreed.

'No, they don't know who you are, right?' said Hook.

Nodding, Brodie smiled broadly.

'And that's because you've given them a false name and address, right?'

The customs man moved his head again.

'What name did you give them, Joe?'

'J. Corbett, I said my name was Mr Jack Corbett,' he said.

Grabbing the bottle of Jack Daniels, Hook poured himself another large one. Gulping it down in one, he shivered as the whisky hit the spot. That was the other thing he remembered about Joseph Cameron Brodie. The man had a weird sense of humour.

Sitting silently the following morning in the six o'clock coldness, one hundred and one thoughts went through his mind as he sat in the middle of snarled-up traffic amongst idling engines and irritating headlights. It had been snowing for most of the night and the city was covered in a fresh blanket of white. Alongside him in the front passenger seat, Goose cat-napped as usual, occasionally yawning, occasionally snoring as Hook's black and orange Sunbeam Talbot saloon stammered and inched its way towards another twelve-hour shift. Once in a while he thumped the car's faulty heater under the dashboard with the side of his fist. Once in a while it came on.

The previous day, cages had all been rattled, rolled and tipped upside down in the city, but the dawn raids on prominent city dealers had been unsuccessful, and that was unusual. It was as if some of the dealers had been waiting for the squad to batter down their doors. Hardly any drugs had been seized, which left Hook with very little to bargain with. A kilo of something class A could be an excellent memory-reviver when information on a city murder was required.

A variety of reasons had been bandied around as to the squad's lack of success. James herself believed that the city was dry because a big bag was due in at any time. How could you seize drugs that don't exist? she had said.

The big shambling Goose had felt that the double murder had unhinged the criminal underworld, sending villains scurrying underground for fear that they could be next on the list for unauthorised surgery. Hook too had a few theories, but one troubled him more than the rest. Someone at Scrubs Lane was talking. He just knew it.

The mobile phone ringing inside Hook's jacket woke Goose up with a start.

'Okay, okay, stay calm and I'll be with you in an hour.'

'Duw, what's up boss?' said Goose, lighting up a cigarette.

'I want you to cover for me at the Chief Super's conference this morning.'

Selecting first gear and acquiring enough engine revs for 80 mph, Hook suddenly slipped the clutch and swung the car completely around, driving straight across the central reservation and onto the other carriageway. Braking harshly by the kerb, Goose's' head clattered heavily against the sun visor, while pedestrian heads turned in curiosity.

'And I want Howard Harvey's house searched again. Floorboards, the lot. We're looking for his little black book where he names names. Slip down to the bear pit as well and see what's happening in Corbett's briefing.'

'Is that all?' Goose replied, speaking through a crushed Marlborough

'No, you can walk from here.'

'I can't open the door, boss,' complained Goose, shaking the handle.

'Kick the bottom panel hard,' suggested Hook, as the passenger door suddenly flew open, causing flakes of rust to flutter away in the wind.

'And if they ask where you are, boss?' enquired Goose, coughing as he stepped gingerly onto a fresh layer of snow.

'Tell them I'm taking my ninety-year-old granny to see her mother in hospital,' he said, as the heater unexpectedly burst into life with a blast of hot air.

'You okay, Goose?' Hook had noticed his colleague's unhealthy pallor, his dark circled eyes.

'Just a few family problems, nothing 1 can't sort, brawd.'

He went on pulling up the collar on a leather coat that hardly fitted anymore.

'Right. When I get back, you and I are going to have a chat, okay?'

Standing at the roadside, Goose watched as the knight in shining armour roared off in his Talbot towards the motorway slip road, its ancient engine leaving a cloud of black smoke all around the constable's new black cords. He knew there was a joke in there somewhere, but it was a little too early for Goose. Lifting up the side of his coat to protect his cigarette from the wind, he lit up quickly and headed for Spandau Barracks.

The pungent smell of commercial disinfectant and boiled cabbage hung in the air, as the old wrought iron lift squeaked and clawed its way to the top of the dark building, before shuddering to a dramatic halt. Rushing out into a white tiled corridor, Hook's footsteps followed him loudly as he headed for Intensive Care. Racing past starched uniforms, white coats and heavily-laden bedpan trolleys, the journey to St Stephen's General Hospital on the mid-Wales coast had taken him two hours, but finally he was there. The depressing scent of overcooked vegetables crucified by steam and water came from a nearby kitchen, as he flipped back his collar and hurried into the ward.

A dozen or so rattling brass curtain rings finally broke the silence, as a sullen faced hospital sister snatched back the curtains to reveal the hospital bed.

Somehow Helen Wainwright didn't look glamorous anymore. Her dark hair was now tied back severely, while pain-filled expressionless eyes continued to soak pale-looking cheeks.

'The bastards,' she said hoarsely. 'The bastards.'

Bending over, he gave her a strong, warm, reassuring hug, the sort her late father had always given her as child. On days when she would climb into the crook of his arm, when a kiss on the forehead would repair grazed knees and many of life's tiny problems. That unmistakable embrace that closed doors on the world and told you everything would be okay.

The heart monitor bleeped intermittently, while the life-support machine and its sophisticated tubes continued to help Helen's mum in her struggle for breath. Evelyn Wainwright had taken a savage beating and was hanging onto life by her fingernails. Both eyes were closed, while her nose, jaw and ribs had all been broken in a display of violence that had pushed her false teeth up through her top lip.

Gently taking hold of Helen's arm, he led her away from the bedside and out to a nearby waiting room, where a young, newly-promoted sergeant who was dealing with the matter joined them. Hook knew from the white gleaming stripes and the neat creases on his tunic that he had probably left the rank of constable just some weeks earlier. The hair was neat and short but the dark fashionable goatee beard remained. Lengthy sideboards, an underlying arrogance and a turned up mackintosh collar told him he had probably been CID. The absence of heavy-duty boots confirmed it. His black slip-on shoes indicated a certain optimism that his return to detective duties was not too far away. No need to waste money on footwear when he was destined for a return to far greater things. A large red shiny nose told you he had only just arrived.

'We found her this morning,' he said. 'She must have been on the floor all night. We think she must have disturbed them. She's had a right kicking'.

In spite of Hook's appearance, Helen still shivered, even though he continued to hold her tightly. During her legal career, she had dealt with many Crown Court briefs that related to violence, but nothing could have prepared her for this. Her world was one of statement bundles, albums of photographs and forensic reports. A civilised and sophisticated existence of nervous witnesses and incompetent juries, where long adjournments and monotonous closing speeches culminates in an end-of-the-day gin and tonic in chambers, irrespective of the verdict. Helen Wainwright had suddenly joined the real world, Hook's world, and she didn't care for it much.

'For God's sake, she's seventy years of age! She's been doing charity work for thirty. All she's ever done is help others. She couldn't spell the word violent' cried Helen.

'Anything gone from the house,' asked Hook of the sergeant.

'Not sure, squire. We think it may be a gang on the Brynglas Housing Estate down in the town, fifteen-year-olds preying on the elderly. They've been targeting isolated houses. It's the third attack this week. It's cash they're after, to buy powder. That's drugs,' he explained helpfully.

'Well why don't you try arresting them, before they kill someone,' Helen said, speaking slowly and deliberately, addressing the sergeant as though he was in a witness box.

'Our CID have. We've had around the clock surveillance, but they change clothes, teams and areas. I don't know if you know anything about the law, but whenever we do bang them up, some smart-arse brief breezes in and flings The Police and Criminal Evidence Act into our face.'

His remarks were spot on. That's exactly what would happen. Hook knew that, yet he felt like throttling this pompous Dyfed Powys prick. And if he continued chewing gum and referring to him as Squire, there was every chance he would.

'Can't you do anything at all?' Helen said.

'No, it's just the rules,' interrupted Hook, 'It's just the bloody rules.'

'We'll need to take samples later on, if that's alright squire,' said the officer, starting to leave.

'Samples of what?' she asked, still distraught by the simple fact that her mother may have been beaten senseless by a team of young thugs, all for the sake of an ounce of amphetamines.

Squeezing her tightly, Hook said,

'Come on Helen, it's just a routine blood sample'.

But as professionals in a violent criminal society, both knew different. He had already spotted the word 'vaginal' on the white form the officer held loosely in his hand. It was a piece of paper the courts were getting used to. This was no straightforward house burglary.

Turning to face them, the Sergeant nervously began to play with the small consent form that required a next of kin signature. Momentarily his arrogance seemed to desert him. Snatching it from his grasp Helen quickly began to read it to herself.

'Blood, vaginal swabs, anal swabs.'

She got as far as pubic hair, when she slumped into a nearby chair. Her heart started to pound, while her lungs seared and her legs advised her against standing. Desperate messages from her mind told her to quit and move outside for space and winter air, where she could regain some composure, where she could vomit alone.

'I'm sorry miss,' the Sergeant said, but we believe...'.

'Yeah, I think we know what you believe,' interrupted Hook, holding a pale-looking Helen in a vice like grip across her shoulders. 'We have to cover every base.'

CHAPTER ELEVEN

Although she was in the early stages of senile dementia, Evelyn Wainwright had accepted Hook like a son, and the condition of the kindly widow with the sunny smile was uppermost in his mind as he supped his first coffee of the morning, laced as it was with a spoonful of whisky. What the hell was happening to society, when kids not old enough to buy fags screw a house for drug money and beat up an old lady for kicks?

Staring blankly out of his office window, he watched as large snowy flakes continued to tumble out of a pewter grey sky. Even the concrete, white-topped architectural nightmares that housed half the community and stretched up towards the skies began to exude a tranquil charm

Professional careers had hindered his romance with Helen and had been put on hold almost as soon as Hook had begun his investigation into her clients. A conflict of interests had reduced it to a few snatched weekends at her mother's idyllic coastal cottage, and the occasional meal at her marina flat. It had to be kept under wraps. Hunter Jarvis would go berserk if he ever discovered that she had been fraternising with the enemy during the investigation and subsequent trial. Particularly if that enemy were Hook. Nobody knew of their liaison, nobody except James.

Bursting into Hook's office, Stobart dropped a small black book onto his desk.

'Tracey Kavangher was right, boss. It was worth searching Harvey's drum again. Found it hidden inside a dummy electrical point in his kitchen.'

Stobart grinned and stood, clearly delighted, like an excited puppy waiting to be patted

Flicking through the pages, Hook could see the names of well-known street city dealers until he came to the back page.

'What's this mean, Eddie? *Read pages 50, 51, 52, 53 and 54* ?' he said. 'Why has he written that? What did he need to read?'

'Escapes me, boss'.

'Right. Go through all his books, everything. See if you can marry these pages up with anything he may have read. Could be important.'

'I have,' he said smugly, trying to make amends for his blunder on the Kavangher warrant. 'But as it happens, it don't relate to anything which could make sense. I've checked all the books at his flat. I can't see what else we can do, boss,' he said.

'Okay. Find out if he was a member of the local library, book club, anything, and check out any books he may have borrowed in the past twelve months. See if these page numbers relate to anything he's borrowed.'

Stobart dropped his head. He could have kicked himself.

'Arsehole,' he muttered as he left the office.

Strolling into the deserted main office, Hook was about to sit down and call St Stephens Hospital to enquire about Helen's mum when the telephone on Stobart's desk rang shrilly, cutting through the silence. Everyone was out working. Quietness was efficiency, he always said. He liked it this way.

'Can I speak to Chief Inspector Stobart?' said the voice.

'I'm afraid you've just missed him,' Hook replied, rolling his eyes. 'Is there a message I can give the chief?'

'Tell him Reg Cawley rang, skip, and I've got that BMW 325 injection that he wanted.'

Hook raised an eyebrow.

'I've always fancied one of those myself,' he lied.

'Give me twenty grand and you can have this one, skip!,' he said, giving Hook the information he wanted before he put the phone down.

Moving to the window, he looked down sadly into the yard at his own unreliable, twenty-year-old saloon. A motor vehicle with a defective exhaust and an odometer whose mileage resembled the winning numbers on the national lottery. It seemed hardly worth the trouble, but he knew sooner or later he had to get an MOT. He had little time to consider

Stobart's impressive taste in cars when the approaching chattering and creaking of floorboards became louder.

Peering around the door, he saw a crowd in the corridor, heading his way. He knew Corbett was in amongst them somewhere; he could see his dorsal fin. Returning to his office he grabbed the whisky off his desk, and dropped it quickly into the waste-paper bin and covered it with a copy of the Western Mail. Popping a polo mint into his mouth, he grabbed a pen and paper and feigned paperwork drudgery.

Television appeals had certainly transformed Corbett's dress sense, and there was something strangely odd about his appearance that morning as he walked into Hook's dingy office, accompanied by Doctor Millie Twist, PhD, a criminal forensic psychologist. Her entourage from the University of Wales, and James, brought up the rear.

Stepping forward, the Psychologist grabbed Hook's hand and began to shake it forcefully until it hurt at the elbow. Throughout she maintained strong unblinking eye contact that showed signs of an underlying arrogance. He wondered if she'd wanted to fight him.

Doctor Twist, thirty-odd years of age, Irish, with close-cropped red hair, sat down opposite Hook in his blue pin-striped suit and university tie. He watched as she confidently pulled a sheaf of papers from her brown leather briefcase. Although not yet officially out of the closet, her obvious interest in James, her love of comfy shoes, and the deep Dr Ian Paisley impersonation when she spoke, hinted strongly at her sexuality.

'I think the man could be sexually repressed, you know' she said in a thick Irish brogue. 'A homosexual, who just cannot come to terms with this fact. He's disgusted and has a hatred of other homosexuals because he cannot form a relationship with any of them. He's probably aged between twenty five and forty five years old, short, physically strong, and every time he gets sexually close to another man, perhaps he cannot follow it through, although he probably wants to. Possibly he goes berserk with a knife when someone touches him sexually, although he himself may have instigated the act.'

Corbett nodded while Hook smiled weakly.

'Then perhaps in psychiatric terms he may be an explosive psychopath,' she went on. 'A state where an individual loses accountability for his actions, a total blanking out of guilt and remorse after each slaughter.'

Corbett nodded again.

'That's it,' thought Hook. 'That's it. Corbett's gone and gelled his bloody hair.'

Gone was the blow dried, wash-and-go style, and in was the new Don Corleone Sicilian slashback. Christ, he'll be having liposuction next, he thought.

'Anything wrong, Inspector?' said Twist, observing Hook's sudden interest in the back of Corbett's head.

'No, no. You carry on, doctor,' he said, already bored out of his mind. Come on Harry, he said to himself, for goodness sake at least try to appear impressed. Play the bloody game. With some effort he tried to smile convincingly but failed. Mumbo fucking Jumbo, that's what this was all about, and he was unable to pretend otherwise.

Psychological profiling had never impressed him, and this Irish academic was no different. Loner, unemployed, average intelligence, history of failed relationships, possesses a vivid fantasy life, loves his mum, hates his dad, blah, blah, blah, have a nice day. Bollocks! Over-worked detectives out on the street would detect these killings. DNA, forensics, a worried mother, a former schoolfriend, a strolling street bobby. Not some bloody empathetic idealist and her books on offender profiling.

'I would say he probably lives alone or perhaps with his mother,' she said giving James another broad smile. 'Someone whom he adores. Maybe he's a lorry driver or some travelling salesman, a job that gives him space, a loner.'

Detecting Hook's continued interest in Corbett's new slimy hairdressing, she tried to regain his attention.

'However, the psychic development of the individual is rather complex so it is, wouldn't you agree, Inspector?'

'I'm sorry?' said Hook, snapping out of his trance.

'I said an individual's psychic development can be complex.'

'Oh, you mean because his internal wiring is buggered, perhaps he isn't a lorry driver or salesman after all, and that he may actually detest his old mum. Is that what you mean, Doctor Twist?'

The psychologist glared back with a look that reminded Hook of his granny's expression when he'd refused to kiss her as a child.

'What the Doctor is saying, Hook, is that she believes I'm looking in the right direction,' interrupted Corbett angrily.

'Offender profiling doesn't aim to identify a criminal, Mr Hook' she said. 'It simply narrows the scope of the investigation by indicating the type of person most likely to have committed the crime, especially when there is no motive.'

'I'm with you,' replied Hook. 'I'm with you. So are we still looking for that lorry driver or salesman?'

Exasperated, Dr Twist began to stuff her file of papers into her briefcase.

It was always a bad sign, as far as Hook was concerned, when Lance Maul was smiling; normally it was an indication that he was about to score some points. Still not having recovered from the mother of all rollickings from the Chief Super about the illegal use of a police vehicle, he was about to bounce right back into Hook's face, and level the scores at fifteen all.

Walking into the middle of the meeting, he handed his boss a few official-looking foolscap forms before settling down in the corner of the room on a broken chair. Sitting forward with his elbows resting on both knees, he stared across at James and winked. The forms had been concealed in his desk drawer for a couple of days, but he had waited for an opportune moment when Hook and many others were assembled. The time for retribution was here, the audience ready, and Hook's neck bared, ready for the axe.

'Copy of McCann's previous, boss' Maul said to DS Corbett.

James looked up.

'We've already got copies in the Thunderbird file' she said.

'No, no, no James. What you've got are the first three pages of Lennie's previous. I've done another check with the Yard see, and he has in fact got four pages.'

James looked confused.

'Well, it's not our fault if they didn't send them. It's an admin problem' she said, already sensing something sinister in the air.

Sadly, Hook could see it all coming, but there was very little he could do. Sitting back, he listened to Maul, and waited for the short sharp pain between the ribs.

'There's only one conviction on page four Super, but I feel it's quite significant,' said Maul staring directly across at Hook and throwing him a sickly smile.

Slowly the Detective Superintendent began to turn a lighter shade of purple, while he quietly read about Lennie McCann's last officially recorded criminal conviction.

It was Hook's worse nightmare; it was trousers down and six of the best time, not only in front of Maul and some of his own staff but also in front of one of the country's leading criminologists.

'Read it' ordered Corbett, throwing the document onto Hook's desk. He picked it up slowly.

'No, no, out loud so we can all hear it,' Corbett said. 'Doctor Twist may be interested in this.'

'Brixton Magistrates Court, 14th January 1993. Grievous Bodily Harm and ...' Hook stopped for a second, then continued. '... Gross Indecency.'

'And the MO please,' said Corbett, twitching in temper.

'The defendant entered a cubicle in public toilets in Railton Road during the hours of darkness with a known homosexual, where after committing an act of oral sex he kicked the complainant unconscious. He served 12 months in Wormwood Scrubs.'

The room was silent. Then,

'Our Mr McCann, it seems, may be batting for the other side' said Corbett still showing his front teeth.

Doctor Twist glanced down at her shoes.

A grin the size of a clown's pocket spread across Lance Maul's face.

'And to think I almost listened to you, Mr Hook,' he said. 'Get a team together Mr Maul, and lift McCann. DNA, forensics, clothing, the works. And don't waste any time on trivialities like alibis.'

Doctor Twist glanced down at her shoes again.

Within seconds of them leaving, Hook was into his first swig of JD. Drinking before ten in the morning normally made him grimace after each swallow. Hook grimaced. Eventually James spoke.

'I'm sorry bach, it's my fault. I should have doubled-checked his previous. Now you've had the blame.'

'If it's anyone's fault, it's the Records Office and I'll sort that out later,' he replied.

'Did you have any idea, it may have been Lennie?'

'He didn't do it,' he said, staring vacantly at the inch of malt whisky that lay at the bottom of his glass.

'But if those pre-cons are anything to go by, he must be a good shout.'

'He didn't do it.'

'But kicking the shit out of a homosexual after having oral sex with him cariad ...'

'He didn't do it. Take it from me.'

He was right, McCann couldn't have done it, that was a certainty. The cockney low life had the perfect alibi, the complete explanation for the first killing of Billy Saduskas. It was a defence that would have withstood the severest of Crown Court cross-examinations. He had been with Hook.

He wasn't someone who involved others in his problems. There was no way he would have compromised James by telling her about it. If the matter did come to light at a later stage she could easily be drawn into a future disciplinary and if James didn't know, she couldn't conspire to help him out.

Even he found it hard to believe what he had done, as he'd staggered towards Helen's flat that night in an alcoholic haze, stumbling along sick and nauseous during his post-trial depression. Resentful, angry, remorseful. But McCann had been laughing and that had made him furious.

The man who peddled poison to the innocent and who had been as guilty as sin at his trial was laughing, laughing loudly at the world as he almost fell out of his taxi right in front of Hook. It was an opportunity Hook just couldn't resist.

It had been roughly ten thirty on the Uxilla Embankment near the river, and he was still wearing his crown court suit; McCann had probably been the only man in the city that evening who had drunk more than him. Lurching around in the roadway as wide eyed motorists swerved wildly to avoid him, McCann couldn't possibly have murdered Saduskas; he was too drunk and had been drinking all night with his brother and other jury members

The acquitted were fully entitled to laugh. It was human nature. But that night he was laughing at the system he had just beaten, laughing at the addicts that he had created, laughing at the all the victims his evil had spawned. Hook could only think of all the individuals throughout society who worked tirelessly, paid or otherwise, who were desperately trying to repair the damage.

He'd been angry all right, but he had been angry at the right time, at the right person, in the right way and in the right place when there were only two of them. Lennie himself had thrown the first punch, and had missed by inches, as Hook had shuffled along the pavement wallowing in self-pity. The counter-punch hadn't travelled far, but had caught McCann on the jaw with sufficient power to render him unconscious. A condition that required he later took all his meals through a health-authority straw at a local hospital. Unfortunately Hook's fist had followed through and smashed against a wall in the darkness, which had caused some grazing and bleeding to his knuckles.

He had no idea whether McCann had recognised him on the dimly lit embankment, and he didn't care. The co-director of Cars International had a reputation for violent interaction with anyone that crossed his path. If anyone so much as looked at him they were in for trouble. If they didn't, it made little difference. However a small hairline fracture of the jaw was hardly suitable punishment for illegal trading in Turkish heroin, he thought.

'Listen, I've got an idea,' he said now. 'Tag along with that gormless erection Maul up to Drugs-R-Us when they pull McCann, and have a mooch around the garage, see if you can find anything interesting in their offices.'

'Up front, warrants, Inspectors Authority and all that stuff?' she replied.

'You're beginning to worry me James. You on HRT or something?'

Watching her leave the office, his eyes began to twinkle. He knew full well McCann could be exonerated by DNA and alibi cronies, but it was the thought of the procedural interaction between Maul and the innocent drug trafficker that amused him most. Both McCanns had a delicate aversion to their liberty being tampered with, and the Scrubs Lane snake-in-the-grass was going to have his hands full. It was a shame he was going to miss it all.

Panting and wheezing like a street musician's accordion, Sergeant Ivor Griffiths breezed into Hook's office, with the crutch of his trousers hanging level with his knees. The sergeant had three weeks to go before retirement; his uniform had retired some years earlier.

With breath like an ashtray full of dead cigars, and the body odour of a dog section, the red-faced sergeant collapsed in a chair, where he slowly began to recover. The custody sergeant had all the appeal of a watercress pasty. Already there were small amounts of saliva beginning to collect in the corners of his mouth. Hook hadn't missed them. Lightening up a small Dutch cigar he said,

'You're not going to believe this, but Jack Corbett's disappeared.'

CHAPTER TWELVE

Falling back heavily, Hook swivelled around in his black leather chair, an item of furniture he had stolen from the office of the Crown Prosecution Service on the ground floor. It was the only way the drug squad could get any furniture. His own broken chair remained in the corner.

'All my shift know about it downstairs. I've just mentioned it to the Chief Super,' Ivor said.

'When did all this happen?' said Hook suspiciously.

'One of my young PCs called at his home about an hour ago. Apparently he packed a suitcase last night and left. His head must have gone.'

Slowly Hook began to smile; he couldn't believe his luck. Had some sort of post-traumatic stress finally relieved him of the one man who appeared intent not only on holding his career back, but also on destroying it?

But the portly little egotistical's head was firmly fixed in place, he knew that. If his AWOL was connected to anything at Scrubs Lane, it had to be with Glenys Cadwalader in the Radio Room. Short and squat and with a few kilos of cellulite to spare, the middle-aged divorcee with bad spelling and equally bad breath had always carried a torch for the head of CID. He had observed a number of their clandestine meetings in out-of-the way country pubs when he was out meeting his informants.

But surely the CID boss hadn't thrown away his entire career on the tart with a heart? The one female civilian clerk everyone avoided at midnight on New Year's Eve?

No matter how much he prayed it was all true, something wasn't right. Surely the man would never leave his adoring public in the middle of a double murder. His desire for media attention was still insatiable, and magazines were already dubbing him Wales' Top Sleuth.

'Corbett,' began Hook, keeping a nervous eye on the mounting spittle only feet away.

'Yes, it's your mate alright,' said Ivor. 'The one that was breathalysed. He's given me a Mickey Mouse and done a runner.'

There was little time to feel disappointed about the senior officer's sudden reappearance. He was already three steps ahead of his colleague and knew exactly what was coming next. In fact he not only had the answer ready, but the look of astonishment as well. Hook was good at astonishment. He could do astonishment.

Pulling a note pad from his coat pocket and leaning over the desk to borrow Hook's biro, the sergeant said,

'What's his real name Inspector?'

With a look that epitomised an elderly spinster observing an elephant's genitalia for the first time, Hook stuttered,

'Christ, I'm sorry sarge, I don't really know! He's an old informant. I've always called him Jock. I hadn't seen him in years. What a shit!'

'All his ID was false,' he moaned, blowing smoke all over Hook.

'Tell you what Ivor,' he replied as he leapt up from his chair and snatched his jacket off the nail in the wall.

'I'll get out on the street right now, and see what I can pick up,' he said, waving as he slipped out onto the blustery iced-up fire escape into a gust that threatened to blow him away.

Hanging onto the wrought iron rail tightly and peering back in through the frozen windows guiltily, he watched his visitor leave. Stepping quickly back into his office, he threw his coat back onto the nail, and took a deep breath. Once again his thoughts returned to Brodie.

Scribbling away in his detective diary, chronicling the events of the day, he jumped as a large brown envelope landed with a thud on his desk. Goose smiled down from above him.

'Latest surveillance photos, brawd, just back from Photography' he said coughing like a colliery horse.

'Christ you sound rough. You're not going sick on me are you?' Hook asked as he tore open the envelope.

Spreading the coloured photographs over the top of his desk, he began placing them in date order when he caught sight of the photograph just beneath his chin. He could only feel embarrassment as he recognised the man that smiled brightly at him in the picture below.

'You alright, boss?' said Goose.

'Why shouldn't I be?' he snapped.

'Duw, you've gone all pale!'

Quickly, Hook checked the accompanying paperwork, but there was no doubt that all the photographs had been taken two days previously. Taken in fact the day before he had met up again with his old pal Joe Brodie. Lennie, his old sparring partner, and his brother Mickey were in the prints all right, but what the hell was the customs man doing shaking their hands? Only twenty four hours earlier the lying Scots bastard had denied knowing them, and here he was at the side of the building days earlier, shaking their greasy palms like an old friend. How the bloody hell could he have been so stupid in trusting a man he hadn't seen for years, particularly when he was employed by an organisation who had more strokes than the British Olympic coxless fours?

His immediate gut feeling told him that the McCanns were also part of some Customs operation and Brodie was still undercover. That's why he had denied knowing them. The sly old devil he thought. However, it was something he could perhaps use to his advantage. He now knew something that Customs didn't. They had no idea Hook was on to them.

'You seen a ghost or something?' said Goose.

'No, no. Just thought I recognised someone, that's all,' he said as he pushed the photograph away,

Many other friends also popped up amongst the collage spread out before them. The Ginger Beast could also be seen calling into their sales office for a cup of tea, while Detective Inspector Lance Maul was caught on camera yet again, arranging for some repairs to be carried out to his precious Vauxhall Omega.

Moving around to join Hook behind the desk, Goose leant over his shoulder and began tapping the photo of a tall elegant; bald-headed man, who wore an expensive white Yves St Laurent mac and black Gucci shoes. He could be seen clearly inside the offices of Cars International, engaged in animated conversation with Lennie McCann. Parked in a nearby side street was his black BMW bearing Dutch plates.

'Henk Leiberman. Fifty. Dutch National. Wanted in Marseilles for drug trafficking,' said Goose.

'Rings a bell,' said Hook, picking it up off the desk before releasing his first smile of the day.

'Thought you might like it,' said Goose. 'I've sent a fax to Interpol for all his details.'

'Interpol don't get back from their Christmas vacation until March' said Hook, rummaging frantically in the top drawer of his desk amongst a disorganised filing system in search of an address. Offering Goose a dusty old polo mint, he said,

'What was the name of that drunken French DI who came over two years ago, chasing that big importation? Remember, he had breath like an African Lion.'

'Sanmartin. From Montpellier, wasn't it?'

Shaking his head, unconvinced, and with a mountain of rubbish and unfiled paperwork on his lap, Hook finally recovered an out-of-date international rugby ticket from the bottom of the now empty drawer. Reading out loud the barely legible scrawl on the back, he said in a dreadful Inspector Clouseau impersonation,

'Haha Cato, Henri Sanmartin of the... Marseilles Drug Investigation Unit.'

'Stick to your day job boss!' said Goose, sitting down.

Watching his boss begin to dial the international number, Goose said,

'Is this a wise move boss, by-passing Interpol? By-passing Corbett? What about the old protocol? Can you trust this frog?'

'Goose my dear friend,' he said. 'How can you trust a man whose country cordially offer us two hundred and sixty five different types of cheese then proceed to kick the living daylights out of us whenever we compete with them at sport?'

He turned his attention to the phone.

'Bonjour Madame, je m'appelle Inspector Hook, agent de police, Pays de Galles, Je voudrai parlez Inspector Henri Sanmartin, si'il vous plait... merci,' he said, impressing Goose with his O level French.

Goose pulled up a chair and sat down alongside him, watching while he sketched Maul's face on the body of a devil on the desk blotter. Sitting patiently, he listened until Hook eventually replaced the receiver.

'They've got half of France looking for Leiberman. Apparently he tried to bring a yacht full of gear into the local harbour about a week ago, but French Customs lost him in the Med. The douane haven't been to bed since.'

Goose could see that Hook's mind was racing on ahead while he stared down vacantly into the yard below. There were even bigger problems on the horizon; he could just sense it.

'How's that?' he said.

'They later discovered a dockside warehouse just up the coast in Montpellier where they think the drugs had been stashed. They found a murdered Algerian inside. Same MO. He'd been slaughtered. I've no idea what slicing open the femoral is in French,' Hook said.

'Christ, is this what Tony Blair meant by European Community interaction?' replied Goose.

Reaching for two cracked mugs and a whisky bottle, Hook said,

'They initially believed there were a thousand kilos of cocaine on board. They now think it could be even more.'

'Bloody hell, we haven't got enough noses in Wales for that lot to go up,' said Goose, holding out his mug hopefully.

'I said they believed. They've done more forensic tests at the warehouse. It's not cocaine,' said Hook, 'I only wish it was.'

Whirling around in his chair, he stopped and poured his colleague a small measure. There was something else on the radar screen, and Goose knew instantly what it was.

'Jesus of Nazareth! It's Babylon, isn't it?' he said. 'Is it coming this way?'

'Your guess is as good as mine. Listen - get an All Ports circulation out on Leiberman. See if we can pick him up before he returns to the continent.'

On his way up to his office the following morning, Hook could hear shouting and arguing in the ground floor interview room. He caught sight of Larry Mulholland and Jack Corbett - the real Jack Corbett - still in their overcoats, collars turned up like two KGB agents, listening with their ears pressed against the badly-fitting sapele door. Spotting Hook's arrival, Mulholland touched his lips with a finger and winked.

Lennie McCann's voice was unmistakable inside the interview room, as he issued some forthright instructions to a member of his legal team.

'Perhaps you haven't noticed, but I've been arrested on suspicion of murder, and it's a load of old bollocks. Now get out there and wiggle your arse and sort out my fucking bail. You're being paid good, good money.'

The three of them stepped back sharply as the door flew open and Helen Wainwright stepped out with a catwalk aplomb. Corbett quickly adjusted his tie while, surprisingly, Mulholland began smoothing down the back of his grey hair. Helen Wainwright had this effect on men.

'Toffee nosed bitch!' screamed McCann as she quietly pulled the door behind her.

Stern-faced, she turned to Mulholland, while Corbett began to assist her with her Dolce & Gabbana black leather coat. He draped it gently over her shoulders.

'I'm afraid we have a conflict of interests here, Superintendent. I absolutely loathe Mr McCann and the feeling is obviously mutual. I'll arrange for someone else from Chambers to represent him. What I can say is that my client appears to be well alibied for both murders, as indeed is his brother. Furthermore, he was badly assaulted on the night of the Saduskas murder on the Uxilla Embankment near the Blue Parrot Club on his way home. Spent the night in hospital, it seems.'

Mulholland's eyes flicked suspiciously towards Hook, who was concealing his bandaged hand inside his jacket pocket. The Scrubs Lane commander hadn't been a top class detective without forming life-long contacts in the criminal underworld, and he knew only too well that his Drug Squad Inspector was never far away from the action. What's more, Hook knew he knew.

'You can bloody well still try and nail him' whispered Helen, who unnoticed pinched Hook's bum as she squeezed past.

Expensive French perfume filled the air as the two mesmerised superintendents watched the elegant barrister head off up the corridor on her way back to chambers. Corbett himself was already lying on a sun-kissed beach in Bali with the attractive limb of the law, drinking pina coladas out of empty coconut shells, while all Larry Mulholland could think of was his wife's curlers and a face embalmed in thick white cream. The lady of the long black robe, whose legs went on forever, was an ageing superintendent's wet dream.

'Nice girl' said Corbett, who was still a thousand miles away in the Indian Ocean.

'Very, very nice girl,' added Hook.

New Year's Eve celebrations were already well underway as Hook wandered about his untidy office in stockinged feet. Gripping the neck of a bottle that hung loosely down by his side, he gazed out over the Docklands through the broken half-closed blinds. The small desk-lamp gave him barely enough light to read, let alone to see the near empty bottle of Jack Daniels he drank from. Although he had kicked the single radiator half a dozen times, it still hadn't come on, while the single bar electric fire in the far corner of his room was about as much use as a French lorry driver in a Calais traffic jam.

Another year was almost over. Another millennium in fact. But nothing had changed for the people of the Docklands over the past decades. Deprivation and unemployment continued to grow like a cancer, while crime was still spiralling out of control. Contrary to what government ministers were saying, the war against drugs had been lost long ago, back when Tony Blair was still reading Peter and Jane books.

Okay, there were still daily battles to be fought, but they were simply papering over the cracks. A takeaway pizza was still likely to appear at your door quicker than a uniformed constable, while his whole squad was sprinting flat-out just to stand still.

Everyone was bobbing about, rudderless, in a sea of apathy. But within a few weeks, Corbett's end-of-year crime report, a neatly typed, cleverly worded document, would kiss and make it all better. A file of massaged, altered and inaccurate statistics on drugs and crime that would indicate, impressively, to his chief constable and then to the Home Office that the Docklands district simply didn't have a problem.

Through the blinds he could see in the distant blackness the tiny headlights that travelled along the solitary road leading from the city into the Docklands community. A long sad concrete artery that led to the end of everywhere.

The general office next door was empty, and he seemed to be making little headway with all the paperwork James had seized from Cars International. Adjusting the desk light, he yawned and rubbed his eyes. Sitting with both hands propping up his face, he looked like a Chinese waiter as his eyes almost disappeared into narrow slits. Nothing was registering with him now. No matter how much he stared at the mountain of paperwork, his brain had called it a day. The offices were cold and depressing, and he was already late for dinner at Helen's. Even James had gone. December 31st had a particular attraction for the majority of people, but Hook was in no mood to celebrate. It had been a bad year. Helen's mum was still in intensive care, and as a result they had both decided to shut out the world for a few hours. Settling for a cosy night at the flat seemed a more sensible way to welcome in the New Year. The new Millennium.

So preoccupied had he been with the mass of international fax messages in front of him that he hadn't heard his office door open, but he soon became aware of the large man standing in the darkness, whose shadow swarmed all over him.

'Christ, you gave me a fright sneaking about like that!'

Placing a large leather briefcase next to Hook's desk, Mulholland slumped down heavily on a chair opposite him. His skin tone showed he was drained and exhausted.

'Can I buy you a quick drink at the end of the street before my son comes to pick me up?'

'No thanks sir' he said, suddenly feeling revitalised at the appearance of some company, someone with whom he could share his thoughts. A meeting of minds.

'I think that Oscar Wilde bloke was probably right. Work is the scourge of the drinking classes,' said Mulholland, sounding a touch disappointed.

'And how is Doctor Mulholland? Busy in Casualty tonight?'

'Yep. Just a few more shifts and then he's off up to Guy's.'

'You must be very proud, having a - what, a surgeon? - in the family?'

'Simon's a good lad Hook. Drinks too much, but he's a good lad.'

Sitting facing the Chief Superintendent, he placed his foot on the bottle of Jack Daniels that lay at his feet under the desk and quietly rolled it back under his seat.

'Any joy?' Mulholland went on, indicating the piles of papers strewn over the desk, while beginning to look suspiciously at the impressive leather chair that his Inspector now occupied. He'd seen it somewhere before in the station. But couldn't think where.

'These faxes we've seized from Cars International, something's not right. I know something's wrong. I'm staring it right in the face, but my mind's gone home,' Hook said, tapping the pile of fax messages with his fingers.

Pushing his chair around the desk, Mulholland sat alongside him and started to scrutinise some of the paperwork himself.

'Bloody Nora, what the hell is that smell!' he said.

'The toilets next door are blocked again' Hook said, grabbing a can of Summer Haze from the window ledge. A few seconds later the offending odour had been camouflaged by a few well-aimed squirts. Minutes later it slipped back in silently through the open door and rejoined them.

'It says here that the McCanns import half a dozen cars every two months or so from Malaga,' he said, resting his chin in the palm of his hand.

'There's a lot of firms doing it,' replied Mulholland. 'High mileage continental fleet cars.'

'Maybe, maybe, but every delivery seems to be accompanied by 50 gallons of petrol,' he said, pushing the fax message towards his boss.

Rummaging in his blue Crombie overcoat for his reading glasses, the Commander slipped them on.

'They probably get it cheap to re-sell over here.'

'They don't sell petrol. They're not a filling station. But – wait!' Hook shouted, knocking over Mulholland's brief case as he rose to his feet.

'Hang on, hang on, I think I've twigged it!'

The Chief Super snatched at his tie and loosened it, awaiting Hook's discovery, whatever it was. Waving the fax above his head, Hook paced around the office. Finally he stopped in the middle of the floor.

'Now, we know the brothers are expecting a big bag in any day now, and my man tells me it's normally fifty kees. This isn't petrol, it's cocaine, this is just a bloody code!' Getting more and more animated, he went on,

'This, Chief Superintendent, is fifty kilos of Cocainehydrochloride.'

'Where do these faxes originate from?' said Mulholland, sliding towards the edge of his seat, as the dark shadow on the wall continued to pace up and down the room.

'A chap called Leiberman from Holland, a known trafficker. They come in from his yacht out in the Med somewhere. I've got him belling the McCanns on the phone last year, during Operation Thunderbird, but we could never get our hands on him. At the moment …'

He stopped in mid-sentence as his fingers began feverishly flicking back through all the faxes he had already studied.

'What's the matter Hook, what is it?'

Finally he found it, and at first, just stared numbly while his aching eyes began to water with fatigue. After some heavy duty squinting he silently began reading it over and over again just to be sure. Slumping back in his chair he began to read it out loud.

'With reference to our previous fax relating to the four Fiat saloon motor cars shortly due to be

dispatched to the United Kingdom. I can now confirm that the 1,000 gallons of petrol that were due to accompany the vehicles will not now be transported as discussed but will be sent via the usual route'.

'Cocaine' said Mulholland, a nervous edge to his voice.

Staring silently at the fax in his hand, Hook's eyes began to widen.

'Hook?'

'I'm sorry Super,' he replied, lifting both hands in an additional apology. 'No, my bet it's the first batch of that new designer drug from the States, and it's bobbing about on the high seas right now, probably heading for the UK.'

'You sure about this?'

'Yeah. Sure as I can be. My bet is that they couldn't run it into Marseilles, so Leiberman and the McCanns are going to flood the market here. This fax was sent three days ago,' he said, pushing the piece of paper across the desk.

'What's their usual route?'

'Come on Super, give me easy ones.'

'This is all very well,' Mulholland said, trying to choose the correct words that wouldn't deflate an inspector who had never quite understood the true meaning of Off Duty.

'But will it take us any nearer to our killer? I mean, these are still murders you're working on.'

'Like I said in your office Super, our man is in this conspiracy somewhere. Whether he's in a different syndicate, been double-crossed or just trying to take over the McCann Empire I don't know. You'll just have to trust me. I just know this is all connected somehow.'

'Scrubs Lane need to detect these murders, Hook. I don't want outside squads taking over from my men if we are seen to be failing, you understand?'

'I can handle this, boss,' he said, a little more forcibly.

'But can you handle this Babylon stuff?' Mulholland said, still scrutinising the fax beneath Hook's desk light.

'Well, if I can't, this city isn't going to have enough mortuaries to cope with it all.'

Wrinkled concern showed on Mulholland's face as he began to digest the seriousness of the information. Hook could see him begin to study the contents of the transcript even more closely, underneath the desk light.

'We definitely haven't got enough mortuaries, Hook,' he said suddenly.

Turning slowly towards his inspector, he repeated,

'We haven't got enough.' He seemed to be slurring his words nervously.

'Chief?'

'You've missed a nought' Mulholland said, before slipping off his glasses and rubbing his tired eyes.

'You've missed a fucking nought.'

It was the first time Hook had heard him use the F word. Snatching at the paper he read it again, this time underneath the light on the desk. Staring wildly he counted once more. His Chief was right. Although somewhat unclear and difficult to decipher, there were four noughts in the message, not three. Adjusting his eyes, he peered again but there it was, an extra nought, and it wasn't going away.

'Christ! 10,000 kilos' said Mulholland in almost a whisper. 'It can't be.'

'Almost 10 ton,' Hook said. 'The country is going to be swamped.'

'I want you to verify everything, ASAP. You and I need to get together.' Mulholland picked up his briefcase as if it weighed a ton. 'And I want you to keep all this to yourself for the moment.'

Hook nodded.

'Listen, I can't see me being able to hold this,' Mulholland said. 'I've got to call in the National Crime Squad. It's all getting out of hand.'

Unable to disguise his disappointment, Hook said,

'Wait Super. Just give me and the boys here one chance. Please. Perhaps the text has a typing error, perhaps it's only 1,000 kilos after all.'

Hook's persuasive attempt had all its normal conviction, yet he knew that it would take more than clenched fists and distorted features to convince his boss.

'The quantity has no real relevance to what we're already doing, other than it brings more pressure to the likes of you and me' he said. 'Nobody knows about this message, only the two of us. We'll find it, sir.'

'The National Crime Squad will bring more men, Hook.'

'But not necessarily more expertise.'

The commander said nothing, but rose and left the office without so much as a seasonal greeting. Hook's mind was all over the place as he listened to the slow padding footsteps of his senior officer making their way along the unlit corridor outside. A few floorboards squeaked, and then he was gone.

With a deadly drug consignment that was about to make the history books, and a serial killer attempting to do the same, how the fuck could the man say Happy New Year, he thought.

Folding the telex message neatly into four quarters, he pressed the creases carefully with his cold fingertips before dropping it into the drawer at the bottom of his desk. Covering it with some old newspapers he pushed the drawer closed with his foot.

The sound of a car pulling up outside had him looking down into station yard. Lazily the automatic gates began to squeak open, before a small dark Mini saloon with full headlights blaring drove in and stopped by the rear doors. Larry Mulholland made his way across the yard, leaving behind fresh footprints in the newly fallen snow. Looking up towards Hook's window on the top floor he waved wearily before jumping into the passenger seat. Hook nodded back.

With a box of Helen's favourite Belgian chocolates under his arm, and another problem to fuel his insomnia, he began to button up his reefer jacket and head for the door, when the phone rang.

'DI Hook' he said, yawning loudly while glancing anxiously at his office clock above the door. The loud music and noise in the background had to be a pub or club, but the voice was unmistakable even though it was being whispered.

'Junction twenty five, first left off the first roundabout and carry on for eight miles 'til you come to that little village just before Tarw Wen Colliery. On the right hand side. We met there in the summer. Remember?'

'Okay. But - Christ, are you sure you want to meet tonight?'

'I think I know who your bent cop is' the voice said, before the line went dead.

Hook's spine began to tingle with that feeling, that vibrating sensation that started in the lower back before gently moving slowly up the spine, and out across each shoulder. The same prickly quiver he'd got when he had first clapped eyes on Helen.

Rushing out of the door, he stopped suddenly before returning to extinguish his little desk light. Racing out through the building, past nodding colleagues and inebriated revellers whose liberty had been temporarily removed for the night, he dashed out into the cold night air. He brushed a layer of snow off the windscreen of his Sunbeam Talbot before leaping into the driver's seat. At the fifth attempt the engine fired loudly, before he drove out through the station gates and onto the dual carriageway. In the darkness, on the corner of an untidy desk on the top floor back at Scrubs Lane, a box of expensive confectionery lay, forgotten.

New Year's Eve revelries were in full swing as he drove through the centre of the city and up towards the dark valleys. But tiredness could be unkind, and he didn't notice the little Mini saloon that had begun to follow him, tracking his every move. During the journey, even James came under suspicion, as did every one of his young hand-picked men. Discovering the identity of the traitor tonight was one thing, obtaining the necessary evidence to rid the force of someone lower than shark's excrement was another. There was no doubt that these rumours were gaining momentum and something had to be done if the reputation of his squad was to remain intact. Whoever the bastard was, he had to be caught quickly. Yawning loudly he shook his head and blinked rapidly to rid himself of fatigue. It didn't work and he yawned again.

Almost forty minutes later and accompanied by Bryan Ferry and Hard Rain, he pulled into the once thriving mining community of Tarw Wen. A run-down district where Thatcherism had not only removed the pit head baths and winding gear, but also the very heart of the little valley village. It was quiet for New Year's Eve, all the grey stone terraced miners' cottages were dark and silent. No-one ever went up to Tarw for a good night out.

Anxiety and Hook had never been sparring partners, yet as he drove at a snail's pace over the thin layer of snow, he found himself pulling sharply into a deserted layby, his car skidding to an abrupt halt. Two hundred yards in the distance on the opposite side of the road, under a damaged streetlight, he recognised the disused roofless gents' public urinal where they had arranged to meet. A rusty padlocked iron gate prevented entry, but part of a wall at the back had been vandalised, and this afforded easy entry. They had used this old red brick building once before. It was quiet and well away from the city, ideal for clandestine meetings between detective inspectors and informants who may have had prostrate problems.

He turned off the car's engine, but with the Roxy Music cassette draining the battery as it pumped out Virginia Plain, he opted to lose the heating. Within minutes the temperature inside began to drop, causing his breath to form pale orange clouds as they soaked up the brightness from the sodium street lights.

Perhaps it was the stillness that had begun to worry him, or the continued belief that one day someone would finally double-cross him. Festive season it may have been, but he wasn't on everyone's Christmas card list. Individuals would pay good money to get him out of their hair, to have him compromised, or have him subjected to some back alley beating that would remove his confidence or something worse.

But if someone wanted to realign his knee joints, a dilapidated piss house on the edge of a tiny village seemed an ideal location, and to make matters worse nobody knew he was there. His own car had no police radio and he had left his mobile phone back on his office desk alongside Helen's chocolates. On the odd occasion, Hook's enthusiasm could cloud his otherwise sound judgement. Tonight was one of those occasions.

Pulling a black woollen hat from his pocket, he slipped it on, tugging it down to within an inch of his exhausted eyes, Sitting like a council estate ram-raider on glue, he did not move, but stared impassively at the ramshackle urinal up ahead. For some strange reason he was feeling uncomfortable and he was conscious that his heart rate had moved up a gear.

When in doubt always pull out was a philosophy of his. He'd preached about it often enough in the office. Perhaps it was just the meeting place that was beginning to spook him, his informant little Billy Saduskas had been carved open in similar surroundings. Maybe it was just the God forbidden time, or even the tranquillity of the place that was giving him that unusual edginess. They were all good bets, but Hook's mind was on the ten ton of white powder that would need the protection of street soldiers and firearms. The McCanns already knew he had their fax messages, but did they know he may have worked it all out?

The ball game was changing. Fumbling with the ignition keys he tried to start the engine, when the passenger door was flung open and the interior light suddenly bathed the car in brightness.

CHAPTER THIRTEEN

The huge face was blue and cold, but the eyes were red and angry. Collapsing into the passenger seat alongside Hook, he growled,

'What the hell's going on? Where you off to? I've been waiting and watching you for fifteen minutes. I said over there,' he shouted, his huge pudding fingers pointing towards the toilet.

Hook's mouth opened but nothing came out.

Frank Maggart's jaw hardened. He was furious, Hook could tell. They had always conducted this part of their relationship in a totally professional manner, and nothing was left to chance. That was one of the reasons why their partnership and strong bond had survived the test of time.

'You've been jerking about in your seat like a boy racer waiting for a Panda car!' Maggart stopped. 'You okay? Because you look bloody awful,' he said.

Shaking his head, smiling feebly, his mind hijacked by fatigued, Hook tried desperately to choose the right words, words that would explain his dilemma. But he failed. Everything went blank, and his only words were stammered.

'You know the score! We never meet in cars! Christ, if I'm seen, I'm history,' Maggart shouted. 'These are multi-million pound organisations we're talking about here. I'm under a motorway for ten grand!'

Extending his hand in an apologetic gesture, Hook remained silent, composing himself, waiting for his friend to calm down. It was a gesture Maggart ignored.

If Hook had a degree in human behaviour and perception, The Beast had a masters. Hook had been unable to conceal his anxiety, with frequent glances out of every window in the car. Maggart watched his friend's uneasy face before glancing again towards the derelict toilets. He could see that the eyes alongside him were pleading guilty, and contact was becoming difficult, and he sensed something wasn't right. There was an odd tenseness about the meeting, and Hook's body language was all over the place.

It would have been futile for Hook to try and lie. Their whole relationship would have ended there and then. Desperately he wanted to explain, but his mouth felt as though it was crammed with pink seaside nougat.

'Look, I …'

'You bastard, you bastard!' shouted Maggart, feeling for the door handle behind his back, his eyes blazing with resentment.

'It's not what you think Frank. Listen, I'm knackered, that's all. I …'

'You bastard, I know why you're sitting up here vegetating on your fucking arse. You thought this was a set-up, you thought that someone who had known you all your life had thrown you to the wolves for a few pieces of silver.'

'Frank, will you just stop for a minute and give me a chance?' pleaded Hook, grabbing his arm in a futile attempt to stop nineteen stone of pure anger from getting out of the car.

Vainly Hook tried to appear relaxed, but the smile was thin and tight, and Frank Maggart was no mug. He felt sure he was going to throw a punch, but the big man simply pushed him off.

'The slate's wiped clean. I owe you nothing.' he said, violently booting the bottom of the stiff passenger door so he could get out.

'You and that bent cop deserve each other, and don't ask me who he is,' he said as the door almost came off its hinges.

Hook could feel things crumbling around him. He was worn out and hadn't had a day off for weeks. Slumping back in his seat he watched as his friend jogged back along the deserted pavement. He heard the sound of a diesel engine start up somewhere in the distance and listened as it became fainter and disappeared. His chin fell onto his chest. Softly he began to mutter every expletive he'd collected since his youth, until finally the list expired. He had to double up on a few. How could he have been so stupid?

When the engine didn't turn over for the tenth time, but simply grunted and apologised, he knew he was in trouble. The snow-covered highway was desolate, and there could have been one of twenty things wrong with the car. There wouldn't be many taxis available in the city on Hogmanay, let alone in a forgotten backwater like Tarw Wen. Scrubs Lane would be having their busiest night of the year, so a lift would be out of the question, and the nearest telephone kiosk was over three miles away.

And finally there was Helen He'd almost forgotten about her, sitting patiently fifteen miles away. Waiting for him to arrive at her flat to see in the New Year together.

His watch showed 11.50 as he set off for the telephone kiosk.

'Come on, asshole, you can still make it' he said out loud, before jogging along precariously on packed snow. The new marina was some distance away, mild depression was a little closer. With excuses at the ready, he stepped gingerly into the darkened hallway, after waving thankfully to the van driver who had stopped and given him a lift. Carefully, he pulled his key from the lock before tip-toeing his way inside. The new year was now two hours old as he switched on the kitchen light and poured himself a treble whisky. A second treble, downed in one, almost scarified his stomach.

Helen's bedroom door was tightly shut, which tended to suggest that the only thing he'd be embracing that night would be one of the five large cushions on her shabby-chic sofa. There wasn't a Do Not Disturb sign on her door, but there might as well have been.

He'd seen the note when he'd first gone into the kitchen, but there was no rush, he had heard it all before. Why didn't you phone? What if I needed to get hold of you? You care more about those bloody drug dealers and your little narks than you do about me. If he'd only realised that his list of previous convictions for letting her down were now reaching double figures, he may have seen it all coming.

It was the coldness in the flat that made him suddenly snatch at the folded piece of paper left on the work surface. The flat's central heating system had been switched off. It was the middle of winter, and that was strange.

Although the writing paper was expensive, and Helen's writing clear and elegant, the message was simple and curt.

'Mum died at 10.45 tonight. Nobody knew where you were. I needed you so badly. But it's the same old story. I'm at St Stephens Hospital. Please don't follow because it's all over between us. We've been treading water for some time and I think it's better this way. Please leave the key I gave you, and close the front door behind you when you leave.'

She hadn't signed her letter, but the tears that had run from the top edge of the paper down to the bottom, smudging a little of her pain, were enough.

It was twenty four hours before Hook turned up in work again, unshaven and shabby, looking like he'd spent his time sleeping with a bottle under a motorway bridge. James watched him slip into his office before closing the door. Ignoring him, she carried on as if nothing had happened.

The office was empty. Twisting around in his chair, he stared at his pathetic little room, but he was still tired. He was tired all the time these days. He still wanted to lie down, catnap, anything that would allow him to close both eyes for a moment. He found himself glaring at things for no reason, staring deeply at the telephone on his desk, the office calendar or the crime files on the radiator, yet he saw nothing, and had little idea of how long he had been sitting there staring. Suddenly he kicked open the fire escape door but again had no idea why. He glanced down the iron escape route that he always used to bypass the bosses. Someone down below waved, but he quickly stepped back inside.

All night he'd dreamt of long corridors with numerous doors, not knowing which one to go through, although he knew one was the door to destruction At daybreak he'd felt his eyes had been open throughout the night, but was grateful they had opened at all.

It was midday before James knocked on his door and went inside. Hook woke up with a start. In anger she threw a white covered book which bounced on the desk before hitting his chest.

'Designer Pharmacology by Professor Baxter of the University of California,' she snapped. 'Stobart traced it to one of the local libraries. It's a book Harvey borrowed once a few weeks ago.'

Quickly he flicked through the pages until he reached the pages mentioned in Harvey's diary. Silently he began to read.

'There's a paragraph here about Babylon' he said, with very little excitement in his voice. 'It's about designer drugs and how they were developed on the West Coast. Looks like Harvey was preparing the ground for the firm's new product. Searching around for info on it. It's even got some sort of formula in here. My guess is that they intended to set up a factory over here, manufacture it themselves. We know Harvey was a chemist.'

Sitting back, she said nothing, but simply watched him, waiting for an explanation.

'Aren't you going to ask me where I've been?' he said woodenly, snapping the book shut.

Kicking his office door so violently that it almost came off its hinges, she leant over his desk towards him, her knuckles white with temper. For the past twenty four hours she had lied through her back teeth to protect him, and now here he was, playing silly schoolboy games, and looking like some down-and-out from Cardboard City. She had never seen him like this before and it hurt.

'It doesn't bother me where you've been boss, it's none of my business' she said. 'But here we are in the middle of a murder enquiry that's putting pressure on everyone, and you decide to go walkabout, leaving me to run the show. Everyone's been chasing you, and I'm sick of lying. Why didn't you answer your mobile? I told Mulholland that you were at a drug seminar up north.'

'I'm sorry' he said. 'It's been a bad year. I just needed some space.'

'The way you're behaving, you're going down the pan, but you're not taking me or this squad with you, do you understand, bach? Corbett's been screaming for you, and it's not my job to circle the wagons.'

Walking over to the window she gazed for a moment through the broken blinds at the backdrop of urban decay that surrounded the station. Taking a deep breath she began to calm down. Sitting on the edge of his desk she said,

'I know this place is the pits, and we're suffocating in a sea of paperwork. I know the McCann trial was hard to take. Christ, the system is letting us down all the time, but we don't give up. you've always preached that to the guys.'

'Helen's mother died on New Years' Eve, he said, rubbing the sleep out of both eyes. 'I should have been with her, having dinner. I let them both down'

'Yes, I know. I made some discreet enquiries over at her chambers and they told me about her mum. I was worried about you, for Christ's sake!'

'But I had more important matters to deal with you see' he went on. 'Detective Inspector bloody Hook went off to see an informant. Just when she needed me.'

'These things happen in our job. God, you should know that by now.'

Leaning over the desktop towards her, sadness engraved on his face, stale whisky accompanied every single excuse. Most of the squad were out on enquiries but some were due back shortly. She had to get him back on track. Trilby James was a Detective and a bloody good one, but she was no social worker or counsellor, and if he was looking for a cup of tea and a Welsh cake, a shoulder to cry on, she wasn't it'

'Nobody forced you to become a policeman,' she said. 'Nobody forced you to become a detective, working twelve hours a day.' There was a hard edge to her voice now, and determination in her blue eyes.

'What's more you're not the first man in this squad to cock things up by putting the job first.'

Slowly he began to look up. He didn't like what he was hearing, but she was right, and it bloody hurt.

'We all know the flack you take for the squad. How you're fighting the bastards out there, and the likes of Corbett in here. So if you're going through hell, for Christ's sake hurry up and come out the other side,' she said. 'Most of the guys joined this squad because of you. You're the only boss we've known who lights the blue touch paper and doesn't retire.'

Jumping off the desk, she said, 'Wait here a sec, boss' as she dashed out into the main office,

He listened to the banging and closing of desk drawers. She returned within minutes, with a bowl of hot water, towel, shaving equipment and a sparkling clean white T-shirt. Everything scrounged from unlocked desks in the general office.

'People have been dumping their problems on you for years. It's not pain you're suffering, cariad, it's nostalgia' she said, tossing him some soap and pulling off his shirt.

Fifteen minutes later Hook emerged into the main office as three frozen surveillance men trooped by, groaning about the freezing conditions behind Cars International. It had been a long cold shift.

'If you have a problem gentlemen, there's three spare panda cars downstairs with three shiny helmets to go with them. Now in my office right away and give me an update.'

Straightening up, they quickly walked into his office. Turning towards James on the phone at the far end of the room he shouted,

'I want an office conference for everyone at four this afternoon. Get it organised.'

James smiled quietly to herself. It was kick-arse time again at Scrubs Lane and Hook was back on the rails.

'By the way' she called back, 'Goose has booked sick.'

The green military night-intensifying binoculars scanned the horizon in the darkness, as the low throbbing sound of the marine diesel engine on the Dutch fishing boat echoed over the water. Carefully it negotiated the deserted entrance to the little west Wales cove, and headed towards some lights on the nearby shore. Only the occasional sound of screaming gulls overhead, and the pounding white surf which seemed to illuminate the whole of the bay, accompanied the two heavily-laden inflatables as they burst through the waves towards the voices in the distance.

Inside a Shogun Landrover two miles away on the cliff top, Mickey McCann dropped the binoculars onto his lap before turning to his brother in the front passenger seat.

'The Eagle has landed' he said, rubbing both hands together. They looked around at the well-dressed man seated in the rear, who seemed unimpressed.

'I think a drink is in order back at your hotel, Mr Leiberman' suggested Lennie, shaking his hand.

'Thank you but no. Tomorrow, gentlemen, I am up early to explore your historical city,' he said. 'Please have your man pick me up outside my hotel at ten.

Down in the cove, countless canvassed packages were already being thrown into the rear of a four-wheel-drive Landover amid whispering voices, while the inflatables swept back out to sea for yet more cargo. Within two hours the Dutch vessel disappeared back into the pitch-black channel on its journey back to the Hook of Holland. Everything had gone to plan, and not a customs officer in sight

In the distance, a grey stone Norman church with its overgrown graveyard gazed down at the lonely whitewashed cottage next door. Below the slate roof, bright yellow kitchen lights burned brightly in expectation as they waited for the whispering voices to arrive. Thirty miles away, Hook slept peacefully in his bed.

Early the following morning and wearing a dark blue Crombie overcoat and black silk tie, Hook stood alone outside the black rusting cemetery gates a short distance from the cortege, and watched sadly as Evelyn Wainwright was lowered slowly into the hard frosty earth. A few minutes earlier he had made efforts to speak to Helen inside the tiny church, but had been waved away by an elderly aunt. It just wasn't the time or place, but he began to seriously doubt if there ever would be. By the time the simple graveside service began to break up, he had already left. Helen, he knew, had already suffered enough pain.

Sitting underneath a striped canopy outside an Italian coffee shop in a city back street, alone with his thoughts, his concentration was fractured by the squeaking wheels of a rusting mountain bike. He watched as it wobbled its way along the pedestrianised walkway towards the inviting aroma of freshly ground coffee. Leaning it against a shop window, which caused a group of pigeons to scatter to the heavens, Joe Brodie walked quickly across the cobbles and joined him.

'Christ, you're taking this drink driving thing seriously' Hook said with very little affection in his voice. 'Thanks for coming,' he added as they shook hands.

'All I've got at the moment are rumours' Brodie said, ordering a cappuccino.

'They'll do' he snapped, trying to keep his emotions in check as the lying Scots bastard sat opposite.

'You okay?' said Brodie.

'Sorry. Just come from a funeral. And I'm having a lot of grief at work.'

'You're going to have a lot more grief when I tell you what the rumours are.'

Hook ran a finger around the inside of his shirt collar before loosening his black tie.

'I doubt it' he said.

'I haven't got a name, but one of your lads is on the take. The talk is spreading like wildfire around the city clubs at the moment.'

'We've had this hearsay gossip around for years, Joe' he said, unimpressed.

'Well, the talk is he was working for the defence in that last big drugs trial. Gave a lot of inside information. That's why it went down the pan.'

'You mean the McCann trial?'

'I don't know. Is that who were on trial?'

'Have you come across the McCanns yet?' he asked, fixing Brodie with a stare. Searching deep for that extra blink or that uncomfortable movement that would give him away. That lack of eye contact or the short clipped sentence that made it easier to lie. He knew he'd already asked him once, but it continued to nag away in his mind, he needed to hear him lie again.

'No, I can't say I have.' Joe Brodie lied like an alcoholic.

If Hook hadn't seen those surveillance photographs of him shaking hands with the brothers, he would have believed him without question. Customs and Excise must run courses and seminars for lying bastards, he thought.

'D'you want me to run their names through our CEDRIC computer, see if any of our lads has anything on them?' he suggested, taking a sip of his frothy cappuccino which left him with a neat white Zapata moustache.

'Thanks, but it's not a problem.'

'Got anything concrete on them?' inquired Brodie, in that matter of fact sort of way, as though he was asking if there was going to be rain later on.

'The McCanns? I don't think they're at it at the moment. Talk is they've put all their money into massage parlours.' Hook could play this game too. 'Tell me, any Customs boys come across this Babylon stuff that's flooding the States?'

'Not yet, but I know our hierarchy have had high powered meetings with the government over it. How many deaths have they had in the States? They tell me it makes crack look like Nesquik' he said.

'You've moved digs, I'm told. Old ones not to your liking?'

'I was upstairs when they called; had a warrant for me for not turning up in court. My old landlady covered for me bless her heart.'

'And now?'

'Sleeping rough in my firm's office at the far end of the docks, till things quieten down. Listen, I anticipate the Colombian job will be coming to a head some time during the next two weeks. I'll be returning to London if we take this team out. You coming up for a weekend?'

Hook smiled and nodded.

'I don't know if this info's sound, but the bloke on the pier who was murdered, did he have a stash, Hook?'

'Harvey? I would have thought so, but we never found one.'

'His house?'

'Negative.'

'Drinking last night in the Docks Hotel, a contact tells me he used to keep it in the old biddy's house next door.'

'Go on.'

'Apparently he'd go up into his loft and remove a loose breeze block in the adjoining attic wall, hide the stuff in next door's attic. Replace the blocks and re-cement it, loosely. Throws some dust over the joint and it's tucked away in next door. Ingenious.'

'She over ninety and bedridden?'

'Exactly.'

'Nice one, Joe,' Hook said grabbing Brodie's hand and shaking it.

Later that morning a collection of Japanese tourists shuffled excitedly over the wooden drawbridge, and into the grounds of the imposing Carreg Castle, a twelfth century fortress that stood proudly overlooking the city centre. Over eight hundred years earlier, descendants of William the Conqueror had repelled local uprisings there. Death was not uncommon in the days of strutting knights, rich tapestries and cobbled courtyards, when it was the smell of woodsmoke and not carbon monoxide fumes that filled the air. The visitors took little notice of a workman in dark stained maroon overalls that strolled casually past, throwing pieces of bread to the pigeons that flew overhead.

Stopping on the drawbridge on his way out, he nodded courteously as they passed; he was in no rush. In fact nobody ever made him rush, he had all the time in the world. But just for a moment he knew he had to linger. Placing a blue toolbox at his feet he leant on the drawbridge, and watched for a moment as some graceful swans swam below in the moat. He looked at his watch but still there was no sign.

The horrified screams of the female castle guide and some of her oriental visitors a few minutes later signalled the return of death to the castle, as they discovered a body, badly mutilated, in one of the lower dungeons,. Endless screams echoed all around the castle walls, reverberating up and over the ancient ramparts and down into the busy city streets. Pulling up the collar on his dark red overalls and straightening his yellow hard hat, there was almost the hint of a smile. There was no need for him to linger any longer.

News placards and fear began to spread around the city like 'flu, as news of Henk Leiberman's demise hit every news programme in the country. The collector of antiques and fine wines was now cosily tucked up inside a plastic body-bag at the city's morgue. A man already erased from the A list of celebrity European drug traffickers.

Meanwhile, between press and TV interviews, Corbett patrolled the corridors of Scrubs Lane like a hostile scrap-yard guard dog. Already a team of puppets was engaged in a mass DNA operation in all the city suburbs, which was a clear indication that the head of CID was beginning to struggle.

The squad office was jam packed when Chief Superintendent Larry Mulholland slipped in quietly and stood at the back. There, he began to listen to

Hook, who had already been on his feet for some time.

No blackboards, flip charts or bamboo pointers; such aids were for members of the training department. People who had opted out of front-line policing for the safer, warmer and quicker route to promotion.

Hook's sharp end was all about bottle, and hard-working dedicated foot sloggers, who were continually being asked to test themselves as professionals in the murky criminal underworld, a criminal arena where rules and guidelines are operated by only one side.

Staring at photographs of the four victims which were pinned to the wall, he slowly paced up and down. Smashing his fist against the first photograph, he said,

'Billy Saduskas. Lorry driver employed by the McCanns with Blackline Transport. Brought the stuff into the country concealed under legitimate cargo.'

'Howard Harvey' he shouted, slamming the side of his fist again at the photograph on the wall. 'Harvey was the run-around, arranged all the big deals in the city for the McCanns, much cleverer than we thought. He may have been setting up a factory to make this Babylon stuff.'

Larry Mulholland listened intently. He and Corbett were due to see the Chief Constable within the hour with an update on the murders, and he needed to be up to speed. Deep down, he knew if these murders were to be detected, it was going to come from within the small L shaped office that was in dire need of refurbishment, a room now totally engaged by the man on his feet.

Banging the third photograph in front of him, this time with the flat of his hand, Hook said,

'Abdul Benazzi, an Algerian. Employed in Montpellier, looking after merchandise, namely …'

He stopped and looked for the green light from Mulholland, who nodded.

'Ten ton gentlemen. Ten ton of Babylon, which Lieberman had brought in and which I think is heading our way.'

This mind splitting revelation plunged the afternoon briefing into total silence. Only a quiet 'Jesus,' and an anxious 'Bollocks' was whispered at the back of the room. Feet scraped under chairs and eyebrows moved while people just stared at the man on his feet. A monastic silence fell on the room. Hook himself remained silent for some time, giving the information time to sink in. After a few moments he spoke again

'Alright. Don't panic' he said, spotting a couple of confused faces near the front 'It's still drugs, the only difference is its weight. We'll still be doing exactly the same things. First chance I get I'll be going over to France for a conference on the

Benazzi murder. It's believed their man was a small time thief who was simply guarding the merchandise in a back-street warehouse.

'And finally, gentlemen, Henk Leiberman himself. Although not nominated for this year's Nobel Peace Prize, definitely one of Holland's finest exports. Presently resting on a stainless steel examination table in the city morgue, not knowing whether he was able to cause mass devastation on our country's streets after all. Common denominator?' said Hook

'They all have a connection with the McCanns,' said James.

'Correct. We think they are all involved with the McCann organisation somewhere, and they were all killed in the same brutal way. So give me a motive,' said Hook

Raising his hand Stobart said, 'Simple. The McCanns have upset a bigger team, trod on toes, double-crossed another large syndicate big time, upset someone, and it's pay-back time.'

'Okay,' said Hook. 'So why haven't the brothers themselves been taken out? Why murder the foot soldiers?'

They looked blankly at each other, some shrugging their shoulders.

'Perhaps this other syndicate is trying to spook the brothers, a sort of 'you're going to be next' scenario,' chipped in Stobart again.

'Right then, so who are we actually looking for?'

'He's a guy either employed by another organisation, or someone has simply enlisted him to take out some of the McCann team. A hit man. Maybe the McCanns are next on his list' put in James. 'They can't operate without a team anyway,' she said. 'Perhaps that was the intention.'

'Possibly, but if he is an outsider, how does he know so much about their organisation and its members?' Hook asked.

'Because this other syndicate dealt with them regularly, knew all their moves' said James. 'Perhaps he used to work for the McCanns.'

'Perhaps so' Hook said, ' So - what about the murder scenes,? Where were they all murdered?'

'A public toilet, a public pier and a castle, all places visited by the public' suggested someone from the back of the room.

'So why were they all killed at these locations? ' he said, pushing on.

James raised her hand slowly.

'Because they were fairly quiet at this time of the year; they were out of the way places.'

'But if they were all prepared to meet in fairly quiet places, they must have been fairly happy about him' he said. 'Anyone got any theories?'

'What about the McCanns themselves?' said James. 'Perhaps they killed them because they were being ripped off. What if Saduskas and Harvey were running a scam with Leiberman, and ripping off the brothers ?'

'Whatever's gone on, we're in dire need of a motive,' said Hook.

Larry Mulholland remained standing at the far end of the room with his arms folded, his eyebrows arched.

'Whoever they are, they're out in the city right now,' said Hook. 'Listen, the puppets aren't going to detect this. It's going to be down to one of you lot. But if there is another victim, gents, they'll start calling in outside squads, and we'll all be pulled out and replaced. Please, don't give them the chance.'

He paused again for a moment as he always did at times like this, to allow his comments time to register, while his eyes scoured the men and women before him, fixing them each with that stare. It was eye contact they recognised instantly. Once or twice a year they all got the old 'brown eyes'. It meant he was depending upon them. It was as simple as that. No need for any macho chest thumping or any flamboyant Gung Ho rhetoric that moistened eyes. There was no need for anyone to go running through brick walls for him, not unless the killer was on the other side.

'Yet again, perhaps the guy's functioning on the fringes of society. Perhaps he's holding down a normal nine-to-five job, or has some successful professional career. Let's not pigeonhole him yet' said Hook. 'Whoever he is, these murders have little effect on him. I think each one makes him stronger. But he's going to make a mistake, have no worries. Everyone makes one mistake.'

'How does this madman manage to sever the arteries up in the groin?' Stobart said. 'Wouldn't he have to overpower them first, boss? It can't be that easy, particularly if they struggled.'

'I'm convinced he knew his victims. He must have an exceptionally strong upper body, and possibly he took them by surprise' said Hook. 'They just weren't expecting it. When surgical shock sets in and they bleed to death, I think he rips off a leg of their trousers and stuffs it in the mouth. Either to muffle their groans or for simple humiliation.'

'Perhaps he's a police superintendent' Stobart called out, but nobody laughed.

Hook gave him a look that forced his chin onto his chest. The bollocking would come later. A few heads glanced around slowly, but fortunately Mulholland had slipped away.

'I want around the clock surveillance on the McCanns to start in the morning' Hook said.

'What about tapping all their phone lines again, boss?' a voice shouted out from the back of the room.

'I'm afraid the Home Office have turned me down. They're inundated with jobs involving the

IRA and some other mob, so that's a non-starter' he said.

Hook was lying. A point had now been reached where he trusted no-one at Scrubs Lane. If there was corruption in the ranks, the telephone facility he had obtained could well prove to be his trump card. However it was times like this that he hated himself the most. Deceiving men who gave him every single ounce of loyalty didn't come naturally. But if there was duplicity, it had to be this way. If wheels were to come off and heads were to roll, he knew his would be the first

'One more thing, gentlemen' he said, raising his hand to stop everyone leaving.

'One last thing, and it doesn't go outside this office. Now 1 know most of you have contacts with Customs at some of the ports, but you don't discuss this enquiry with any of them.'

Loud murmurs, accompanied by the movement of chairs as people continued to leave, had him raising his hands again.

'And that's not a suggestion, it's a bloody order,' he shouted.

The exodus halted.

'The McCanns are still flagged to this office, but I believe Customs underhandedly may also be watching them and may try and steal the operation. They have no idea I'm on to them. Trust no one.'

Racing around city back streets in a CID car, with a stomach full of pie and chip marinated in fizzy orange drink was always unpleasant. But riding in the passenger seat of James's Citroen 2 CV, as it star-jumped its way over the city's cobbles, was like riding in a wheelbarrow when you were a child.

'Pull over, pull over!' yelled Hook, suddenly yanking at the steering wheel and causing James to brake sharply. They skidded to a halt outside Sexarama, a brightly painted sex shop.

'Now, you don't look left and you don't look right, you just stare straight ahead' he said, adjusting the rear-view mirror, which came off in his hand.

Stuffing his half-eaten chicken pasty into the glove compartment, he watched as, through the rear window, he saw the man that was leaving the Gents across the road. He eyed up the figure as he paused for a second outside the convenience, fastening up the buttons on his white mac, while his brown leather briefcase rested on the pavement. Eventually he bent over and picked it up, before moving off.

A huge smile broke across Hook's face; it was moments like these that sometimes made the job worthwhile. Why would a man who wore Gucci shoes stop for a public piss, when the Crown Court was just around the corner? Because that was where he was heading. Tingling, the prickly heat slowly advanced up his spine. The feeling was back.

'Who is he, what's going on?' she complained, still staring diligently ahead.

'He's been bloody cottaging, that's what the perverted little Queen's Counsel has been up to. I … Oh no …' Hook said, as he watched Hunter Jarvis skip in and out of the traffic, jogging across the road directly towards them.

Hook pulled up the collar on his reefer jacket and turned to face James. There was nothing left for them to do, but a bit of surveillance improvisation. Forcing himself against her, he grabbed James in a tight lovers' embrace that startled her for a moment, but she knew instantly what was required and didn't complain.

'I want you to clock his briefcase as he passes,' he whispered in her ear.

It was the nearest she'd ever been to Hook's dark brown eyes and the thick dark curls that crowded around his collar. His aftershave had a slight hint of musk, and she prayed Jarvis would take his time. Perhaps stop and wait for a bus, or even do some window-shopping. She began to wonder how Hook himself was feeling, as she pushed her chin softly into the side of his neck as though she was about to play a violin.

Inside the sex shop window a large fully inflated blow up doll, complete with dubious hairstyle and thick red lipstick, gazed across at them both. The mouth was open wide as though she was singing. For some reason it reminded Hook of an old Sunday School teacher. Her right leg had a small puncture and the limb had completely deflated. The breasts were uninspiring.

Relaxing, James twisted and stroked the tiny curls. Peeping over the top of his collar he watched as the barrister finally strode off into the distance. Levering himself back into his seat, James began to rearrange her hair.

'How was it for you Inspector?' she sniggered.

'It will be a lot better if you just tell me if there was anything on the side of his briefcase' he said.

'Nothing' she replied, 'Apart from his initials. HJ. What's going on?'

Harry Hook smiled quietly to himself, and watched as the expensive white raincoat disappeared around the corner. He'd never been an eye-for-an-eye man, but the odd occasion did throw up openings, which he found difficult to ignore. Moses the caretaker had described how an elegant man in a white mac had visited the toilets on the night of the Saduskas murder. He'd seen him in there on other occasions. His only mistake had been the initials on the leather briefcase, he'd got them the wrong way around. HJ.Hunter Jarvis QC.

Detective work could be bizarre. One minute it was squeezing your scrotum, the next it was ruffling your hair.

CHAPTER FOURTEEN

Jumping straight out of the car Hook, headed for the Crown Courts, waving frantically for James to join him. Out of breath, she finally caught up with him on the pedestrian crossing outside the Crown Court building. In the council car park across the road the driver of a dark Mini watched them, unnoticed.

Marching on through the Crown Court corridors past waiting witnesses, he nodded to solicitors, ignoring her pleas to slow down.

'Okay, okay' she panted when she caught up with him. 'So that pervert Moses said one of the last guys he remembers seeing was tall, wore a white mac and had a brown briefcase. So?'

'It's him, James.'

'But Moses said he thought the initials were JH. He's not even sure' she said.

'It's him, James,' Hook said again, racing on ahead. 'He got the letters the wrong way around, that's all.'

'Hang on a sec boss. The mans a Queens Counsel, he's a personal friend of our assistant chief. He goes to garden parties and things. He's got Rt Hon in front of his name.'

'I'm not particular, I'll speak to anyone,' he said sternly.

'No, be serious.'

'I am serious James. He was in those Kingsway toilets the night Saduskas was killed, mark my words,' he said, knocking loudly on the door to the barrister's room at the far end of the corridor. 'All I want to know is what he was doing there.'

'Christ, can't a silk pop into a gents for a piss without you crawling all over him? This isn't personal is it, cariad?'

'James, we're investigating a triple murder here, not scrounging raffle prizes for the police ball' he said, breathing heavily as he struck the door again.

Detectives' stomachs were as important to criminal investigations as any DNA sampling. Nagging gut feelings that vibrated whenever you smelt a clue. Uncanny perceptions and hunches that set murder incident rooms cheering and champagne corks popping. That flair and experience that got others promoted. Hook had such a stomach.

Sidney Moses had not only described the man as posh, but had also said he had been a frequent visitor to the toilets. It was nothing personal, but Hook had always suspected Jarvis of being gay. Affluent barristers who lived in Vale of Glamorgan mansions and who charged £250 pound for a ten minute consultation didn't usually visit smelly underground piss-holes for a bit of social chit-chat. Jarvis had been playing doctors and nurses without the nurses.

When no one responded to his knocking, Hook slowly pushed down the door handle, breathed in deeply through his nose, and slipped inside. Sitting alone at an impressive oak desk in the corner of a large room, a wigless Jarvis, surrounded by a small library of legal books, sat examining a mountain of documents. Sweet smoke from a King Edward cigar filled the air, while a cut-glass Waterford decanter, half filled with what must have been an expensive Port, stood on the corner of the desk. A brown leather briefcase and white raincoat lay on a chair nearby.

Clearing his throat loudly, Hook winked at James while she apprehensively peeped over his shoulder with her fingers crossed. It came as no surprise when Jarvis ignored them.

'Inspector Hook and DS James, from Scrubs Lane, sir. May we have a word please?' he said firmly.

Jarvis never looked up but replied,

'Busy. Middle of a fraud trial. Make an appointment with Chambers. Good day.'

Moving across the highly polished block floor until he stood in front of him, Hook said,

'I'm afraid our enquiries are somewhat urgent, sir.'

'Urgent or not, they are going to have to wait. Now shoo' the barrister replied.

'This is a Murder enquiry, and I have to ask you if you visited a public convenience at approximately 9pm on Thursday the 23rd of last month. The one in the Kingsway.'

'Our body is a magnificently devised, living breathing mechanism' said Jarvis. 'Yet yours appears to have developed a hearing defect. Close the door on your way out.' The brief was becoming annoyed.

Tugging at Hook's sleeve, James attempted to pull him away, but he was beginning to enjoy this confrontation Over the years Jarvis had generally held the upper hand in Crown, regularly forcing Hook onto the legal ropes in the witness box as he ducked and weaved around the rules of evidence. Some Recorders would even allow the ayatollah of arrogance to ride roughshod over witnesses in packed courtrooms.

And there was nothing Jarvis liked more than taking a policeman apart, piece by piece, before a crowded audience. But things had suddenly changed. Circumstances had now dumped the QC out into the unprotected world. A world where he couldn't bully and intimidate others, a place where he couldn't claim the law of privilege.

Placing both hands on the desktop, Hook slowly leant forward to within two feet of counsel's face, where he spotted small beads of perspiration begin to gather near the barrister's hairline. It wasn't the room's temperature that was causing Jarvis to perspire. Hook continued to watch, as one of those beads began to slide down the man's heavily-creased forehead. Round one was just about to end.

'Did you visit them, Mr Jarvis?' Hook said raising his voice just a little, as the single bead of sweat stopped abruptly above the silk's eyebrow.

Slowly the Head of Chambers lifted his eyes, moving them over the top of his gold designer reading glasses. In a show of arrogance and an attempt to intimidate his visitors, he replied,

'You may be able to browbeat some ten-year-old glue sniffer down at that police station of yours, but breezing in here and attempting similar tactics may give you cause for regret, Inspector.'

'The question is a simple one' said Hook. 'It's either yes or it's no.'

Helen's sudden appearance as she stepped into the room momentarily took the wind out of Hook's sails. He hadn't spoken to her since New Year's Eve and all the emotions came flooding back. Jarvis began to smile with relief, as he regained some much-needed poise.

'You ready, Hunter?' she said coolly, ignoring both his visitors.

'Helen, my dear girl' he said, beginning to collect up his paperwork while clenching the cigar between his teeth.

'Would you contact Mr Peter Quelch, the Assistant Chief Constable, and inform him that I wish to complain most strongly about the conduct of one of his senior officers.'

Trilby James felt nothing but despair. The new year was only days old and here he was, about to collect his first official complaint for the new millennium.

Waiting until she had reached the door, Hook called out from behind a cloud of smoke,

'On your way back, Miss Wainwright, would you inform the Recorder in number one court that Mr Jarvis here is assisting the police with a murder enquiry.'

Hook threw Jarvis a big look and raised both eyebrows.

'It was the one down in those old toilets in the Kingsway' he said.

'Sit down, Inspector' Jarvis said, giving Helen the slightest of nods to leave. 'Your fortitude is something to be admired, but of course these things do have the nasty habit of bouncing back on oneself when one least expects it.'

Jarvis had an infuriating habit of avoiding eye contact, by glancing over the top of the head of the person he was addressing, as though he were speaking to someone just behind. Now, twisting around in his leather-padded chair, the QC gazed out through window blinds that actually worked, looking down into the bustling city centre. Rolling the cigar back and forth in his mouth like a New York boxing promoter and, deliberately ignoring Hook, he finally turned towards James.

'Now what is it exactly you want to know, dear? If I visited those toilets in the Kingsway on the 23rd of last month, is that it?'

'You heard the question, counsel, because you just repeated it. Now answer it please, and cut all this crap' he said. 'This is a murder investigation.'

'Am I a suspect, Inspector?' he asked.

Leaning forward again in his search for the whereabouts of the little bead of sweat, he said,

'Well, I've got my suspicions, but I don't know if it's reasonable as yet. Let's just see how things shape up, shall we sir?'

'Alright. Let me see. I left chambers that evening at roughly eight forty five. There was a cold chill in the air and I was caught short. I parked my car near a public convenience, and in the confident knowledge I was not committing any misdemeanour known to the British criminal justice system, I went inside.'

'Did you see or hear anything suspicious?' Hook said.

'It was all very quiet. I saw the caretaker as I went in, if that's what you call suspicious. I could hear some poetic drunk in the end cubicle.'

'You went into one of the cubicles?'

'Yes, the one next to the drunk, but I was away from there in minutes.'

'Poetic?'

'I could barely hear him, but he was babbling on about the heart being like ice. I'm not sure, what he said exactly. It was all so incoherent and none of my business. My own hands and feet were certainly like ice.'

'Please try' said Hook.

Pondering for a few seconds while deliberately blowing wreaths of smoke in Hook's direction, Jarvis finally replied.

'I'm sorry, he just seemed to be mumbling. It certainly wasn't T.S.Elliott.'

'And you definitely saw no one else?'

'Apart from the caretaker, no.'

'Could you describe this voice you heard? The accent, for example?'

Jarvis slowly shook his head.

'Why are you so sure he was drunk.'

'Sitting alone in a cold public convenience reciting bilge! What else could he be, Inspector?'

'This is important sir. If you remember anything else, would you please ring me immediately?'

He had already sensed that Jarvis was becoming a little uneasy, his eyes occasionally vacant while he spun slowly round in his chair with very little eye contact. The barrister had something on his mind, Hook could just sense it. They were about to leave, when he called out,

'*Sweet darkness is only moments away,* Inspector.'

'I beg your pardon?' Hook said, turning in puzzlement as the QC poured himself another drink. Taking a generous swig Jarvis said,

'I remember now. It was something like, *The heart will feel like ice... ... .* yes that's it... ... ..*like ice.... but don't struggle ...darkness is only moments away...* no ... *sweet darkness is only moments away.* It was all so bizarre.'

Marching out of the room, Hook called over his shoulder,

'I'll send someone around to Chambers tomorrow to take a witness statement.'

'There was more than one person in that cubicle next to me, wasn't there, Inspector?' he inquired, while he replaced his wig.

Nodding once, Hook and his sergeant stepped out of the room. Quietly he pulled the door closed behind them.

CHAPTER FIFTEEN

O'Malley's Tavern in a cobbled back street was crammed with off-duty police, mingling and chatting about results, promotion boards and villains in the frame. Alongside the jukebox, half a dozen fresh faced probationers stuck to the station's new WPC like shit to an old army coat, amidst clouds of smoke and the sound of Irish folk music.

Hook sat morosely next to Goose and James in the corner, in a mist of liquor. Fighting to stay awake, he occasionally sipped quietly on his Jack Daniels and ice. Goose was now back in work and celebrating the occasion by downing copious amounts of Drambuie and lemonade, which resulted in his chin spending the greater part of the evening resting on his chest. He'd been drinking heavily for months and there was talk his marriage was in trouble. Hook himself was hardly in a position to lecture anyone about the evils of alcohol, but Mr Reliable was beginning to worry him.

Senior Officers' promotion dos bored Hook rigid, particularly when the recipient of the selection process was unworthy in his eyes. Listening to bull-shit speeches that normally elevated the officer to the status of some Hollywood super-cop was bad enough, but smiling and applauding, pretending it was all true, he found nauseating. Awaiting the statutory stripogram was even worse. Unfortunately heads of department were expected to attend, and his appearance was necessary. But this gathering of ranks had a special interest for Hook. Somehow tonight he felt like a losing Oscar nominee who had to smile and feign delight when the winner was being announced.

'So, what you think?' slurred Goose.

Considering for a moment, he said,

'The bastard wants every victim to suffer. He's not just content to kill them outright. He wants them to feel every bit of pain and fear that death can bring. The guy's so evil he's even talking them through their last few breaths.'

'No, no, no, I mean this shit do. This crap job,' Goose stammered, his eyes starting to bulge in his effort to focus on Hook. 'The whole crappy promotional circus shit.'

Looking up at the huge banner overhead that swept across the entire room, Hook smiled at the felt tip scrawl above: *Congratulations on your promotion to Chief Inspector. Well done Lance.*

He wasn't that disappointed. With a sponsor like Corbett and the full backing of the lodge, Maul had always been assured of the inside trap.

'Gutted' he laughed, emptying the last half-inch in his glass. 'I feel like I've been playing musical chairs and I'm the one who's ended up without a seat,' he went on. 'Same again boys?'

He dropped a fistful of change onto the bar, and picked up another three Jack Daniels and ice before the bored-looking peroxide barmaid with the braided hairdo winked at Hook and nodded towards the Snug bar behind her. She wobbled away unsteadily on brand new heels, carrying two of the glasses with her to the pair still sat in the corner.

The sheer madness of a man wanted on warrant for breathalyser offences, drinking alone twelve feet away from sixty off-duty policemen, wasn't lost on Hook.

'I see stupidity isn't confined to the police service' he said, joining Brodie in the crowded Snug. 'Your governors know about the shit you're in yet?' he said, trying to make himself heard above the noise and live music, while scanning the bar for faces he'd seen in the Police Gazette.

There was anxiety written on Brodie's face and dark shadows beneath eyes that looked concerned for the first time since they had met up again. He'd never have taken Brodie for someone who worried.

'You haven't told anyone at Customs I've been bagged, have you? You promised Hook. This operation is important to me.' Hook could sense the anger in his tone.

Slowly he shook his head.

'Calm down. No, I haven't.'

After discovering the surveillance photo of his friend shaking hands with the brothers, he wondered why. Whatever Customs were up to, he was more determined than ever to find out. However, chatting to Brodie in the middle of a busy city pub surrounded by an armada of policemen, when the man was the subject of an arrest warrant, was about as unprofessional as a detective could get.

'Listen, bugger off Joe, before I get pulled with you for conspiracy' he laughed.

'One minute Hook. I'm reliably informed that your friends the McCanns are expecting a big bag some time during the next day or two, possibly coke. That's why I'm here. I rang the station and they told me where I could find you.'

Although he still appeared cheerful, Hook felt uncomfortable. There were too many prying eyes. When a DI spoke to anyone in a pub, punters' ears began to move.

'Listen, give me a bell tomorrow,' he said, turning away to rejoin the celebrations next door.

He was halfway along the tiny dark corridor that connected the two bars, squeezing past the arriving stripogram dressed as a traffic warden, when Brodie called after him.

He knew the Drug Squad boss was giving him the brush off, and that his colleague probably already knew of the McCann's new consignment. Under normal circumstances he would have firmed up a little more on the other piece of information he had for him, but he was angry. He was being treated like some run-of-the-mill police informant and not the old friend he really was. It was something Joe Brodie wouldn't tolerate.

'Your buddy Stobart is as bent as a meat hook, my friend,' he shouted after him, his voice echoing all along the corridor.

Hook stopped in his tracks. He felt as though he had been exploring the inside of an extinct volcano when he had heard the first hint of a slight rumble. Turning on his heels, he returned and grabbed Brodie roughly by the arm and barged him out through a side door into an unlit yard at the back of the pub, an exit normally used by after-hours drinkers to escape unannounced police raids. It was a door Hook knew well.

'What's the matter with you, Joe? Keep your bloody voice down! There're boys from the complaints department in the bar next door' he said, releasing his grip on Brodie's arm. He was annoyed.

'Okay, okay I'm sorry. I'm told the brothers knew Stobart when he was a DC in Clapham. My man tells me it sounded as though they knew each other very well. They apparently referred to him as Eddie. It all sounded very cosy.'

'But Stobart worked at Clapham CID. How far is that from Brixton, where the McCanns lived?'

'Right next door' Brodie replied, beginning to relax.

'But he's only just transferred to south Wales, he hasn't really had time to be bent here.'

'Someone said his misses actually moved back to Wales almost a year ago, and your Eddie has been commuting.'

'Christ, who's this nark of yours Joe?' he said, slumping down on a cold aluminium keg, trying not to look too suitably impressed.

Casually winking, Brodie slowly began to tap the side of his nose conspiratorially. It was always pleasant when Customs gained the upper hand over the police.

'Well if they lived near his patch up the smoke, of course he'd know them,' said Hook, on the defensive. 'He's probably arrested the bastards.'

'Oh, he arrested them alright. Our Eddie lifted them right enough. An armed Supermarket blag.' said Brodie. 'But witnesses disappeared, and the evidence was watered down to such an extent that when the file of papers reached the CPS it didn't get past go. They kicked it into touch, and the brothers walked. But he's probably told you all this' he added with that Customs smugness.

Hook didn't reply.

'The fucker's bent, Hook.'

'Don't beat about the bush, Joe.'

'You may jest, but my man actually thinks the brothers may be bringing in a huge consignment of that new designer drug Babylon, and not coke. Talk is they intend flooding every Council estate within a hundred miles of the city.'

But Hook wasn't really concentrating; half his mind still lingered on the squad's latest acquisition from the Met.

'Areas of high unemployment, deprivation and drug taking' continued Brodie enthusiastically. 'Swamp the areas with cheap Babylon, get the kids addicted and comer the market. That's their plan.'

'I'm impressed Joe, nine out of ten,' replied Hook as the customs investigator began to lift the rusty latch on the gate in the yard.

'By the way, any progress on the murders?'

Shaking his head Hook replied, 'I was hoping you had some news for me.'

'I have, but you're not going to like it,' he said as the smile left his face. 'The latest rumour circulating the Docks' pubs is that it's a copper' he said, disappearing up the street. 'I'll be in touch,' he called back over the wall.

Standing alone in the centre of the yard, surrounded by aluminium kegs and the smell of burst bin bags, he watched the full moon begin to muscle its way past heavy white clouds, while the late evening wind continued to ruffle his hair. That's all he needed now, he thought. A murder suspect who was working alongside him at Scrubs Lane.

Just for a moment he thought long and hard about the gravity of such a statement, while he searched his pockets for a late night smoke. He'd appreciated Brodie's frankness but after a while decided to push such absurd information to the back of his mind. Well, somewhere near the back anyway. A killer wearing blue? Surely not.

What he couldn't dismiss, was the fact that Customs also knew about the possibility of the first consignment of Babylon hitting the shores of the UK. Now Customs were aware, it was human nature it would be uppermost in Brodie's mind. Most detectives would have wanted to score maximum points for their own organisation. He would have done exactly the same thing. Although he had never played ring-a ring-a-roses with Customs, he had always trusted Brodie, but now he was beginning to have doubts. Perhaps Brodie had been working on the Babylon operation all along.

Was there really someone bent in the office, working alongside him over the years? There weren't too many of his squad who hadn't had the finger of corruption waggled in their direction at some time or another. Innuendoes and smear campaigns came with the job, he tried to convince himself. False allegations intended to hijack a trial, or spurious dealer claims in the hope that an officer would be suspended and banned from their door. These were all par for the course. But tonight the feeling about Stobart in the pit of his stomach began to suggest something totally different.

A huge cheer from inside signalled the appearance of the female artiste, who was just about to remove her fixed penalty ticket for the newly-promoted Chief Inspector at Scrubs Lane. All evening he had been putting it off, but as he was about to make his way back to the lounge, he realised what had to be done. Whether he liked it or not, at some stage during the evening he would now have to shake hands and congratulate Lance Maul on his advancement, a gesture that the man would milk for all its worth. It was something Harry Hook could take in his stride, he thought. But how the hell could you shake hands with something that normally rattled before it struck? Taking a deep breath he squeezed the latch quietly on the yard gate, pulled up his collar and slipped away into the night.

He made his way along the wet pavements through condemned streets of derelict terraced houses built in the twenties. Only a stones- throw away from Scrubs Lane, he had already decided to sneak up the fire escape and spend another night of uncomfortable insomnia in the black leather swivel chair. It was an early start in the morning.

Cutting across his face like a rusty razor blade, the icy wind almost forced him to a standstill, as the little French car skidded out of the dark; a handful of icy sludge flew up from the gutter and splattered his trousers.

'Sorry cariad,' she yelled. ' Jump in.'

He climbed in thankfully and sat back as the little car drove off, swerving around soggy burst sofas and rusting shopping trolleys that lay overturned in the middle of the street.

'Thanks. You're a nice girl, James.'

'Nice girls do things for you. Bad girls do things to you. Curry?' she suggested.

'Is Goose okay?'

'Yeah, I've got Ivor Griffiths to give him a lift home.'

Kensington Lane, and the surrounding rabbit warren of streets, bustled with multi-cultural pedestrians and boisterous youngsters who staggered from wine bar to fun pub in search of a good time. Most of the noisy amusement arcades in the side streets were packed with kids who should have been getting ready for bed, while a couple of Rastafarians dealt a little happiness from a darkened doorway.

Driving slowly along the lane, they passed an unlit alleyway alongside a Cantonese restaurant, where, in the middle of a heap of rubbish bags, a destitute bundle of humanity lay on the ground enjoying his amphetamine rush. A hypodermic syringe still hung from his arm.

Hook scowled.

'And they want to legalise it' he said.

Most of the city's nicer restaurants were in this area. Fashionable yuppie refreshment places where the plates were big and the portions small. Brasseries where people ate dishes they couldn't pronounce. Stopping by the kerb, she was about to switch off the headlights when he walked right in front of them

'Christ, it's him,' she said. 'What the hell's he doing around here at this time of night?'

Still wearing his shell suit, they watched as Sidney Moses, carrying a brown carrier bag, stepped into the car's dipped headlights, almost falling over the bonnet in his eagerness to make progress. Rushing along under the lane's colourful neon lights, he dodged through the traffic and crossed briskly to the other side of the road, before disappearing into some public conveniences.

'Does he still work in those other toilets, down in the Kingsway?' she said.

'No, he never went back after the murder.'

Although there was an absence of any shivering near Hook's spine, he nevertheless had a feeling that something wasn't right. It was the brown carrier bag that concerned him.

'When he comes out, let's give him a pull, eh boss?'

Adjusting the interior mirror, he moved his head in agreement, sat back and folded his arms. Five minutes later two young girls, who looked as though they were still in the local comprehensive sixth form, skipped out of the conveniences and joined the moving masses. Both wore thick leather belts which doubled as mini-skirts, high heels, and legs that could have made a top-shelf magazine. Hook gave them the once over. Probably no homework tonight, he thought.

'Down boy, heel!' James said.

Heavily painted, the fat lady that followed the girls out and up onto the street had to be a Tom, up from the Docklands for richer pickings. Wearing shiny high heels. she wobbled away along the opposite pavement into the night, searching for new punters with feeble eyesight. Her dark bushy Tina Turner wig and tight fitting clothes did little to disguise the advancing years. Redundancy couldn't be far away.

'Jesus, do men actual pay for things like that, bach?'

'Search me' he replied, shrugging his shoulders and yawning. Cupping his cold hands together he blew in some warm breath, still staring intently at the toilets in the rear-view mirror. Impatiently he looked at his watch as more people went in and out. Moses was still inside after twenty minutes. The glances they began to draw from the three Rastafarians who were still dealing in a little ganja had him pushing open the passenger door.

'Come on, let's get him.'

Standing in the centre of the grey tiled floor surrounded by empty flushing urinals and unoccupied well-disinfected cubicles, he glanced up at the glass skylight. Mystified he began to scratch his head.

'He's not in there, he's disappeared into thin air. The ladies next door perhaps?' he said to James after returning to the pavement outside.

'I've just been in there, it's empty too. The skylight?'

Hook shook his head.

'Well we've clocked everybody that's gone in and out,' she went on. 'So what now?'

Returning to the car, Hook lit his last cigarette of the night before turning in his seat to face her. Inhaling quickly he said,

'You first.'

'Okay. The only way out was the skylight and he certainly couldn't climb of it, it was too high. No back entrance. Bottom line, we've just gone and missed him. Our view of the entrance wasn't brilliant. We've blown it.'

But they hadn't missed him, he was sure of that. Pulling the brown carrier bag he'd found in the gents from inside his coat, he threw it onto her lap. At the bottom of the bag she could see a small cheap lipstick. Taking it out of the bag she began to screw it around until the pink head began to rise out of the tube. She looked across at him, frowned quizzically and began shaking her head. He muttered something under his breath.

'Okay, go on.'

'I think Sidney Moses is wandering around our city dressed as a woman,' he smiled.

From the moment he had seen her muscular calves wobbling away unsteadily on high heels, he knew something hadn't been right. Women, especially Toms, didn't walk like that. She had trudged along the pavement like a Welsh hill farmer visiting the Inland Revenue. Mr Moses, he was convinced, had gone into the toilets a man and come out an ageing, fat, bushy haired prostitute.

The following morning Hook sat with both buttocks perched firmly on the comer of a desk in the main office, having spent the early hours fruitlessly searching the city for Moses. It was something that needed further attention. Giving his early morning briefing, he stopped when Maul poked his head around the door.

'Larry Mulholland's office, two minutes' he said before disappearing.

That morning he'd been too busy to notice the four shiny prestige motor cars, each accompanied by a smartly-dressed chauffeur, which were parked in the layby at the front of station. Shiny motor cars were an unusual sight around the Docklands, but their presence would have prepared him, because Chief Inspector Maul certainly wasn't likely to give him an advanced warning.

Walking into the Oval Office, as the men referred to Larry Mulholland's room, with a mouth stuffed full of toast, while tenderly carrying three other heavily garlic-buttered rounds on a paper serviette, wasn't the entrance he would have wished for. A room full of distinguished short-clipped grey hair or seriously-receding hairlines almost made him choke.

His own Chief Constable, Charles Jones, sat deep in thought at the side of the desk, with his left hand wrapped tightly around his mouth as though he'd just been punched by one of the others. Moving one of his fingers, he pointed to a chair.

'Sit down and relax, Mr Hook' he said, removing his hand. 'We are all former CID officers here, and fully appreciate the occupational hazards of trying to combine a crime investigation with meal breaks.'

Swallowing hard and standing erect, he awkwardly offered everyone present a piece of his breakfast. They all refused but it seemed to break the ice. Taking his seat like a quiz show contestant, he sat back and tried to relax. Sitting amongst all that impressive serge and scrambled egg made him feel a little uneasy.

'Chief Superintendent Mulholland here has appraised us of your confidential information on Babylon,' said Jones, 'and how you're running part of the murder enquiry alongside this drug investigation.'

Hook replied with a nod.

'I think everyone in this room is painfully aware of the serious implications this new designer drug will have on the young in our society, if dealers do market it in this country,' he went on. 'That's why I've asked every chief constable in Wales to this meeting. This is no PR exercise Inspector, there's a social holocaust on the horizon just waiting to blow up in our faces.'

Hook nodded again as he continued to struggle with a mouthful of brown toasted bread. He had always liked Charles Jones. He was a plain-speaking man with few frills. A vastly experienced policeman who had worn the T-shirt on operational matters, not someone manufactured at the Bramshill Police College with a course photograph on his office wall and a jazzy brass nameplate on his desk. Many Chiefs were just a Jack-of-all-ranks yet master of none, but Jones had footslogged the back streets of the city and, in CID parlance, had 'done the bizz.' Someone with actual ability who had come up the hard way. If Hook had even thought of bullshitting the top man, Jones would have torn him up for ACPO arse paper.

Looking fiercely over the top of reading glasses that had started to slide down a bulbous perspiring nose, George Gardiner, the well-padded head of North Wales Police, left his seat like a great shaggy dray horse that had just climbed a hill. Pouring himself another coffee from the nearby trolley and seizing yet another chocolate digestive, he turned to Hook and growled,

'Do we know, Inspector, why this new substance is so lethal?'

Hook had to think for a while.

'The probability is that it reacts so that chemicals in the body combine in such a way that the body is unable to tolerate the drug. What chemicals combine and why, they still don't know. How it affects the body will depend on the genetic make-up of the individual.'

Quickly observing the vacant expression on Gardiner's sixty-year-old face, Hook continued, paraphrasing.

'In simple terms, sir, Mr Mulholland's body, for example, could possibly tolerate it, but yours possibly wouldn't. Why? Nobody seems to know. Babylon seems an appropriate name. In some cultures it refers to the police.'

'And do you think it's arrived yet, Mr Hook?' he said, inserting the first cigarette of the morning into a grimly turned down mouth.

'My guess is it has.'

'How is it taken?'

'Orally. It seems a lot of people in America remove the filling of a sweet, like a sherbet lemon, and fill it with Babylon. They can suck away at their leisure. Snorting's popular too. Users who inject have described it as three-day walk through paradise. Many return in a box.'

'Its chemical make up?'

'Like a lot of designer drugs, very little research has been done on it. Take ecstasy for example - we still don't know what the long term effects are. One report from the States suggests it contains opium derivatives such as heroin and morphine, mixed with stimulants like amphetamines, ephedrine and cocaine hydrochloride. We know it gives you a heavy duty rush.'

Folding his arms, Hook watched the wrinkled brows on the heads of the hierarchy.

'And are you aware of the principal players?' asked Jones.

Pausing briefly, he knew he was on new territory here. He didn't normally have to discuss his operations with such exalted ranks in the organisation. This wasn't the time or place for clever smart-arse operational appraisals, or simple guesswork in an attempt to impress. This was the heavy artillery, and the examination paper looked pretty stiff.

'I think so. I believe we are heading in the right direction,' he replied with a confident honesty in his voice. 'All I need is just a little more time. It has to be connected with Cars International, sir.'

Pulling his chair even closer towards Hook, a concerned Gardiner frowned.

'If 1 were a drug user in some disco, Mr Hook, what would draw me towards this Babylon stuff, when there are already so many other illegal substances available?'

The thought of George Gardiner snorting Babylon and boogying-on-down in a rainbow of fluorescent laser, clad in a pair of tight leather pants, tickled Hook, but he kept his composure and carried on.

'It releases to the brain similar chemicals to that of a Pitbull terrier when fighting,' he said. 'It gives the user a feeling of unbelievable physical invincibility, and a huge increase in one's confidence. There's a similar increase in one's energy levels and a vast increase in one's sexual libido.'

Gardiner slowly raised an eyebrow. Hook went on.

'It's addictive, like heroin, and there's no lethargic come-down after it wears off. It's sixty per cent stronger than cocaine,' he continued. 'If this drug does take a foothold the consequences are horrendous.'

Twisting the ends of a thick white moustache, the formidable Gardiner growled on.

'So why are we all so concerned about this drug, Inspector?'

'In America, one in every five hundred people who have taken it so far have died.'

The room went deathly quiet.

'This drug - in the States, do kids - I mean school and college kids - take it?' said Gardiner eventually.

'Everyone takes it,' replied Hook, who was now starting to relax.

'But aren't young school kids going to find this stuff expensive?' said Gardiner.

'Not as expensive as their funerals,' said Hook. 'What's more, gang violence would increase in our cities, as crime organisations jockeyed for supremacy. This drug is taking over from where crack left off in the States. According to the FBI, it's the drug the world's been waiting for. Initially, it's going to be very cheap to buy.'

'And apart from the obvious reasons Inspector, why has this drug become so lethal in America?'

'It seems that some sort of religious cult on the west coast who are making it, are also alternating its purity. For example some batches will be ten percent, twenty percent pure; others around fifty to sixty. Occasionally they'll slip in a batch that's a hundred. A hundred percent. One minute your tolerance level is happy taking the twenty percent gear, which in itself is good stuff. Then one day unknown to yourself you do some hundred percent powder and bang, it's goodnight Vienna. Nice people.'

'Why *Babylon*?' Charles Jones asked.

'Well, in biblical times, Babylon was a strong, powerful place, but corrupted and immoral' replied Hook. 'Today's Rastafarian communities hate any kind of oppression and it seems they're using the name Babylon as a reference to any governments that they feel oppress the poor. They hate the police. And China, America and Russia. They want Ganja and other substances legalised. Rastafarians don't want to be told what to do - they want to be left alone.'

'If this consignment of Babylon has arrived on our shores, how long would you estimate it would take for the main dealers to get it out onto the streets?' asked Gardiner.

'Well, the network's already in place, so no more than a week' replied Hook.

The concern on their faces was clear and their expressions grim as the four ACPO officers huddled together, forgetting Hook and Mulholland for a moment. Hook's mind nibbled away at the outcome of this meeting. There were a number of scenarios available. This no run-of-the-mill drug importation. It simply depended how strong as a foursome they were going to be. Calling in the National Crime squad to take over the enquiry was a favoured possibility, as was the setting up of a special task force. But there was one thing that worried him most and he knew instinctively it would be brought up. Brushing cigarette ash and some biscuit crumbs from the front of his tight white shirt, the red faced Gardiner, with some effort, slowly got to his feet.

'If this stuff hasn't arrived as yet, I think we should pass the investigation over to Customs and Excise' he said. 'They are the first line of defence in this country after all, and probably have a more superior intelligence network. We could work alongside them. '

There were too many heads wobbling for Hook's liking, and he began to panic at the thought of Lies-R-Us being given the seal of approval to take over his squad's latest operation. Turning towards Mulholland, he looked for support but his immediate boss was well outranked and all of a sudden appeared lightweight by comparison to others in the room.

Mulholland had already anticipated his Inspector's next move. Scowling, he shook his head slowly to warn him off. But Hook was having none of it.

'Look,' he said, interrupting their discussion. 'Customs may be the first line of defence in this country's battle against drug trafficking and have an outstanding information network world-wide. But my boys have an operational experience in this city they could never match. Day in, day out, they work in the very heart of the community. They have their fingers on the pulse. They know where it ticks and how it ticks. Flood it with Customs and a host of new faces, and these villains may well panic. I just know Customs will introduce their own brand of mushroom investigation and cause no end of problems.'

Sinking back in his chair. he glanced at the elderly faces around him, and knew immediately he had been too rash, and probably somewhat rude in disturbing their deliberations. Criticising another drug enforcement agency wouldn't have gone too well either. He had spoken too quickly and hadn't thought it through. In his anxiety, he even forgot exactly what he had said. It had been a pathetic, piss-poor attempt to secure their confidence and retain the investigation. The smile that was leaving his face was replaced by one of wrinkled self-disgust.

'Your Chief Constable tells us that you're expecting a thousand kilos, is that correct, Mr Hook?' Gardiner said.

Swallowing hard, Hook felt a rough lump turn up in his throat while the inside of his mouth started to feel like a piece of fresh blotting paper. He started to cough, but he had no idea why. Lying had never before been this difficult.

'Yes that's right,' interrupted Mulholland quickly. 'The evidence we have suggests it's a thousand kilos.'

Hook slipped a finger inside the collar of his tight black T-shirt and moved it around a little, feeling the dampness that the previous lie had generated. Slowly his breathing returned to normal.

Twenty minutes later it was all over, as the four Chiefs began to rise and throw on their expensive black Gannex coats.

Tapping him on the shoulder, Charles Jones said,

'Good luck Mr Hook.'

'Thank you sir, I'll do my best.'

'You'll have to Mr Hook. Failure is not an option.'

Getting to his feet, Hook smiled apprehensively before shaking the hands of all the hierarchy as they left the room. The handshakes made him feel important, they were warm yet strong, each accompanied by firm eye contact that implied trust and confidence. It must be like this when officers received the Queen's Police Medal at Buckingham Palace, he thought. As he came back down to earth, Gardiner poked his head back around the doorway and said,

'By the way, what exactly is a Customs Mushroom Investigation, Inspector?'

'They'll keep us in the dark and feed us bullshit,' answered Hook.

After the door was closed he thought he could hear Gardiner chuckling in the corridor as he walked off, but he wasn't sure.

'Don't let me down, Hook' Mulholland said.

CHAPTER SIXTEEN

It was past three when he and James finally drove out of Scrubs Lane. The shift had gone well. Seventy kilos of cannabis resin had been seized from a house in Vintin Lane, next door to the home of Howard Harvey, and everyone was impressed. The unreliable Joseph Brodie was working well, and it was time to relax.

He hadn't eaten properly for over a week, his mind and didn't seem to have the time. But after the meeting with the chief constables, the thought of a quiet chicken biryani and something that vaguely resembled a glass of Beaujolais Nouveau at the quiet Light of Bengal in Sullivan Street suddenly fired him up. Within minutes they were pulling up outside the restaurant but watched in dismay as a crowd scene began to develop in the street.

They could see that a youth had been stabbed and his trousers were saturated in blood, a vivid redness that had also stained the cold grey pavement he had collapsed on. Although his body was blocking the entrance to the tiny curry house, his head and unconscious eyes hung limply in the gutter.
They watched from the other side of the road as blue lights from nearby Panda cars flashed their emergency reflections in all the surrounding shop windows, while the ambulance siren in the distance began to get louder. Sullivan Street a

neighbourhood where you wouldn't let your mother do her Christmas shopping.

Peering through net curtains that were in desperate need of a swill, James could see the body of a second man lying prostrate under an overturned table inside. He too appeared unconscious. Grubby white shirts with frayed collars were everywhere as Indian waiters excitedly chased their shadows, while the overhead shorting neon light hummed and crackled at will. Sometimes the guest list at the little restaurant could contain the unsavoury, and violent altercations were as common as the stained tablecloths inside. People didn't normally visit the Light of Bengal if there was something else open.

'We can't even have a quiet meal these days. Shall we clear off?' said James hopefully.

'No, let's give the boys a hand. Perhaps it's just a bit of Curry Rage' he said

Hammering on the passenger window, the little Bengali manager, wearing a bright blue bandleader's tuxedo three sizes too big for him, pleaded for their help.

'Calm down Mohammed' said Hook, alighting quickly. 'Now tell me, slowly, what's happened, as though you're back learning English in night school.'

'They men who are injured over there, Mr Hook, they pick all night on the man that have scarpered away. They take his food off his plate and humiliate that man. That gentleman that run away has enough and leaves my restaurant quietly but they jump him. But then he stabs one with his knife and punches one then runs away.'

'Fixed penalty justice,' James said.

She pushed her way through the small crowd of drunks that had gathered on the pavement to watch the injured being tended by arriving paramedics. Taking notes at the scene, the young probationer constable, who looked about fifteen, acknowledged Hook with a respectfully nod.

'Better show the flag' he said. ' Let's give the boys here a hand.'

The unlit lane at the rear of Sullivan Street was an area of wheelie bins and burnt-out cars, where used syringes and the strong smells of multi-cultural food wafted from the endless fast-food takeaways that stretched along the decaying thoroughfare; seedy properties concealed hot-oil or talc establishments, that nightly produced endless smiles and bin bags stuffed with used tissues; countless foreign dialects screamed from inside opened windowed kitchens, as late night revellers sought refreshment.

'I'm bloody starving, cariad' whispered James, working her way around the refuse, as chef-like screams and wok-like flames reverberated into the night.

'I could murder a bag of chips. '

The sound of a car door being slammed shut in the distant darkness alerted them as they stepped out of the concealing shadows. Pure instinct had him picking up a nearby house brick, which he began to toss up and down in his hand as his eyes strained in the dimness to identify the small dark outline of a motor vehicle whose engine idled quietly at the end of the lane. Experience told him that the car had no intention of stopping, as its full headlights were activated and that sudden, unmistakable sound of grinding gravel as its wheels spun. warning him that the car was accelerating along its escape route towards them.

He didn't need to be a mathematician to work out that the width of the vehicle wasn't that much narrower than the laneway itself, and there were immediate calculation problems to be considered if he and his partner were to survive. James' eyes widened, the lane's unevenness bounced around the car's headlights as it raced towards them with its engine screaming. Squinting against the brightness, she stood her ground, determined to move only at the last moment in a futile effort to recognise the driver or perhaps the number plate, or even both. But peering through half closed lids at three fifteen in the morning in a pitch-black lane, she couldn't judge the speed and approximate distance of a getaway car. She was fortunate, because Hook could. And did.

She had no answer to Hook's thirteen stone as he hit her upper body like an All Black number eight, sending them both crashing down a short concrete incline, as the Mini saloon bounced past at high speed. Noisy dustbins overturned and bin bags rolled in all directions as they both ended up outside the back door of a noisy Chinese takeaway. The two stray cats seated on a neighbouring wall seemed unimpressed.

Peeping out of a kitchen window, the small oriental face watched as both emerged from beneath a pile of split rubbish bags, scrambling to their feet.

'You wanna food you come to front of shop like everybody else, so,' he complained.

She wanted to laugh but a couple of her ribs cancelled the idea.

Surrounded by a yoghurt-purple wallpaper and repetitive sitar music, reminding Hook of a Welsh harp being played by a drunk with a saw, it was almost an hour later that both finally finished eating. Mohammed and his smiling waiters yawned in the background, occasionally checking their wrists for the time, but always smiling.

Details of the dark coloured saloon had already been passed over to uniform, but they were both disappointed that they hadn't done better. A dark saloon in an even darker lane wasn't likely to make Crimewatch, or end up anywhere near the front pages of the evening Echo for that matter. Description of driver: not a bloody clue.

'I've got a feeling,' she said, 'that there was something hanging in the back window of that car. I'm sure I saw something swinging around as it turned out of the lane.'

'Keep thinking. It may come to you later.'

'Yeah. Anyway, thanks,' she said raising her glass as she finished off the bottle of cheap house red, compliments of the management for their earlier efforts.

'What for?' he said, snapping the last poppadum.

'You know what for' she replied, rubbing her grazed knees under the table.

'It's okay ma'am, I'm a cop, I'm just doing my job,' he said without any expression.

She began to laugh when suddenly, without warning, he pulled out the pin and dropped the grenade into her lap. He wanted to see her reaction. That's the way he did things.

'Who's bent? In the Squad? Any idea?'

Choking back a mouthful of warm wine, she coughed and struggled as the alcohol made its way back along her throat, spilling down her chin and onto the front of her pink shirt.

'You what?' she spluttered.

Tossing her his handkerchief, he said,

'My sources are normally spot on. Most of the warrants on the big dealers have been negative - it's almost like they were waiting for us. It's becoming the talk of the pubs.'

She didn't like what he was saying, but she knew he wouldn't have said it unless it was kosher. If she was just learning about it, she knew full well Hook had been keeping it under wraps for a lot longer, until he'd felt sure. Naming names wasn't her style, but corruption in the workplace was a little different.

'Are you a hundred per cent? I mean, someone in the office? Working with me? Bent? No, I don't believe it. What for? Money?'

'All things can be corrupted, all you need is a perverted mind,' he said.

'I can see it in your eyes. You know already who it is. It's Stobart isn't it? Go on. I'm listening' she said, leaning over the table little closer. It had to be something connected with the former London bobby. Everyone else in the department was like a brother.

'It seems Eddie Stobart knew both McCanns when he was a DC in the Met' he said. 'It appears that he watered down an armed robbery they were involved in, so that the CPS had little option but to offer no evidence. Usual thing - missing witnesses, missing exhibits and poor statements,' Hook replied. 'He also lives in a £250,000 house and has just ordered a £25,000 BMW. But of course I could be wrong.'

Rubbing her pale hands up and down her equally pale complexion until both cheeks began to regain some colour, she stared for a moment across the brown blemished tablecloth towards him. Expelling air through puffed-out cheeks, she slowly shook her head. If she was feeling demoralised, what the hell was going on inside his head, she thought. The office had been his life for the past three years. A department that he had raised, nurtured and protected like a Godfather. He had pulled it up out of the gutter, dusted it down and rebuilt it into a formidable unit, much to Corbett's annoyance. And now here was someone about to destroy it.

'But he's only just been transferred to us,' she said.

'Apparently he's been commuting. His wife moved back to Wales a year ago.'

James wrinkled her nose and ran the fingers of both hands slowly through her fluffy blonde hair, indicating some further evidence would be required if she were going to accept that Stobart had really become the office Judas.

'When I met him that first day' he went on, 'I knew I had seen him somewhere else, but I just couldn't remember where. It's been bugging me. Then when I began checking the first surveillance photos we ever took at Cars International, I found

Stobart in one of them.' James made a face again. 'He was talking to the McCanns outside their office.'

'So why didn't we ID him earlier?' she said. Glancing over at the yawning waiters, Hook smiled back at them and waved. Pulling a black and white surveillance photograph from the inside pocket of his jacket, he pushed it across the table towards her. Studying it for a moment ,she shoved it back angrily.

'The bloody shit,' she said. 'He's got long hair and a full beard, no wonder we didn't pick him out. Perhaps he was there on a legitimate enquiry for the Met.'

'Perhaps my arse is a banjo, Miss James,' he said.

'But knowing it and proving it are two different things' she said. 'It's still all circumstantial. He's not going to admit it, is he?'

'I could check his bank accounts I suppose, but Stobart's not stupid. I've been watching him recently' he said.

Sitting in the corner of the darkening restaurant, the lowering lights gently hinting that Mohammed and his staff were now on overtime, she watched him for a moment, his strong face stained by worry now, shaded by fatigue.

'You're coming home with me tonight ,cariad' she said, beginning to throw on her coat.

'You're having a good few hours' sleep and a full Welsh breakfast in the morning.'

Arguing would have been pointless. Anyway, he didn't have the energy.

'Can I ask you something?' she said. 'I mean, these murders - I know you believe that the murders and this big consignment of Babylon are in some way linked. I mean, what I am trying to say bach is... ' she didn't finish.

'What you're trying to say,' he interrupted. 'is - do I actually have any idea at all who's actually responsible?'

She half smiled and nodded her head. There was nobody else in the world that Hook would have admitted it to, but James was different. She was - well, she was just James.

'To be perfectly honest, I haven't got a bloody clue' he said, shrugging his shoulders before slipping on his jacket.

Shaking each waiter's hand for the fourth time, while James went to fetch her car, he began to probe a little deeper into the fracas that had disturbed the peace earlier. After being given a free bottle of wine and a late Christmas card with the meal, he felt obliged.

Nobody at the premises could ever remember seeing the assailant before, until an ageing chef poked his dark hairless head and black fiery eyes through the small serving hatch opposite.

'The man you look for come here once before, for a meal.'

Stretching his chin forward so that he could do up the top button on his reefer jacket, and still only vaguely half interested in an incident that would probably end up another undetected crime statistic, he turned towards the old man and said,

'When was this?'

'The same night as that murder sir, in those toilets.'

Suddenly he could feel it returning again, that warm tingling sensation that crept along his vertebrae.

'How are you so sure it was the same night?' he said, offering the little Asian cook one of his French cigarettes from the packet.

'Because a Policeman come in later that night for some egg curry and chips for his shift and tell me about the terrible killing. It would be a Thursday night, yes?'

'Yeah it was. What time did this man leave your restaurant that night?' he said, as James began blowing the horn outside.

'About eight o'clock,' said the old gent. 'He use that telephone behind you, sir, before he leave.'

'I don't suppose you know what number he rang' he said, lighting up the man's cigarette with his lighter.

Puffing away with some gusto like a schoolboy behind the bike sheds, the little man turned his head politely and blew a huge cloud of smoke towards a large metal rice container on the nearby cooking range. He watched for a moment as the smoke drifted up towards the yellow-stained ceiling that hadn't been painted in a decade. Hook's mind turned briefly to hygiene - he wondered if all Asian chefs smoked as heavily. There wasn't an ashtray in sight.

Turning back to Hook and lounging casually on the shelf of the serving hatch, he said,

'Do you know, Inspector, that Humphrey Bogart also smoke these wonderful French cigarettes in Casablanca?'

Loneliness was a terrible thing, thought Hook. Sleeping upstairs, working downstairs every day, with little time for conversation or anything else. No wonder he was enjoying his moment in the spotlight.

'Well, well, I never,' Hook replied. failing to sound interested in the history of the cinema, though not disabusing him of the difference between a Gitanes and a Gauloise.

'But do you know what number he rang?'

'It was a number in the city, sir. He wrote it on the wall behind you.'

Turning sharply, the sight of over two hundred hand-writing samples near the telephone quickly reduced his chances of solving yet another violent city crime. The scribbled telephone numbers scrawled by inebriated jotters caused his sudden surge of tingling in his vertebrae to subside. Seedy pinned-up calling cards offering massages or French lessons; taxis or a gay friend he didn't need. What he wanted was the telephone number the lone diner had rung.

'How do you know?' said Hook, turning back to the chef. 'That he rang a number in the city. I mean?'

'Because sir, he get the number from that lady in the enquiry, and he borrow my pen to write it down on that wall.'

Hook was missing something here. Again he concentrated on the endless figures that had been pencilled, biro'd or inked all over the orange emulsioned wall, penmanship scratched by bladdered punters chasing a lift during the early hours.

'I still don't follow,' he said. 'There's bloody hundreds of numbers here.'

'There, in green ink,' said the Bengali, proudly pulling a green felt-tip pen from the top pocket of his brown coat. 'There in front of your eyes, in green' he shouted excitedly.

The green felt-tipped numbers almost leapt off the wall and seized Hook by the throat. Something was beginning to develop here for sure, as the tingling returned with some vengeance, screaming up his spine before tearing across each shoulder. Central 500005 was an easy enough number for him to remember. There was no necessity for him to write it down.

'Listen, are we sure about this? 1 mean one hundred per cent sure?'

'Of all the joints in all the world you will be having to be coming into mine' the little Asian muttered, allowing the cigarette to hang limply on his wet lips.

'Yes, yes, Casablanca, I know!' he said, 'But for Christ's sake, are you really sure about this?'

Somewhere behind the clouds of smoke the little chef nodded enthusiastically.

Shaking everyone's hand for the final time. Hook jogged out and along the red-stained pavement blemished by the evening's violence ,and jumped into the waiting Citroen, which was colder inside than out. Colour had now returned to his cheeks and some sparkle back into his eyes.

'What's up?' she said, aware of the sudden resurgence of energy that now sat bubbling alongside her.

'The driver of that Mini tonight, it's got to be the same bloke that sorted these blokes out. I've got a telephone number he rang when he was in there a few weeks ago. He had a meal there the same night as the murder in the Kingsway. It appears he rang Central 500005.'

She seemed unimpressed.

'I'll check the number tomorrow and pass it over to uniform. Can't fault you bach, detecting a GBH and a Dangerous Driving all in one night'.

'No need to' said Hook. 'I've rung it hundreds of times myself. Its Billy Saduskas's flat.'

Just then Hook's mobile rang.

'It's PC Bowen sir. I'm sorry to trouble you, but I thought you might want to know about the two lads assaulted earlier at The Light. They're both good Section Eighteens. Still no sign of the saloon, but the second lad was stabbed in the groin. He's lost a lot of blood but is out of danger now. It looks as though his femoral artery may have been nicked. Good night sir.'

'Good night constable' Hook said. 'And thanks for ringing.'

'Are you thinking what I'm thinking?' she said.

He didn't answer. His mind was miles away. He knew at last things were beginning to move in his direction and that the pace of the enquiry would now start to take off. He'd had an element of luck, he knew that, but by helping uniform to deal with a late night assault he had helped to make his own luck. And that's exactly what good detectives did. At last it was the breakthrough he had searched for. Whoever had carried out that violent attack at The Light earlier, had clearly been provoked into doing so. But whoever he was, he had rung the first victim, little Billy Saduskas, at his flat an hour before he had been murdered.

'Who the hell is this bloke?' she said, as a passing panda car driver waved to them.

'He's a prime suspect for the murders, that's who he is' he replied.

He was right, but that was the easy part. Now all he had to do was find him.

Early morning sleet lashed the side of the mountain while mist began to descend from the snow-capped peaks above, wrapping itself like a tourniquet around the little Citroen as its engine continued to grit its teeth in the battle towards the summit. Only the occasional sound of a stray cow moving aside on the narrow icy track told than that they were heading in the right direction.

It became increasingly difficult for Hook to recognise the landscape as the one he had visited as a child, when he had played with short-trousered friends in golden fields of uncut barley. During days when it had been far easier being a general in charge of two friends against an unseen enemy than a drug squad inspector hunting down a serial killer.

'If we go on any further, bach, we'll be in England,' moaned James.

'This car got angina or something?' he asked as she changed down yet again to a lower gear.

Their two-hour marathon journey finally seemed at an end as barking dogs in a nearby barn announced their arrival, while a low white cottage emerged out of the mist. Hammering on the door with the side of his fist, Hook waited as a brass storm-lamp creaked outside on a rusty bracket. Slowly the door began to open, and the glow of the lamp framed the face of a small bespectacled man with a head of thick uncombed grey hair. Kind blue eyes brightened, and a sunny smile began to light his face as he recognised one of his visitors. Seizing him by the arms he squeezed Hook warmly before taking James's arm and leading her inside, towards a huge log fire crackling noisily in an inglenook fireplace. Pointing to two battered leather armchairs, both visitors sat down either side of the roaring fire, while the old man perched on a tiny wooden stool.

Long and oak-beamed, the room was adorned with sepia photographs in silver frames, lined green velvet curtains and a black pebble doorstop. The curling candlesticks antique and the warming pans that hung nearby were genuine brass, and clearly still in use. But most of the room seemed sad and undusted and there was a feeling that people were missing from there. The place had the smell of a damp Welsh chapel.

'Jacob' said Hook, 'I want you to meet a good friend of mine. Trilby James. We work together.'

The old man glanced over the top of his tiny reading glasses and grasped her hand warmly.

'I am pleased to meet you. My name is Jacob Saduskas' he said.

Within minutes, they were drinking tea at the fireside, as the flames danced among the restless logs.

'Billy often spoke of you, Harry, and how well you were doing in the police. I have been hoping upon hope you would come and see me. You see, I didn't know the other policemen that called,' he said. 'They say you watch toilets, and don't really investigate Billy's murder.'

Arching his eyebrows, Hook glanced over at James.

'Did you know my son, Billy?' he asked James, beginning to pour her more tea. She shook her head.

'They say he was a drugs dealer in the city, but did he deserve to be murdered, Harry?' he said, his eyes filling with tears.

Placing his cup on the floor, Hook leant forward and grasped the old man's hands.

'Listen Jacob,' he said. 'No, Billy didn't deserve to be murdered. He got mixed up with a bad crowd. But we need your help to find them.'

The little Jewish engineer who had survived eight decades and the holocaust began to sob quietly.

'In Dachau they inject us with drugs every day, their experiments kill many hundreds of people. And now my son is involved in selling them. He must have been evil, Harry.'

'Did many of his friends call here?' said Hook, avoiding an answer that would have added to the father's pain.

'Billy would stay occasionally, then disappear as quickly as he came. He was always back and fore. I did notice many months ago, after his mother died, everyone wants Billy. The telephone is always ringing and he has to go out late at night in his lorry.'

'Did you see any of his friends?'

'They do not come into my home, but sometimes he takes them into the barn' he said, pointing out across the yard. Wiping away some tears with the sleeve of his badly ironed shirt, he said,

'Come Harry, I'll show you.'

The old white-washed barn was warm and dry, and they were greeted by the old man's canine alarm system which indicated, by sets of flashing white teeth and deep throaty growls, that the method was in excellent working order. The building was full of sparkling tools and naked internal combustion engines, chains and grease, and smelt of a man who knew how they worked.

Nosing around, Hook could tell that the place was clean, and there was no further need to embarrass Jacob by carrying out a full search. After all, Billy Saduskas was nothing more than a small time street dealer, a street soldier who had been headhunted to drive Blackline lorries full of dope.

'There is no need to look any further Harry, I have already searched myself.' smiling briefly.

Hook nodded, but like James, seemed absorbed by something at the far end of the barn, something that was covered by a huge green tarpaulin, and bales of hay. The old man smiled wryly as he watched their interest grow. Tugging away at the green sheet, which caused the bales to roll around the floor at their feet, he finally exposed a compact motor car.

'A Mini saloon' exclaimed James, her blue eyes widening.

'A dark Mini saloon,' added Hook.

Proudly, Jacob strolled around the little car, patting it affectionately on the roof as though it had just completed the Monte Carlo rally. Jumping into the driver's seat, he said,

'I did it up for Billy, but then when I finished it, he seemed to lose interest.'

'That's children for you' said James, keeping a watchful eye on the audible alarm system that was growling nearby.

'He wanted one just like his friend, then when I finish, he decides he wants a sports car instead.'

Getting into the passenger seat of the little black saloon, Hook sat alongside Jacob, his back already beginning to tingle.

'What friend? What friend of his had a Mini, Jacob?' he said, twisting the gear stick playfully as if the question itself was irrelevant.

'I never saw him, but they came in here a few weeks ago, perhaps a few months even. It was getting dark. Anyway, after his friend left, Billy asked if I could do up this old Mini as he fancied one like his friend. He was always changing his cars, Harry, you should know that.'

Taking a deep breath, Hook put his arm around the old mans' shoulders.

'Now listen Jacob, this is very important. Can you describe the car that called here? Please take your time.'

After a little while he said,

'I'm sorry, I didn't take any notice. It was a dark colour I think; it was parked right down near the entrance. My eyes are weak, Harry. The number, I'm afraid, no. It has a radio ariel on its roof.'

Disappointment was etched on Hook's face as he levered his frame out of the car. Slowly both detectives nervously edged their way past the snapping jaws of Jacob's companions when the old man called over to them.

'Wait a minute.'

'We'll wait in the yard if you don't mind, Jacob,' called Hook spotting too much slack in the dogs' chains.

A white sprinkling of snow covered their heads like Muslim prayer caps as they waited outside in the storm. Shivering, they watched the old man lock up the barn.

'It had one of those bouncy things, Harry, it had one of those bouncy things hanging in the back window as it drove off. I remember now,' he said as they headed back through knee-deep snow towards the warmth of the cottage.

James' recollection began to kick in. and she nodded her head. Clenching both fists excitedly. she said,

'You mean a sort or mobile? Like a kid's toy, on elastic?' she said, as man nodded his head.

'What sort of mobile was it, Jacob?' Hook asked gently.

CHAPTER SEVENTEEN

'A Spiderman. Believe it or not, the Mini's got a bloody Spiderman bouncing up and down on a piece of elastic in the back window' said Hook as the office listened.

'We haven't got an index, but his little mobile should make it easier to identify. We need to find it ASAP. If this was the car that nearly ran us down at the back of the Indian, I want to know why the driver was ringing Billy Saduskas a short while before he was murdered.

Just then the telephone rang. Hook answered it, snapping his fingers to James who threw him a biro. Slowly everyone began to slip on their jackets. It was something they recognised instantly, it was one of those calls, unplanned, unrehearsed and unexpected. Hook's voice had that excited edge which had them snatching at ignition keys and covert radios. Frenetic mayhem, suddenly replacing a calm professional briefing. There were always days like this, when operational briefings went out of the window and things were played off the cuff. It was moments like this that Hook loved. Improvisation. Scribbling away, he said,

'Yeah, yeah, got that, brilliant. Yes, yes, I owe you one.'

By the time he had slammed down the phone, everyone was on the starting grid. Heading towards the door he suddenly came to an abrupt halt in the middle of the office.

'Hold on. I need someone to man the phone in the office in case my man rings me back,' he said. 'A Blackline wagon has just left Dover and should be with us in three hours.'

Both Goose and Stobart volunteered as James looked on suspiciously. She hadn't taken her eyes off Stobart since her conversation with Hook at The Light of Bengal.

'I want you on my team Goose; you keep an eye on the office, Eddie' shouted Hook as he made for the door with his beloved reefer jacket dragging along behind him.

'Would there be any chance of you giving us a rough clue, boss?' panted Goose, trying to light up a Marlboro on the run as they tore down the station stairs.

'Yeah, sorry - there's three hundred kilos of cannabis on board' he grinned.

The savage wind raced down from the top of the Bwlch Mountain, bending the sharp tussock grass flat against the ground as Hook watched Goose gamely urinate against a tall Norwegian pine for the third time. Tapping his fingers anxiously against the steering wheel, he gazed down from the forestry at the lines of neatly parked lorries below. The Blackline Yard seemed quiet and deserted.

'You want to get that prostate examined,' he said, as Goose joined him in the car.

'Nobody even wags their finger in my face, Inspector,' Goose replied, smiling as he zipped up his trousers.

They watched as a man secured the yard with a heavy-duty chain, padlocking the high security compound, while the floodlights surrounding the premises flashed on dramatically. Things began to look bleak.

'Shit, it's not coming' said Hook, as he got out of the car and began stabbing away at the digits on his mobile. 'I'll give my man a ring,' he said. Goose watched him carefully.

'It's been bloody diverted to Liverpool' he shouted, diving back into the car. 'Call the troops back to the office, Goose' he said, as forestry gravel peppered the underside of the car like a burst of machine gun fire.

Trooping dejectedly back into the office, everyone slumped down at their desks, cold and miserable. Suddenly monotonous success was replaced by what-might-have-been and it showed.

'I'll get the coffee on,' called Goose, leaving the room. 'We can't win 'em all, chaps,' he shouted.

Coats were dejectedly thrown aside and cigarettes popped into down-turned mouths. Some watched as Hook sat at James' desk in the corner, a blank disappointed look on his face. He was good at disappointed. Pushing aside some of James' paperwork, he lit up a cigarette before seizing a small portable tape recorder, which had strangely been left running under a pile of files. Pulling the little silver machine towards him, he pressed a button and waited for it to rewind. Inhaling deeply he sat back and began to blow a long plume of smoke towards the stained ceiling, pressing the 'On' button with a casual stab.

Gradually people began to take interest, as the tapes in the tiny cassette began to whirr. He across at Stobart and then back at the machine. Normally it was used in undercover work, or to tape police informants. On this occasion things were about to take a dramatic twist. This informant was working for the bad guys.

Everyone was silent now, as familiar voices burst forth into the office. Everyone was heard leaving earlier. A short silence was followed by the telephone on James' desk being lifted, while Stobart – the only man left in the office - tapped out an eight-figure digit. His voice sounded urgent.

'Listen, it's me, Eddie. I ain't got long. You'll have to call it off. I said, there's a change of plans. Now don't be stupid, you'll have to. I don't give a monkey's - call the bloody thing off.'

Hook's eyes flew across the room towards Stobart, whose brow looked confused. The tape continued.

'Look, they're only neighbours! Well I can't help your flamin' profiteroles!' Slamming down the receiver Stobart still wasn't finished. *'Bloody women'* he grumbled.

Waiting for an explanation, Stobart glared at Hook, not knowing if he'd been the subject of some silly wind up, or if this was all part of some juvenile Welsh Drug Squad initiation ceremony. Nobody appeared to be laughing.

While Hook was seriously thinking about his next line of dialogue in an effort to extricate him from further embarrassment, the tape burst back into life with a vengeance. The sound of the office door being opened was unmistakable.

'Left my fags here somewhere' Goose was saying, followed by the sounds of a drawer being searched. *'Hey Eddie, why don't I keep an eye on the phones while you pop into the canteen to get yourself some sandwiches? They're still getting the cars out downstairs, they'll hang on for me. They know about my prostate!'*

Hook raised his eyebrows and moved uneasily on his chair. Glancing about the room he looked for Goose, but he was still out making coffee.

It was like listening to a radio drama. The sounds of a door being opened and closed again, and a telephone being used, were very clear. Hook felt a nauseous foreboding in the pit of his stomach.

The voice was different this time. It was quiet, whispered, but Hook turned up the volume. It was something they all needed to hear. It was a moment they would never forget. It was going to tear the department apart.

'Mr McCann please, quick. Mickey, it's Goose. The boys have just left for Blackline, the DI here has had info about three hundred kees of blow due in from Dover shortly. Okay, okay I'm only telling you what they're doing. Okay, if it's a load of balls you haven't anything to worry about then. No, I don't know who his nark is. But it's a false alarm, that's the main thing. Listen I've gotta split, they're all downstairs waiting for me. Cheers'.

Assorted coffee mugs and plastic beakers trembled on the small tin tray that Goose held in his hands as he stood in the doorway. James rubbed her eyes in total disbelief, while others just turned away in shock. Nobody, it seemed, could look at him. All went deathly silent - the lack of sound was deafening. Briefly life stood still as Hook's career began to flash before his eyes, while Goose stood rooted to the spot, head bowed, trying to hold a tray, now flooded in coffee, that must have felt like a ton.

It seemed appropriate that Stobart should be the one that broke the silence. Shouting, he ran towards Goose, raining blow after blow into a body that refused to defend itself.

'You fuckin' bent bastard, no wonder we can't win 'em all!' he yelled, throwing wild punches into Goose's pale swollen face. Eventually Goose collapsed onto the floor soaked in blood and hot coffee as people tried to pull them apart.

Holding onto Stobart as the tray and mugs bounced and smashed all over the office floor, Hook shouted to James, who was also struggling to pull him away.

'Get everyone up to the canteen now James. Out, the lot of you!' he cried.

His colour was already that of an angry puce when he pulled his colleague up off the floor by his lapels before jostling him into his office and depositing him on a chair. Kicking the door shut behind them, Hook sat down. On the other side of the desk, bloodied and dishevelled, Goose began to weep softly. Neither spoke as he nervously twisted a pencil until it snapped. He interlocked his fingers, then, shivering, fidgeting with his nails. Gripping the sides of his chair, Hook's jaw tightened.

'Why?' he said.

There was a long silence, before Goose began to stammer out short, incoherent sentences of apology that meant nothing, while the tears and the tremors continued. The occasion probably demanded some sharp self-righteous rhetoric that would strip Goose of any remaining dignity, but Hook knew that would come later, in interviews and court appearances. For a moment he almost began to feel sorry for a friend who had always been the backbone of the office. Using dirty tricks to catch out one of his men left him with an overwhelming feeling of guilt, planting hidden tape recorders and creating bogus operations to flush out the rotten was causing his stomach to ache.

The phone on his desk was only inches away, yet he looked at it for a long time. His eyes moved over to the window and out into an evening that had also turned to black, but there was only one thing he could do. For a few moments he watched the concrete artery with all its traffic and headlights, and then back at his colleague crying opposite, but the problem was still there. Taking a deep breath, he quickly picked up the receiver and said,

'Message for Superintendent Powys, Complaints and Discipline please. Ask him to meet me in my office ASAP. You had better ask Mr Mulholland to attend as well' he said, before slamming down the phone.

'Please don't, Harry,' cried Goose. 'I couldn't handle it inside. Please, I don't want to go to prison. Let me go and I'll apply for a transfer.'

Hook watched as his right hand man came apart before him. There was much he wanted to say, but at that very moment his mind not in a good place. He didn't know where to start. He was Godfather to his kids, had often stayed with his family in the city suburbs. Now he was going to be instrumental in taking their father away from them. What's more, Goose had been doing it under his very nose, when people like Joe Brodie and others had warned him continually. Perhaps he should have acted sooner. Now it was all too late. He just wished the man would stop crying.

Pushing his chair away, Hook got to his feet and headed for the door. He was unable to stand it any longer.

'Wh … where you going boss?' he stuttered.

'To spew,' whispered Hook.

Late the following afternoon, the Marina looked peaceful and tranquil. Creaking yacht timbers bobbed up and down in the swell. Sitting in the little Citroen, Hook and James watched in silence as dusk began to fall. It must have been his twenty fifth cigarette of the day as he lit up one more, while James tossed her half-eaten cheese roll to the awaiting gulls.

Inside he was stripped of every feeling except loss, bare of any emotion except grief. Exposing his colleague as bent to everyone in the office was one thing and was bad enough. Turning him in, and destroying a whole family, was another, and was worse. Regret had already kicked in.

'I know what you're thinking boss, but he was having a grand a month. How do you say no?' she said, looking for words that would help ease his pain.

'You move your fucking head from side to side, James,' he snapped.

'Okay, okay he fooled us all cariad, and all the squad get tarred with the brush of corruption. But it's not your fault. Anyway, where is he now?'

'Out on bail for a month. They've suspended him,' he snapped.

'That moment, that very minute a policeman decides to become bent' she said. 'Why do you think it happens?'

'That's simple,' he began. 'One day the force doctor tells you your heart is getting worse and he suggests that you may have to retire on medical grounds. You keep everything to yourself. Dark sleepless nights are spent worrying about triple by-pass operations, about money, about your kids, and you panic. Every minute. every hour of the day, every day of the week, the very disease that killed your old man terrifies you.'

Flicking his half-finished cigarette out through the open passenger window to join a small heap outside, he went on.

'All you need then is a DI who is so absorbed in everything else that he doesn't see it coming, although it was clear in his eyes every single day. He was ripe and an easy touch for the McCanns. Goose hasn't been right for months.'

He was about to light up yet again when he suddenly stopped and slapped James on the knee. Blowing out the flame on his lighter he stared across to the other side of the marina. It was the smoke from the twin exhausts coming from the rear of the dark blue saloon that he saw first, about a hundred yards away. The car's engine was idling lazily while it remained stationery, parked between two ocean-going yachts which had been pulled out of the water.

'Over there, over there,' he said, pointing. James squinted desperately in the failing light.

'You see Helen's flat? It's parked about ten yards away to the right' he said. She looked again and then saw it. It was impossible to recognise its driver but both of them clearly saw the masked face of the Spiderman mobile that hung chillingly in the back window. Gently it moved back and forth as the sea breeze blew in through the driver's open window.

'It's him alright. Yep, that's our Spiderman guy' she said, trying to control the excitement in her voice while she adjusted her binoculars.

'G-golf, eight eight one, Alpha Tango Hotel,' she called out calmly. Snatching his radio off the back seat Hook repeated the registration number to the control room.

'It's an urgent vehicle check WR, location of suspect vehicle the marina complex, over.' He had barely finished speaking when the saloon suddenly sped off at a high speed, swerving in and out of iron capstans and other small craft towards the marina entrance. Both watched as it bounced over the quayside cobbles before disappearing.

'Christ, what the hell's going on?' cried James, starting up a car that would have had difficulty in pursuing a cement mixer.

'He's got a scanner, he's listening to our broadcasts,' he shouted, as James vainly attempted acceleration. 'He knows we're checking him.'

Speeding back towards the city centre in the middle of rush hour traffic, James' radio crackled into life. *'Reference vehicle check Golf 881 Alpha Tango Hotel, the index is allocated to a Daimler Jaguar saloon car, owned by the Metropolitan Police and allocated to Assistant Commissioner Anthony Drysdale, over.'*

'God, he's got false plates. Christ, is that a coincidence, that it's allocated to a police vehicle?' she said, still scanning the four lanes of grid-locked traffic ahead for any sign of him.

'It's got nothing to do with coincidences James, the man's taking the piss,' he growled.

Moments later she pulled up behind a large shiny milk tanker and watched her reflection in the huge aluminium container on the back of the lorry, its air brakes hissing aggressively as though she were getting too close. She wasn't that sure at first but after checking her nearside wing mirror she quickly turned to Hook who was shaking an empty cigarette packet in his search for another smoke.

'He's not just taking the piss bach, he's about ten cars behind . . . .now he's started to follow us.'

Resisting the temptation to turn in his seat and give the game away, he casually pulled down the passenger vanity mirror, which was now filled by a huge green bus directly behind, full of noisy new-age travellers.

'Shit, I can't eyeball him. Which lane is he in, for Christ sake?'

'He's following us now in the inside lane, just behind that Landrover, nine or ten cars back, but I still can't see his face, the street lighting, it's too shadowy.'

'I can't see bugger all' he shouted. 'You sure it's him?'

'I'm fairly sure' she yelled as traffic began to move off.

Eventually the vehicles up ahead began to slow as a red set of traffic lights loomed up in the distance.

'If this bastard wants to start playing mind-games, I'd better go and introduce myself' he said, removing his bulky reefer jacket and starting to open the door.

'Be careful boss' she said. 'For Christ's sake be careful.'

He was already beginning to curse his overindulgence in tobacco as be hit the ground running, totally ignoring the V sign from the new-age bus driver behind. The importance of identifying the driver seemed to increased his leg speed, as he sidestepped his way between an armada of dipped headlights and aggressive horn blowers, sprinting towards the inside lane in the semi darkness. Slapping and banging the approaching bonnets in frustration, he unsteadily changed direction, racing over the wet road surface. His heart was racing.

But all his ungainly athleticism had been observed long before he had got anywhere near the Mini. Out of breath, he could only watch from a distance, as it suddenly reversed up and onto a grass verge, before accelerating and swerving away across a council-owned rugby pitch towards the distant blackness. Collapsing over the bonnet of a silver Mercedes, he appealed to the startled driver as the traffic slowly began to move off again.

'Did anyone see the driver of that Mini? Can anybody describe him?' Desperately he tried to re-inflate lungs that felt as though they had just been scoured with a pumice stone.

'I think he must be one of those new age travellers' a voice called out from inside Merc, as the driver almost ran over Hook's feet in his efforts to get home from the office.

Standing alone in the centre of the carriageway, he watched as the tiny rear brake lights of the Mini momentarily came on as it stopped on the halfway line, about eighty yards away. He listened as its engine revved noisily, tempting him, almost baiting him to continue with the chase. Within seconds it was off again, escaping into the distance.

'Bastard' he muttered as he went to search for James. 'Double bastard.'

Scrubs Lane was slowly coming to life the following morning as the bleary-eyed night staff prepared to hand over their shift. Overweight station cleaners in overalls and curlers buzzed in and out offices while enormous silver machines hurtled on ahead like R2D2. The whole station began to smell clean again after another twenty four hours.

Hook hadn't slept much, barely two hours; the face was unshaven and his eyes looked like piss holes in a sandpit, as he slipped in quietly through a side door. It was five fifteen.

Normally he distrusted police coffee in paper cups, but it was free, sugared and unattended in the empty inspectors' office as he breezed past and scooped it up. It looked like the stuff they used to unblock drains, and tasted like the stuff it unblocked.

Sipping away cautiously he made his way up to the top floor.

Stepping into his office, the man was sitting behind his desk, waiting for him in the dark. He'd been there most of the night.

'You're in early' Hook said, sitting down opposite him. The big black swivel chair whirled around in anger.

'I came here for a new start. Okay, I'm not everyone's cup of tea, but I thought you were different,' said Stobart, with the volume turned up.

'These are difficult times,' Hook said calmly, seeing Stobart's application for a transfer facing him on the desk. 'I had to make a decision and I got it a little wrong, but I think you need to fill in a few blank spaces before I express some regret.'

'But you thought I was corrupt, yes?'

'Too bloody royal' said Hook. 'I'm not bloody Mystic Meg. Why the hell didn't you tell me you already knew the McCanns when you were up in the Met?'

'Yeah, it was stupid, I know. But I wanted to put them away, to impress you.'

'Well we all want to be super cops, but you're playing a dangerous game.'

'I know everyone here thinks I'm a bit of a geezer, loud and all that, but I just wanted to make an impression. Make no mistake, I can do this job, no problem.'

'So could Dennis Neilson, Eddie, before he resigned from the Met and started boiling heads.'

'I'm not bent, boss. Never have been.'

Rummaging in his reefer be finally found a half-finished cigarette he'd nipped earlier the previous month. Lighting up gratefully, be inhaled slowly, the flame momentarily illuminating his own trench-fatigued face. He never took his eyes off Stobart for a moment. The Londoner was doing same.

'So is that it?' enquired Hook, with just a hint of sarcasm.

Fidgeting with his watch. Stobart's eyebrows knitted together.

'Bullshit-free zone, Eddie.'

'Okay, okay. I'd been trying for years to get onto the CID and when I finally did, I found half the squad on the take. I refused point blank to take the brown envelope and just turn a blind eye. Anyway, I'd been after an Alfa Romeo for ages and one of the lads said he had this ace contact in some car auctions. Well as it happens, as it goes, I bought one for ten grand.'

'Go on.'

'Well it turns out that he hadn't bought it from the auctions as promised, but from McCanns Car Sales. That was the name of their firm. They set me up.'

'You're losing me a bit,' said Hook.

'The Alfa was actually more like twenty grand. I'd had no idea, but the lads in the office then had something on me. If I bubbled them, they said I would go down with them. My cheque was made out to the McCanns. It looked bad. Paid ten grand for a twenty grand motor.'

'That it?'

Stobart started to nod, but suddenly stopped as Hook's dark brown eyes continued to stare.

'Bullshit free zone?' said Stobart meekly. Hook nodded.

'Okay, up front. The McCanns were in the frame for an armed blagging, big supermarket, East End. I was the officer in charge, but exhibits went missing. Statements the boys took for me were shit, and my DI watered everything down. The station janitor could have submitted a better file. I made a few waves but they blew me out of the water. I was transferred onto a surveillance squad by the end of week.'

'And our photos of you looking like Jethro Tull? Talking to the brothers outside Cars International?'

'Oh that was ages ago boss. I was down with the wife, visiting her parents - they're quite wealthy, own a big garden centre - anyway, I knew the bastards had moved down to your patch. Pure coincidence, I happened to pass their garage one day and I couldn't resist it. I went in and mouthed off about them doing the supermarket job and that I wasn't bent, and that one day I'd eventually pot them.'

'What did they say?'

'They told me to fuck off or I'd end up in a scrap yard crusher.'

Picking up Stobart's transfer request, Hook squeezed it into a ball and tossed it into a wastepaper basket under his desk.

'I apologise, Eddie' he said. 'Let's make sure you stay out of that crusher.'

'You believe me, boss?' he asked

'Sure' he replied, dousing his cigarette in his cup of Mr Muscle.

'Cheers,' he said, forcing a weak smile.

'It's all right Eddie. I checked with an old mate of mine in the Met last night. Tea or coffee?' he called as he went to put the kettle on.

CHAPTER EIGHTEEN

On the fifteenth ring James finally accepted that it wouldn't go away. With her head buried face down in the warm crumpled pillows, after a night on Beaujolais Nouveau, her arm stretched out across the shadows towards the little pine bedside table. Grabbing the handset roughly, she pressed it somewhere near her right ear and grunted. Her bedroom was warm and dark and her shift was still three hours away.

She recognised the voice immediately and she sat up abruptly, naked. Swinging both legs out and onto the cold floorboards, she searched frantically for the switch to her bedside light. Slowly she opened her eyes.

The voice sounded angry and bewildered and came straight to the point.

'Someone's pinched our Heroin. Twmpath Beach, twenty minutes.'

The line went dead.

James sat alone in her car in the early morning gloom, waiting patiently. She watched the cold crashing surf as it pounded in towards the deserted cove like white shrouded hands, snatching and grabbing at rocks and pebbles, before retreating back towards the heavy swell, only to try again. Turning off the radio she sat back in her seat and began to listen to the rhythmical sound of the shifting shale, when she heard a noisy exhaust in the distance.

One pound of top grade Turkish heroin worth ten grand on the streets was missing, and this was going to take some explaining. Skidding to a halt on the wet sand next to her, Hook pushed open the passenger door and called her over.

After brushing a pile of chip papers and empty coke tins off the seat, she slipped into the front of his car alongside him. Wearing a ten-year-old grey duffle coat, red bobble hat and Telly Tubby slippers, she looked tired.

'Just tell me this is a dream, and you're making it all up' she said, sticking her hands tightly under her armpits in her search of some early morning warmth.

'It's no dream,' he replied.

'Are we talking about the last batch of heroin we seized from that kebab house?'

He nodded, watching her early morning reaction.

'You mean someone's taken a pound of smack from our stores, next to your office, under our very noses?'

Shaking his head, he said,

'Not taken, Trilby. Stolen.'

'Hang on a sec, cariad. I did a stores check the day before yesterday. It was there then. In fact it was there yesterday as well. I don't get it.'

'Oh, it's there now okay, on the top shelf. Exhibit bag, exhibit label, but it's not heroin. The bag's full of bloody glucose. It's been switched,' he said, still on the lookout for any piece of body language that might put her in the frame for a theft that was likely to secure someone a lengthy term of imprisonment

'Cut it out bach. I know what you're doing. I'm having the old Hook once-over.'

'Sorry.'

For a moment she stared out to sea gathering her thoughts. She began to move about in her seat, restless, but little to do with the early morning cold. Straightening up, she turned towards him.

'Look boss, it's got to be one of our squad, let's get that out of the way. Nobody in uniform would take a chance coming into our office,' she said. 'There's only one key, the place is alarmed. You got any clues?'

'Stobart perhaps, or even Goose,' he said, 'if you want me to name names. But it needs to be sorted quickly before Corbett finds out. Funny, my horoscope yesterday said that a guardian angel was watching over me and that I had to be philosophical, strong and brave, and that happiness would come my way.'

'Perhaps he took today off,' she said. ' What are we going to do?'

'About what?'

'This stolen Heroin.'

'What stolen Heroin?'

'Noted,' she said, with a perceptive look at him. 'See you back at the Station later then.'

Back in her own little car, she waved half-heartedly across at him, before her engine exploded into life and began to pull away up the rough single-track incline that led away from the beach.

Closing his eyes for just a moment, Hook sat back and listened to the moving shale a few feet away. There was no doubt that if rumours of the missing heroin hit the corridors of Scrubs Lane, his whole department would be back in uniform by two o'clock, and if it were discovered he was concealing a theft of ten grand's worth of H, the result would be even worse. Nothing seemed straightforward any more.

But James was right. The stores near his office were alarmed, and there was only one key, so it had to be one of his staff. Eddie Stobart was the newcomer, the unknown quantity. He could easily have switched the powder when James was back and fore, checking the stores. In fact anyone could have stolen it, but his money was on the firm favourite, the man from the Met.

The tranquillity of Twmpath beach wasn't lost on Hook. Moments like this were few and far between. Places where craggy breathtaking landscapes merged with vocal masses of surf that momentarily put things into perspective and oscillated the mind's pendulum from distress to composure. Looking into the rear-view mirror, he caught sight of the gaunt face that stared back at him. Stretching out his chin, he stroked and scratched his dark stubbled throat and started to notice the leanness that pressure had brought. Vainly ransacking his reefer for his first smoke of the morning, he finally gave up with an early morning curse. Pulling up his collar he quietly folded his arms and closed his eyes on the world. With some effort he pushed all his problems towards the back of his mind, and began to listen to the retreating pebbles, as they wrestled with the oncoming tide. His eyes were heavy, and quietly he fell asleep.

Later that morning he drove into the back of Scrubs Lane and deliberately pulled into the parking space allocated to the station's new uniform boss, Chief Inspector Lance Maul. He was in that sort of mood. Already he had decided against informing the station's hierarchy about the missing heroin, preferring to keep it in-house until he'd got to the bottom of it. The grumbling in the pit of his stomach reminded him he was taking one hell of a chance.

Glancing up he saw Corbett, standing at his window on the second floor, claws extended. Wiggling his index finger, he beckoned to Hook who moved his head in acknowledgement. Consulting his watch, he began to wonder what was in store, as he ran up the stairs. It seemed a bit early for lines and detention.

Knocking twice, Hook took a deep breath and went inside. Corbett kept him waiting, as he normally did to everyone who went into his office, pretending on this occasion to look for something on his desk drawer. Standing before him, Hook had already rehearsed an excuse for the misappropriation of the class A drugs. Corbett finally looked up and spoke to the weary-looking man before him.

'You look as though you could do with some annual leave, Hook' he said.

'I had some five years ago sir,' he replied. Corbett ignored him.

'That bent bastard has gone missing.'

'I don't follow, sir.'

'Mrs Jane Gander rang HQ this morning. He hasn't been home for two nights, and she's worried sick'

'I'll get the men out straight away, give the city a sweep. Hotels, flats, relatives, the lot.'

Rising from his chair, Corbett walked slowly across to the window and lowered the blinds. Some important issues were going to be discussed, Hook knew. It was always like this when the blinds were lowered. Corbett must have seen it in a film somewhere.

'Technically, Constable Gander is no longer a serving police officer. His actions, although not yet proven, are nothing short of disgraceful' he said. 'That man has put a huge question mark over your future in the squad.'

'Yes sir.'

'Neither you, nor any member of your team, will search for him. Understand?'

'Yes sir.'

'In fact, nobody at this station is to have any contact with him, unless he fails to answer his bail later this month, in which case he will be arrested.'

'Yes sir,'

'And this information is classified, Inspector.'

'Classified, sir. Yes sir.'

Most of the Squad were already leaving the office when Hook strolled in and summoned them back. Posting a guard at the office door, he said,

'Goose has done a runner. He hasn't been home for the last few nights. Now this isn't an order because I know what the general feeling about him is. But I'm asking you if you can keep an eye out, and let me know if you locate him.'

Ignoring some feeble mumblings of protest behind him, he said loudly,

'Please.'

Turning to the blackboard behind him, he straightened the little model of Spiderman that someone had brought in from a child's nursery. It was pinned against the board with a staple pin through its neck, intended as a humorous reminder of the squad's top objective. When it was put up, there hadn't been much laughter. Written in pink chalk underneath the ten-inch toy with the masked face was the word *suspect*.

During great wars in history, Generals would often have a picture of their opponent hung on the wall. Some felt it was a way of getting to know them. Observing the red and blue figure closely, Hook began to feel exactly the same.

'Who are you, you evil bastard?' he said, pushing the staple even deeper into the miniature neck, drawing a small bead of blood from his thumb.

Breezing into the office with a handful of mail, James began tossing envelopes into baskets on each desk, when she stopped and stared at the holiday postcard from France in her hand. She smiled knowingly.

'Postcard here addressed to Detective Inspector Edward Cedric Stobart,' she said, throwing it onto Stobart's untidy desk

'Been telling your friends porky pies again, Edward?' she laughed, as a red faced Stobart snatched it up in embarrassment.

Hook, who had been busily scrounging a cigarette from an unattended desk, looked over his shoulder with a startled expression.

'What did you say?'

'Been telling porky pies again... ... '

'No, no, the name, the name?'

'Detective Inspector Edward Cedric Stobart' she replied.

For a moment he looked as though he was in the early stages of Alzheimer's, staring around at everyone before scratching the back of his neck. Glaring across at Stobart and then at the postcard he held in his hand, he said,

'My office, Cedric, immediately. You too, James.'

As if in a daze, he walked back into his office, shaking his head, as a nervous Stobart followed dutifully behind. But it wasn't Stobart's efforts to infiltrate and impress the higher echelons of society that he was interested in. And it wasn't the holiday deceit that concerned him.

'Nice name, Cedric, very nice name,' he muttered to himself before slumping down at his desk. 'It has a sort of computerised ring to it.'

He stretched the skin of his face with his fingers, exasperated at his earlier failure to spot the obvious. James just shrugged her shoulders as she followed him into the office.

Bloody Cedric. The acronym CEDRIC. A Customs and Excise computer up at New Scotland Yard. Modern technology that contained the names and addresses of every drug operation in the UK or overseas that Customs ran. It included the name of every user, dealer, trafficker, or snippet of intelligence known to the organisation. The Police of course had their own PNC computer. In fact Joe Brodie had offered a number of times to check people for Hook on the Customs and Excise Drugs Recording Information Computer, better known as CEDRIC. Except it wasn't called CEDRIC any longer. Customs had changed its name over eighteen months ago when the system had been overhauled. So why had he got it wrong?

'What's the name of the Customs computer up at the Yard?' he said, resting back in his chair and pointing to James.

'Can I phone a friend, boss?' she laughed, then spotting the annoyance in Hook's eyes, she went on seriously, 'It's changed. They changed it ages ago to … FREDRIC, wasn't it?'

'Tell me Eddie. It's an acronym for what?'

'About two years ago some boffin in central London changed the data base to the Foreign Recording... ..um... .. Evaluation of Drugs... ..um... ... Regional Information Computer.'

This computer was the Customs bible. What the hell was going on? Why hadn't Brodie been calling it by its correct name?

'Listen boss, I may have told one or two people I met on holiday …' began Stobart, still looking slightly embarrassed.

Raising his hand, Hook stopped him.

'This is important, Eddie, and I want you to listen carefully. I need you to go undercover, down in the docks, immediately. I want you to locate a Joe Brodie. He may be using the name Corbett. He's an undercover Customs man working as a labourer on the Colombian boats so be very discreet. I don't want you to blow his cover. When you find him tell him I need to see him ASAP.'

'Sure thing boss.'

Later that morning, balancing two cups of coffee unsteadily on a plastic tray and carrying a report in her mouth, James went into Hook's office and sat down.

'Another sighting of the Spiderman guy last night,' she said. 'The night shift at Central saw him, drove off before they could get to him.'

Sitting low in his chair with his shoulders hunched up around his ears and both stockinged feet on the radiator, he stared out of his window, totally unimpressed. Lazily he pushed off against the radiator and swivelled around to face her.

'It's the third sighting this week,' she went on.

'Bet you a week's wages they didn't get a description' he said, picking up a set of darts someone had left on his desk before launching them with some venom into the back of his office door.

'Well no, they didn't bach, but it shows he's still around' she said, bending back sharply as a dart flew over her shoulder. Still disinterested, he said,

'Did they clock him anywhere near a police station, by any chance?'

'Aye, across the road from the Reuben Street nick, by a bus stop as it happens.'

'Don't worry. He just craves excitement, he simply wants to adjust the game, make it more stimulating, more exciting.'

'Am I missing something here, bach?' she said.

Pulling on his coat, he looked unconcerned at the report she handed him, dropping it into his bottom drawer, a drawer now packed with unsigned paperwork.

'He's stopped outside a city police station. He's playing with us. He's getting bored.'

'How can you be so sure?'

'Can anyone describe him yet?'

'Well no, nobody's got that close, you and I have probably been the nearest and even we can't describe him. The night shift thought the Mini had darkened windows.'

'That's all we need.'

Buttoning up his reefer, he kicked open the fire escape door and cautiously made his way down the iron stairway. Holding tightly onto the rail, he moved like a man who had once fallen. Alcohol may have played its part.

Grabbing her duffle coat, she trotted after him for yet another trawl of the city streets, in search of the elusive Spiderman guy.

'Who the bloody hell is he boss?' she said as he started up the Sunbeam Talbot in the yard below.

'Who the hell is he?'

Bursting into life, the misfiring engine brought inquisitive faces to the second floor windows, while excessive decibels disturbed the typing pool on the ground floor. Peeping through his office blinds on the second floor, Jack Corbett shook his head and silently mouthed an expletive.

Proudly accelerating out of Maul's parking spot and through the station gates, Hook said,

'He's a crackerjack of a psycho. Callous, confident and egotistical, he's intelligent and physically strong, and murder has little effect on him,' he continued. 'I don't think he works for anyone and I think he has a psychological hatred of people connected with drugs. We're nowhere near him at the moment and he knows it. He's getting bored. He wants to play.'

'You sure about that?' she said.

'Not really' he said, as they stuttered along the dual carriageway, holding up traffic. 'But it should keep Corbett off my back for a few days.'

Two days later, clutching his hand luggage, Hook made his way through the city's international airport and out through the automatic doors to the drop-off zone, where James awaited in her CV Saloon. Throwing his luggage onto the back seat, he gave a huge sigh of relief as they accelerated away in the fading evening light.

Two days in a land which had the hardest toilet paper in Europe, and unhelpful Gendarmes who always seemed to talk when there was nothing to say, had been tiresome.

'How was Montpellier, cariad?' she said, as he tossed her some duty-free perfume.

'My counterpart had garlic breath, and all they did was eat.'

'And the murder in the warehouse?'

'Same MO as ours. The femoral artery was severed and he bled to death.'

'And were his trousers cut off and stuffed in his mouth?'

'No, that was the only difference. Benazzi was wearing shorts.'

'He was lucky then' she said.

Hook rolled his eyes.

'The French are chasing their tails at the moment, but he's our man alright,' he went on. 'I'll fill you in later with the details. Brodie been in touch yet?'

With his arms folded and his head nodding at intervals, Hook struggled to stay awake. Pulling up at a set of traffic lights opposite St Mary's Roman Catholic Church, which stood nobly on top of a small grassy knoll overlooking the dual carriageway, James began to drum the steering wheel with her fingers in her impatience.

Suddenly one of the huge oak doors of the church began to squeak. At first she didn't recognise the man who shuffled out and tottered down the steps unsteadily. He looked haggard and drawn. Long flowing hair had now been replaced by a shaven white skull, while his filthy chino trousers and raincoat pointed to nights of isolation on hard park benches. Despairing eyes told her of the black unrelenting depression that had been his only companion, while the neck of a bottle hung precariously out of his coat pocket.

'Jesus Christ,' she cried 'It's Goose.'

They clambered out of the car, leaving it abandoned at the traffic lights. But he had seen them, and in no time had disappeared into a small housing development behind the church. Within minutes Hook had given up the chase and returned to the church steps, where James sat alongside a smashed bottle of dark rum.

'Good God boss, he looked terrified,' she said.

Pushing open the heavy oak door just enough for him and James to squeeze through, they both stood for a moment in the dimness on the black and white chequered floor that stretched all the way down to the altar. A considerable white crucifix above the altar drew their eyes towards the ceiling.

Shafts of red and yellow light gently tainted their faces, as the sodium streetlights outside burst through leaded light windows all around. Fussing around with two burning altar candles at the far end of the church they could see the figure of a small man in the darkness. Hook could see he wore a large black trilby hat, grey double-breasted overcoat and a brown scarf, with the slightest hint of a clerical dog collar showing. It was early closing time at the house of God.

Together the two made their way along the central aisle, past the now empty pews, when James touched Hook's arm and pointed to the open door on the confessional box a short distance away. Hook had hoped that Goose was using the church to escape the elements, but somehow the open door left too much of a clue. He knew Goose was attempting to crawl out of a deep black abyss that was beginning to close at the top. Wondering if a friend ripped to shreds by remorse would make it, made his conscience shiver.

Stopping at the foot of the altar, a small notice affixed to the grey marble plinth caught Hook's eye.

In heavy black print it said, *Alarm. The Sanctuary and Tabernacle are both Alarmed. Please Keep Out.*

'Crime prevention eventually comes to the Papacy. Is nothing sacrosanct, Father?' said Hook, turning to the cleric, his voice echoing around the church.

'Instant gratification, that's all the youth of today want,' grumbled the ageing Irish priest. 'They want everything straightaway, nobody waits anymore,' he said, still leaning over the altar. 'Last week I found used syringes in our font. I have to lock up every night.'

Flashing his warrant card Hook said,

'A good friend of ours and a member of this church, Max Gander, has just left here in a hurry. We're worried about him.'

Pulling a torch from his overcoat pocket, the old man switched it on and pointed its beam at the tiny plastic wallet that Hook held out before him.

'Yes, we have spoken,' he said. 'But of course our dialogue has to remain private and secret.'

'Listen father,' pleaded Hook, 'I respect the laws of religious confidentiality, but I need to speak to Max. I need to know if he's alright.'

'I'm afraid, Mr Hook, that's impossible. The confessional is between Mr Gander and his spiritual director and no one else. I just hope you can understand that.'

'The guy's in a mess for goodness sake. He has a wife and three kids, as you probably know, and I think he's in dire need of help. Wouldn't you agree?'

As the three began to make their way back along the aisle towards the door, outside shafts of light which spread across the pews began to light up the priests face. James eyes began to brighten.

'Wait,' she said 'This is all rather hypocritical, doesn't religion have anything to do with common sense? All the Inspector and I wish to do is help Max.'

Rushing on ahead, Father Callaghan had quite clearly made up his mind and had little else to say. '

I'm sorry,' he called back. 'It's confidential.'

'Do you know the definition of confidentiality, Father?' said James with a little forcefulness in her voice.

Suddenly the little man hesitated before turning around sharply. Under the brim of his trilby he appeared angry. Hook bowed his head, but he knew James well enough to know that her knowledge of definitions was generally pretty sound. The majority she'd made up herself.

'It's when two police officers feel that when they arrest a man of the cloth for indecency in a public toilet, he should be given a chance. If they feel it would be of more benefit to everyone concerned, including his parishioners, if they let him off with a caution and kept an eye on him rather than totally ruin the rest of his life.'

'Isn't this blackmail, miss?'

'You can call it what you like, I call it common sense,' she said. 'We're here to help.'

Hook suddenly recognised the ecclesiastical groper in the darkness.

'His mental state' he said. 'Is Max in danger?'

The Priest nodded quickly, clearly embarrassed by this untimely reminder of his sexual antecedents.

'And how long have we got to find him?'

'He seems to have abandoned all hope,' the Father replied sadly.

'How long?' said Hook, beginning to lose patience. 'How bloody long?'

'Forty eight hours' said the priest.

Sitting at a corner table in The Red Balloon cafe near the dock gates, Hook's fingers began to squeak on the window as he rubbed a small inquisitive hole in the condensation, before peeping out impatiently towards the docks entrance. It was early afternoon the following day and he'd been searching for most of the night. Still there was no sign of Goose.

He watched as, at the far end of the café, a small weasel of a man in his late fifties, with out-of-date sideboards but an up-to-date criminal record, begin to unzip a red training bag full of stolen cigarettes. Furtively he began selling cartons to the unshaven Greek proprietor behind the counter. Hook himself had already turned down two hundred. With a heavily-lined face, a thin pencil moustache and wearing a small brown trilby, Hook wondered if he'd been one of the Great Train robbers.

He watched the little thief disappear through the door, took a last good look at him and photocopied the man's face in his mind. There would be another time. But there just wasn't enough time in the day any more to deal with two-bit villains; there were more important matters at hand. Preserving his job had to be one.

Smashing crockery after a meal at The Red Balloon generally had little to do with Greek culture or tradition. Plates were normally thrown against the wall following complaints about the food. Pushing away his plate of autopsy and gravy, he sipped cautiously on his mug of tea when the skinny, middle aged waitress, with hair like lacquered candyfloss, returned to his table. He put her about forty five, divorced, and had about as much sex appeal as a fire hydrant. Staring at Hook's lunch, she pulled the cigarette from her mouth and leant over his table. There were two buttons missing from her white low-cut blouse. If she'd had a cleavage at one time, it wasn't there now. Not enough time in the mirror, thought Hook as the smudged lipstick moved in closer.

'You haven't touched your food, luv' she said, touching his shoulder gently. 'Anything the matter?'

It had been a long time since Hook had been pulled, and he was flattered.

'No, no,' he replied. 'I probably should have had the moussaka.'

'You did have the moussaka, lovely,' she said.

Just then a frozen Stobart rushed into the busy café, out of breath.

'Sorry I'm late' he said, pulling up a brown wooden spoon-back chair and sitting down.

'Right' Hook said quietly, before resting his folded arms on the table. 'When is Brodie going to ring me.?'

Stobart appeared tense as he leaned across the soiled gingham tablecloth.

'He's not, boss. He doesn't work here' he whispered.

Irritated, Hook began scratching the back of his neck. Glancing around the busy cafe for prying eyes, he glared back across the table once more.

'Corbett. Jack Corbett. I told you he may be using the name Jack Corbett.'

'I've checked both names thoroughly. I've got friendly with a girl in the Docks office whose got access to the computer here. Your man doesn't exist, boss' he whispered again.

'Right, well, if the computer says he isn't working down here, that's it then' Hook muttered sarcastically. 'You telling me you've spent two days chatting up some bird, while the enquiry has been done by computer technology?'

There was concern on his face and Stobart could see it. It wasn't in Hook's nature to be sarcastic with any of his staff, but he was tired. So much to do, so little time.

Stobart had checked, double-checked and re-checked every single employee at the docks. Even when his shift had finished he'd spent the remaining hours keeping obs near the docks entrance, or visiting the rough dockside pubs in search of the elusive Joe Brodie. He knew his boss would have trouble accepting the news, and Hook's body language told him he was right.

'God's honour boss, a month's pay, the guy's not working here.'

'Perhaps he's casual labour, off the books, off the bloody computer, working for some small time firm nobody knows about. Perhaps he's hiding from the Social.'

'Listen boss, I know what he looks like. Don't forget I've got the photo they took at the nick after he was bagged. There are thirteen Scotsmen employed down here and I've personally checked every single one. One is in hospital, which I've checked, and another dropped dead on the job two days ago.'

Hook's eyes almost showed signs of optimism, but Stobart shook his head quickly.

'Sorry. I've been down the morgue boss' he said. 'It's not him.'

'Colombian iron ore boats, he's working undercover on a big job' he pleaded, but Stobart moved his head from side to side.

'If Customs say they're working on a big cocaine job, they must be down here somewhere.'

Eddie Stobart smiled weakly, he looked pale and ill at ease.

'Okay, okay Eddie what is it. Spit it out.'

Pulling his chair up closer to the table, Stobart quickly checked the cafe behind him. He cleared his throat nervously as he leant across the table and stared directly into his inspectors eyes.

'They haven't had a Colombian boat in here for three years.'

Not too many people got one over on Hook, and the gnawing truth for him, as the enormity of his problems began to mount, was that Customs had done exactly that. They had made him look a prat. The bastard Brodie was working on a big job alright. But could it be Babylon.

'Okay Eddie, thanks' he said. 'You've done well.'

Dropping some cash alongside his plate of untouched wet dough, Hook got to his feet and brushed himself down.

'Okay if I pick the restaurant next time, boss?' Stobart called, as the DI opened the door to leave.

Stepping out onto the dank terraced street, beneath gigantic overhead cranes that seemed to stretch out forever, the wind flew directly up the street towards him, causing his face to sting and his eyes to water. Sheltering in the doorway of a funeral parlour, he cupped his cold hands around a cigarette, and lit up quickly. For a moment he began to enjoy the warm phosphorus scent of the match that filled his nostrils, while he seriously began to consider if there ever would be a next time.

Later that same afternoon, the phone rang on Hook's desk. The voice came from a telephone kiosk somewhere near the city's railway station, he knew. He could hear shunting trains and a British Rail announcer in the background.

'I understand you've been looking for me.'
'Don't you think we need to talk?'
'Where?'
'You like French films?'

An hour later, Hook, with an upturned collar and black scarf that hid most of his face, hurried along Quilp Street, a dingy area at the far end of

Kensington lane. Occasionally he stopped, checking on reflections in shop windows to see if he was being followed, before quickly moving off again like an agitated pimp, with his head down. Stopping again outside a closed antique shop, he glanced along the street again before disappearing through the double swing doors of the Bijou cinema next door. He hadn't been followed.

A tall, thin man in his sixties, with glossy slashed-back hair, a shiny dinner suit, a dickie bow and brown shoes, watched him suspiciously as entered the foyer. Hook guessed, by the huge brilliantine quiff that rose at the front of his head like a great bow wave on a cruise liner, that in a former life he'd probably been a Teddy Boy. He had an air of management about him. Hook nodded his head politely.

The airless, decaying picture house smelt of cheap deodorants and ice cream. Searching for some money in his coat pocket, he approached the glass box office that was the size of a large freezer and seemed just as cold. The surrounding walls were covered with large black and white photographs of dead Hollywood movie stars, all of them in a lopsided pose as they stared out from their portraits and up at the ceiling. An overweight Bette Davis look-alike occupied the box office and appeared jammed inside. Bug eyed and heavily made up, her severely permed wavy hair didn't move an inch as the gusting easterly wind accompanied Hook inside. Moving like a stiff-backed guardsman, the manager stepped forward and sharply pulled the doors shut. Hook nodded again.

'One single, downstairs' he said, pushing the money through a hole in the glass.

'Upstairs is closed due to house renovations anyway luv' she said, shoving a small blue ticket towards him. 'And our usherette is off sick so you'll have to find your own seat. The main feature has started.'

Pulling at his scarf so it hung loosely on his neck, he made his way through the swing doors into the darkened auditorium along a dark red carpet that felt as though he was walking on freshly laid tarmac. Sitting in the empty back row, the whole row of dusty seats squeaking under his weight, he glanced at his watch, sat back and waited.

At the far side of the cinema he watched two blonde spiky-haired men in their late twenties kissing and giggling as the black and white images of the naturist film rolled on towards the intermission. He pulled back his sleeve and studied his watch again. He knew he had to be out of there before the lights came up. Seated down at the front, a bald-headed man moved his hands in his pockets suspiciously quickly.

Hooks eyes began to feel heavy, bored by the celluloid nakedness that jumped, dived or swam all over the screen before him. Sitting comfortably was the kiss of death for an overtired detective; even the tanned pendulous Parisian breasts failed to energise him. Pulling a cigarette packet from inside his coat, he popped one into his mouth and sparked up. Now, how was he going to play this?'

The row of pull-up seats began to vibrate as someone made their way towards him. Slumping down alongside him, Brodie held out his hand.

'Sorry I'm late,' he said.

'Thanks for ringing me.'

'No problem. A contact in the docks said someone had been enquiring about me. I thought it was you. I thought I saw you leaving the docks café.'

It was too dark to check the look in Brodie's eyes, to see if the bastard was lying again. It was just his voice he had to go on. Brodie's breathing was fast and deep. He had either been running or he was becoming a little nervous.

'Forget the job for a moment Joe. Just tell me, as a mate, why you lied to me.'

'Just listen Harry. I've only got a few minutes. I'm due to meet someone urgently. Yes, I'm undercover and have been for twelve months. I'm not actually working out of the docks all the time and I'm not looking at the McCanns, though they're on the periphery of the enquiry. I should have trusted you Harry, and I apologise. Can I just say there's a top cabinet minister involved? Westminster. You know what I'm saying.'

'You Customs boys never change, Joe' Hook said, still trying to finds Brodie's eyes in the dimness.

'End of the week Harry, I'll ring you and fill in all the blanks. I promise.'

'Cross your heart and hope to die?'

Brodie laughed and lent forward. Talking quietly he said,

'Now before I go, this may be something or nothing so don't get excited. I'm back and fore the docks and I've got friendly with a second engineer on the SS Arianna out of Buenos Aires. Anyway, one of the chefs on board went AWOL just before Christmas and still hasn't returned. They haven't told the authorities as yet. The captain's afraid they'll impound the ship.'

'Name?'

'Hector Barrantes, approximately thirty six years old, homosexual, born Maldonado, Argentina. Released Maracaibo prison, served fifteen years for murdering his boyfriend in a Buenos Aires dockside bar where they worked.'

'Description?' said Hook his eyebrows raised, almost touching his hairline.

Brodie seemed to think long and hard. Staring at Hook, he eventually whispered,

'Six one, athletic build, normally unshaven, thick black hair, untidy, swarthy complexion. Last seen wearing jeans and black donkey-type jacket. Listen,' he said getting to his feet. 'I'll have more for you by the end of the week. I've got to rush.'

'This second engineer, I'll need to speak to him.'

'Leave him to me for the moment. It's confidential and he doesn't want the police involved. They're hoping Barrantes will return shortly. Let me work on him.' He patted Hook on the shoulder.

'Hang on. How'd he kill his boyfriend, Joe?' Hook said, getting up.

'Stabbed him with one of his kitchen knives, somewhere near the stomach area. He bled to death before he reached the hospital.'

After watching Brodie burst back out through the swing doors and into the foyer, he sat back down and began to smile. A south American merchant seaman floating around the city with previous convictions for murder with a knife. Lighting up another Gitanes cigarette, he sat back and began to enjoy the tingling in his lower back.

CHAPTER NINETEEN

It was just before seven the following morning when Hook walked into the busy charge-room and threw Harry Griffiths a packet of duty-free cigarettes. James almost bumped into him as she ran through the unit out of breath.

'Twmpath Cliffs - there's a guy in a car up there, the caller thinks he's got a shooter. Anyone fancy it?' she said.

'If I wasn't stuck in this bloody pit, I'd love to,' lied Griffiths, as Hook chased after her

'When I returned to the station last night there was a message on the answering machine for you' she said, still panting.

Pulling out the choke on her little Citroen parked in the station yard, she went on,

'I tried to ring you but your mobile was switched off.'

The engine fired into life like a Suffolk Punch lawn mower. Hook yawned and muttered something incoherent, which sounded like 'Sorry'.

'Anyway,' she continued, as he yawned again. 'He had a Scottish accent and said he enjoyed the film. Said he'll be ringing you shortly with some info that should please you'

Hook's forehead creased as the automatic gates began to open, very slowly, in front of them.

'Say anything else?' he said, still appearing unconcerned.

'Yes, gave us the number of a red ford transit van leaving the docks at midnight with ten grands worth of cocaine. A couple of the lads arrested three men from Liverpool. Nice little tickle, bach! You got anymore informants like him hidden away?'

Hook stared across at her and raised an eyebrow.

Driving hesitantly along a narrow icy lane that lead to the cliff tops five miles outside the city, James' concentration increased dramatically as the roar of the channel, hundreds of feet below, greeted them. Ploughing cautiously along the winding coastal road, with her nose almost pressed against the windscreen, the wind buffeted the little Citroen around like a fairground ride. Occasionally they caught sight of the grey mass down below, as it continued to batter away furiously at the foot of the cliffs.

Approaching a dry stone wall with an entrance just big enough for a car to drive through, a grim-faced armed response officer in a black baseball cap waved his MPS submachine gun from behind the wall, bringing the Citroen to a sliding emergency stop.

It didn't take Hook long to spot the rest of the armed teams concealed behind silvery bending trees and snow-capped stone walls, brandishing an assortment of firepower that pointed directly towards a red car parked in the centre of the cliff top. He could see that deep tyre tracks led to the stationary Audi saloon, now surrounded by a foot of thick white snow that glinted as dawn began to break.

Motionless at the wheel of the car, the driver sat crying, fifty yards from the cliff edge. They couldn't hear a great deal in the howling gale but the smoke from its exhaust told them the engine was still running.

When the number plate came into view, Hook's stomach began to turn cartwheels. There was no need to ask. He knew who was at the wheel.

Crouching, they ran to the wall where Chief Inspector Lance Maul sat shouting instructions into his radio. There was urgency and barely-controlled panic in his voice as he struggled with the extra responsibility promotion had brought. His puffy face was now blood-pressure red. He looked as though he'd spent a night in a coracle in the north Atlantic.

'I require a trained negotiator at the scene immediately' he said, shouting even louder into his radio. He threw Hook a steely glare, reminding him who now had that extra pip on his shoulder.

'Why do you want a negotiator?' called Hook, slumping down on the icy grass alongside him, while the primal scream of gale-force winds turned dialogue into a shouting match.

'I said - why do you want a negotiator?' he shouted again, nudging him earnestly with his shoulder.

'An old lady walking her dog asked him if he was alright. He told her to piss off. Something was pointed, she thinks it could be a handgun' Maul shouted back, holding onto his new black and white checked baseball hat that rested comically on slightly protruding ears.

'But she's not sure.'

'No.'

'So why don't you just ask him if he's armed. Speak to him, he won't bite.'

'My concern is the safety of others, Hook, not just him.'

'What others, for God's sake? If you all fuck off and leave him, he'll be okay.'

'You know the score regarding ACPO procedures relating to firearms incidents, I take it.'

'Oh I know the score alright, Lance. He's not parked over there watching the wildlife, the man's in a crisis. Any second now, he's going to drive over the fucking edge. He's not here to shoot anyone, and you bloody know it.'

Hook paused to allow the words to sink in.

'Listen Hook, I'm the Operational Commander here, and I'm suggesting the two of you return to the Station. I've got all the advice and manpower I need.'

Pulling up the hood on her duffle coat, James began to get to her feet when Hook pulled her back roughly, causing her to slump down awkwardly against the wall. She cursed, and blamed herself. She should have known her boss wouldn't go quietly.

'Goose isn't armed, Lance. He's living in his own world of desperation, he's unbalanced. Let me have a word. All these guns are going to do is spook him.'

Tugging again on the peak of his baseball hat, which the gale continually threatened to dislodge, Maul never moved an inch.

'Watch my lips, I'm the OIC here. Now the negotiator will be here in about twenty five minutes, so I want you both to return to Scrubs Lane, understand?'

'By that time it could be too late' said Hook.

'That's not my problem. Max Gander, it seems, has already been parked here most of the night. Half an hour won't make that much difference.'

Sitting with her arms folded and her back tight against the wall, James began to consult her watch. It was only a matter of time before Hook gave up on Maul and committed his first disciplinary offence of the morning. By her reckoning disobedience to orders was about twenty seconds away.

'Look' he said impatiently, 'this silence, this quietness, nobody saying anything, nobody doing anything - there's no dialogue. For Christ's sake, this isn't tactics - it's sheer bloody incompetence!'

'Ten seconds' she whispered, looking up at the sky, as the sea hit the foot of the cliffs with a deafening thud.

'You have a responsibility towards Goose as well as the safety of others, Lance. Don't allow your own prejudices to influence what needs to be done here. You've got to help him, Lance.'

Turning slowly to face him, Maul fixed Hook with the slightest hint of a contemptuous grin.

'You talk about incompetence? When you and your squad's reputation is in tatters?' he screamed into the wind. 'Now I'm only going to say this once more. I want you off this plot.'

'Will you please, please allow me and James just five minutes with him? Just a few minutes?'

It was Hook's last attempt at mannerly common sense.

'Please.'

'Just two minutes, Inspector. I'm giving you and Sergeant James just two minutes to withdraw from this plot, and that's an order.'

Folding her arms even tighter, James rolled her eyes and threw a glance up towards the heavens while she waited for her inspector's final reply. She had a fair idea that it wasn't likely to be some eloquent prose.

'It beggars belief how someone like you ever got to the rank of Chief Inspector' Hook shouted. 'Because you're an arsehole. You always have been an arsehole and you always will be an arsehole' he yelled, their noses almost touching.

James looked across at her boss. She'd heard worse descriptions.

Clambering over the dry stone wall, Hook ignored several requests to stop and began to jog towards the car. He began to wonder if he had done the right thing, as the wind buffeted him and the cliff edge came suddenly into view. He hadn't realised it was that close.

Shouting instructions into his radio, as baseball hats and the barrels of submachine guns popped up and down over adjoining walls like ducks in a shooting gallery, the Operational Commander could only watch in vain. With the front of her grey duffle coat flapping about like the wings of an aggressive swan, James scrambled over and ran after her boss.

Out of breath, she finally caught up with him, standing twenty yards from the Audi. The engine idled quietly while Goose sat, staring out at the channel, with the driver's window halfway down. Dark shadows under heavy half-closed eyes and a huge grin across a pasty face greeted his colleagues, as he changed his emotions in the blink of an eye.

'Well, well if it isn't my old dependable friend, Mr Harry Hook,' he slurred. 'What kept you?' He chuckled like a baby. 'The inner voice of conscience keeping you awake at night, Harry?' he shouted, revving the engine until it squealed like a slaughtered pig.

Trying to remain upright in the middle of the cliff top was like trying to stand in a small rowing boat on a choppy sea. Hook and James interlocked their arms, while the surrounding armed officers watched them carefully.

'Well, that's solved the mystery of the missing heroin' Hook said. 'He's bloody full of smack, he probably thinks he can fly off the bloody cliff edge.'

Lifting a bag of white powder from inside the car, Goose waved it laughingly at them, like a naughty schoolboy.

'A hundred doses of happiness, just a little pick-me-up to help me towards the edge this morning, Inspector,' he called, scattering fine grains of diamorphine out to the wind.

'Listen Goose, just switch the engine off a moment, let's talk about this,' he yelled. 'I don't think I've got much time. Lance is on the warpath.'

'You let me down Harry. You didn't have to do it, you know you didn't. You finished me, Harry.'

His cold cheeks were stained by a night of tears.

'Don't fool about, Goose. They think you've got a gun.'

'How else would I have got you up here?' he shouted, pulling his daughter's toy water pistol from the glove compartment.

Squeezing it off in Hook's direction, he shouted, 'Bang, bang, you're dead, Harry!' as the wind pushed the jet of water back into his face.

Fifty yards away two high-powered velocity rifles gripped by grim-faced snipers continued to aim their tiny red laser spots that moved discreetly around Goose's chest.

'Don't piss around with that water pistol Goose' shouted James. 'You're not flavour of the month with some of these armed response boys you know. Just give us five minutes.'

'I may not have that long left. I've got a dicky heart you know' he said, beginning to sob.

'We know,' she shouted. 'Just a few minutes, Goose. Think of the family, your kids. Think of the future' she went on, moving closer to the car.

As if in a warning that they were getting too close, Goose let the handbrake off slowly, causing the cable to whine noisily as the car's weight strained for a moment under the tension. Moving steadily, it began to gain momentum down the small incline towards the cliff edge. Although the gear was in neutral Goose continued to rev the engine furiously, before snatching up the handbrake, bringing it to a sliding halt twenty yards from the six hundred foot drop. Arm in arm, they quickly followed.

Screaming wildly with other allegations of betrayal, his emotions turned on their head again as anger suddenly replaced blubbering distress.

'I asked you for a chance Harry, but you threw me to the lions. You've taken my family, my dignity, my life, everything.'

'I'm not letting you go, Goose' shouted Hook. 'You're not fucking nailing me to the cross, not until we have a talk.'

With the sea winds nudging them dangerously towards the edge, James held onto her boss's arm tightly while someone began shouting his name in the background. She knew exactly who it was.

Leaning across the passenger seat Goose forced open the door, which the gale almost ripped off its hinges. Patting the leather passenger seat with his hand, he called out, 'Okay Harry, let's talk.'

James felt an even colder chill move up her back, a chill that had nothing to do with the weather or the wind. She knew this wasn't Goose any more. This was no standard cry for help. She could almost feel his determination.

Hanging onto Hook's arm tighter than a kid at the dentist, James shouted, as she felt him begin to move.

'Don't you bloody dare boss, don't you bloody dare! We've lost him and we're not going to get him back. This is all about retribution and vengeance!'

Hook's mind scrambled around in confusion while he stared for a moment at the empty passenger seat twenty feet away. There was nothing about incidents like this in the police training manual.

With a mixture of tears and laughter, Goose's rantings became almost incoherent as he continually invited Hook to join him in the front of the car. There was little Hook could do, other than stand and watch, as the early morning tension tightened to a conclusion that was inevitable. Hook could already sense that Goose was a clean white sheet away from a Co-op funeral.

'The way down to hell is easy, Harry,' he cried, the cold tears streaming down his unshaven cheeks. 'Getting into the front here with me is the awkward bit.'

'Don't Goose, don't do this! It doesn't have to be like this!' Hook screamed, still fighting to remain upright as he and James held onto each other tightly.

With one eye on the cliff edge, Hook looked on hopelessly as the rear wheels began to spin savagely, throwing up icy crusted earth, while the engine revved wildly. James seized Hook's arm so tightly it was beginning to bruise, but they could only watch as the waving detective with the lopsided grin accelerated the Audi into the vast grey space of infinity before him. Although he seemed to be smiling, his eyes were already dead.

Four and a half seconds later the vehicle fractured into a hundred pieces as it bounced around on the rocks below.

James clenched her jaw as she struggled to hold back the tears. There was no way a male armed response team, let alone Maul, was going to see her break down. While the stand-by ambulance and the armed teams headed down to the beach, he tugged on her arm and pulled her away from the edge.

'Let's get out of here,' he said.

Heading back along the M4 Motorway towards Scrubs Lane, he was ready for the *you're becoming a loose cannon* speech from Corbett. Goose was now just another Coroner's statistic. The feeling that everything had been his fault continued to eat away at him.

James could see the trouble features sitting alongside her, so she veered into a service area for coffee and an informal de-brief. They needed a little space.

'You okay?' she said as he continually tapped his little plastic spoon on the sugar jar, staring down at the busy motorway.

'The thing is, are you okay?'

'Aren't I always? Don't I always survive?'

Sitting in a quiet corner of the cafeteria, he nodded.

'Yep, you always do.'

'Listen cariad, this is not your fault. It's not anyone's fault.'

'But he engineered it all. He knew an armed incident would get me there. He wanted me in that car.'

Whispering, she replied,

'Let's get this straight - he was depressed and he took his life. But whether he was unstable, frightened or plain greedy, he became the traitor, not you or I. It was an uncontrollable set of circumstances.'

'That's it then,' he said sarcastically.

'No, it's not actually. It may not be the right time to mention this, but I ran into Helen in a wine bar in town yesterday.'

Hook dropped the plastic spoon.

'Give her a call, boss. She wants to talk to you.'

'I will' he said. 'But there's one quick call I need to make first. I've got to get to the bottom of this.'

She watched with interest as he began tapping out a number he had written down on the back of his hand. He lifted the mobile to his ear, scanning the cafeteria instinctively. Planting the first French cigarette of the morning between his white dry lips, he acknowledged and smiled genially at a passing waitress who was old enough to be his mother.

'My God, you have missed her' she said, leaning over and pressing a button. 'I find the reception is better with it switched on, bach.'

Hook made a face.

While he slowly redialled the number he said,

'I need to find out what Joe Brodie's investigating. I think it could involve Babylon and maybe some top government minister. But I'm not happy, don't ask me why, but I'm not.'

'Customs and Excise Drug Investigation Department' said a deep cockney voice on the other end. 'London Division.'

'Morning squire, I need to speak to Joe Brodie urgently,' said Hook

'Who?'

'Customs investigator Joe Brodie. I used to nark for him ages ago. I got something tasty.'

The sound of the handset being dropped like a hot potato and chairs being scraped on an office floor caused his eyebrows to meet. But he just had to find out what Joe Brodie was investigating.

'Who is this?' grunted the second man.

'Just tell him it's the Fatman, he'll know,' he said in a fake cockney accent.

Shaking her head, James just sipped her coffee quietly.

'Where are you speaking from? Give me your address? How can we meet?'

'Hang on a second squire, that's three questions all in one. Now I'm not some two-bit grass, you understand? But it's urgent I speak to Brodie. I only deal with him when I get this information. Now is he there or what?'

Covering the mouthpiece, he sat and listened to the noise of more chairs being quickly moved, and the muffled chattering of urgent voices in the background. Dropping his cigarette into the ashtray his brow wrinkled again, when a third and even more articulate voice came on and addressed him. It had to be the top man.

'Good morning sir, may I help you?' said the voice.

'Christ almighty, I hope some bugger can!' he said. 'Now I haven't spoken to Mr Brodie for a long time, but there's a thousand keys of 'puff coming through one of the ports in the morning and I need to speak to him fast.'

'Would we be talking about cannabis, sir?'

'Well I ain't talking about the magic dragon, squire.'

'Where exactly are you calling from, sir?'

'Fucking hell, I'm handing you a two million quid job on a plate and you're doing some sort of moody on me. I take it he does still work for your empire?'

'Well we do require to know who you are, before we disclose that kind of information, sir.'

'If I ring back tonight, eight 'o'clock, will you give me a number where I can reach him?'

'Would you be prepared to let one of my men in the office here deal with you sir? You'll get quite a substantial informant's fee of course.'

'No, it's okay, sunshine. I'll ring the old bill instead and speak to one of their police horses,' he jeered. 'I'll probably get more bloody sense out of them.'

'They're playing silly buggers' he said, cutting them off. 'There's something up alright. There's no way Customs would turn down two million quid's worth of cannabis. They're no different to us; they'd have a way of contacting him in an emergency. There's something strange going on. I'm not happy.'

'So - is your mate still with Customs?'

'He's got to be. Perhaps his undercover is so tight they can't pull him out. But we're going to find out for definite.'

'We off up the smoke then? Will I need an overnight bag, Inspector?' she replied, fluttering her eyelashes mockingly.

'Get a life, James' he said.

Standing tall and erect on a disgustingly cheap carpet remnant, Hook began to think of Helen with her big brown eyes and laughing smile. It had been a long time since the thought of a cosy dinner at her flat had happily dominated his thoughts. Outside a small robin landed on the snow-covered window ledge, desperately searching for food, while Corbett sat before him droning on about loyalty and discipline.

Every five minutes thoughts of Goose returned.

The words 'loose cannon' figured frequently in his ten minute diatribe as he had expected, as did the words reorganisation, respect and corruption. Clenching his jaw, Hook successfully stifled a yawn. He'd been here before. Watching Corbett's face was like panning for gold – every time you looked, it was always the same, the expression surly. It never changed.

But nothing seemed to matter now, as again thoughts of Helen began to return. How she smelt, the warmth of her embrace, the fullness of her lips … He forced his interest back to the tiny bird, flying from sill to sill, refusing to give in, scratching, scavenging for survival, when suddenly the very word rocked him back on his heels. Uniform.

His eyes didn't actually bulge, but they did a close impression. It felt as if Corbett had deliberately urinated over his shoes in the gents.

Uniform. Oh no. There was no way he was going to spend the next fifteen years in an ill-fitting NATO pullover, with the constant reminder of who he worked for emblazoned across his chest. Visiting pubs to ensure everyone was the right age or signing the time sheets of senile lollipop ladies on rainy afternoons.

Wet-nursing probationer constables who hadn't yet started shaving was as important as any other job in the force. But detective work had been his whole life, his very existence, since he'd chosen this career, and here, with one foul sweep of Corbett's cheap biro, it was all going to end. It was a seasoned and passionate detective's worst torment, a sideways move back to street duties in a silly hat.

'Why?' said Hook. 'Uniform?' The very word almost stuck in his throat.

'A week Monday, and your enquiry regarding Babylon will be taken over by your replacement. The chief constable has been appraised of the transfer. Jeopardising an armed operation was the last straw.'

Corbett smirked.

'I didn't endanger anything!' Hook shouted. 'Sir' he added, lowering his voice.

'DC Gander was waiting for me to appear. He wanted me to see it all. In fact he was looking for a co-driver to go over the edge with him. And he wanted it to be me.'

'That's not Chief Inspector Maul's version of events.'

'Has Chief Superintendent Mulholland sanctioned my move?'

'He's on annual leave.'

What a coincidence, though Hook.

'I take it you'll want me to work under Chief Inspector what's-his-name downstairs' he said, not hiding the contempt in his voice.

'You know his name, Inspector, and you've got it in one' snapped Corbett with a game-set-and-match smile. 'Yes, you'll be working under Chief Inspector Maul.'

Leaving the office, he could feel his mouth drying up, while Corbett's grinning smirk appeared to grow wider by the second. Just as he was about to open the door, he turned back to face the Superintendent.

'Headquarters have asked me if I would personally inform DC Gander's wife of his death. Like me to offer your condolences, or shall I leave it? Sir?' he said, slamming Corbett's door so violently that the glass decanter rattled loudly in the cabinet next to his desk.

A short while later, as Hook and James drove out of Scrubs Lane through ankle deep slush in a brown Drug Squad Ford Escort van, four smartly dressed men in expensive-looking suits drove into the yard in a black BMW. As it pulled in through the gates, it caused Hook to brake sharply to allow them right of way Arriving like the Mafia at a meeting of the families, the driver appeared to nod in Hook's general direction. The others ignored him. He knew they had all been made an offer they couldn't refuse.

'It's the National Crime Squad' he growled, as the gates slowly closed. Looking into his rear view mirror as they pulled into a parking bay, he said,

'Corbett and Mulholland have lost their bottle.'

'You disappointed?'

'I tell you what I am disappointed in. Every time I bump into the Crime Squad, I seem to be driving this heap of shit and they're driving some prestige top-of-the-range stuff.'

'All our cars are out on jobs boss, this was the only one left in the pool' said James.

'They looked at us as though we'd just emptied a septic tank.'

She chose to ignore that.

'So what do we do now?' she said.

'Let's get out of here before they officially pull us off the case.'

'You think that's really going to happen then?'

'Well, the past twelve months has been a touch *annus horribilis* for the squad.'

'But what about all the seizures, the arrests, the long hours, the chances we take?'

'We aren't exactly squad of the year you know' Hook said. 'We have got a bit of previous for corruption, alcoholism, and now suicide.'

Slipping off her red fleece and turning up the van's heater as they headed for the M4, she turned to face him and frowned.

'Your predecessor, DS Bell, let us all down by screwing a tom in a massage parlour, don't forget' expanded Hook. 'And now Goose has put the tin hat on it.'

Still not fully understanding, she said, '

And the alcoholic?'

'Eddie Stobart. Didn't I tell you? It was on his personal record from the Met.'

The Motorway was relatively quiet, and Hook completed the journey with James in two and half hours, arriving in central London by mid-afternoon. He had kept the earlier conversation with Corbett to himself; his mind still lingered on Goose's death. Corbett and any impending transfer to the uniform branch didn't matter anymore; he'd made up his mind to resign from the force the moment Goose had hit the vastly deep briny.

The visit to London would also give him a little space after his friend's suicide. He knew the tabloids and their reporters would lay siege to Scrubs Lane until they got the story they wanted. Gossipmongers at Scrubs Lane would be holding an open day. And of course there was the arrival of the National Crime Squad. Prior to leaving, he had left details of Hector Barrantes, the missing seaman, with the incident room at Scrubs Lane. It would be up to them to find him.

'Right, we'll play this one by ear. We're nothing to do with drugs, remember' he said.

They hit heavy traffic in central London, a city now swamped by a January sale epidemic.

'If they think we're Drug Squad, they'll give us bugger all. I'll throw Brodie's name into the ring and just see what happens.'

'You really are unsure about Brodie, aren't you?'

'First, he was undercover in the docks, working on some Colombian job,' he said. 'But that was a load of crap. At a guess I think he's still under cover, possibly he's infiltrated the McCann organisation and he'd chasing down that load of Babylon. Getting customs to admit that, I think, is going to be difficult. These guys have diplomas for lying.'

Arriving at the headquarters of Customs and Excise in Lincoln Gardens, they went up to the sixth floor, where they were met, and led into an immaculate office of ankle-deep carpets and expensive furnishings.

'It's got the edge on your pit' she said, pointing to Big Ben and the nearby Houses of Parliament.

He wasn't someone who was easily impressed but he could see that there wasn't a plastic coffee cup or stale half-eaten sandwich to be seen, nor an old newspaper to read in the toilet. In fact ,the office had its own ensuite bathroom. It also smelt very nice.

In the far corner of the room stood an expensive antique French buffet hutch, crammed full with elegant coloured spirits, while a hand-carved box of Havana cigars graced a small marble Italian coffee table in the centre of the room. Just behind the door Hook spotted a beautiful antique French hat stand in dark oak. He wondered why. He'd never observed anyone in Customs wearing a hat.

'Try not to look impressed' he whispered.

Eventually, Senior Customs Investigator Julian Aldermartin breezed into the room, followed by a tall, slim secretary with blonde hair that needed colouring. She reminded Hook of Miss Moneypenny.

Carrying a file of papers, which she left on his desk, she bestowed a weak smile on Hook as she left, giving his reefer jacket and jeans the sort of glance reserved for visiting relatives who brought dog shit into your lounge on the heel of their shoe.

Stretching over his desk, almost as an afterthought, Aldermartin shook them both by the hand, and welcomed them to London. He made them feel as though it was their first time out of the valleys, and they were on some kind of Jim'll Fix It trip with the choir. Hook just smiled; he never trusted people who stared him straight in the eye and whose handshake seemed to go on forever. He immediately recognised Aldermartin's voice as the important-sounding man he had spoken to earlier.

Both he and James settled themselves on a hide Chesterfield sofa that seemed the length of a supermarket aisle.

'Yes I had your call. You are Superintendent Hook, I take it?'

Hook smiled reassuringly, while James raised an eyebrow and threw him an exasperated look. Sometimes she just wished he would prepare her for these moments. It was simply that the Customs head of drugs investigations needed to be outranked if they were going to make any headway with this organisation. Elevating himself when home advantage had been sacrificed tended to help when dealing with Customs.

Still trying her best not to appear inspired by the surroundings, she spotted St Pauls Cathedral in the distance and sighed quietly.

With the fingers of both hands steepled together supporting his double chin, Aldermartin glanced for a moment at the file of papers before him. Hook wondered if the Hugo Boss suit was his everyday wear, or if he had just returned from an important wedding. The Peter Smith shirt was white, crisp and silk, and the tie was Eton. The Knightsbridge haircut wouldn't have given him much change out of sixty quid, and caused Hook to start fidgeting self-consciously with his own unruly curls. A pair of black Italian shoes, probably hand-made, had him slowly rubbing his own badly scuffed footwear slyly up and down the leg of his jeans.

But a poorly-grown thin moustache failed dismally in its efforts to make Aldermartin look older. Hook put him in his early thirties. He spoke like an TV news reader. Hook noticed the heavily nicotine stained second and third fingers on his right hand and doubted if he was as confident as he appeared. There were obvious signs of stress, and he even wondered if the guy had ever worked at the sharp end. Highflyers normally didn't have the time. People like him normally left each department before they were found out

There was no doubt that Aldermartin was being fast-tracked for the higher echelons of the organisation, and equally there was no way he was going to do anything other than by the book. But like all Her Majesty's Customs' men, the bastard was smug.

'Would you explain exactly why you're interested in Joseph Brodie, Superintendent?'

Settling down comfortably on the chesterfield and crossing his legs to appear relaxed, Hook said,

'It's just that he's been clocked near the Docklands down near us by some Murder Squad boys. Someone mentioned he was a Customs investigator so as I was in London today on other enquiries, I thought I'd just check him out. He's not a suspect or anything. This is just a routine check.'

'I'm afraid all the information on Mr Brodie is classified, Superintendent. What I can divulge is that I terminated his contract two years ago, but he never actually returned his ID papers. He just disappeared.'

Hook's stomach began to churn.

'Classified. Of course' replied Hook.

'Is this anything to do with your importation, Superintendent?'

'This is a murder enquiry. I'm sorry, what importation would that be?'

'Come come Superintendent. Marseilles, Babylon, due in the UK shortly.'

'Someone been peeping into our computers again Mr Aldermartin?'

'You must be aware, Superintendent, that Her Majesty's Customs and Excise is afforded pole position in all information relating to drug importations into the United Kingdom, a law dating back to the days of smuggling and piracy.'

Retaining his composure whilst listening to this Customs bullshit was always going to prove difficult, but he needed to stay in control if he were going to stand any chance of getting the information he wanted. Aldermartin had to think he was the guy wearing the big white hat.

'Drug investigation isn't really my speciality, Mr Aldermartin, but I take your point. It may be something our own Drug Squads need to take on board,' he lied.

'Could you tell us why Brodie was sacked?' James asked.

'I'm afraid his medical records are confidential, but as you are aware Superintendent, there is an avenue open if you require sight of them. An official written request from your Chief Constable will suffice' he smiled, shuffling Brodie's papers tantalisingly in front of them.

'Medical records' repeated Hook. 'Was Brodie injured whilst on duty or something?'

'All I can say, Superintendent, is that until we have an official written request from your organisation, Joseph Brodie, in keeping with the highest standards of Her Majesty's Customs and Excise, was an excellent investigator.'

'Of course' he said. 'Of course. Have any of your people had any intelligence on him since his disappearance?' Hook asked casually.

'Some months after we'd dismissed him, someone apparently saw him in a bar on the Costa Brava with two south Wales dealers, but it was never confirmed.'

Big Ben struck three o'clock and Hook began to smile, basking in that warm tingling feeling as it began to stride deliciously along his vertebrae towards the back of his neck.

Of course. The McCanns and Brodie. Yes, he should have known. Those photos. Some partnership. Some team. No wonder they had been difficult to nail. Even drug organisations had their own spin-doctors now, he thought.

Still sitting with his head resting on his interlocking fingers, Aldermartin smiled grandly.

'When you locate him next, let me know.'

Hook nodded politely, while a little voice at the back of his mind was yelling 'bollocks!' through cupped hands.

The meeting over, both rose to leave when Aldermartin took Hook by the arm and pulled him gently towards the buffet hutch. Throughout the meeting he'd been waiting patiently for this moment and was well prepared. He was just beginning to wonder why it had taken so long. He knew it had little to do with alcohol and hospitality.

'If I could digress for just one moment, Superintendent' he said, adjusting the silk handkerchief in his top pocket.

'This job your force has going on Babylon, do you think Central Wales Police would consider a joint operation with Customs? We already have a fair amount of intelligence on it, you know.'

Scratching his neck, Hook looked pensively out across central London. He could do pensive. His delay brought a sparkle of anticipation to Aldermartin's eyes. He glanced across towards James, who had been listening throughout.

'To be perfectly honest,' he began.

James rolled her eyes and brushed some fluff from her jeans.

'And in the strictest of confidence, it's now out of our jurisdiction. We believe it's being landed in a remote island off western Scotland' he said.

James looked away and squinted rapidly as though someone had just thrown a tray of cat litter in her eyes.

'In confidence, of course' said Aldermartin. 'But could you divulge where exactly it will be landed? This is just for our files, of course.'

Flashing his eyes over to James, he flicked them down momentarily to Brodie's file that lay invitingly open on the desk before them. He moved back towards the window with Aldermartin in a leisurely manner. It was a signal she had seen before. With their backs turned and whispering out of the side of his mouth, he said,

'Trawler, three weeks' time, McGonacle Bay, Western Isles of Scotland.'

An elated Aldermartin sighed contentedly, while Hook watched James reflection in the window, silently rummaging through Brodie's personal record.

Aldermartin was beginning to turn around too quickly for Hook's liking. He gripped his host's arm firmly and pulled him back towards the window.

'Tell me, how far are we from the Millennium Dome?'

'Any luck?' he asked as they descended in the lift a short while later.

Offering her hand, Hook looked at the inked address on her palm. Grinning he read,

'Doctor Garth Penry-Ellis, 20 Bredenbury Gardens, Notting Hill. Okay let's get out of here and see if we can find out why they got shot of him,' he said.

'Better still, let's get out of here before we get arrested' she replied.

Travelling through the back streets of Notting Hill in search of Doctor Penry-Ellis, she suddenly pointed to a large detached Victorian property, surrounded by overgrown laurel bushes. It was the sort of building one could easily miss. In fact it was the sort of building you wanted to miss. The house itself was dark and appeared in need of repair, while internal wooden shutters were closed on every ground floor window. He began to wonder if those who went in ever came out again. Only a large brass sign on an equally large gatepost told you who was at home.

Accelerating through the entrance and along a gravelled drive, Hook braked suddenly without warning, throwing James against the dashboard, as chippings and wet leaves rattled against the underside of the car. Reversing slowly back towards the entrance, he stopped for a moment and looked at the fading brass nameplate partially covered in moss. Dr Garth Penry- Ellis was a consultant psychiatrist.

'Come in bach, come in' said Dr Ellis, shaking their hands warmly, as a shower of sleet began to bounce off the doorstep outside. Taking their coats, he led them past a smiling receptionist into a warm comfortable office, which had a roaring coal fire.

Bespectacled and bearded, Ellis was as broad as he was tall, and had probably been a loose-head prop when in training. He hadn't trained for a long time though. A framed photograph taken of the St Mary's Hospital Rugby third fifteen in 1965 confirmed it.

'My next appointment is in fifteen minutes, so I've got a little time' he said.

Looking across at the leather couch under the window, Hook began to wish he'd made the visit alone. Perhaps the dumpy little West Walian could explain the long dark corridor that was keeping him awake at nights, and interpret the significance of the six doors he had to choose from whenever he fell asleep.

'We've just spoken to Julian Aldermartin of Customs and Excise' he said, holding out his warrant card which the doctor appeared to scrutinize. 'I appreciate you seeing us at such short notice but it's of paramount importance that we have some background on Joseph Brodie, a former employee of theirs.

'Duw, Duw, is it bloody hot in here boys or is it me?' he said waving, his hand across the front of his face and loosening his tie. 'Want me to open a window?'

James shook her head.

'Aldermartin has probably given you most of the detail regarding Mr Brodie' he said.

Hook replied with a serious nod. It was almost five o'clock in the evening and he was still telling lies.

'I've been following it most nights on TV up here. Seems like you've got a man intent on cleansing the Land of my Fathers of the criminal element, and probably saving the tax payer thousands.'.

'Oh the murders! Yes, well, all the victims were villains all right, but our man's by-passing the legal system and re introducing capital punishment' smiled Hook

'And you think it could be Brodie?' he said turning to Hook.

'Oh no, no. To be perfectly frank it's something else I think he's up to. But he's in the capital, acting a little strangely' he said, refusing to give too much away.

'Why, you don't think he's capable of killing someone, surely?' James interrupted sharply.

'Contrary to what the commandment tells us, young lady, I believe that everyone is capable if the circumstances dictate' he said. 'The most pacifist people in the world have been known to kill for various reasons.'

'What did you think of him, Doctor?' Hook asked.

'In confidence, he came here five times. In layman's terms, he was suffering from a chronic form of clinical depression. Suddenly he just stopped coming; I rang Aldermartin who told me he had disappeared and was probably abroad.'

'Joe and I go back a few years' said Hook. 'He always struck me as a mentally tough man, a terrific investigator, big family man. Depression? That surprises me.'

'Then you know about the family I take it.'

'Met them a few times in the past, great kids. Liz is doing well up at Oxford and Sally is doing her A levels according to Joe.'

Penry-Ellis looked across at Hook curiously, a look of dark concern washing across his bearded face.

'You mean you have no idea what's happened to his family? Aldermartin didn't tell you?'

Sitting up straight, Hook leant forward, his eyes narrowed and his forehead creased. Scratching the back of his neck he shook his head. Walking over to the fire, the doctor spoke quietly.

'I'm afraid Elizabeth overdosed on Heroin. it was the first time she had tried it during her first year up at Oxford. Sally died at an illegal rave in Hackney. Ecstasy. She was thirteen years old. The man lost two daughters within six months. It totally destroyed him.'

Hook's jaw dropped as he realised what they were beginning to unearth. For a few moments he was unable to speak or formulate any sort of dialogue. James too appeared stunned. Finally he spoke.

'His wife?'

Pushing a falling log back into the burning coals, the doctor went on, 'Divorced him after Sally died. Re-married, living in Australia. It seems she blamed him.'

Hook's few seconds of sadness were suddenly replaced by a guilty feeling of anticipation, as Brodie's psychotic plight broke out into the open. Something special was unfolding, and you didn't need to be Holmes or Watson to see it. That instinctive moment in every murder investigation when you know beyond a shadow of a doubt that you're about a foot from the back of the killer's neck. That split second when criminal logic and gut reaction merge into a jelly-like sensation that sends your guts spinning like a tumble dryer. That moment was now seizing Hook.

Slumping back in his chair he began to fumble in his jeans for a cigarette which he quickly lit. Drawing slowly and thoughtfully, he began to blow clouds of smoke towards the elegant cornice that decorated the high ceilings. Pangs of guilt momentarily began to confuse him, not knowing whether to celebrate or commiserate, anger and sympathy embraced while he slowly began to take it all in. Trying to harness his increasing excitement, he began to admire all the art that surrounded them on the white emulsioned walls. Black inked impressions of old colliers at the coalface scraping a living thousands of feet underground. Charcoal sketches of long winding valley streets filled with people who had aged before their time, during days when drugs were things found in Hospital cabinets.

'How long ago was all this?' he asked finally.

'Must be 3 years now.'

'Doctor, is it possible he could have infiltrated a drug organisation by some means or other, and is systematically killing each member? He obviously has a deep hatred of drug dealers. I think he may have become a vigilante. Doctor Ellis, does that fit?'

'Well, he had an enormous love for his family, that I do know. And yet I believe he was a man capable of extreme violence. The death of his children and the loss of his wife destroyed him, pushed him over the edge. He had raging demons inside him which I failed to get near.'

'But does this all fit?' said Hook impatiently.

'Possibly. As a drugs officer, I know he believed he'd let his kids down. At the inquest, I understand the coroner blamed the dealers and drug traffickers, describing them as a cancer on society. They were never caught and that didn't help.'

'Each murder victim was tortured, Doctor Ellis. He bled them slowly by cutting an artery. He even talked gently to them as they were dying.'

The kindly doctor was silent. Then he answered.

'Perhaps it had some connection with his time at Tree Tops, a children's home in Glasgow,' said Ellis browsing now through Brodie's dossier.

Moving even closer to the edge of his seat, Hook said,

'Children's home? I didn't know.'

'Yes, his parents died when he was young and he had a bad time there during his adolescent years.'

'Child abuse?'

'That's right. He was regularly assaulted by one of the male staff, both physically and sexually, as a child.'

By the very thickness of the file the Doctor was perusing, Hook had a fair idea that Brodie's infancy had been spent in terror, a childhood nightmare that never ended A huge lump lodged tightly in his throat.

Reading upside down was something that Hook had perfected during his schooldays. The majority of the time it was nothing more than a useless party piece, occasionally useful when you sat before the bosses. Staring at Brodie's file he began to read the thick, black, pathetic, weak and corrupt words stamped across the pages. *Insufficient Evidence.*

'I can't put this any other way' said James, 'and I have a reason for asking. But - what do you consider the worse part of his ordeal at the home? Did he ever say?'

'Most of all this came out in hypnotherapy, when he was regressed' Ellis said. 'He continually referred to one of the carers there, a big man who would come to his room late at night and have sex with him. Rape him. He became so terrified he would excrete in his pyjamas as soon as he saw him. In his temper, this man would sometimes tear off Brodie's pyjama trousers and stuff them in his mouth to stifle the screams, while he interfered with him in the darkness. Brodie was seven years old.'

The room was silent.

'Did they ever do the bastard? I'm sorry, Doctor. I mean, was he convicted?' James said in a whisper.

'No, I don't believe the matter ever went before the courts. No corroboration, I understand.'

'Did you yourself ever find out who this man was?' Hook said. 'Did he identify him? Is his name in that file in front of you?'

There was now some concern beginning to show on the portly psychiatrist's face. They had already been there for more than the allotted fifteen minutes. He began to move around the room like an expectant father in a maternity ward. Breaching the rules of confidentiality didn't come naturally to him, and visions of an uncomfortable witness box ride began to disturb his thoughts.

'Am I legally bound to tell you, Inspector? I mean we do have the rules of privilege to observe here. I think I've already stepped out of the bounds.'

'Would you consider bending those rules minutely, just for a moment, Doctor Ellis? Your nation back home is having enormous problems at present.'

Hook's almost childish, pleading voice and puppy-dog eyes had James gently shaking her head. She wondered if he'd ever studied drama at school.

Scratching both sided of his greying beard roughly, while resting both elbows on the desk before him, Hook watched as the craggy little therapist appeared more and more concerned as the interview proceeded. Everyone had their problems, Hook thought, as Doctor Ellis began to brush his bristles with the back of his fingers, causing flakes of dry skin to float softly onto his waistcoat.

Hook's eyes gleamed with impatience, while the little psychiatrist wrestled in this professional tight corner with all his nationalistic principals and morality. All the laws of confidentiality appeared weak by comparison.

'In confidence' promised Hook anxiously.

'In confidence' the doctor stammered.

'We haven't been here Doctor Penry-Ellis, I swear,' he said, emphasising the 'not' quite fiercely.

'Okay, okay,' he said quickly. Consulting his notes, he went on.

'The assaults went on for years. During regression he wouldn't say the man's name. This carer had tattoos on his chest - *LM loves JB* - and across his abdomen, just under his belly button, he had the words *Welcome to Hell*. I assume JB was Joe Brodie.. Who LM was, I have no idea.'

The evening skies of north London began to darken like a huge black tarpaulin. Sitting motionless for a few minutes, they watched the blackness reduce the moon to a narrow curve of silver. Finally she grabbed his hand.

'Well done boss' she smiled. 'Scrubs Lane, we have ignition.'

'It's okay ma'am, it's my job, I'm a cop. Good guys like me, bad guys hate me. That's why I'm here ma'am' he said with a straight face. Solving murdes had a strange effect on some people; Hook's dreadful impression of American detective Joe Friday was just his way.

Already mind-altering chemicals were taking effect – the natural kind - and the endorphins were already pleasuring his brain. Not only did he feel he could have jogged back to south Wales, but he actually wanted to. That's how the supreme prize of detecting murders affected him.

He began tapping out the Scrubs Lane telephone number on his mobile while the sensations continued to increase. His teeth gripped another burning French cigarette. Seconds later he was through to the incident room, which as usual sounded busy in the background.

'Where are you, Hook?' shouted Mulholland with some irritability. 'We've been trying to get hold of you all afternoon.'

'Hello Super. I thought you were on leave. I'm up in London. We've just spoken to a psychiatrist about a Joe Brodie who use to work for Customs; cut a long story short, I think he's our Spiderman guy. I believe he's been working for the McCanns, but it looks as though he's been taking out most of their organisation. He lost two daughters through drugs,' said Hook, stopping for a moment to draw breath. 'He's a vigilante, boss. The McCanns have got to be next' he said. 'We should …'

'Get back here as soon as possible' interrupted Mulholland. 'The McCanns are not next on the list. We've found another body this afternoon.'

'Jesus Christ Almighty, who's he done now?'

'Listen to me Hook. I want you back here straightaway.'

'Okay, okay Super. James and I are going to grab a quick bite to eat, and we'll be with you by about nine.'

'I said straightaway' shouted Mulholland, before Hook was cut off.

'What the hell's going on boss?' James said.

'There's been another murder' he said tensely. 'The Chief sounds as though he's really under pressure.'

'Who is it?' she asked.

'No idea. He slammed the phone down on me, but a penny to a pinch of shit it's someone connected to the McCanns' he replied, sounding a touch deflated at Mulholland's response.

They circled the dark wet streets of Notting Hill, looking for some sort of rough clue or traffic sign that the Royal Borough of Kensington may have erected to assist the Celts in returning to their native country. After circling Hyde Park four times, they eventually found what they were looking for. Accelerating up the slip road towards the M4, James said,

'McGonacle Bay, Western Isles of Scotland. Sounds rather remote. Customs could take weeks to find it.'

'Shouldn't think so. I made it up' he said.

'So where does this put our serial killer from the pampas, Hector Barrantes?'

'He doesn't exist.'

'How?'

'Brodie's description of the Argentinian always worried me.'

'Why?'

'He described him as thirty six years old, six one, athletic build, unshaven, thick black untidy hair, swarthy complexion, wearing jeans and a black coat.'

'And?'

'He was describing me James, he was describing me. I also backpacked around south America after Uni. Maracaibo Prison is in Venezuela, and Maldonado where he was allegedly born is in Uruguay, not in Argentina. Olay! He gave me a load of crap.'

Patting him firmly on the back as he accelerated into the fast lane, she said,

'So who the hell is LM?'

Tired and hungry, they finally arrived at Scrubs Lane, driving quietly into the rear station yard. They had made good time, it wasn't yet eight o'clock.

Immediately he could see something was up. Chief Superintendent Mulholland stood alone in full regulation uniform outside the back door, waiting. Others, including Corbett and some of his senior puppets, appeared to be peering out of upstairs windows; in fact there was a strange air about the place. James herself had never seen so many journalists milling around the station entrance.

Holding onto his hat as he rushed out into the wet windy yard to join them, Mulholland motioned to his own Peugeot and they both jumped into the back.

Sleet continued to hammer down, spewing unsparingly from the broken roof guttering that surrounded the mortuary. Within seconds they were soaked but the cold icy water bruising Hook's head and shoulders it had little impact A balding man with a deaf aid and strands of wispy grey hair, lashed down over the top of his head with hairspray, opened a side door to let them in. Stepping into the longest corridor in the city, they followed the limping mortuary attendant, along the depressing white-tiled passageway, ignoring the dimly lit Chapel of Rest on their right. Hook was now pale and gaunt, his lips were cold and dry. Halfway down the passageway the smell of surgical disinfectant and sudden death hit them head on.

Double metal doors at the far end of the corridor were slightly ajar when he saw her. Where Helen was lying, she had a large red towel wrapped around her middle and legs. There was very little white left. Stopping alongside the trolley, he gazed down at her and felt sick. He wanted to scream, to call out her name, but his jaw just shivered. She looked as though she had just stepped out of a shower. Her face appeared calm, while her open eyes hinted little at the carnage that lay beneath the towel. Leaning over, he gently brushed her lids with his thumbs and closed them tightly.

She had drip marks on her arm, where resuscitation had been attempted and blood on her teeth where a ventilation tube had been roughly inserted. Grabbing a nearby robe he angrily covered her bruised breasts, swearing at nearby attendants under his breath, even though he knew mortuaries and dignity had very little in common.

Softly he took her hand and lifted it off the trolley. Her palms were still warm and comforting, yet her fingers were cold and stiff. Letting go, he knew, was going to be impossible. Taking hold of his arm, James started to pull him away, but he wouldn't let her. He knew it would be the last time he would see her, and already the picture in his mind of how she used to be was fading fast.

Out of the corner of his eye he could see the open fridge door and the red stained unzipped body bag that had brought her there. Again he wanted to scream, although he knew he wouldn't. James watched as he grasped Helen's wrist. She knew he was searching for a pulse, but she said nothing.

The room began to move around him and the strength had gone from his legs, but he was still aware of Professor Woolfe, the Home Office pathologist, in the corner, wearing green gumboots and a large plastic apron. Everyone was dressed in theatre green.

Under the harsh fluorescent lighting, he watched and listened to the suctioning squeal of the rubber gloves as Woolfe struggled to pull them on. The noise seemed deafening. Sticking out of the professor's top pocket, he could see the scalpel in its sheath, the instrument that would take her body apart. The government's licensed butcher, with his indifference and lack of sensitivity, had already reduced her to just another violent city crime statistic.

When the Professor began to hose down a nearby stainless steel table, the walls began to rush in and he needed to get out. He wanted to scream 'leave her alone, for fuck's sake, please God, leave her alone!' but nothing came out. Nearby, Mulholland stood erect with his head slight bowed, holding his hat tightly in his hands, as though he was already standing by her graveside.

There was little he could do about the tears in his eyes, but he pulled himself up, turned to the mortuary staff and whispered,

'Yes that's her. That's the body of Helen Wainwright.'

Pushing the advancing Mulholland away roughly, he turned and barged his way through the double doors and back along the corridor alone. Tugging at her sleeve, Mulholland shook his head as James attempted to follow. Heavy footsteps and incoherent shouting ricocheted back along the passageway. The ID was over.

Sitting with the Chief Superintendent in his car at the side of the Mortuary, James listened to the relentless sleet as it continued to hammer on the sunroof in the dark.

'Perhaps I should have told him when you were up in London' he sighed, fiddling with the ignition keys.

'Yeah, and he would have driven back like a madman, sir' she replied. "No, I don't think there was a best way.'

'She had complained to people in Chambers that she thought someone had been following her' he said.

Her mind drifted back to the occasion at the marina when she and Hook had spotted Brodie in the Mini not more than ten yards from her flat, but she said nothing. Failing to identify what Brodie had been doing near her home and possibly alerting her to the danger, she knew would be rampaging around in Hook's conscience and already pulling him apart.

'They found her in Chambers, down in the archives, this afternoon. It's our Spiderman guy again. A typist remembers seeing a workman wearing maroon overalls and a yellow hard hat leaving the offices, but that's about it. There's building work going on everywhere around there, so it could be nothing.'

'Who found her, sir?' she asked.

'Hunter Jarvis. He's a gibbering wreck at the moment,' said Mulholland.

'I bet he is.'

Starting up the engine, Mulholland began to head back to Scrubs Lane, with a policeman's suicide and yet another undetected murder weighing heavily on his shoulders. His mind like his driving was chaotic, as he drove through heavy city traffic like a provisional licence holder.

'Don't worry Super, all we have to do is find Joe Brodie' she said, throwing him a line of encouragement.

'You both a hundred per cent it's him?'

'My DI is, and that's good enough for me, sir.'

'He's already been circulated as wanted throughout the country, all the ports have been alerted. Let's hope he hasn't left the city.'

'It's become a big game to him. He's still around alright.'

'Miss Wainwright lost her life because Brodie thought that, as a member of their defence team, she was responsible for the McCanns acquittal in Crown. He couldn't have been further from the truth.'

Activating the security gates at Scrubs Lane they sped through the slush and into the rear yard, when cameras and people began shouting in their direction. Crowds began rushing towards them from the direction of the Station entrance, as they recognised Mulholland's blue Peugeot saloon. Flash bulbs illuminated the evening's misery, while others began to shout his name. James herself could never remember such a number being assembled outside for any previous murder.

'Bloody morons' he said.

'Christ, there must be half of Fleet Street out there! What the hell's going on?'

'They believe Goose was the Spiderman guy' he replied, pulling into his allocated parking spot.

Switching off the engine, he said,

'A press release went out this afternoon about the suicide, and they've put two and two together and come up with five.'

'Goose, the Spiderman guy?' she mumbled as she stepped from the car. 'Goose. Interesting theory.'

Walking over to her Citroen tucked away in the corner of the yard, the Chief Superintendent called across to her.

'There's a briefing at 0600 hours tomorrow. We need him there, James' he said.

Driving across to the Marina to look for him, she guessed right first time. Bouncing over the wet dockside cobbles that glistened with rain, she could hear the hollow flapping of mast on rigging, floating across the yacht-infested water. Pulling up behind

Hook's Sunbeam Talbot she stopped. Just for a moment she sat listening to the water lapping the stone steps nearby, while it gently heaved around in the harbour below.

On the other side of the brightly-lit anchorage, faint popular music emerged from inside the marina disco, while outside young people kissed and hugged in the rain.

Hook could see them too. Sitting alone, he stared at Helen's flat above, chain smoking his way through another packet of French cigarettes. He had a powerful urge to go inside just once more, just one last time. There was an overwhelming need to smell her coats in the hallway, feel the soft luxury of her bathroom towels, recapture that same passionate and emotional warmth he always felt when she opened the door and kissed him. With a voice that was as rich and seductive as the single malt whisky they often shared. Just one last night alone on her shabby-chic sofa, just a few final hours with the everlasting memories.

Jumping into the front seat she said nothing, but gazed with him up at the dark empty flat. What the hell could she say?

'I haven't got a key to the flat any more, ' he said, his eyes fixed in a trance, soaked by an hour of tears.

'I really don't know what to say. I wish I could think of something that would help, but I can't.'

'That afternoon you and I saw him in the Mini down here. My bet is he was watching her flat, and I couldn't even put two and two together.'

'The man's a psychopath, he's unpredictable, nobody could have foreseen that coming. You're a half-tidy detective bach, but you're not that bloody good. Listen, stay at my flat tonight. '

'Thanks, but don't worry about me, I'm not going to fold like some picnic table. I'll get it all together by tomorrow. Helen would have expected me to. I just want one last night in there, alone.'

'Good, because tomorrow you and I are going to start looking for him. You and I are going to find him. You and I are going to arrest him, not Corbett or any of the puppets. Not the National Crime Squad. You and I are going to trawl the bloody gutters bach, until we find that raving Scots psycho.'

With his chest pressed against the steering wheel and his nose almost touching the windscreen so he could gain a better view, he mumbled

'If you say so, Sarge. '

Pulling a half bottle of Jack Daniels from her pocket, hurriedly bought from a nearby off-licence, she placed it on the dashboard.

'This should help you sleep. I'll pick you up here at half five in the morning, alright?'

Softly she pulled his hand away from the steering wheel and pressed a small brass Yale key into the palm of his hand.

Tucked away in a small country lane hidden by bushes and trees, not more than ten yards from the junction of the main A2229 that led towards the city centre, a white Jaguar saloon stood parked out of sight with its lights switched off. Its driver George Pugh watched with heavy eyes the occasional traffic that passed him, heading into the city. It had been one of those quiet shifts with no shouts. A passenger dozed quietly alongside.

Sitting back comfortably with his fingers interlocked over a rising and falling girth, Constable Pugh sucked quietly on a polo mint, occasionally balancing the tiny disappearing sweet on the end of his tongue, before withdrawing it suddenly like a south American tree lizard. It had been that sort of shift. Pulling up the collar on his patrol coat, he watched with interest as frost began to creep over the bonnet of the car. Normally on such occasions he and his elderly companion sang a medley of their favourite Rolling Stones songs to break the monotony, but an out-of-tune duet of Jumping Jack Flash earlier seemed to have dampened their enthusiasm.

The 4.2 litre engine purred silently, while it kept the internal heater blowing warm air around the occupants' feet A tiny dashboard clock showed 3.29am.

Only another six shifts and George Pugh would be retired, after 30 years. He was fifty five years old, with greyish white hair, eyes that laughed and a frame that was three stone heavier than it should have been. It was difficult for him to remember the last time he had reported a speeder. He had cautioned many and had daily bollockings for not doing more. But PC138 Pugh was an advanced driver par excellence, who could make a car talk. Very shortly, he would make the police Jaguar natter one last time.

He heard it in the distance heading their way, faintly at first, a car making early morning progress, a car in a hurry. Elbowing his observer in the stomach, PC Morris sat up with a start as though he'd had a bad dream, pretending as usual that he hadn't been asleep. Almost fifty four years of age, small and thin, with more nasal hair inside his nose than on his head, he and Pugh listened for a moment before casually buckling up their seat belts.

The approaching engine began its roar of intent, increasing gradually, now racing out of the early morning darkness, disturbing the morning's tranquillity. Loosening his tie and flexing his fingers as though he was about to give a piano concerto, Pugh touched the accelerator sensitively and waited. He enjoyed these little vehicular altercations; the cut and thrust of boy racers in hot hatches kept him young, made the night shift go that much faster. Once again he wasn't going to be disappointed.

The rear end of the Jaguar jumped around friskily on the wet laneway as it tore out of its hiding place, throwing up gravel against the underside as the early morning speeder flew past. Within half a mile, as the sodium streetlights overhead flashed by, Morris spotted it in the back window, smirking at them, as the Mini negotiated a roundabout on two wheels.

Braking smoothly, the bonnet of the Jaguar rose and fell on its front suspension, its full headlamps illuminating the masked face of the Spiderman toy.

'It's him George, fucking hell it's him!' Morris shouted, grabbing the radio handset. 'We're going to need help' he said anxiously as his colleague pushed the Jaguar broadside around the roundabout, it's headlights bouncing around in the Mini's interior mirror, as it tried to get away.

While illuminated public buildings, impressive historical monuments and expensive city restaurants long since emptied, flashed by at over a hundred miles an hour, both patrolmen were already considering the outcome of the chase. Snotty nosed fifteen year olds having an illegal drive in Papa's new Renault Turbo was one thing; pursuing a psychopath wanted for four savage city killings was quite different.

Morris' voice broke the silence that had descended on the control room at HQ and boomed out across the airwaves. Slowly people stopped talking, half-knitted jumpers were dropped, cups of hot coffee slowly lowered.

Pursuits were nightly occurrences in the city, and experienced wireless operators barely raised an eyebrow while listening to the noise of screeching tyres and racing engines, as chases began to develop. Most people knew George Pugh and there was little chance of anyone eluding him. Even Schumacher would have had problems staying with the tubby father of five in busy city traffic. Burnt-out Astras abandoned by the glue-sniffing unemployed, and overturned Mondeos left spinning by speed freaks, were as common as the nightly stomach content on the grey city pavements. But the driver ignoring the blue flashing light tonight was in a different league.

'Tango Whisky fifty following suspect vehicle Austin Mini saloon car, registration number Golf 881 Alpha Tango Hotel, towards Boulevard de Leon and the city centre at speeds of ninety to a hundred miles per hour. Driver believed to be Joseph Brodie, I repeat Joseph Brodie, wanted in connection with the city murders,' barked Morris.

A selection of emotions appeared on people's faces under the dimmed control room lights, ranging from anxiety to distress, as the two ageing constables pursued the mentally disturbed speeder.

'For Christ's sake get them some assistance' someone shouted.

Mulholland answered the phone as though he were still asleep. The sergeant's voice from headquarters was both urgent and agitated.

'Sorry to trouble you Super, but Tango Whisky fifty is in a high speed pursuit. They're chasing Brodie in the Mini, he's doing over a hundred miles an hour through the city centre.'

'Right, I'm on my way in.'

'Hang on sir, hang on, the suspect has just stopped for the boys in Arlington Gardens, near the Odeon cinema.'

'Get an armed response team over there ASAP' shouted Mulholland, slamming down his phone.

The two unbuckled their seat belts, and fingering their truncheons, stepped from the Jaguar and approached the Mini from the rear. Hesitating slightly, Pugh lowered his voice into a deeper, more authoritative tone. Shouting in the stillness, he called for the driver to switch off his engine.

Rubbish and litter flew around their feet as the wind began to blow the Mini's exhaust fumes up towards the grey skies. Without warning, it reversed violently, its engine screaming as it smashed into the front of the Jaguar saloon. Both patrolmen jumped clear; slipping on the frosty road surface, the mini's rear wheels missing Morris by inches, before tearing ahead once more. Racing back to the patrol car with the sound of broken glass crunching beneath their soles, they roared away from the Odeon cinema immersed in both fear and exhilaration.

'Talbot Roundabout the wrong way, heading towards the Kingsway, he's just forced an articulated lorry off the road. Mini travelling at over ninety miles an hour' shouted Morris, as the Jaguar hit a patch of black ice causing the back end to wiggle about in delight

'Kingsway dual carriageway, travelling the wrong way up carriageway towards Banwen Industrial estate, vehicle is all over the road,' shouted Morris, as Pugh began to smile to himself.

Within feet of the rear of the badly damaged Mini, the Jaguar dropped back again, before Pugh slipped into a lower gear, effortlessly racing up behind his quarry again. Pushing, prompting, annoying its driver as the powerful headlight of the police car bounced around behind. Occasionally he would ease off deliberately, dropping back some distance, giving Brodie a false hope of escape, before accelerating right up behind him again, while they pushed him on to even faster speeds. All they needed now was a nice tight bend.

Although he was still a hundred and fifty yards away, George Pugh had already seen him, standing unsteadily on the nearside pavement outside Debenhams, taking deep breaths as he decided whether or not to step onto the crossing. George Pugh's blood pressure increased significantly as the late night reveller stepped shakily onto the crossing. An Austin Mini saloon missing you by six inches while travelling at a hundred and five miles an hour appeared to have the same effect as six cups of hot black coffee. A police siren travelling a little faster on the wrong side of the road sobered him up immediately.

With the last of the sodium street lighting now left well behind, both vehicles headed into the countryside darkness on full headlights, racing towards the industrial estate. The warning sign tucked away in the hedgerows indicated clearly that the bend was ahead, and that the hazard was sharp and dangerous. Travelling along doing a ton on a road surface prone to skidding, while being chased by the law, gave Brodie little time to adhere to the Highway Code.

Slipping into third gear, Pugh pushed right up tightly behind the little Mini one last time, almost cremating him with the cars powerful lights. Then fifty yards from the approaching hazard he stood on the brakes, fighting with the steering wheel as the rear end of the car threatened to overtake the front.

With his backside moving around in the seat like a jockey in the saddle, he watched as Brodie was pushed far too fast into the approaching bend. Braking too late, the Mini hit the bend like a highspeed train.

    Skidding broadside, it spun around in the road ahead of them, bouncing over onto its roof, its headlights pointing skywards like searchlights, as it crashed down a small grassy embankment. Rolling over a half a dozen times it finally came to rest on its roof. With the wheels spinning wildly, both constables scrambled down the embankment towards the mass of tangled metal.

CHAPTER TWENTY

Pulling into the marina complex later that morning, she could see him waiting in the front seat of his car. He'd been waiting most of the night. Although he had already started on his first cigarette of the day, he had that 'good 60 minutes sleep' complexion, but after a night in the front seat of a Sunbeam Talbot, his body felt as though it had slept on a dozen sacks of grain. He slipped into the front seat of her car alongside her, and handed her back the Yale key. There was no going back. Helen was dead and the flat was history. The eyes gave everything away, and she could see he was consumed by grief. Inside he was hurting like hell.

Driving through the slowly awakening city streets of litter and a chasing wind, milkmen and window cleaners, he made small talk, the odd joke about the weather, but Helen was never mentioned. A muted grunt was his only response when Goose's funeral had been mentioned. There was room for one thing in his head at the moment. Joseph Cameron Brodie.

He had little idea of how he would react if he arrested him, what he would say or how he would conduct himself At the moment he pretended he didn't really care A psycho killer Brodie may have been, but a small part of Hook felt he had only been doing something that his squad had failed to do:

removing part of an international drug organisation from society.

Then he had killed Helen, and that changed everything. His own mind was still in casualty, and any sympathy he'd had for Brodie had all but disappeared. But Brodie was mad, and there seemed little point in thinking about wild instant revenge.

Keeping cool and professional was paramount; nurturing a deep, almost psychopathic hatred of a man that had become ill through the loss of his whole family, would do little to alleviate his own sorrow. Wounds needed to heal, not be allowed to fester. Keeping contact with external realities and fending off feelings of impending psychosis as far as Brodie was concerned needed a strong will.

Driving slowly through the automatic gates into the wet station yard, his revulsion suddenly returned with a vengeance when he saw it at the far end of the yard.

'They've got him, James. Someone else has got him' he said.

Inside a garage with its up-and-over door open, and a Scene Of Crime *Do Not Touch* sign displayed outside, he spotted the dark blue Mini on the back of a small, rusty low-loader. Or what was left of it.

Peering inside the crushed and mud-spattered write-off, he could see particles of smashed windscreen glass, blood and hair, and began to wonder if death had offered the Glaswegian a timely alternative to a life of imprisonment. If offered the choice, he knew which one Brodie would have selected.

'Bastard!' he cried.

Touching James' shoulder, he pointed to the toy Spiderman that slowly swayed around in the early morning breeze, its masked face covered in the debris of the early morning chase.

Without warning Hook suddenly smashed his fist through the already cracked and broken rear window. Startled, James watched as he ripped the doll from inside and stuffed it angrily into his jacket pocket. Grabbing his arm, she pulled him back. His hand was bleeding.

'What the hell are you doing?' she said.

'Don't worry.' He smiled grimly. 'I'm simply going to shove it down the bastard's throat if he's still alive.'

'You sure you're okay?' she asked.

A ripple of polite applause broke out in the incident room as both Hook and James walked in. James' neck flushed and she smiled self-consciously, accepting the early morning accolades for a job well done. Already in interview mode, Corbett, with a brand new suit and shirt, pretended he hadn't seen them. Sitting at a table composing his victory speech for the press and TV, he eventually gave them both a curt nod with his heavily gelled head as they passed. Hook ignored him and continued to push his way past the puppets who moved their heads slightly in recognition.

Eventually they reached Larry Mulholland who was sitting on the edge of a table amongst a crowd of Drug Squad men at the far end of the room. They could see he was chatting, animated, laughing. Hook breathed a sigh of relief; he could already sense it. Brodie was still breathing.

'Congratulations, Inspector. Nice work. We've got him.'

Hook smiled painfully as Mulholland shook his hand vigorously.

'Are you okay? I mean, why don't you take some time off, now that we've got him? You know, after Helen's …'

'Murder. After Helen's murder you mean, sir' he snapped.

'I am truly sorry' Mulholland said. Then, 'Brodie was arrested two hours ago.'

'So we gathered' he said, clearly disappointed not to have been the one to take him into custody.

'Traffic chased him all over the city. They pushed him off the road out in the suburbs. They've patched him up in hospital and they've just released him. They're bringing him back any moment now.

Apparently he won't talk to anyone. Took four officers to cuff him and bring him in after they pulled him from the car.'

'And he's fit to be detained and interviewed?'

'According to Doctor Simon Mulholland in Casualty, yes' smiled Mulholland.

'Three cheers for Doc Mulholland' said James dryly.

'The car?' said Hook

'Stolen from the west end of London. False plates we believe, we're still checking. But wait for it, there was a home-made knife under the spare wheel in the boot Although it's only about eight inches long, they tell me you could shave with the bloody thing. Scene Of Crime think there are traces of fresh blood, although minute, near the handle. Although it's early days and it's been wiped, they think it's been used recently.

A feeling of nausea gripped Hook, and his stomach felt as if he'd swallowed a ball of nettles. Of course there was blood on it. It had been stuck deep enough into Helen's body, for God's sake. Christ, Mulholland was becoming as insensitive as bloody Corbett.

Nearby Scene Of Crime men watched Hook carefully as they bagged some exhibits. They could see he couldn't take his eyes off the polythene exhibit bag and the short rough knife it contained. Noting

Hook's concern, one of them picked up the bag and pushed it into a nearby drawer.

Although he could hear everyone talking, it was as if they were underwater and nothing made sense. He could feel the over-powering anger returning, and when he saw the bags that contained her clothing, he lost all colour from his face. He could see Helen's pin-striped skirt, a bloodied garment that the knife had torn to shreds. Tights, red panties, red brassiere and a red blouse were all there. He knew they'd all been white when she had bought them.

'Anything else?' he snapped

'A diary containing among other things the names and addresses of all his victims, and ferry tickets over to Calais, with hotel receipts which put him in Montpellier on the day Benazzi was murdered.'

'Right.'

' Scene Of Crime have also recovered a blood-stained boilersuit from under the spare wheel in the mini. Brodie's knackered. We've got him trussed up like a Christmas turkey.'

Just then the room exploded into noise as a dozen disc drives on the HOLMES computers awoke, signalling the dawn of a brand new day. Looking around him, Hook could see that everyone, including Mulholland, had already forgotten Helen in the euphoria of success. Three empty bottles of Famous Grouse whisky and twenty one plastic cups on a nearby desk confirmed it. Rejoicing murder incident rooms were no place for a grieving lover.

Only seventeen hours earlier, Helen Wainwright had been butchered to death. The one person in the world he had loved. And now people had already pushed her to the backs of their minds, forgotten like old Christmas paper. Corbett, the fat bastard, hadn't even offered his condolences. That was the way murder enquiries were, that was the way detectives could be. The only thing that mattered above everything and anybody else was the result. As long as that tick went in the detection column on the right-hand side of the Crime Register, everything was hunky-dory.

A tired-looking female public relations officer, unused to rising at such an ungodly hour, tapped Hook on the shoulder.

'Will you stand against that wall? I want an up-dated photo of you for this evening's Echo' she said.

'Piss off' he said, without looking at her.

Lakes of cables and cameras began to flood into the incident room as television personnel pushed desks and chairs aside to accommodate the lighting equipment. Ignoring everyone, top-of-the bill Jack Corbett pulled down his tight-fitting waistcoat and ogled his reflection in a nearby dirty window. For 0600 hours he looked pretty good, he thought. Downstairs, local journalists were already being herded into a side interview room while they waited for a fresh pack of tabloid boys to arrive from Fleet Street.

Staring at the paper in his hand, Corbett rehearsed away under his breath, brushing past Hook and James as he went to meet his audience.

'I want to interview him, Chief' Hook said to Mulholland.

'That's impossible. There's a clear conflict of interests here.'

'But I need to speak to him.'

'The defence at his trial would rip you apart,' Mulholland said, with one eye still fixed on the TV crew nearby. 'I agree with Mr Corbett on this one. Detective Sergeant Bluck of the National Crime Squad has been allocated to the task. For Christ's sake, how could we let you interview him, when he's … when he's … Helen... Miss Wainwright …'

'You mean murdered, you mean because he's murdered Helen' he said, helping the Chief Superintendent with a verb that appeared to be giving him no end of problems.

'You know what I mean Hook. Just get a grip' he said, looking over the top of his detective inspector's head as he kept his eye firmly fixed on the position of the TV producer opposite. The man now in charge.

Watching Mulholland eagerly walk away into the blazing TV lights, Hook felt like a child lost on a beach during a Sunday school outing. Even the top man was beginning to suffer from the intoxication of success. That vanity and egotism that sometimes seized a senior officer when a serial killer was apprehended. When that thin veneer of respect begins to peel back like soaked wallpaper, as the gates of opportunity squeak open again. Offering perhaps one last unexpected promotion, one last pension increase. It was always sad when a man whose reputation was once unshakeable, a man who had once inspired you, suddenly abandoned his iron principles.

For a moment he watched as both Corbett and Mulholland flirted with a teenager from the TV make-up department. Gently, she patted the bags under Corbett's eyes with foundation powder, before starting to take out the rough edges on a shiny face that would need a little work

With the ground floor resembling Wimbledon on finals day, Hook began to head for the highest part of the building. He had a feeling the make-up girl was going to be some time.

Ten minutes later, sitting alone in the main squad office, with stockinged feet resting on a radiator while James went to fetch some coffee and toast, he looked out of the window and up at a bleak grey sky. Tiny yellow lights awakened under rows of slanting tiled roofs that stretched as far as the eye could see, while small globules of unkind icy rain began to pepper the glass, before racing each other down towards the windowsill below. And everyone at Scrubs Lane was happy.

The hierarchy at the station could now relax and bask in the glory achieved by others. The media had got their story, and for the next few weeks would squeeze every drop of drama out of the demise of others. The city's residents were no longer tormented by fear. Off-duty detectives would be bragging in their local that they had been the arresting officer. And Helen was dead.

Briefly the Docklands picture outside became distorted as James appeared in the glass reflection before him, racing along the corridor behind him with her blonde hair bouncing like a runaway pony. She was shouting something he didn't understand. She was waving to him, but he didn't know why. Mild depression still suffocating any positive thinking, and it continued to peep over his shoulder as his thoughts went back to the mortuary.

Out of breath, she slumped down alongside him. Shaking his arm feverishly, she panted,

'It's not... it's not... it's not him, boss!'

Although he knew exactly what she had said, it took a little time for it to sink in. Stupidly he said,

'What do you mean?'

'Brodie, Joe Brodie! That's not Brodie they've just brought back from the hospital!'

He jumped to his feet, heart racing.

'You sure?' he said.

'Christ bach, I met him that night with you, when he was breathalysed. His head is all bandaged but it's not him' she went on, struggling for breath.

'What's Corbett said?'

'I haven't told him' she confessed.

Within minutes, he was unlocking the door to a small medical room just off the custody suite, which smelt of antiseptic and cleanliness, a strange fragrance for Scrubs Lane. Opening the door, Hook went inside, followed closely by James. He stared at the heavily bandaged, dark haired man seated on the green leather examination table. The uniformed constables guarding him leapt to their feet as he entered. Smiling, he motioned to them and they sat back down.

The man in the white paper-thin boilersuit, still handcuffed, jumped to his feet and asked the first question.

'Who the fuck are you?'

Shaking his head almost apologetically, Hook began his exit stage left, walking backwards out of the room.

'I know who I am, squire, but who the hell are you?' he said, as he pulled the door tightly behind him.

Moments later he arrived outside the incident room. The entrance was crowded with officers who pushed and jostled, trying to get a view inside as Corbett and Mulholland were about to make the front pages. The room itself had been emptied, the corridor was full. He could see the blinding lights inside and could hear people already talking.

Shouldering men aside he finally reached the entrance, where a young television assistant placed his clipboard limply across Hook's chest. His attempt to halt him failed dismally.

'Get ready to roll' barked a tall man with unkempt hair and a khaki body warmer, as Hook burst through the double swing doors and stepped into the middle of the media circus

'What the bloody hell's going on?' a cameraman shouted.

'I'm sorry about this chief' he said to Mulholland in whispered tones while Corbett listened in, 'but it's not Joe Brodie you have downstairs. Don't ask me why or how, but it's just not him.'

Snapping his window blinds shut after putting on the lights in his office, Mulholland bent over and ignited his antiquated gas fire, which responded with a loud bang. Both Corbett and Hook occupied the same cold Chesterfield. There was a first for everything.

'Listen to me Inspector. Just answer this for a moment. Forget the man, whoever he may be. Are all the facts in relation to Brodie correct, yes or no?' enquired Mulholland, who's calmness was now a thing of the past.

'Yes sir, he's our man.'

'Is that the Mini he's been using in the yard?'

'Yes sir.'

'And you're absolutely sure, beyond a shadow of a doubt?'

'Yes sir.'

'So who the bloody hell have we got downstairs, Hook, tell me?' shouted Corbett, jumping to his feet.

Here was a marble-hearted man whose resentments expanded daily. And a superintendent who had just seen the glittering prize of front-page fame ripped from his grasp.

'You have as much idea as I have,' he said. 'Like me to ask him?'

Inside the interview room, Hook slipped the cassette into the tape machine while James formally cautioned the man in the white boiler suit, who smiled broadly. For a moment Hook said nothing, but just removed the white plastic clock from the wall before slipping it into the bottom drawer of the desk. No sense in giving the accused something to focus on, something to study when the questions commenced. Interviews of this nature required a blank canvas. Bare faced walls, all ready for bare faced lies.

'Well fuck me, its Sony and Cher again!' the man said with some arrogance.

Similar in build and colouring to the real Mr Brodie, he sat cleaning his fingernails with a small paper clip he had picked up in the medical room. Sutured and roughly bandaged, his head and nose were now twice their normal size. Tattoos adorned his hands and throat, and the accent was definitely local. A muscled neck and powerful sloping shoulders told you he lifted weights, and had probably never said please as a kid. Hook guessed mid-thirties, with a shed full of form, the majority for street violence and robbery. The suspect had been around the track.

Eventually Hook decided to speak.

'Tell me, why won't you tell us your name?'

Menacingly, the man leant over the desk, and pointing at them with the index finger of his right hand, he shouted,

'Listen, you pair of tossers, you've informed me of my rights and I wish to uphold those rights, okay?'

Picking up his chair, he turned it around and sat with his back to them, staring at the dirty beige wall. Folding his arms and crossing his legs, he began to whistle *The Green Green Grass of Home.* Perhaps he didn't know the words, thought James.

Hook knew that silence, to a suspect, could be of great comfort or of great pressure, depending on the circumstances. Get it wrong and the interview was over. If the defendant was going to dominate these proceedings, he and James might just as well have joined in with the whistling.

'Okay, okay so you work out and you like Tom Jones, but if you're trying to antagonise us you're wasting your time' said James. 'I've got the CD.'

She paused.

'The car you rolled this morning has been nicked from London. It's got false plates. We'll know who you are within the hour, when we send your prints away' she said.

He started to whistle the second verse.

Whinging about his early morning shift and arthritic knees, Sergeant Ivor Griffiths knocked loudly on the door and disturbed an interview that was going nowhere. Carrying an old Worthington beer tray with three mugs of coffee and a cracked bowl of sugar, he placed them with great care on the desk before them.

'Hello Iggy' he said casually, pushing the coffee towards the white boilersuit. 'How's your old man?'

Leaning backwards over his chair, Hook grabbed the coughing sergeant by his arm as he began to leave.

'Friend of yours, Ivor?' he asked coolly.

'Not really' he replied. 'But I used to know his old man. Iggy Jackson, isn't it? I mean - Jackman. Yeah, Jackman. Still on the scrap is he, Iggy.?'

Spinning round to join them, Jackman leapt to his feet and began to clap mockingly.

'Brilliant, fucking brilliant' he said, beginning to laugh. 'I was arrested two hours ago and it took an old grey-haired pig to crack it for you. Brilliant!'

Chuffed and smiling, Griffiths slipped out of the interview room and closed the door behind him; it was always nice to get one over on the CID.

Pulling his chair closer to the desk, Hook stared directly into the eyes opposite. He needed Jackman to look closely too, he wanted the defendant to see so many things, but above all he wanted to show there was no fear, no respect from the other side of the desk.

But Hook saw problems there too. A closer inspection of the man in the white boilersuit showed dilated pupils, a skin that was perspiring, a complexion that was clammy, and an agitated mind. It was anger that put the strength into the arms and fists, and Hook considered moving his chair back a touch. He knew there was an unknown powder in Jackman's system, probably speed, that was making the interview difficult. Moving his chair away from the table and out of Jackman's face would be conceding some of the high ground. Lifting his chair he pulled it right up tightly against the table, and smiled engagingly as their knees collided underneath.

'What's so funny about being implicated in four murders, Iggy?' he said, referring to Jackman's sickly smirk. 'Not to mention the one in France'

'France! Christ forbid! I'm from a fucking children's home' he said, his eyes darting from one interviewing officer to the other. 'I didn't go to the seaside 'till I was twenty. France! I grew up in places where kids cried all night and pissed the bed. France! You gotta be desperate if you're trying to pin a take-and-drive on me!'

'This is no con trick, Jackman' James said. 'That Mini's a bigger problem than you can imagine.'

'Look sunshine, I've been interviewed and lied to by cretins like you two since I was ten years old, but okay, just listen up, and then piss off' he said. 'Bottom line, I borrowed it off some geezer I met in a pub. I can't remember his name and I can't remember the pub. Now you can't keep me here forever, I've got to walk eventually. It's the rules, sunshine' he laughed loudly. 'It's just the wonderful fucking rules.'

During an interview where there were desperate probing questions but no answers, Hook watched the hands of his watch push forward. In another half-hour it would be daylight The one thing he felt confident about was that Brodie wouldn't have had anything to do with a two-bit hoodlum like Jackman. The car was stolen, it had to be. How else could he have got it? But from where?

'Hang on a sec' Hook said, turning to face James. 'We're not thinking straight here. Logic is what normally finds the truth, good old fashioned logic. Right, so he fails to stop, drives like a maniac and assaults policemen as though there was a prize at the end of it. All for a tuppenny-ha'penny theft of a conveyance.'

'I didn't steal it! And I legged it 'cos I was worried about the breathalyser.'

'No, no. They bagged you at the hospital and you were clear' Hook said. 'But of course, your life did depend on it, didn't it Jackman? Get up. I want to search you.'

Getting to his feet, Jackman slowly pointed to his accusers.

'Put one finger on me and you're fucking history, sunshine.'

It was the sort of remark Jackman regularly made to policemen. When you were six four, it was the sort of statement you could afford to make.

'Well, it's going to get done one way or the other' Hook replied, also beginning to stand.

'I've been searched' he growled, sitting back down.

'Not properly you haven't' he said, giving him a hard unblinking stare, as thoughts of Helen came flooding back.

'Want me to call the police surgeon, boss? Full internal, rubber gloves, the works?' James said enthusiastically, catching on to Hook's way of thinking.

The words *rubber gloves* seemed to have a strange effect on the accused, who returned to his feet and snatched angrily at his zipper. Slowly he peeled off the boiler suit as requested. He'd had the rubber glove treatment once before during a prison search and like a lumber puncture, it was something you didn't volunteered for.

'You a dyke or something, love?' he said, as the suit floated to the floor exposing tattooed buttocks, and a firm naked body that caused James to raise an eyebrow.

Rummaging around in the creased white suit that lay at Jackman's feet, Hook knew there was little time to waste. It happened so quickly that even James, who was finishing her coffee while politely looking away, didn't even see the hand that thrust between Jackman's legs. Hearing a complaining yell, she glanced around in time to see him snatch a small bag of white powder that had been taped between Jackman's legs just behind his testicles.

Wincing as the length of sticking plaster tore away some pubic hair, Jackman pulled on the boilersuit once more, and finally slumped down on the chair.

'Okay, big deal, I'm on a bender. With my record, I'll be out in two' he smirked.

'Where did you take the car from, Jackman?' Hook said sternly, but the defendant began whistling again.

'It's important I get hold of the owner. It's the key to everything.'

Jackman just winked.

Opening the polythene bag of powder on the desk before him, Hook touched the end of his tongue with a few tiny crystals, in an unofficial testing procedure.

'And you really think I'm interested in two ounces of Charlie? When that Mini contains enough forensics to give you five life sentences?' he said.

Getting to his feet, Jackman's movements became erratic. The thought of becoming yet another prison statistic caused him to move around like an expectant father in a maternity ward. Although he and Hook had never previously met, the man was beginning to worry the shit out of him; he'd always found it relatively easy to intimidate policemen, but this guy wouldn't stop staring and was sticking to him like a limpet mine.

'Forget the window, Jackman, we're on the top floor and there's one hell of a drop' Hook said, as he spotted the defendant giving it the once over.

All the agitation wasn't lost on Hook, but time was running out, dawn was about to break.

The thought of eating meals again in a stale grey atmosphere of boredom and stench, where lunch and dessert were all lumped together on one metal tray, had Jackman starting to nibble on dirty fingernails.

Carefully, Hook began emptying the polythene bag and its cocaine contents into his untouched mug of coffee; calmly, he began stirring away. He never took his eyes away from the prisoner for one moment, as Jackman's eyes snapped open as if spring loaded. Looking on in disbelief, he watched as all the evidence for possession of a class A drug with intent to supply finally dissolved into a white lumpy sludge.

Trying her best to disguise her shock, James looked on, as if destroying prime evidence was an everyday occurrence. She'd never seen him destroy prime evidence before, but she knew roughly what he was up to. Tapping the spoon on the edge of the mug, he walked over to a suspect who now nervously leant against the wall. Pushing his face to within inches of the bandages, he said coldly,

'And you think I'm interested in this junk? You think we're bullshitting? You think this powder is some big deal?'

Opening the window, a sudden burst of cold winter wind brushed across his face as he casually poured the adulterated Maxwell House out and down into the yard below. Decaffeinated cocaine splashed all over Chief Inspector Maul's Vauxhall Omega.

He glanced at his watch again. It was almost too late. If Jackman had stolen the car from somewhere in the city, from under Brodie's nose, from outside Brodie's address, they needed him to give them that address before Brodie discovered the Mini missing. There was no doubt in his mind that Brodie would do a runner if he awoke to discover that his car had been taken during the night. Everyone in the country was becoming affected by crime. No-one was immune, even serial killers. With all his customs experience he wouldn't have too much of a problem in leaving the country,

Hook was determined that he should be the one that placed his hand on Brodie's arm, not the Met or some overseas police force in the distant future. The very idea that his Customs friends at one of the ports might seize him as he left on an easily-obtained false passport made him shiver. There was a score to settle. As the grief and hatred returned with a vengeance, he even began to think about killing him, but quickly dispensed with the notion.

'And you really, really thought that was all the evidence we had against you, Iggy?' laughed Hook 'You're out of your league pal' he said, switching off the tape machine, signifying the conclusion of the interview.

With his nerve ends rattling and the end of his tongue almost immobilised by the powder, he and James began to walk smartly towards the door, with a confident synchronised look in their eyes. The confident look was as important as anything. Jackman needed to see that look.

Watching the door slowly closing behind them, Jackman, who was now moving around the room like a horse in a stable fire, desperately called out.

'Wait!' he shouted. 'Just wait a mo!'

CHAPTER TWENTY ONE

The rough grey sea hugged the winding Welsh coast, roaring up over large deformed rocks that stood like medieval effigies, sculpted by thousands of years of rampaging channel tides. A hundred yards away Caravan Q109 stood buffeted by a boisterous north westerly, as flying sand tormented a few early morning walkers, and a dozen plastic litter-bins bowled around the site in a break for freedom.

The drawn green and white checked curtains fluttering in a draught, and a full Calor gas bottle underneath, appeared the main evidence that someone was in residence in the caravan. Deep tyre marks where a car had once stood at the side were now partially covered by sand; the impressions were narrow which indicated the car had been small. Black wrought-iron steps outside the caravan door was also an indicator that someone was at home. Only a few residents occupied the site during the winter months. the other six thousand mobile homes at the Sunshine Valley Caravan Park appeared to be empty.

It was half seven when the first armed response officer crawled nervously on his belly through the sand, and slipped quietly underneath Caravan Q112. Slowly he took aim at the pretty green and white curtains opposite, but the swirling sea spray and moving sand was affecting the telescopic sight on his Heckler and Koch carbine. A clear shot was going to prove difficult. Within thirty seconds another twelve men from the armed response unit were also in position, swarming towards the target premises like the black death. Encircled by enough firepower to hold up a Chinese army, Brodie, unless sensible, was heading for a body bag.

Caressing two high-powered rifles a hundred and fifty yards away, two police snipers lying on the roof of the camp laundrette steered their guns towards the door of G109, a powerful insurance policy against any last minute hiccups.

'We'll sit tight, Chief' said Corbett. 'Let's wait until it brightens up a little, give the firearms boys a better chance.'

'I'm hoping it won't come to that, Jack' replied Mulholland, throwing him a stern no-nonsense look.

Inserting his binoculars delicately through the closed blinds in an upstairs storeroom three hundred yards away, Corbett observed the developing drama down below.

'And you're sure it's Brodie's caravan?' he said.

'No what I said was, Iggy Jackman is adamant he pinched the Mini from outside that caravan at about three o'clock this morning, and camp records show that a J.Brodie is renting that van. I'm assuming it's got to be him,' replied Hook morosely.

'You okay, Hook?' asked Mulholland.

Hook nodded with unconcerned indifference.

'I know you're not happy with the situation, but common sense tells me you stay away from Brodie. Neither Mr Corbett nor I are totally happy about having you on plot.'

Hook turned away.

'Did you draw firearms,' said Mulholland.

'Mr Corbett told me not to, sir' he said.

'What the hell was Jackman doing down here in the first place?' asked Corbett.

'Trying to put together some drugs deal with someone on site' Hook replied. 'Just stole the car to get home.'

'Did he actually have any drugs on him, do we know?' said Corbett

'No, clean as a whistle sir' he said

Sitting quietly on a box of crisps at the back of the storeroom, James' hand shot up quickly to her mouth and she coughed loudly. Watching Corbett shout instructions into his radio almost a quarter of a mile away from the action zone brought a wry smile to her face. The rank of Superintendent brought other advantages apart from the pay scale, she thought. Self-preservation had to be top of the list.

Sitting at a small table in the middle of the room an elderly constable sat writing, logging each radio transmission, while another constable sat watching him.

Lowering his binoculars for a moment, Mulholland turned to Hook and said,

'There's a telex on my desk for you when we get back, from an Aldermartin chap at Customs. His men have had a sighting of Lennie and Mickey McCann day before yesterday at a villa in Malaga. Thought you should know.'

'Deserting rats from the preverbal sinking ship, no doubt' said Corbett. 'If they're wise they'll stay abroad.'

The voice sounded excited as it crackled out over the radios. Everyone crowded around the table and listened.

'Yankee Foxtrot 20 to control, confirm target on premises, target on premises, over.'

Turning to Mulholland, Corbett said,

'Over to you Mr Starter'

'Let's have him, Jack' said Mulholland, again peeping through the blinds.

'Zulu Alpha 2 to all units... '

'Hold on Jack' shouted Mulholland. 'Stand by, stand by, there's... . . . . '

'Christ Almighty Chief, what's going on?' groaned Corbett, lowering his radio.

Quickly adjusting his binoculars, Mulholland watched as a young girl, a child, wandered past caravan number Q109, her blonde hair blowing about her. Her dressing gown flapped open in the wind, revealing a short pink nightie. She ambled slowly along carrying a small red towel and soap.

Caravan residents sometimes took a short detour to look at the sea as they visited the conveniences prior to breakfast. But it wasn't that often they walked into the middle of a full-blown armed siege. Suddenly the door to G109 squeaked open, and something in a cup was thrown to the wind. Armed officers with twitching heart rates could only watch tensely as she unexpectedly pulled open the door which was still slightly ajar, and uninvited, stepped inside.

A dozen sub machine gun barrels followed her in, before being lowered slowly towards the sand. It was time out at Sunshine Valley.

'What the bloody hell's happening now Chief?' shouted Corbett, trying to squint through a gap in the blinds.

'Well if we do a show out now, Brodie's got himself a ready-made hostage. How the fuck did she get through the cordon, Jack? I thought this place was supposed to be deserted!'

'Who is she?' said Corbett.
Mulholland's mind was in turmoil. He was a trained negotiator; and had sat exams and attended courses on the subject; he had even lectured to police recruits. But what if the child were used as a human shield?

What if he were armed and began firing at random? What if he asked for transport to take her away? The scenarios were endless and he wasn't sitting in a warm classroom. What's more he knew that the tabloid presses had already been switched on and were waiting patiently for a headline. Hook could see that his complexion was slowly turning bone white.

'Chief' snapped an irritated Corbett, 'who is she?'

'Christ, it looks like a bloody ten year old kid Jack!' he replied, scratching his chin nervously, peering out through the blinds again. Lounging casually in the comer on a couple of multi coloured beanbags, Hook listened to the early seeds of panic as the top brass began treading water, awaiting each other's comments. Inside the storeroom the tension grew.

As the beanbags scrunched noisily on the hardwood floor, Hook could feel something itching under his arm. Searching inside his reefer coat, he adjusted the nylon strap until the shoulder holster became a little more loose.

'Quiet, for God's sake' whispered a testy Mulholland. 'Bloody sound carries like the wind this time of morning.'

Levering himself up off the floor, Hook walked over to the window and looked through the blinds.

'Want me to get over there and see if there's a chance to snatch the kid, chief?' he said, as though he was offering to pop out for a paper.

'You stay right where you are' grunted Corbett.

The old leather suitcase that lay open on the unmade bed had travelled through the majority of European airports, and as Brodie stuffed it full of dirty shirts and shaving tackle, it was about to take off again. Patting the inside pocket of his long grey overcoat to check for a passport and single air ticket to Spain, he jumped when he saw her, standing motionless, just inside the door. He hadn't heard her come in.

'Hello madam!' he said, calmly continuing with his packing. 'And what can I do for you.?'

'Could I have a drink of squash please?'

For a second he half smiled at her youthful precocity. Moving over to the fridge he pulled open the door and poured some juice into a paper cup. She was the sort of kid you saw every day in TV adverts, the one that stood by the sink with her mum. Pure blue eyes looked up innocently at his tense, unshaven face while he handed her the cup.

She sat on the bench. The cheap pink nylon nightie she wore had been ripped, and her slippers were badly worn. Items that should have been replaced at Christmas. Something told him she too had her problems.

The likeness was startling, and it stirred him. He was about to brush the fringe from her eyes in an old gesture, but he pulled his hand back sharply. Those days had gone. Studying her as she drank, he said,

'Listen, promise me you'll stop visiting strange men in strange caravans. Okay? Not unless your mum is with you.'

'My mum's in bed with her boyfriend' she said matter-of-factly.

This was going to take just a little time. He wanted to rush off, but he guessed that's what everyone always did in this little girl's life. His own childhood memories stirred quietly in the dark recesses. Money for sweets and familiar hands that ruffled short hair, all beneath stale beer breath. Fridays nights never changed. It was always the same man that climbed into his bed and hurt him.

Gulping down the squash that left an orange ring around her mouth, she belched, before politely returning the cup with both hands.

'My mum thinks you're strange, cos you don't speak to anybody around here.'

Pulling a sad face, he pretended to bite his lip.

'And what's your name then?'

'Mandy Jenkins' she said, her attention now taken up with a small silver picture frame that had been placed on the top of the suitcase. It was a colour snapshot he'd looked at every single one of the one thousand and eighty nine days since they'd gone.

'You do ask a lot of questions, miss' he said, picking up the picture before sitting down beside her. It was something he did most days, a commemorative ritual that never diminished his anguish. Staring miserably at a frozen reproduction of a happy father with two laughing daughters on a warm Brighton beach. The sensitive stirrings never went away, and hung onto his body like terminal cancer.

Almost mesmerised by her likeness, his thoughts returned to days of primary school tears and bicycle rides in all-day sunshine, when the little girl began to tug at his arm.

'That there, what's she got there?' she said, pointing enthusiastically to one of his daughters in the photograph.

Peering closer, he could see Sally clutching it in her hand. He'd never forgotten how he had bought it for her on the seafront at Brighton that summer. Sally too had been tugging away at his arm before he'd given in and paid the £2.75 the shopkeeper had demanded.

'That's Spiderman.'

'Why Spiderman?'

Getting up, he pushed the silver frame inside the suitcase and slammed it shut. Thinking for a moment he said,

'Perhaps because Spiderman's young. He's fast, and strong, and climbs up walls. Why not Spiderman?' he said, laughing. The sound was strange in his ears. Throwing the empty cup into a waste-paper bin, he said,

'Now off you go, back to your mum before she comes looking for you.'

Gently, he guided her tiny shoulders towards the door where she turned and flashed her eyes once more.

'I'd like a Spiderman.' she said.

With one final check around G109, he lifted the suitcase. It was time to go. He'd been hanging about far too long as it was, his flight was due to leave. Heaving it towards the door, he stopped abruptly as she stood there. He slowly lowered the suitcase, and looked down at his smiling visitor. Perhaps he should take her with him, he began to think; perhaps Sally had been returned to him after all. If only the headache would go away, the tight skull, the incessant dark clouds of despair. Some people called it stress. Doctor Penry-Ellis had called it his psychopathic personality. But what did he know?

'Hang on a sec young lady, I think I know where I may be able find one. Now close your eyes and I'll be back in a minute.'

Leaving his case, he pushed the door open and stepped into a flurry of sand outside, as the wind threw the door against the side of the caravan with a resounding bang. Squeezing both eyes tightly shut, his excited little neighbour sat quietly on the bench. She never saw him again.

With his back against the caravan window and the sand whipping up in his face, he barely had time to realise that his car had gone, when a high pitched Welsh accent cut through the wind.

'Armed police, armed police, Joseph Brodie you are now totally surrounded by armed officers, stay exactly where you are.'

Raising his head, he could see immediately that he was faced with six heavily-armed members of a firearm team. He knew there must be others. The first three appeared young and cocky, new to front line work, having been plucked from street duties because, under controlled training conditions, they could shoot straight. Brodie was glad; he wasn't likely to suffer.

One wore his baseball hat back to front, which did little to impress him. He was clearly under stress and showed no discipline. Number four had a fashionable cropped haircut and a neatly trimmed goatee beard, fashion statements that he had hoped would make him look really tough, but succeeded only in making him look gay. Too many Bruce Willis movies, too much talking down the pub, he thought.

Watching the man's jittery feet position continually change, he knew he wasn't tough.

His eyes quickly found the inspector, who continued to yell instructions from just yards away. They couldn't miss. Standing erect with his feet apart, the man looked new to the rank, confirmed by a complexion as fresh and rosy as a spring morning, his features as yet untainted by stale grey skin that evidenced long stressful shifts with a gun. This man had determined fear in his eyes.

Broken red facial veins highlighted the face of the last officer, short and overweight with body armour that hardly fitted. He had that contented gaze of a man who knew he held the aces. A constable in his thirties, probably ex-army, who had served his time in the Falls Road. The eyes that swivelled under the dark peak of his cap were clear and brave. Brodie watched, as he coolly rolled a spent match back and fore along his stained teeth. Although one out of six wasn't bad, he knew they were all empowered to kill him.

Through his binoculars, Mulholland watched as an ARU officer ran from the caravan, carrying the little blonde visitor kicking and screaming into the distance.

'She's out' he shouted.

'What's happening now chief?' said Corbett.

'He won't put his hands up' he said. 'Brodie won't put his bloody hands in the air. What's he playing at?'

'Does he understand the instructions?' queried Corbett, rushing to the window.

'Christ Jack, how the fuck should I know? I'm up here!'

'Hold on - the bastard's dipping his hands into his pockets. Perhaps he's got a shooter Larry!' Corbett said, squinting through a second pair of binoculars.

'What the fuck are the armed response boys up to? It's getting a bit hairy down there. What the hell's he up to, Hook?' Mulholland asked.

'It's very simple' Hook replied, foraging inside his coat for a stray cigarette. 'He wants them to shoot him.'

Astounded, Mulholland looked at Corbett, who stared back blankly and muttered something obscene under his breath. Getting up from the beanbags, Hook began brushing some dust from the legs of his Levis.

"He's trying to get them to panic and kill him' he said, yawning, as he opened a packet of crisps.

Pondering their next move, the Scrubs Lane top brass chatted quietly in the corner while the armed teams below awaited instructions. Mulholland's advice to the firearms tactical support officer of 'stand by' appeared appropriate, yet somewhat unhelpful if you were facing a man who had Just won the country's 'serial killer of the year' award by a mile.

Whilst the bosses discussed Plan B with the tactical officer over the air, Hook slipped unnoticed out of the room and walked silently down the stairway towards the foyer. Carrying a pile of sandwiches in an old box James barred his way

'What the hell are you doing James?' he whispered, trying to squeeze past her outstretched arms.

'Was it the tuna and mayonnaise or the cheese and pickle you ordered, bach?' she said quietly.

'Don't be fucking stupid James. Get out of my way.'

'Let's have it, boss' she said, holding out her hand. He tried to push past her again but her arms returned to the wrought iron handrail.

'Give me your Smith and Wesson boss. You don't need it. Brodie's going down, not you.'

'Get out of my way' he said angrily. 'I just need to speak to him!'

'You move an inch past me with that shooter and I'm going to make such a din on my radio, you won't get past first base. You're not thinking clearly. You think Helen would want you to do this?' She was pleading desperately. Placing the box at her feet, she held out her hand

'Please, hand me the gun.'

Running through the deserted camp centre that was boarded up like a ghost town, he passed shuttered shops and iced up kiddies' rides. Lactic acid started to build in his legs while the sand running introduced some tightness to his chest, as he dashed in and out of the caravans towards Q109. There was an urgency to confront him; the need to face him one last time, a powerful urge to stand toe-to-toe with the man that had taken her away; just one last chance before police firearms split open his chest.

He ducked under a huge billboard that advertised the previous summer's donkey derby, fancy dress competitions and bingo. He could see an announcement about the knobbly knees contest, but nothing about armed sieges.

The wind carried the ARU inspector's hoarse instructions bellowing towards him like a tannoy system as he tore through the site towards then There was a frightening and unmistakably threatening tone to his voice.

'Joseph Brodie, I am giving you one final warning. I want you to slowly remove your hand from your pocket, keep looking towards me Brodie … keep looking into my eyes … don't take your eyes off me Brodie … don't walk towards us … Stop! Stop! We will open fire if you continue, Mr Brodie!'

Sprinting towards the voices, Hook eventually stumbled past the Armed Response Unit and into the half-circle that had ensnared him. Half marathon runners looked fresher. Raising his arms, he signalled to Brodie, who stopped dead in front of him, halting his stroll towards the uniformed shooting gallery and suicidal oblivion.

Brodie wasn't frightened, he'd always decided that leaving the planet was a far better option than being incarcerated on it. But his right hand was still thrust deep into his double-breasted overcoat

When he finally stood in the sand before him, Hook's expression was one of fury. Plunging both hands deep into the pockets of his own reefer jacket, he stood opposite the former customs officer, a man now stripped to the bare bones of any dignity, respect, or hope. He'd caught up with him at last.

'I knew you were in this scenario somewhere, Hook' he shouted, a huge smile breaking over his face.

Hook said nothing; he stood quietly, staring at the man that had made criminal history in the city. Overhead a crowd of scavenging seagulls shrieked and swooped towards them, squawking angrily in a feathered protest at the absence of winter food. Within seconds they were swiftly heading back out towards the sea. Heckler and Koch submachine guns had a funny effect on some wildlife.

'Hector Barrantes, government ministers ... Any more... ..?'

'I had to try anything, Hook.'

'Born Maldonado ... Maracaibo prison ... geography's not your strong subject, Brodie. You blew it. You've lost your touch.'

'Nobody destroys my family with impunity, Hook.' It was an almost apologetic tone. 'The people who violated my kids, and the feeble laws of the land, they had to pay dearly.'

'Inspector Hook, I am ordering you to withdraw, you will step back immediately' shouted a voice from the shooting gallery behind him.

Now standing fifteen feet apart, Brodie, with his hand still thrust out of sight, began running on the spot. Hook didn't know if it was anxiety or the early morning chill seeping through his coat. He didn't care. Brodie had already started to make admissions about his crimes.

'Still upsetting the top brass I see' Brodie went on. 'Now if you're not supposed to be here, intuition tells me that you're not armed like the rest of those very nice gentlemen behind you.'

With both hands still inside his jacket pockets, Hook shouted back,

'Don't count on intuition any more. It's over, Brodie.'

'You and I, we could have been such a good team. They're parasites, you know. We could have cleaned up the city. You're a good man, a clever man Inspector' he continued, eyeing Hook's concealed hands suspiciously, and the bulge in his right-hand coat pocket.

Butchery to bonhomie all before breakfast. Psychology could be a confusing subject, thought Hook.

'If you're trying to appeal to my intellectual vanity, you're wasting your time' Hook shouted, spitting out some sand which had blown into his mouth.

As if the armed confrontation was beginning bore him, Brodie began to kick sand around aimlessly, although his eyes never left Hook's face. Slowly but surely, through his on-the-spot running, he had deliberately moved a couple of feet closer. Hook hadn't missed it.

He also became aware that they were both wearing similar dark coats, and a dose of apprehension kicked in when he spotted two police snipers on a nearby roof fifty yards away. One wrong move and it was all over.

They were top specialist firearm officers, he reminded himself. They were the pick of the team, and top marksmen like them never made mistakes. Moving a little to his right and a touch closer to the caravan, he crept out of their line of fire. He began breathing correctly again.

'Joseph Brodie, take your hand away from your pocket. Slowly. You are totally surrounded. Let's do it all peacefully. Inspector Hook, I am fucking ordering you to step back quietly, do you hear me?'

'Frightened, Hook?'

Smiling generously, Hook shook his head.

'Psychology was always one of your strong points, but I don't think you're carrying' said Brodie, loud enough for Hook to hear. 'You see, you're in their line of fire so they won't shoot.'

With his hand still concealed inside his pocket he slowly raised the front of his coat.

'I could kill you right now, and you wouldn't feel a thing.' His mood was now beginning to change.

In the distant backdrop Hook could see the miles of rolling sandhills that swept up towards the floating grey clouds moving quickly along the coastline, and felt the salty taste of the sea stick to his tongue. While the wind gently flattened his hair, he knew there were worse locations to fall, mortally wounded.

'You wouldn't shoot me Brodie. You don't kill people wearing blue.'

His voice sounded unconvincing; just for a split second the dryness held it back in his throat. Listening to the warnings and the threats, the sounds were beginning to disturb some scar tissue in his memory, producing flashbacks of a drugs raid that had gone wrong. The terror, the plume of smoke, the terrifying crack, followed by a demolition ball smashing him in the chest, then darkness. Hook had been lucky, but he'd seen enough Westerns to know that some cowboys never got up. On that occasion he had frozen. He wasn't about to freeze again. Get it sorted, he said to himself.

In the background he could hear the familiar sound of helicopter blades whirring in over the sea. He hoped it was the police chopper and not the paramedics, ominously arriving early with their words of comfort and saline drips. Staying calm was of paramount importance. If Brodie should see that he was frightened, his respect for him would dissolve. Just the slightest hint of falsetto and the ball game could completely change.

'Policemen are like wild badgers, Hook. You're right, they need to be protected. We're so alike you and I.'

'We're both men, Brodie. That's where the similarity ends.'

'But I respect you. Christ, did a young generation perish in the Flanders mud so these bastards could corrupt and poison another generation? For God's sake, I'm on your fucking side man!'

'You were never on my side. Scum who poison society are one thing, but Helen Wainwright

'… you got it all wrong Brodie, you screwed up. She wasn't part of some big legal conspiracy that helped acquit the McCanns. Society found them not guilty, not Helen Wainwright. She detested them more than anyone. You stupid sick bastard.'

Even in anger, Hook couldn't fail to observe the bewildered expression that registered on the face of the man in the sand. A vigilante who now only found peace while slaughtering others.

'Joseph Brodie, this is one final warning. Now I want you to slowly remove your hand from your pocket, very slowly. Inspector Hook, place both hands on top of your head. Do it, do it, fucking do it now.'

There was a frightening firmness in the Inspector's voice. It wouldn't have been the first armed incident that had turned pear shaped. Hook knew that police history was littered with them.

But both men had now come too far, and they ignored him.

'I know there's a category for people like me, but she was one of them, Hook' he said sadly, still oblivious to all the screaming in the background.

The very mention of her name diluted any fear he may have had. Buffeted by the wind he struggled over the soft sand and walked right up to him.

'Don't try and intimidate me with that gun, Brodie. I'm not into this Russian roulette thing. You may happy to be removed from a world that carries on without you, but I think I'll stay around a while. Make up your mind, what's it to be? Stick or twist?'

Moving back sharply, the Scotsman frowned Shouting like a spoilt child, he said,

'But she was part of their organisation. They did get to here. She did launder their money, I swear it.'

He could feel nothing but hatred generating in his guts. He felt like punching his face numb then and there. But the man was unstable and detached from his mind. A psychopath in dire need of help, something he'd brutally refused others. Defiling her memory may have been his way of easing some of his guilt, Hook didn't know.

'It's a neurotic fantasy Brodie. You're a sick man.'

'Whatever I am, I'm not lying, Hook. How would I know the two of you were an item? How would I know they gave her the Cabriolet for free? She never paid a penny, the paperwork is still in their office.'

'You're a liar, Brodie!'

'She owned her mother's cottage in west Wales. How would I know it's called Slate Cottage? That it's next to a churchyard? Check, for God's sake. She owned six properties in Edinburgh. Christ, she went up there over Christmas to finalise the seventh in Argyle Gardens.'

His whole career had been spent listening to lies, but something told him that everything he was being fed contained a sickening truth. He began to feel cold while more revelations of betrayal spewed from the Scotsman's lips. The startling disclosures continued to squeeze the very strength from him. He felt he might fall onto his knees, but he knew he couldn't. Not here. Not now.

'Check all the deeds on those properties. Her marina flat, she bought it cash, hundred and twenty grand' he went on. 'No mortgage. What the fuck do you think I was doing outside her flat that day, when you chased me? I was delivering an envelope for Lennie. She's a junior barrister not the fucking Lord Chief Justice, Hook. Get your Drug Profit Confiscation boys to check her bank accounts. Trust me.'

Hook was already starting to pull his right hand out of his coat but Brodie beat him to it. Empty handed, he withdrew both his gloved hands, throwing them up towards tha response team sigh in unison.

He watched as Hook called his bluff, slowly drawing the toy Spiderman from his own coat pocket.

'Nice one, Hook' he called, starting to lower both hands. 'I'm impressed. One-Nil.'

Holding the toy directly in front of Brodie's face like a gun, Hook said,

'If you haven't the guts to top yourself, don't ask someone else to do it, Brodie.'

Oblivious to yet another final warning which screamed over the sand, Hook slowly turned and walked towards the uniforms that whispered petty insults as he approached. The word 'lunatic' appeared popular as they allowed him to pass.

Calling after him as he left the circle, while his imminent death loomed ominously, Brodie's final disclosure hung in the air like a thick channel fog.

'For fuck's sake man, they were landing the gear down west! Her mother's cottage was the safe house!' he shouted, racing after Hook.

Moving quickly the men from the Armed Response Unit quickly and efficiently pulled him, struggling, to the ground, like a pack of hyenas would an antelope on the Serengeti.

'They kept the gear there before they brought it up into the city. Who the fuck do you think beat up and killed the old lady?' he spluttered, as a powerful forearm pinned his neck to the ground.

Stopping suddenly, with his back to all the shouting, Hook gazed down at the shifting sand and listened, rooted to the spot while every sickening word hit him like a freight train.

'Lennie McCann of course' Brodie gasped as the silver-coloured handcuffs tightened, cutting the skin on his strong struggling wrists. 'The old lady had no idea what was going on. She caught him checking the cellar one night. The man's an animal.'

With relative ease Brodie lifted his head up and away from his captors' hands, to watch the back of the man that was leaving. There was nothing much left to say.

'Good luck Hook!' he yelled.

It seemed a long way back to Scrubs Lane, and the weather forecast had given more snow. With both hands tucked deep inside his reefer pockets and his shoulders hunched against the wind, he decided to walk a while, taking a scenic route along the coast before he would join James on her way back to the station. There was little point in rushing, so he made his way alongside the ancient sea wall that stretched for miles alongside Sunshine Valley.

Stopping momentarily, he stared down at the crashing surf forty foot below as it thundered against the sea wall. For a second he looked out at the horizon and then at the rocks down below. He felt dizzy as huge clouds of spray softly soaked his hair. Slowly he began to unbutton his jacket.

Pushing his hand deep into his inside pocket, he pulled out the Spiderman toy, before buttoning up again. Expressionless, he dropped it into the sea as a couple of early flakes landed on his shoulders. He felt nothing and didn't bother to watch as the little figure in the red mask bobbed about in the surf before floating, face down, out to sea.

After scrounging a cigarette from a road sweeper on the edge of Sunshine Valley, he set off for the city. Although he had tolerated the hole throughout the summer months, his suede boots had now decided to let in water. A few armed response vehicles passed him on the way back to the station; one or two waved, but no one stopped. It didn't matter. James would wait for him. Others would now interview and deal with Brodie, and there was no need to hurry.

The defendant had been deprived of his clothing by the time Hook arrived back at Scrubs Lane. Alongside a young duty solicitor, he sat in a side interview room, handcuffed, wearing a sparkling clean white boiler suit and paper shoes. Hook didn't return his glance as he went into the radio room directly opposite.

Leaning on the windowsill in the corner talking to the chief constable on the phone, Corbett basked in self-glorification, clearly attributing the operation's success to nobody but himself. Admiring his window reflection, he was saying,

'I agree with you sir, he almost wiped out the entire organisation. Thank you sir, that's kind of you to say so. We'll put him before the court tomorrow.'

Putting down the phone, Corbett said,

'My office nine o'clock tomorrow morning' as he left the room. He didn't give Hook a second glance.

'Anyone seen Trilby James?' asked Hook, slumping down wearily on a chair, before pulling off his wet shoes and socks.

'She's gone to give the boys a hand with a burglary at Cars International. The intruder is still believed to be on the premises' replied the female operator, adding 'and would you please take your socks off the radiator, sir!'

An irate sales manager and two young probationer constables stood surrounded by a fleet of cars on the front forecourt of Cars International (Wales) Limited when James arrived. On the outskirts of the city, the impressive motor sales business stood surrounded by a high security fence, which also enveloped administrative offices and a large sprawling car showroom, which housed a hundred more cars.

'I don't care if there is anyone inside, wuss. Nobody goes trawling about on some fishing expedition until Lennie McCann or his brother arrives' said the man with a lilting Cardiff accent.

'And you are?' snapped James jumping from her little Citroen.

'I'm the keyholder, Steve Savage. Assistant Sales Manager. Why?' he said, smoothing down a stained brown shiny tie that hung from a frayed white collar. His shoes were white slip-ons, and didn't inspire confidence. The trousers were beige cargo pants that his ten-year-old son should have been wearing, and seemed a strange fashion mixture for a man in his forties who was trying to sell you a top of the range BMW. The small swallow tattooed on his neck may well have been the company's logo, she thought. He was the sort of serial deceiver you wouldn't have bought a mud flap from.

'You goes anywhere near those offices, darlin', before them McCanns arrive, and the shit will really hit the fan.'

'That's lovely' she smiled, pushing him aside as she walked towards the back of the building with her two colleagues.

'Nice tie. Llandovery?'

Watching them run off, he quickly rang the brothers on his mobile.

She followed the two constables to an open window, just slightly ajar, in the wall of the toilets at the back of the offices.

'Alarm?'

'Looks as though it didn't activate. Savage arrived earlier, saw the open window and heard noises inside' one of the officers said.

'Right, I want you both to keep watch out at the front. If there is someone in there, they'll never get out of this compound.'

After they had given her a bunk up, she sat unsteadily for a moment, balancing on the windowsill, before swinging her legs down through the window and inside the Gents. Holding tightly for support onto a Durex machine fixed just inside the window, she bent her back, before sliding quietly through, as the machine tore away from the white tiled wall. Angrily she uttered an expletive in Welsh as it clattered onto the wet floor. So much noise, so little protection, she thought, as she looked at the broken condom machine at her feet. If the intruder hadn't been aware of her presence at first, he certainly was now.

Systematically she made her way towards a faint sound of music, peeping nervously into some small offices as she went. Opening the double doors that lead into the main showroom, she stopped abruptly by a silver BMW. Crouching down, she dropped out of sight. There were people in that showroom, she could just feel it. She had no idea where, but they were in there all right.

Looking through the back window of a Mercedes saloon, she could see the pride of the Cars International fleet, a gleaming blue Rolls Royce Silver Shadow, elevated on a red carpeted platform that slowly rotated in the centre of the showroom. She wondered if the music was coming from its car radio. She also wondered if she should have called for some back up.

Creeping slowly closer, she could hear the finely precisioned Rolls Royce engine idling quietly. Although it was surrounded by a hundred vehicles, someone had started it up. It had to be one of the two men that sat on the back seat, talking. The music from the Rolls' push-button radio was Beethoven, but she couldn't remember which symphony.

Hooks voice sounded a concerned as it came over the air.
 'WL to Delta Sierra 30, you okay up there James?'
 Turning down the volume on her radio, she whispered back,
 'Stand by, boss.'
 It was a simple remark but her tone said there were problems, and she was missing her partner.

She could now see they were sitting upright together in the back seat, yet there didn't appear to be any dialogue between them. Nobody was talking. Everything was far too quiet, apart from the sombre music. Perhaps things had been said already.
 Still crouching, she moved silently up alongside a yellow Mazda still some distance away from the showroom showpiece, when she recognised the two men. Managing directors Mickey and Lennie McCann had been there all night. Death hadn't come easily.

Jumping up onto the revolving podium and moving even closer, she looked uneasily through the rear passenger window at their cold, expressionless faces, still being white-washed by the early rigor mortise which had already seized their jaws and necks. Bruised and wounded faces stared back.

Lennie's mouth was filled with a grey cotton material; she could see the half-inch turn-up that appeared to spew out from inside his mouth. His brother's mouth was wide open, screaming, his last piercing request for mercy, flatly refused.

Blood splattered a number of nearby car bonnets, indicating the brothers' demise had occurred at different locations in the showroom some hours earlier, at different times. Re-uniting them in style for the final judgement seemed a nice touch.

She remembered then that the music from the car radio was a movement of Beethoven's Eroica symphony. The funeral march.

White crystallised powder filled the inside of the car and covered both brothers up to the neck. Only their heads were on show. She'd remembered burying her father in a similar way on a sandy Porthcawl beach when she was a child. Carefully she opened a rear door, releasing a mountain of powder that flowed around her feet in a mini avalanche. White chemicals with a sprinkling of scarlet that had been twenty four hours away from the city streets.

'WL to Delta Sierra 30, are you receiving me over? Are you okay, over?' shouted Hook, urgently seeking reassurance regarding her welfare.

Lifting the radio slowly to her mouth, she composed herself.

'Delta Sierra 30 to WC, I'm inside the showroom, with the bodies of Lennie and Mickey McCann, and I've found a consignment of Babylon. Assistance, I need assistance boss, can I have some assistance' she pleaded.

Rushing from the radio room, Hook could see that the interview room opposite was now empty, and that Brodie had been taken away. Pushing people aside, he ran across the station yard and into the cellblock in time to see him being led silently away in handcuffs, down a poorly-lit cell passageway that reeked of the body odour of thousands of prisoners. Banging loudly, the gate to the corridor slammed behind him, when halfway down Brodie stopped for some reason. It was as if he sensed Hook was standing there, watching him. Half-turning his head, he nodded in the dimness, staring at Hook one last time.

He gave a self-satisfied grin and a slow, deliberate wink, before bending down and disappearing through a tiny iron door that slammed behind him with a deafening finality. They both knew they would never set eyes upon each other again.

CHAPTER TWENTY TWO

Sitting on a kitchen stool in James' modest kitchen, Hook gazed down from the bay window at the swollen river Morlais. Reaching over the work surface, he watched the water flow majestically towards the splendid city bridges in the distance. A week was a long time in a murder investigation. He sat quietly among the copper pots and pans, and the ropes of garlic and peppers, like a misplaced appendage after holy wedlock. He showed little interest in the party that raged in the next door room.

The thick, fat rat that sat watching him from the opposite riverbank was a lot smaller than the one that had suspended him from duty seven days earlier, for jeopardising yet another armed incident. His permanence in the youthful yet successful Drug Squad was already the subject of hierarchy discussion; his investigative immobility now down to the grudge-bearing king rat himself, Jack Corbett. Somehow he knew that the Superintendent wouldn't let him stay for the sake of the kids.

Surprisingly, Mulholland had also put a little distance between himself and his Drug Squad inspector, disappearing quicker than a desert sidewinder in shifting sand.

Carefully caressing two inches of Jack Daniels that served to anaesthetize a mind that was still in intensive care, he bolted it down, as fragmented images of Helen began to scramble out of the dark recesses of his mind. There was little doubt she was coming and going as she pleased, and even the single malt whisky was having problems intercepting her.

The belated squad Christmas party raged in the lounge next door and people had been in and out all night chatting; sympathy and liquor were in abundance. Entering the warm pine kitchen, the hostess sat down beside him.

'Penny for them' she said, starting to fill his empty glass.

A half smile began to break across his face, and he squeezed her arm affectionately, before returning his gaze to the river. The rat had now disappeared.

'Cariad, stop beating yourself up over Helen. Listen, we're all shocked. She laundered the money for them, remember? Okay, she paid a high price for her deceit – the highest price - but you weren't to know' she said.

'I'm a detective, and she used me. She didn't just defend the McCanns, she worked for them, don't forget' he said, tossing a salted peanut into the air which he failed to catch in his mouth.

'You're not a bloody clairvoyant!'

'You know what, we stopped a couple of times at her mother's idyllic cottage, where in an idyllic cellar they stashed idyllic drugs. Perhaps she thought I was an idyllic touch.' He drained his glass once more. 'I know the defence is always on these day's about more police co-operation, but this was ridiculous.'

'You nailed him, just you, and don't you ever forget that. So what's going to happen to him?'

'A plea to diminished responsibility. Rampton for life. I think he'll die in madness, not too far from hell.'

'And you?'

'My madness will be pushing paper in some office if they keep me' he laughed. 'They've already served notices on me. I didn't realise there were so many disciplinary offences for being successful. I'm thinking of putting my ticket in after I get six of the best. When police work becomes just a job, James, it's time to move on.'

Just then the kitchen telephone extension jingled next to the bread bin and Hook picked it up.

'May I speak to acting Detective Inspector Trilby James please?' the voice said with some authority.

Handing her the phone, he watched as his understudy's pale face looked embarrassed, her smiling eyes confused. He'd never heard her stammer before.

'You're, you're positive, positive then?' she said as Hook's eyes continued to search for the rat.

'They've found another body, about an hour ago' she said, replacing the handset slowly.

'You – what?' he said stupidly, although he'd clearly understood her the first time. It was the sort of thing stressed-out suspended detectives seemed to say in moments like this, particularly after a long evening with Jack Daniels.

'Another body, another body, bled to death. They want me and the rest of the squad in at six in the morning.'

'Where?' he said, beginning to hiccup.

'One of the flats in Seville Villas.'

Sliding swiftly off the stool, he snatched at his reefer jacket which lay folded on top of the fridge, and nodded towards the front door.

'Oh no, oh no, I'm not driving over there with you, and that's final.'

'Please.'

'They've served you with a regulation nine notice. That, amongst other things, means you go nowhere near police stations or speak to another police officer. You shouldn't even be here, boss.'

As they sped across the city through late night traffic in the little Citroen, she said,

'What the hell's going on bach? Brodie's in custody. This is all getting a bit complicated for me.'

'

'Don't worry, it's just the epilogue' he said.

'Do you think it's your dad, boss?' she said quietly.

Hook shrugged his shoulders.

Slowing down near the junction with Seville road, they could see a heavy police presence about halfway down the road, outside the flats. An elderly grey-haired constable smiled and waved them through towards an alternative route, while in the background a fragile blue and white police cordon tape fluttered defiantly in the night wind.

He knew there was no way Corbett would let him within twenty miles of another murder scene. Trying to get past uniform staff whilst suspended was going to prove a little awkward He knew he was leaving himself as wide open as a book of remembrance, but he needed just a few seconds with the victim.

Pulling into a nearby cul-de-sac, she shook her head as he pulled his reefer tightly around him. Turning up his collar, he began rummaging in his pockets for one last late night smoke.

'What's the point, boss? You're in enough shit as it is.'

Jumping from the car, she watched as he scaled a high boundary wall, giving her the thumbs up sign before disappearing towards the Seville Villas under the cover of darkness. Switching off the headlights, she crossed her fingers, sighed and waited. She was going to miss him.

Sneaking through the back gardens of low class suburbia, over wet mattresses and around unsociable mongrels, he scrambled towards the bright lights and the throbbing din of the lighting generators at the back of the flats. He'd never seen so many houses without curtains. If there had been a competition for detecting dog shit during the hours of darkness, Hook would have run away with the final.

A kitchen light was on inside his father's flat and he could see a number of plain clothes policemen inside, some pointing. Police arc lights lit up the side of the flats where Scene Of Crime men scavenged for clues, while silver fingerprint powder had already been brushed tenderly around some ground floor windows.

Picking up a partially-buried old black wellington from the top of the gardens, he lowered his head as great flurries of snow blew all around. As he passed a group of clue-searching constables, Hook grunted from behind his turned-up collar and moved past with his exhibit. They showed little interest as he headed towards the flats.

The young policeman at the foot of the stairs leading to the first floor was far too interested in his pretty female uniformed companion to notice him, as he slipped by and strode up the stairway, dropping the boot on the steps. With his heart hammering and the strange smell beginning to get worse, the appalling odour rose like an Hawaiian wave to greet him on the landing.

'You're debarred, Hook,' Maul grinned, placing his arm across Hook's chest like a night club bouncer. 'You don't have the authority of a school crossing patrol at the moment.'

The loud unmistakable voice that had both their heads turning sharply came from the other side of the landing.

'Let him through' ordered Mulholland, who stood chatting to a grim-faced Corbett and a couple of Scene Of Crime men.

Out of breath, he began to explain the reason for his presence before they had a chance to verbally lash him and tell him to piss off, but the Chief Superintendent raised his hand in front of him.

'It's alright Hook, just explain what Brodie's up to here.'

The door of number 5A was open, and he could see down the hallway opposite. Once again, he could almost taste the scent of foul decaying flesh that had already started to rot on the week-old corpse.

'I've got a theory, sir,' he said. 'I just need to look at the body. I may be totally wrong.'

'But a toilet attendant who was just a witness? Is there a connection? With the McCanns?

With drugs?' said Corbett, with troubled eyes that could see the neat packaging of the city murders start to unravel rather untidily.

'Just a quick look, sir. Two seconds' Hook asked.

Snatching a pair of cold white overalls from a Scene Of Crime man, he slipped them on and pulled up the hood.

'If I may help a little …' said the officer, slipping him an extra-strong mint and a white facemask.

Walking into the hallway he was aware of the smell of perspiration that hung around the flat like a prison gymnasium.

Inside the lounge, Professor Woolfe's eyes acknowledged him over the top of his glasses, before they returned to the small dictaphone in his hand. The Edinburgh-born pathologist with kindly green eyes and centre-parted hair looked like the sort of man you would have bought a bible from on your doorstep. The man who studied the science of disease always reminded Hook of the white-haired granddad from numerous Disney films, yet he was capable of removing major organs from inside a body with the ease some men grind a cigarette into gravel.

He could see that other men in white overalls were in many parts of the brightly lit room. Another was quietly taking photographs that would end up in thick grotesque albums that would eventually turn jurors' stomachs.

Passing a Scene Of Crime bag, he picked up a small plastic hand torch before stepping over a pile of dog shit and making for the kitchen.

'I wouldn't go in there, laddie, it's in real bad shape' the Professor called.

Tentatively he pushed open a badly scratched sapele door which had a broken handle, and stepped cautiously into the dark unhappy kitchen. Nudging the door shut behind him, he stood alone for a second in the darkness with his back against the door, fidgeting nervously with the torch in his hand, desperately trying to switch it on. It was a long time since he'd heard himself breathing so rapidly.

Finally the weak beam lit up part of the room. In the middle of the floor he could see a small rusty picnic table, on which was a carton of sour milk. Underneath the table he could see small black pellets of rat shit and he shivered. A solitary blue hand-painted wall cabinet with an open sliding glass door contained nothing but out-of-date butter and a tin of powdered milk. An overturned box of Coco Pops that lay on the floor appeared to be the man's only extravagance.

Under the cabinet he could just about make out the outline of a body that was sitting on the floor, with its back propped up against a filthy electric cooker. Moving closer he began to squint in the dimness. Suddenly the beam of the torch lit up a grey frozen face, an image that caused him to fall back heavily against the kitchen door.

'Jesus Christ.'

Staring up at him only feet away, with eyes and mouth twisted and distorted, Moses sat heavily made-up in a long black ladies' wig, thick pink lipstick, bronze blusher and dark false eyelashes. The gold hooped earrings he wore were large and vulgar.

'Didn't they explain to you outside?' Woolfe called out from the lounge.

Following the light of the torch, Hook's eyes moved slowly up and down the body. Low priced brown checked curtains and a plastic curtain-rod were still held tightly in his hands, violently ripped from above the window after a last attempt to get to his feet. His head, partially covered in wall plaster, was tilted back and silently frozen, screaming for forgiveness. Hopelessly the victim stared up at the damp flaking ceiling, searching for clemency perhaps from the higher court, as the coldness and sweet darkness of death were patiently explained. Leniency had clearly been refused.

Blood covered most of the bare black floorboards, and had dried like a sticky red tar. Fatty acids also leaked from the decomposing body, samples of which would later help Woolfe to give the exact time of death. Both his hands had defence wounds and were badly cut.

Something told him that Brodie had spent a long time alone with Moses before subjecting him to the agony of death. There were childhood nightmares to be regressed, skeletons to be removed and mortality to be discussed. Black eye mascara had run distressingly down Moses' cheeks and stained a lot of his lower face. He had cried like a baby just before dying.

A lone fly buzzed annoyingly around Hook's head as though he were intruding. He had no idea if it had managed to survive the winter, or had earlier been one the maggots that now patrolled behind Moses teeth.

It was difficult to establish which groin had been stabbed, but the odd angle of Moses' right foot gave Hook a clue. The leg from a pair of brown tights that Moses had been wearing had been cut and hung grotesquely from the deceased's pink-shaded lips. It was halfway down his throat.

A beige long-sleeved blouse and grey knee length pleated skirt, from a city Oxfam shop, were both saturated in congealed blood. A pair of black sling-back shoes lay close to the body.

'I think he's been dead for just over a week' said Woolfe, opening the door and moving into the kitchen. 'The cessation of life came rather violently to Mr Moses, laddie.'

Hook half-smiled tiredly, admiring the Professors trendy pink and navy polka dot bow tie.

'Christmas present, laddie,' he said, observing Hook's interest.

'Would you mind pulling up his blouse, Prof?' Hook asked, shining the torch again on the body.

'He is wearing some ladies underwear, if that's what's concerning you. He's not wearing pants though, just a suspender belt.'

'No, it's something else Prof.'

Bending over the body, and with his hands sheathed in surgical gloves, the pathologist slowly unbuttoned the blouse that hung over the skirt. Gradually five rolls of expansive white flesh just below the black brassiere were exposed, and slid down towards the deceased genitals like a huge white tumour.

'What are you searching for, laddie?' he said, kneeling down alongside him.

With his lips sucking the paper face mask in and out sharply, Hook grimaced as he seized a disgusting grease-covered spatula from the top of the cooker and began to push it delicately between the rolls of fat in front of him. Cautiously he began to lift some flesh as though he was checking the underside of a well-done omelette.

'Stab wounds, are you looking for incision marks Inspector?'

Shaking his head, Hook began to raise the fourth roll of flab and half- smiled at the tattoo that slowly came into view.

'LM loves JB' an intrigued Woolfe exclaimed, moving in a little closer.

'Leonard Moses loves Joe Brodie' Hook said, slipping the spatula under the last roll of fat.

'I don't follow, laddie.'

'This, Professor, is Leonard Moses,' Hook said. 'Over twenty five years ago he was employed by social services in Surrey as a carer at the Tree Tops children's home. This is the reptile who, over many years, tarnished forever a seven-year-old kid named Joseph Brodie Someone whom he should have protected, someone he should have loved. Perhaps all that harm has been undone now.'

'And what's under that last roll?' the Professor asked keenly, as Hook started prodding away again.

Lifting the flesh and holding the rolls of fat apart for a moment, Hook smiled sadly at the second tattoo.

'Welcome to Hell?' said Woolfe whose eyebrows dipped sternly towards a pair of confused Scottish eyes.

'A paedophile with a dark sense of humour' Hook said, rising stiffly to his feet. 'Hope you have a pleasant evening with his stomach content, Prof' he added, shaking Woolfe by the hand before handing him the spatula.

Outside on the landing, the divisional commander patted Hook vigorously on the back as he stepped out of his white overalls while vividly describing the contents of the kitchen. Corbett, with a strange flash of what seemed like sincerity, grabbed Hook's hand and shook it once. Jack Corbett was like those actors in films who bent over and loosened the shirt and tie on people who had already been fatally shot. It was always too late.

Making his way down the stairway, he pushed Maul aside brusquely in search of the journalists outside. Spotting the media circus at the end of the street behind the police cordon, he waved grandly and headed in their direction.

Deepjoy, it was all sorted.

'So you think Brodie first recognised Moses when he went into those toilets to meet - and murder – Saduskas?' asked Mulholland.

'Yes. I'm told Moses left the children's home before the balloon went up. I think he travelled the country before ending up in Wales. He'd already changed his first name from Leonard to Sidney to throw people off the scent. From the moment he recognised him behind the chicken wire, Moses was placed on the shopping list. It was nothing to do with drugs, but everything to do with the terrible abuse he'd suffered at the children's home.'

'What else has Moses been up to during the last few years, I wonder?'

'God knows. He's got a few previous for indecency. Every sexual offence on the statute book I shouldn't wonder. We know he dresses up as a woman.'

'Yes, why is that?'

'Christ, how should I know, Chief?' said Hook throwing his commander a baffled stare. 'But I think Moses was probably dressed up and ready to go out on the town when Brodie called to murder him. He was the last one that was killed.'

'After Brodie disappeared from his job at Customs, how did he manage to infiltrate the McCann organisation?'

'Met the brothers by chance. They were on holiday in Spain, Brodie was just bumming around Europe after his kids died and his marriage broke up. They were out there doing drug business, he just sussed them out one night. Plenty of drink, and Lennie couldn't keep his mouth shut. Brodie introduced himself at the hotel and impressed them before talking his way into a job. Bob's your uncle, a grieving father became a psychopathic vigilante, and decided to rid us of our top drug organisation.'

'So what was his actual job with the brothers?'

'Just a sort of run around, collected debts, drove a bit of dope here and there when others couldn't do it Just a bit of extra muscle who stayed in the background' said Hook.

'The brothers just liked him' he went on. 'But all along, his intention was to find out all about the organisation and to systematically take them out. The death of his kids on drugs pushed him over the edge.'

'Who is that behind you, Hook?' the Chief Superintendent whispered.

Standing on the doorstep outside number 5B, the elderly man just stood and stared across the landing at them both. Neatly trimmed hair above a clean shaven face, a red V-neck pullover with shirt and tie, and grey pressed M&S trousers had transformed the appearance of a man already influenced by visits to AA.

'I'll see you, Chief' Hook said.

Making his way across the landing towards him, he could see the hope and remorse in the man's eyes, while the trembling outstretched blue-veined hand was still troubled by alcohol, or the lack of it. Ignoring the greeting, Hook simply squeezed past him and stepped into the unlit hallway, before making his way towards some unforgettable furniture in the lounge.

'Merry Christmas, Harry' the old man said.

It was a start.

THE END

Acknowledgements

There are a few people - friends, and of course my family - I would like to thank for helping me get this book written, finished and published. I won't name them for fear I leave someone out, but you know who you are.

And to the South Wales Police force who have, albeit unwittingly, provided me with such a rich seam of history, activity, facts and stories. Thank you.

Printed in Great Britain
by Amazon